# Psychological Aspects of Women's Health Care

## The Interface Between Psychiatry and Obstetrics and Gynecology

### Second Edition

# Psychological Aspects of Women's Health Care

## The Interface Between Psychiatry and Obstetrics and Gynecology

### Second Edition

Edited by

NADA L. STOTLAND, M.D., M.P.H.

DONNA E. STEWART, M.D., D.PSYCH., F.R.C.P.C.

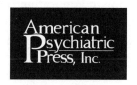

American Psychiatric Press, Inc.

Washington, DC
London, England

**Note:** The authors have worked to ensure that all information in this book concerning drug dosages, schedules, and routes of administration is accurate as of the time of publication and consistent with standards set by the U.S. Food and Drug Administration and the general medical community. As medical research and practice advance, however, therapeutic standards may change. For this reason and because human and mechanical errors sometimes occur, we recommend that readers follow the advice of a physician who is directly involved in their care or the care of a member of their family.

Copyright © 2001 American Psychiatric Press, Inc.
ALL RIGHTS RESERVED
Manufactured in the United States of America on acid-free paper

04 03 02 01   4 3 2 1
Second Edition

American Psychiatric Press, Inc.
1400 K Street, N.W.
Washington, DC 20005
www.appi.org

**Library of Congress Cataloging-in-Publication Data**

Psychological aspects of women's health care : the interface between psychiatry and obstetrics and gynecology / edited by Nada L. Stotland, Donna E. Stewart.
—2nd ed.
    p. cm.
  Includes bibliographical references and index.
  ISBN 0-88048-831-X (acid-free paper)
  1. Gynecology—Psychosomatic aspects. 2. Obstetrics—Psychosomatic aspects. I. Stotland, Nada Logan. II. Stewart, Donna E., 1943-
RG103.5 .P7725 2000
618'.01'9—dc21

00-033141

**British Library Cataloguing in Publication Data**
A CIP record is available from the British Library.

Cover image: Digital Imagery © copyright 2000 PhotoDisc, Inc.

This book is dedicated to Harold, Lea, Naomi, Eve, and
Hanna Stotland and to
Eileen Stewart, Andrew Malleson, M.D., and Michael Malleson.


The editors wish to thank Janet Dalzell, Jennifer Wood, and the staff at
the University Health Network Women's Health Program,
who made this book possible.

# Contents

## Pregnancy

## II

### Gynecology

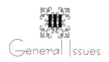

## General Issues

# Contributors

Barbara L. Andersen, Ph.D.

Departments of Psychology and Obstetrics and Gynecology, Ohio State University, Columbus, Ohio

Sheila B. Blume, M.D., C.A.C.

Former Medical Director, Alcoholism, Chemical Dependency and Compulsive Gambling Programs, South Oaks Hospital, Amityville, New York; Clinical Professor of Psychiatry, State University of New York at Stony Brook, Stony Brook, New York

Olga Brawman-Mintzer, M.D.

Associate Professor of Psychiatry, Mood and Anxiety Program, Department of Psychiatry, Medical University of South Carolina, Charleston, South Carolina

Linda Hammer Burns, Ph.D.

Licensed Psychologist; Assistant Professor, Department of Obstetrics and Gynecology, University of Minnesota Medical School, Minneapolis, Minnesota

Melanie L. Carr, M.D., F.R.C.P.C.

Department of Psychiatry, University Health Network, Toronto, Ontario, Canada

Corinna E. Dan, R.N., B.S.N.
Community Health Nurse and Program Coordinator, Department of
 Adolescent Health/Health Education and Outreach, Erie Family Health
 Center, Chicago, Illinois

Diana L. Dell, M.D., F.A.C.O.G.
Assistant Professor, Departments of Obstetrics and Gynecology and
 Psychiatry, Duke University Medical Center, Durham, North Carolina

Jennifer I. Downey, M.D.
Associate Clinical Professor of Psychiatry, Columbia University College of
 Physicians and Surgeons, New York, New York

William B. Farrar, M.D.
Department of Surgery, Ohio State University, Columbus, Ohio

Mindy Thompson Fullilove, M.D.
Associate Professor of Clinical Psychiatry and Public Health, Columbia
 University; Research Psychiatrist, HIV Center for Clinical and Behavioral
 Studies, New York State Psychiatric Institute, New York, New York

Paula J. Adams Hillard, M.D.
Professor, Department of Pediatrics, Children's Hospital Medical Center;
 Professor, Department Obstetrics and Gynecology, and Director of
 Women's Health, University of Cincinnati College of Medicine, Cincinnati,
 Ohio

Margaret F. Jensvold, M.D.
Senior Scientist, Institute for Research on Women's Health, Washington, DC;
 Center for Life Strategies, Bethesda, Maryland

Irving G. Leon, Ph.D.
Lecturer, Department of Psychology, University of Michigan, Ann Arbor,
 Michigan

Laura J. Miller, M.D.
Associate Professor and Chief, Woman's Services Division, Department of
    Psychiatry, University of Illinois at Chicago, Chicago, Illinois

Jan Moore, Ph.D.
Division of HIV/AIDS–Epidemiology Branch, Centers for Disease Control
    and Prevention, Atlanta, Georgia

Michael F. Myers, M.D., F.R.C.P.C.
Director, Marital Therapy Clinic, Department of Psychiatry, St. Paul's
    Hospital; and Clinical Professor, Department of Psychiatry, University of
    British Columbia, Vancouver, British Columbia, Canada

Carol C. Nadelson, M.D.
Clinical Professor, Department of Psychiatry, Harvard Medical School;
    Director, Office for Women's Careers, Brigham and Women's Hospital,
    Boston, Massachusetts; and President, CEO, and Editor-in-Chief,
    American Psychiatric Press, Washington, DC

Malkah Tolpin Notman, M.D.
Clinical Professor of Psychiatry, Cambridge Hospital, Harvard Medical
    School; and Training and Supervising Psychoanalyst, Boston
    Psychoanalytic Institute, Boston, Massachusetts

Robert O. Pasnau, M.D.
Professor Emeritus, Department of Psychiatry, University of California–Los
    Angeles School of Medicine, Los Angeles, California

Diane A. Philipp, M.D., F.R.C.P.C.
Staff Child Psychiatrist, Hinck's and Dellcrest Treatment Centre, University
    of Toronto, Toronto, Ontario, Canada

Gail Erlick Robinson, M.D., D.Psych., F.R.C.P.C.
Professor in Psychiatry and Obstetrics/Gynecology, University of Toronto;
    Director, Programme in Women's Mental Health, Department of
    Psychiatry, University Health Network, Toronto, Ontario, Canada

Marcia Russell, Ph.D.
Senior Research Scientist, Prevention Research Center, Berkeley, California

Kathleen Blindt Segraves, Ph.D.
Associate Professor, Department of Psychiatry, Case Western Reserve
    University; and Director, Behavioral Medicine Service, Department of
    Psychiatry, Metrohealth Medical Center, Cleveland, Ohio

Robert Taylor Segraves, M.D., Ph.D.
Professor, Department of Psychiatry, Case Western Reserve University; and
    Chairperson, Department of Psychiatry, Metrohealth Medical Center,
    Cleveland, Ohio

Barbara B. Sherwin, Ph.D.
Professor, Departments of Psychology and Obstetrics and Gynecology, McGill
    University; and Co-Director, Menopause Clinic, McGill University Health
    Center, Montreal, Quebec, Canada

Dawn K. Smith, M.D., M.S., M.P.H.
Medical Epidemiologist, Division of HIV/AIDS Prevention–Surveillance and
    Epidemiology, Centers for Disease Control and Prevention, Atlanta,
    Georgia

John F. Steege, M.D.
Professor, Department of Obstetrics and Gynecology, University of North
    Carolina, Chapel Hill, North Carolina

Donna E. Stewart, M.D., D.Psych., F.R.C.P.C.
Professor, Departments of Psychiatry, Obstetrics and Gynecology, Anesthesia,
    Surgery, Medicine, and Family and Community Medicine, University of
    Toronto; and Lillian Love Chair in Women's Health, University Health
    Network, Toronto, Ontario, Canada

## Nada L. Stotland, M.D., M.P.H.

Professor, Departments of Psychiatry and Obstetrics and Gynecology, Rush Medical College; and Chair, Department of Psychiatry, Illinois Masonic Medical Center, Chicago, Illinois

## Anna L. Stout, Ph.D.

Associate Professor, Departments of Psychiatry and Behavioral Sciences and Obstetrics and Gynecology, Duke University Medical Center, Durham, North Carolina

## Margery S. Sved, M.D.

Chief, Adult Psychiatry Service, Dorothea Dix Hospital, Raleigh, North Carolina; Adjunct Associate Professor, Department of Psychiatry, University of North Carolina School of Medicine, Chapel Hill, North Carolina; and past president, Association of Gay and Lesbian Psychiatrists, Philadelphia, Pennsylvania

## Carole Warshaw, M.D.

General Internal Medicine and Primary Care, Cook County Hospital; and Clinical Associate Professor, Department of Psychiatry, University of Illinois, Chicago, Illinois

## Katherine L. Wisner, M.D., M.S.

Assistant Professor of Child Psychiatry, University of Pittsburgh; and Medical Director, Pregnancy and Infant/Parent Center, Pittsburgh, Pennsylvania

## Kimberly A. Yonkers, M.D.

Associate Professor, Department of Psychiatry, University of Texas Southwestern Medical Center, Dallas, Texas

# Foreword

ROBERT O. PASNAU, M.D.

This book is the long-anticipated sequel to the first edition of *Psychological Aspects of Women's Health Care* written almost a decade ago. In this edition, the authors continue the tradition of writing and speaking plainly about the fascinating, and at times baffling, relationships between women patients and their obstetrician and gynecologist physicians. As the authors note, the field has changed dramatically since the first volume was published. The major forces leading to these transformations have been the significant medical and surgical advances in clinical practice and the prevailing attitudes toward health care influenced by managed care. These transformations also reflect the growing awareness that the interface between psychiatry and obstetrics/gynecology is more than the old psychosomatic study of disease and symptoms. It now encompasses the behaviors and attitudes surrounding reproduction, human sexuality, and abuse.

The present book follows closely the outline of the first edition. Drs. Stotland and Stewart have solicited chapters from major leaders in the specialties of psychiatry and obstetrics/gynecology covering every major area of contemporary concern, and they set a very high standard indeed. The first section is devoted to pregnancy. As the authors explain, over the past 10 years scientists have developed methods of genetic testing for preimplantation embryos and for gene mutations responsible for some ovarian and breast cancers. Sextuplets have survived to full gestation. Research on the use of psychotropic medications during pregnancy has also been more fully developed and standardized. The second section covers gynecology. Again, the progress in the past decade in the management of HIV/AIDS and pelvic pain and in the psychiatric aspects of the menopause are extensively reviewed. In the final section, "General Issues," the editors have been particularly effective in providing widely ranging but fair reviews of subjects that include eating disorders, sexual dysfunction, and violence against women, to mention only a few. Of significant value is Dr. Stotland's chapter on the provision of consultation-liaison services to obstetrics/gynecology services. This chapter, as is true for all those preceding it, is well written and referenced and the style is free and readable. The approach continues to be eclectic in the style of contemporary clinical psychiatry. The editors and the contributors have done their parts in producing a useful, valuable, and scholarly book.

I recommend this volume for medical and nursing students, residents in obstetrics/gynecology and psychiatry, and for all practicing clinicians working in the area of women's health.

# The Interface Between Psychiatry and Obstetrics and Gynecology

## An Introduction

NADA L. STOTLAND, M.D., M.P.H.
DONNA E. STEWART, M.D., D.PSYCH., F.R.C.P.C.

Since the first edition of this book was published, scientists have devised techniques for genetic testing of preimplantation embryos and for the gene mutations responsible for some familial breast and ovarian cancers. Sextuplets have been brought to term. Knowledge of lesbian health and health care has grown. HIV/AIDS has continued to spread disproportionately fast among women, especially African-American women. The provision of health care and the relationships between patients and health care professionals have been drastically altered by managed care entities. Increased and better screening has minimally decreased breast cancer deaths. Fewer women have access to abortion services. We thank the chapter authors for bringing the results of several years of new findings to this compendium of issues at the interface of psychiatry and obstetrics and gynecology.

This interface may be conceptualized narrowly, as a subspecialty of the psychiatric study of somatic symptoms and diseases (Alexander 1950). From another perspective, however, psychosomatic obstetrics and gynecology includes a realm both broad and deep that begins with men's and women's feelings and behaviors related to female reproductive physiology (Benedek and Rubenstein 1942). It ranges from the events surrounding conception–or its frustration—to reactions to terminal gynecologic malignancies. It encompasses the joyous embodiment of romantic love and the enactment of the most brutal victimization. Although only a small percentage of psychiatric and other mental health professionals explicitly devote their clinical or academic practices to this area, virtually all encounter these issues in their work with patients and their families, with medical students, and with residents.

Although many organ systems and their pathologies are associated with psychologic meanings, dynamics, conflicts, and symptoms, the relationship between psychiatry and the reproductive system is especially rich. *Hysteria* originally designated a psychiatric illness caused by the wanderings of the uterus from its proper site in the pelvis. The term was coined over 2,000 years ago and was still in use in the late twentieth century (Pomeroy 1975). Long after dissection had demonstrated the realities of the anatomy of uterine connections, Sigmund Freud linked hysteria to forbidden sexual wishes and sexual frustration (Freud 1931/1961).

In 1891, *JAMA* published an article titled "Can the Gynecologist Aid the Alienist in Institutions for the Insane?" (1891/1991). Portions of this article were reprinted for historical purposes in 1991. The author or editor, who is unnamed, cites the work as alleging a link between the functions, dysfunctions, and removal of the ovaries and uterus and psychiatric illness and treatment. A quote from the article asserted that "oophorectomy may be relied upon generally to cure insanity limited to the menstrual period" (p. 3230); this statement presaged attempts a century later to treat premenstrual symptoms. Other recent controversies are also foreshadowed. Bemoaning the "indisposition of alienists to accord the gynecologist a place in cooperation with them" the article explains,

> there was said to have been too keen a desire to try oophorectomy as a panacea for all kinds of insanity in women. There was also an effort made to introduce female physicians upon this tide of so-called necessity, and thus were blended disadvantageously questions of public policy, or expediency, with what should have been scientific inquiry. ("Can the Gynecologist Aid the Alienist in Institutions for the Insane?" 1891/1991, p. 3230)

Clinical work and experimental studies performed in the years after Freud's major contributions have disproved some of his assumptions about female psychosexual development, sexuality, and psychopathology. At the same time, new facets of patients' sexual histories prove to be as important in the etiology of psychiatric illness as those asserted in the past, albeit in a different way. Many patients with personality disorders, posttraumatic stress disorders, and other diagnoses have histories of sexual and physical abuse.

Sexually transmitted diseases and new reproductive technologies challenge the psychologic coping mechanisms of patients and the skills of their psychiatrists today.

AIDS has introduced the possibility of a serious illness or a lingering death into many sexual encounters (and into gynecologic care). The discrepancy between knowing the methods by which disease transmission can be reduced and implementing those methods in interpersonal behavior remains unresolved. Women and children are the fastest-growing populations infected with the virus. In order to design and implement strategies to reduce the transmission of HIV, public health workers must be informed of the psychology, sociology, and anthropology of female reproductive behavior (see Chapter 16). Breast and pelvic malignancies raise other psychosocial issues. The exchange of knowledge between psychiatrists and obstetrician/gynecologists (OB/GYNs) may improve the diagnosis and effective treatment of breast and gynecologic malignancies by identifying the factors that deter women from self-examination and regular medical screening. An awareness of these factors will help the psychiatrist enhance patient compliance by helping patients understand and cope with their fear of pelvic examinations, and it will help gynecologists adapt examination techniques to minimize emotional distress.

In other areas, improvements in outcomes and discoveries at the cutting edge of theory and practice may have paradoxical effects. Among the middle and upper classes, maternal and perinatal mortality rates have decreased and anesthetic techniques have improved. Parents-to-be are informed of and participants in obstetric decisions. Thus every couple demands to have a perfect childbirth and a perfect child, and failure to meet those demands has, at least in part, contributed to 80% of obstetricians in the United States having been sued at least once for malpractice (Charles and Kennedy 1985).

These demands for perfection often begin not only before birth but also before conception. Astounding, previously unimaginable developments in reproductive technology seem to offer the possibility of biologic parenthood to every infertile woman or couple (Christie and Pawson 1987). Yet these developments pose a host of problems, the resolution of which will require knowledge of biology, psychology, sociology, anthropology, ethics, and law, but the clinical dilemmas face psychiatrists in the field right now (Dickstein 1990). At what point in the diagnostic and treatment process for infertility do continued expense, life disruption, and bodily intrusion constitute an obsession? How can the psychiatrist help the patient and the treatment team make prospective policy and ongoing decisions? What ethical and psychiatric issues are raised by the voluntary and paid donations of gametes, embryos, and gestational services of one woman to another (Lantos 1990)? What roles, if any, should psychiatrists play in screening, support, and treatment? Unprecedented family constellations could offer us the opportunity to discern how family dynamics and psychologic development are shaped by genetics and by the environment.

The dialogue between obstetrics and gynecology and psychiatry, and among OB/GYNs, patients, and psychiatrists, is interwoven with social change (Stotland 1988). Tensions are reflected in language: *doctor* and *patient*, with their rich mutual obligations founded in age-old relationships, become *provider* and *consumer*. *Primum non nocere* ("First, do no harm") becomes *caveat emptor* ("Let the buyer beware"). OB/GYNs are often women's primary care physicians and the experts on their most intimate bodily parts. As such, they become the object of the strong negative and positive attitudes of their patients; they are transferentially endowed by their patients with magical technical and emotional powers. In turn, most obstetricians' offices are bedecked with photographs of infants they have delivered, testimony to a mutual emotional investment in their patients that goes beyond the skills of the accoucheur.

Women have also reacted with vituperation to the actual and perceived arrogance, insensitivity, psychologic ignorance, and authoritarianism of OB/GYNs. Laypersons and medical gadflies have published books with titles such as *Male Practice: How Doctors Manipulate Women* (Mendelson 1982), *Seizing Our Bodies: The Politics of Women's Health* (Dreifus 1978), and *Immaculate Deception: A New Look at Women and Childbirth in America* (Arms 1975) alleging and sometimes documenting negative physical and emotional effects of gynecologic interventions, some of which are unsupported by scientific evidence. The book *Our Bodies, Ourselves* (Boston Women's Health Collective 1984) conveys the message that the self-esteem and physical health of women can be improved by knowledge about their own anatomy, physiology, pathology, and treatment—that this knowledge need not remain the arcane preserve of physicians.

Social scientists and other professionals have documented physicians' demeaning attitudes toward women patients in articles such as "A Funny Thing Happened on the Way to the Orifice: Women in Gynecology Textbooks" (Scully and Bart 1973) and "The Training of a Gynecologist: How the 'Old Boys' Talk About Women's Bodies"(Hellerstein 1984). In some women's consciousness-raising groups, women examined their own and each other's bodies in a more prosaic and immediate attempt to demystify, inform, and accept themselves. Self-help groups teaching and performing menstrual extraction and suction abortions as well as routine examinations moved into the previous professional preserve. Other self-help or consumer groups continue to focus on providing information, support, and preparation for reproductive experiences such as infertility, pregnancy, childbirth, and breastfeeding (Bing 1973; La Leche League International 1987; Seiden 1978). Today's "alternative" approaches include baby massage and prenatal yoga.

In this environment, OB/GYNs practicing in good faith have been hard put to fathom the skepticism, rage, and litigiousness of their patients. Few, if any, specialties require such mastery of a combination of ever-increasing scientific knowledge and technical skills in addition to long hours, legal liability, and exposure to clinical situations of overwhelming emotional intensity (Friedman 1986). Training programs in obstetrics and gynecology include little instruction in psychodynamics, psychopathology, and interpersonal skills either in formal didactics or by example. Often, the patient population in teaching hospitals consists of disadvantaged women whose social circumstances distance them from the upper-middle-class doctors-in-training, prevent them from seeking timely care, disincline them to complain about their care, and interfere with the pleasures of a successful outcome (as when a resident delivers a baby to an overwhelmed young teenager who will take it home to a dangerous housing project). Trainees are brought face to face with the medical outcomes of social problems, such as domestic violence, rape, incest, and sexual abuse, that they do not have the time, knowledge, support, or resources to address (Adler 1972). These factors conspire to increase their focus on the cognitive knowledge and technical agility that their mentors reward.

The changing circumstances of medical practice further erode opportunities for doctors and patients to get to know and trust one another. Managed care, with choices of plan made at the employer rather than consumer level, inhibits or obliterates patients' choices of physicians. Patients make frequent geographic moves. Doctors have little motivation to understand their own responses to patients and medical situations, to examine patients' responses to them, or to develop skills that put patients at ease. Physicians practice in groups and subspecialties, both of which decrease continuity of care. In fact, it might be said that the sicker and/or more distressed a woman is, the less likely it is that she will obtain care from a physician who is familiar with her personality; defenses; usual responses to illness; family, religious, and social supports; and other coping mechanisms. The psychiatrist's role in providing this sort of information and enhancing these skills is ever more important under these circumstances (Dunbar 1954; Karasu et al. 1979; Lipowski 1986; Stotland and Garrick 1990).

Contraception and induced abortion are areas in which personal feelings about sexuality, reproduction, and gender roles as well as religious and cultural rules and values color and politicize medical practice. Contrary to popular belief, abortion has been practiced throughout recorded history and was permitted until a few centuries ago by the Roman Catholic Church (Newman 1991). New physicians, sworn by the Hippocratic and other oaths to protect "life," are arrayed opposite each other as they define life and the priorities of one form of life over another. Legalization and the improvement of medical techniques have reduced the gynecologic complications of induced abortion to a small fraction of those of childbirth. The same is true for major psychiatric sequelae. The decision to terminate a pregnancy is a weighty one, however, necessarily made under the pressure of time and best made with support and without coercion in either direction. Governmental restrictions on abortion limit the options for poor and psychiatrically ill patients and the professional autonomy of psychiatrists and gynecologists to discuss those options with their patients (*Webster v. Reproductive Health Services* 1989).

This volume is a clinical and theoretic sourcebook for the practitioner facing the many universal and specific issues of obstetrics and gynecology that arise in psychiatric practice. These issues may include presenting symptoms, as when a patient is referred for care after suffering a rape or being diagnosed with infertility or malignancy. In other cases, the role of the obstetric/gynecologic event or condition in the psychiatric illness is not volunteered or even recognized. Sexual abuse, a frequent feature in the history of patients with several major psychiatric disorders, may require particularly informed and expert diagnostic skills or several years of building trust in a psychotherapeutic relationship to reveal itself. The fact that a psychotic, manic, or depressed inpatient is postpartum may be apparent only when one learns her children's ages from the family or reproductive history. Feelings about a hysterectomy or the loss or termination of a pregnancy may play a role in the dynamics of a current conflict. Women also have questions and concerns about the psychiatric aspects of menstruation and menopause. We hope that this work will remind readers of the many rich connections between psychiatry and obstetrics and gynecology and will inform their research, teaching, and clinical work.

The choice of topics to be addressed in this book was determined by three guiding principles: 1) What issues specific to women are encountered by psychiatrists and other mental health workers? 2) What psychologic issues should be considered in providing women's health care? 3) What are the special problems seen in a consultation or liaison service to an obstetric/gynecologic program? Notman and Nadelson's (1978) pioneering work in the area of women's health is an excellent starting point, but the past two decades have seen rapid technologic and theoretic developments. Thus, a fresh look at some of the old issues and an attempt to explore some of the new dilemmas are required. Nowhere is this more apparent than in the rapidly developing field of new reproductive technologies. We have tried to emphasize those topics in which new developments have occurred. We have been guided in our choice of subjects by our clinical work, in which we daily see women referred by physicians for problems specific to their gender. Our research in psychosomatic obstetrics and gynecology and our teaching of medical students and residents has helped to focus our attention on those issues that are most common and problematic.

This book is divided into three sections: "Pregnancy," "Gynecology," and "General Issues." The "Pregnancy" section consists of seven chapters covering topics ranging from the psychology of normal gestation to physical and psychiatric complications during and following pregnancy. Robinson and Wisner's chapter on fetal anomalies (Chapter 3) addresses the new prenatal diagnostic techniques as well as the management of dynamic issues that emerge when abnormalities are detected. In Chapter 5, Stewart and Robinson discuss the use of psychotropic drugs and electroconvulsive therapy in the pregnant and lactating patient. Dell's chapter on adolescent pregnancy (Chapter 6) explores the etiologic factors and treatment strategies for this population. Leon's chapter on perinatal loss (Chapter 8) describes the emotional reactions of parents bereaved by miscarriage, stillbirth, or neonatal death and suggests approaches for treating clinicians.

The "Gynecology" section consists of eight chapters dealing with both common gynecologic problems and some of the more controversial issues such as induced abortion and the new reproductive technologies. In Chapter 9, Jensvold and Dan explicate the role of the menstrual cycle in exacerbating as well as precipitating psychologic symptoms in biologic and social contexts. Sherwin gives a comprehensive account of the psychiatric aspects of menopause in Chapter 12 and reviews the sometimes confusing literature on exogenous hormone administration. In Chapter 13, Steege and Stout discuss the assessment of chronic pelvic pain and its management by the gynecologist and/or mental health professional. In Chapter 15, Burns presents a thoughtful overview of the psychosocial concomitants of gynecologic malignancies as well as the emotional demands on the oncology team itself. Finally, in Chapter 16, Moore and Smith consider the special meanings and implications of HIV/AIDS for women.

The "General Issues" section addresses several timely topics. We have tried to present a broad and balanced picture. A psychodynamic perspective on reproductive choices and development is offered by Notman and Nadelson in Chapter 17. Segraves and Segraves, in Chapter 18, offer the latest wisdom on sexuality, sexual dysfunction, and sex therapy. Substance abuse (Chapter 20) and eating disorders (Chapter 21) are other issues too frequently overlooked in obstetrics and gynecology practice and are discussed here by Blume and Russell and by Stewart and Robinson, respectively. Andersen and Farrar's chapter on breast disorders and breast cancer (Chapter 22) is especially important in this era when uninformed fears of breast cancer influence women's compliance with medical recommendations and considerable controversy about diagnosis and treatment persists. Violence against women, in the form of spousal abuse, rape, and incest, has a major impact on their physical and emotional health. Recent findings have altered both diagnostic and treatment approaches, as discussed by Warshaw in Chapter 23. Sved, in a chapter new to this edition (Chapter 24), discusses the special and insufficiently acknowledged health care issues for lesbian patients. The rapidly changing health care scene adds new ethical and legal issues, discussed by Nadelson in Chapter 25, to the already complex world of women's health. In Chapter 26, Myers addresses a topic often missing in works of this kind: the reactions of men to women's reproductive events. In Chapter 27, Stotland addresses the provision of psychiatric consultation and liaison to obstetric and gynecologic services. Finally, Fullilove addresses the meaning of minority status in Chapter 28.

This book can be used for teaching medical and other health care students, as a reference for residents in psychiatry and obstetrics/gynecology, and to inform the clinician who is working to improve the care provided to women patients.

# References

Adler G: Helplessness in the helpers. Br J Med Psychol 45:315–326, 1972

Alexander F: Psychosomatic Medicine, New York, WW Norton, 1950

Arms S: Immaculate Deception: A New Look At Women and Childbirth in America. Boston, MA, Houghton Mifflin, 1975

Benedek T, Rubenstein B: The Sexual Cycle in Women (Psychosomatic Medicine Monographs, Vol 3). Washington, DC, National Research Council, 1942

Bing E: Six Practical Lessons for an Easier Childbirth. New York, Bantam, 1973

Boston Women's Health Collective: The New Our Bodies, Ourselves. New York, Simon & Schuster, 1984

Can the gynecologist aid the alienist in institutions for the insane? JAMA 16:870–873, 1891, reprinted in JAMA 265(24):3230, 1991

Charles SC, Kennedy E: Defendant. New York, Free Press, 1985

Christie GL, Pawson ME: The psychological and social management of the infertile couple, in The Infertile Couple. Edited by Pepperell RS, Hudson B, Wood C. New York, Churchill Livingstone, 1987, pp 35–50

Dickstein LJ: Effects of the new reproductive technologies on individuals and relationships, in Psychiatric Aspects of Reproductive Technology. Edited by Stotland NL. Washington, DC, American Psychiatric Press, 1990, pp 123–139

Dreifus C (ed): Seizing Our Bodies: The Politics of Women's Health. New York, Vintage Books, 1978

Dunbar HF: Emotional and Bodily Changes: A Survey of Literature on Psychosomatic Interrelationships. New York, Columbia University Press, 1954

Freud S: Female sexuality (1931), in The Standard Edition of the Complete Psychological Works of Sigmund Freud, Vol 21. Translated and edited by Strachey J. London, Hogarth Press, 1961, pp 223–243

Friedman EA: The obstetrician's dilemma: how much fetal monitoring and cesarean section is enough? N Engl J Med 315:641–643, 1986

Hellerstein D: The training of a gynecologist: how the "old boys" talk about women's bodies. Ms 13(5):136–137, 1984

Karasu TB, Plutchnik R, Conte H, et al: What do physicians want from a psychiatric consultation service? Compr Psychiatry 18:73–81, 1979

La Leche League International: The Womanly Art of Breastfeeding. Franklin Park, IL, La Leche League International, 1987

Lantos JD: Second-generation ethical issues in the new reproductive technologies: divided loyalties, indications, and the research agenda, in Psychiatric Aspects of Reproductive Technology. Edited by Stotland NL. Washington DC, American Psychiatric Press, 1990, pp 87–96

Lipowski ZJ: Consultation-liaison psychiatry: the first half century. Gen Hosp Psychiatry 8:305–315, 1986

Mendelson R: Male Practice: How Doctors Manipulate Women. Chicago, IL, Contemporary Books, 1982

Newman LF: Historical and cross-cultural perspectives on abortion, in Psychiatric Aspects of Abortion. Edited by Stotland NL. Washington, DC, American Psychiatric Press, 1991, pp 39–49

Notman M, Nadelson C (eds): The Woman Patient: Sexual and Reproductive Aspects of Women's Health Care. New York, Plenum Press, 1978

Pomeroy SB: Goddesses, Whores, Wives, and Slaves: Women in Classical Antiquity. New York, Schocken Books, 1975

Scully D, Bart P: A funny thing happened on the way to the orifice: women in gynecology textbooks, in Changing Women in a Changing Society. Edited by Huber J. Chicago, IL, University of Chicago Press, 1973, pp 283–288

Seiden A: The sense of mastery in the childbirth experience, in The Woman Patient: Sexual and Reproductive Aspects of Women's Health Care, Vol 3. Edited by Notman M, Nadelson C. New York, Plenum, 1978, pp 87–105

Stotland NL: Social Change and Women's Reproductive Health Care. New York, Praeger, 1988

Stotland NL, Garrick TR: Manual of Psychiatric Consultation. Washington, DC, American Psychiatric Press, 1990

Webster v Reproductive Health Services, 109 S.Ct. 3040 (1989)

# Pregnancy

# Normal and Medically Complicated Pregnancies

DIANE A. PHILIPP, M.D., F.R.C.P.C.
MELANIE L. CARR, M.D., F.R.C.P.C.

The miracle of pregnancy and the transformation of women into mothers has fascinated people from antiquity to the present. However, it is only during the past century that mental health professionals have begun to contribute to our understanding of the psychologic aspects of pregnancy and the psychosocial phases that women pass through on their journey into motherhood. Although this century has seen tremendous strides in the field of obstetrics, including the management of formerly nonviable high-risk pregnancies, there is a lag in our understanding of women's psychologic adaptations to medically complicated pregnancies. In this chapter, we begin by exploring the psychologic aspects of normal pregnancies, particularly in first-time mothers. Next, by providing a brief overview of medically complicated pregnancies, we create a framework for examining current understanding of the psychologic adaptation of pregnant women to their high-risk status. Finally, we consider the role of the psychiatrist consultant to obstetrics and gynecology.

## The Psychoanalytic View

The psychoanalytic movement was among the first to consider the psychologic meaning of pregnancy to young girls and women. Although Freud's theory regarding pregnancy is now viewed as antiquated, it bears brief mentioning because it was the dominant view for much of the twentieth century. Freud understood the female wish for pregnancy by adapting his notion of the Oedipal conflict to girls. He believed that young girls, in coming to terms with the absence of a penis, initially blamed their mothers for their "castrated" bodies and turned to their fathers to replace the "lost" penis. Freud viewed the final resolution of this phase as a replacement of the wish for a penis by the wish for a baby (Freud 1933/1964).

As more women began to offer their perspective in the psychoanalytic arena, the emphasis began to shift away from this notably phallocentric explanation. Influential in finally breaking with the older view, Benedek (1970) saw pregnancy as a basic biologic drive in women, not merely a substitutive function:

> Thus motherhood is not secondary, not a substitute for the missing penis, nor is it forced by men upon women "in the service of the species," but the manifestation of the all-pervading instinct for survival in the child that is the primary organizer of the woman's sexual drive, and by this also her personality. (p. 139)

These ideas have been developed in more recent reports by authors who have seen the wish for motherhood as based not only on biologic drive but also on an identification with what is essentially female. Several therapists have noted a richness in themes of identification with the woman's own mother (Kestenberg 1977; Lester and Notman 1986; Pines 1972, 1982). Over the course of the past century a shift has occurred in the psychodynamic conceptualization from viewing pregnancy as a wish for a penis like the father toward an acceptance of the importance of an identification with the mother.

## Psychologic Stages of Normal Pregnancy

In the late 1950s, Greta Bibring set out to do a longitudinal study of normal pregnant women using a multidisciplinary team of mental health and health care professionals (Bibring 1959; Bibring et al. 1961). As a result of her observations, Bibring postulated that pregnancy, "like puberty or menopause, is a period of crisis involving profound psychologic as well as somatic changes" (Bibring 1959, p. 116). Further elaborating on the analogy to puberty and menopause, she noted that these are all biologically mediated transitions from which there is no return. Once one becomes a mother there is no returning to the previous childless stage (Bibring 1959). We would add that the advent of effective contraception and the legalization of abortion have placed pregnancy in a unique position; it is the only developmental stage that may or may not be embarked upon depending on a woman's choice and her cultural milieu. Bibring was perhaps the first to describe normal stages of psychologic development in pregnancy (Bibring et al. 1961). Numerous other investigators have provided greater detail about the phases of pregnancy; we attempt to synthesize the various perspectives in this chapter.

Although most authors view the psychologic stages of pregnancy as beginning with conception, we find it more useful to use a broader context and consider the development of mothers as beginning in childhood and continuing well into the postpartum. Girls can be observed preparing for motherhood by trying on the role in play. As Morris (1997) pointed out, a familiar scene is that of young girls fighting over who will play the mother in a simple game of "house." Stern (1995), writing from the perspective of an infant psychiatrist, suggested that long before conception occurs, the young girl or woman imagines herself as a mother as well as imagining her infant and child. When the woman finds a partner, these "representations" and "schemas," as Stern calls them, undergo further elaboration because she now has new information about the child's future father. Once pregnant and into the postpartum, the woman is faced with increasing information about the fetus, herself, and her husband, and so the internal representations of these individuals evolve (Stern 1995).

Once conception has occurred, there are three distinct psychologic phases that most women pass through during their pregnancies. These stages roughly correspond to the three trimesters of pregnancy and appear to be triggered by various psychologic, biologic, and cultural influences. The first stage of pregnancy is usually thought to begin when the woman realizes she is pregnant and to last until she experiences quickening (fetal movements), at approximately 4 1/2 months. During this stage, as new and often uncomfortable physical symptoms develop in the expectant mother, ambivalence about the pregnancy is common. Ultimately, in a wanted pregnancy, the fundamental task of this first stage is the acceptance of the pregnancy (Sandelowski and Black 1994). Women struggling with this task may show behavioral signs, such as denial of the pregnancy or unusual reactions to bodily changes (Cohen 1979).

Several other psychologic changes begin at this time. In the clinical literature, "psychologic slippage" or forgetfulness has been described (Raphael-Leff 1991). Only recently has this notion been examined empirically, in a cross-sectional study of memory in pregnancy (Sharp et al. 1993). This study confirms women's subjective experiences—over 80% of the pregnant women studied perceived their memory as impaired compared with only 16% of non-pregnant control subjects. On objective measures of memory, the pregnant subjects were significantly impaired in comparison with control subjects in their recall of lists of words. Because no differences were found in the performances of women among the three trimesters, the authors concluded that no single hormone could be singled out as causative. Certainly one might have expected that the rising levels of estrogen in pregnancy would, in fact, be protective because estrogen has been found to heighten verbal memory in women (B. B. Sherwin 1998). Nevertheless, beginning in the first trimester and continuing into the early postpartum period, a woman's memory may be somewhat compromised. This change can become clinically significant in situations in which patients are given large amounts of information to retain.

The predominant fear expressed by women in the first trimester of a wanted pregnancy is a fear of miscarriage (Leifer 1977). Other themes of this stage include increased emotionality, preoccupation with bodily needs (particularly food), and an obsession with her "secret" (Raphael-Leff 1991). Many women continue to keep the pregnancy secret until they have passed into the second trimester. As the viability of the pregnancy seems more ensured, the mother embarks on the telling process. She typically progresses in a hierarchic order from those closest to her outward (Raphael-Leff 1991; Rubin 1970).

The second psychologic phase of pregnancy was historically thought to be initiated by quickening and the undeniable realization that life exists within. With the advent of fetal ultrasound, the progression into this next phase of development may be accelerated for some women (Raphael-Leff 1991). Regardless, with the reduction or disappearance of many unpleasant physical symptoms, the second trimester of a woman's pregnancy is a time of relative peace and fulfillment. The most important tasks for a woman in this stage are initiating an emotional affiliation with, or attachment to, the fetus and recognizing the fetus as a separate individual contained within her (Bibring et al. 1961; Cohen 1979; Leifer 1977; Lester and Notman 1986; Pines 1982; Raphael-Leff 1991).

In his work, Stern (1995) pointed out that from about "the fourth to the seventh month there is rapid growth in the richness, quantity, and specificity of the networks of schemas about the baby-to-be" (p. 23). This is apparently heralded by either quickening or by fetal ultrasound. Also at this time, signs of "motherliness" or a wish to nurture the infant become apparent (Lester and Notman 1986). Leifer (1977) identified several behaviors indicative of attachment such as talking to the fetus, calling the fetus by a pet name, and maneuvering the fetus so that the partner may observe movement.

Hormonal correlates of maternal attachment were examined in a large, multicenter study of pregnancy. Fleming and colleagues (1997) used both cross-sectional and longitudinal data and found that attachment to the fetus significantly increased between the first and second trimesters. However, no correlation was found between the hormonal changes of pregnancy and the measures of maternal attachment assessed during pregnancy. Interestingly, an increase in the estradiol to progesterone ratio (E/P) through the course of pregnancy was consistently related to stronger feelings of attachment in the postpartum. Therefore, hormonal factors may contribute to attachment, particularly in the early postpartum.

With the sensation of fetal movements, the mother begins to recognize the fetus as a separate entity. Issues of separation and individuation from her own mother may be triggered by this process. In addition, it is during this phase that the woman may have anxieties about identifying with, or becoming like, her own mother (Morris 1997). The typical resolution of this period is a reworking of previous attitudes that helped the young woman separate from her mother in earlier developmental phases. Ideally, the pregnant woman develops a new-found appreciation for her mother and the mothering role in general (Bibring et al. 1961; Cohen 1979; Morris 1997; Pines 1972, 1982). According to Cohen (1979), unresolved conflict with one's own mother is more stressful than marital conflict and is a predictor of maladaptation to pregnancy. However, in the study by Fleming et al. (1997) no change was found in mothers' relations with their own mothers, although it is unclear how this relationship was measured and if questions of separation and identification were examined.

As expectant mothers come to accept their fetuses as separate from themselves, they may also develop new feelings of ambivalence toward the pregnancy. For many women, the stage after quickening brings relief that there is indeed life within as well as a sense of fulfillment (Leifer 1977; Rubin 1970). However, it is not uncommon for women to harbor feelings of resentment toward the fetus (Benedek 1970; Pines 1972; Trad 1991). Around this time, a woman begins to "show" and thus loses control over who knows of the pregnancy (Rubin 1970). The mother may feel treated as a "pregnancy" and not as a person. Consequently, she may have an increasing sense of aloneness, which may be exacerbated if she has predominantly childless, nonpregnant friends (Raphael-Leff 1991) or if she continues to feel ambivalent or negative about the pregnancy.

The third and final psychologic stage of pregnancy begins when physical discomforts again predominate and the mother has a sense of her infant as viable (Lester and Notman 1986; Raphael-Leff 1991). During this stage maternal–fetal attachment is expected to be at its highest, and "nesting behavior" is occurring—that is, preparations for the baby's arrival, such as purchasing furniture or selecting a name (Leifer 1977). The absence of this nesting behavior at this stage may indicate a maladaptation to pregnancy (Cohen 1979; Leifer 1977). Thus the predominant themes during this time center on preparation for the baby's arrival, somatic concerns, and worries about the delivery.

According to Stern (1995), the elaboration of schemas about the expected baby declines beginning around the seventh month. The image apparently becomes less clear than previously. Fleming and colleagues (1997) described a similar phenomenon and reported a slight decline in positive feelings about the fetus in the weeks immediately preceding the birth. These may be protective functions on the part of the mother, to ward off any potential feelings of disappointment should the real baby differ significantly from the fantasized one (Stern 1995).

During this final stage, expectant mothers again focus on bodily sensations, and appearance may become an increasing concern. In a survey of obstetric patients at 36 weeks' gestation, Hofmeyr et al. (1990) found that although 20% of the patients reported feeling more attractive, more than 50% felt less attractive and 60% had a decreased interest in sexual relations with their partners. This sense of being unattractive appears to increase throughout the course of pregnancy but actually peaks in the postpartum (Berk 1993; Leifer 1977).

At this time in the pregnancy, anxiety about the delivery increases (Leifer 1977). Fears tend to group around several themes. Worry about the health of the baby often ranks highest (Kestenberg 1977; Neuhaus et al. 1994). Pain and loss of control during delivery are other major concerns (Mackey 1995). Antenatal classes have attempted to address some of these fears. Unfortunately, to date only a limited amount of research is available regarding the efficacy of prenatal classes in improving psychologic outcomes for women, and the results of this research are conflicting (Nichols 1995; Zwelling 1996).

With each developmental milestone of the fetus, the sense of the unrelenting push toward separation is reinforced (Trad 1991). At no point is this more true than with delivery of the infant. Delivery is a profound culmination of much of the physical and psychologic preparation of the mother and her partner. In one brief moment, two become three, and the course of their lives is set on a new, unalterable path. Postpartum issues are discussed elsewhere in this volume (Chapter 7), but it is important to reiterate that development of the mother continues after the birth as an interactive process between the woman and her baby (Bibring et al. 1961; Stern 1995).

## Medical Complications of Pregnancy

The notion of high risk can be broken down into both medical and psychosocial categories (L. N. Sherwin and Mele 1986). In this discussion we primarily consider the former; the latter is covered elsewhere in this text. The designation of *high risk* is given to approximately 30% of pregnancies in the United States, and these pregnancies account for 50% of perinatal mortality. Complications may develop at any stage of pregnancy as a result of preexisting or emergent maternal disorders, obstetric difficulties, or fetal compromise. A cursory overview of these medical complications follows, to set the stage for discussion of the psychologic aspects of high-risk pregnancy. A more detailed description is beyond the scope of this chapter, but appropriate references are included. It behooves the psychiatrist working at the interface of psychiatry and obstetrics to have a working knowledge of the medical complications that can develop in pregnancy in order to have a full appreciation of the patient's course and to provide an effective liaison service.

Maternal factors associated with increased risk during pregnancy include hypertension, diabetes, cardiovascular disease, renal disease, malignancies, and HIV. Some of these present for the first time, or only, during pregnancy. For example, hypertension is a complicating factor in approximately 5%–10% of all pregnancies (Sibai 1992). Preeclampsia, a disorder specific to pregnancy, is characterized by hypertension, edema, and proteinuria. It accounts for the majority of hypertensive gravidas and develops with increasing frequency after the twentieth week of gestation. Eclampsia is preeclampsia with convulsions. The only specific treatment is delivery, but temporization with bed rest, medications, and careful monitoring may be justified if the patient is remote from term (Mabie and Sibai 1994). The remaining minority of cases involve chronic hypertension. Management of this latter group is controversial; many experts now recommend not treating mild elevations in blood pressure. The benefits of treating severe hypertension in pregnancy appear to outweigh the risks of the medications used, however, because maternal and fetal morbidity and mortality are significantly reduced with treatment (Sibai 1992).

Since the introduction of insulin, fetal and neonatal mortality in pregnancies complicated by diabetes has reduced from approximately 65% to 2%–5% (Landon and Gabbe 1992). Strict glucose control, both preconception and prenatally, appears to further reduce the risk of congenital malformations in the fetuses of diabetic women (Palmer 1994). As with hypertension, the vast majority of cases of diabetes (90%) develop during pregnancy as gestational diabetes (Landon and Gabbe 1992). For some of these women, however, that diagnosis intrapartum may foreshadow a diagnosis of non–insulin dependent diabetes later in life (Palmer 1994).

Cardiovascular disease complicates 0.4%–4% of pregnancies and is the most frequent nonobstetric cause of maternal mortality (Biswas and Perloff 1994). The effect of cardiac disease on the pregnancy differs depending on the severity of the underlying disorder. With close monitoring and management, women with other medical illnesses such as mild to moderate renal disease, blood disorders, seizure disorders, multiple sclerosis, and even certain cancers in remission are increasingly able to have a successful pregnancy outcome. It is only when these disorders are severe that the prognosis for mother and fetus may be compromised.

In the past two decades, HIV has increasingly complicated the pregnancies of young women. In an extensive review, Fowler et al. (1997) reported that of the estimated 30 million individuals infected with HIV worldwide, 11 million are women and 3 million are children (90% of whom were infected perinatally). It is notable that in women of childbearing age, risk factors that prompt HIV testing are frequently underrecognized by clinicians (Schoenbaum and Webber 1993).

Pregnancy does not appear to affect the progression of HIV (Hoyt 1997). However, treatment for HIV-related conditions may be delayed because of risk to the fetus (De Ferrari et al. 1993a, 1993b). In terms of HIV's impact on the pregnancy, North American studies comparing HIV-infected women with healthy control subjects have demonstrated no significant differences in obstetric complications or birth outcomes (Minkoff et al. 1990; Selwyn et al. 1989). Many factors are believed to increase the risk of transmission of HIV from mother to fetus; however, new retroviral treatments administered during pregnancy and later to the neonate can reduce the risk of perinatal transmission from 25% to 8% (Centers for Disease Control and Prevention 1996). Knowledge about risk reduction in HIV-infected pregnancies has given new hope to HIV-infected women considering their reproductive options.

Obstetric factors that increase risk in pregnancy include habitual abortion, multiple gestation, placenta praevia, and abruptio placentae. Miscarriage is a common problem in pregnancy, but most women will go on to deliver a healthy baby in a subsequent pregnancy. A small subset of women, however, will repeatedly lose their pregnancies, a condition known as *habitual abortion*. Possible contributing factors include chromosomal abnormalities, dysfunction of the maternal endocrine system, infection, structural anomalies of the reproductive tract (e.g., cervical incompetence), and underlying maternal disease (Pernoll and Garmel 1994). Treatment of habitual abortion, therefore, is aimed at the underlying cause.

With the increasing numbers of women delaying childbearing and the new reproductive technologies, the number of multiple-gestation pregnancies has increased substantially in the past two decades (Bowers 1998). It is well known that the presence of additional fetuses increases the risk of complications for the mother and the fetuses. Ideally, early diagnosis with ultrasound allows for increased surveillance and improved outcomes. Unfortunately, not all cases are diagnosed antepartum (Palmer 1994).

Of all pregnancies, 2%–3% are complicated by serious hemorrhage, often in the third trimester (Pernoll 1994a, 1994b). Placenta praevia, which occurs in 1 of every 200 pregnancies, is a major cause of such bleeds. Placenta praevia is the implantation of the placenta in the lower segment of the uterus so that the placenta extends to the margin of the internal os of the cervix, partially or completely obstructing it. It presents as painless vaginal bleeding, and diagnosis is established by ultrasound. Management depends on the amount of bleeding, gestational age, fetal well-being, and presentation.

The other major cause of third-trimester bleeding is abruptio placentae, in which the placenta begins to separate from the interior uterine wall too early in gestation. In 20% of cases this bleeding is contained within the uterus, behind the fetus, resulting in a "concealed" abruption. Close monitoring of both mother and fetus is essential if abruption is suspected, because both are at serious risk of significant morbidity and death.

Fetal complications that cause a pregnancy to be designated as high-risk include intrauterine growth retardation (IUGR) and intrapartum fetal distress. IUGR complicates 3%–7% of all pregnancies. Many factors are associated with IUGR, including infection, multiple gestation, poor nutrition, eating disorders, chromosomal abnormalities, congenital malformation, maternal hypertension, maternal smoking, and drug and alcohol abuse. Once IUGR is diagnosed, serial determinations of growth are undertaken, and treatment is aimed at contributing factors. After the age of viability, delivery is considered if fetal compromise is evident (Gabbe 1986).

In some cases, complications develop during the intrapartum period in a pregnancy that had progressed smoothly until term. Significant steps have been made in identifying fetal compromise during labor. Lower morbidity and mortality rates have resulted, primarily through the determination of fetal risk for hypoxia. The benefit of intrapartum surveillance is that it allows for confirmation of fetal well-being and may prevent unnecessary obstetric intervention. Unfortunately, false-positive results still occur, and operative deliveries are sometimes undertaken unnecessarily. The advantages of increased technology must be weighed against the disadvantages, including the psychologic aspects of having a monitored labor.

## Psychologic Aspects of High-Risk Pregnancies

Although a vast body of literature exists on the medical aspects of high-risk pregnancies, there is only a small body of knowledge about resulting psychologic reactions. In this section we attempt to explore the meaning of this diagnosis to expectant mothers, the ways in which it may affect the developmental milestones outlined, and some specific issues pertaining to these patients.

In general, it appears that once women are diagnosed with high-risk pregnancies, they struggle with each psychologic stage of pregnancy. The normal ambivalence of early pregnancy may be protracted and therefore may delay acceptance of the pregnancy. After quickening, these women may have greater difficulties attaching to their fetuses. Furthermore, in the final stage of pregnancy, nesting behaviors may be delayed or even absent and dependency may be heightened. Some of these difficulties may persist into the postpartum.

In considering the psychologic adaptation to high-risk pregnancy, it is important to recognize that even women with normal pregnancies may perceive themselves to be "at risk." Marteau et al. (1991) found that a pregnant woman's perceived risk of having a baby with an abnormality did not correlate with her actual risk. In a recent study, Searle (1996) noted that although women tend to underestimate the actual risk of an abnormal outcome, placing it at around 1/1000, most of these women were anxious that their own pregnancy was at risk. Anxiety about the well-being of the fetus ranked highest among their concerns. By far the most important anxiety reducer (for 90.5%) was the availability of routine antenatal screening tests, which provided these women with the "reassurance" that all was well (Searle 1996). One must wonder, however, what role the routine availability of these tests plays in creating a sense of risk and abnormality in the first place.

The high-risk group itself is not homogeneous, and thus it is difficult to draw conclusions about all women with high-risk pregnancies. For example, the patient's reaction to the diagnosis is affected by the stage at which the pregnancy is identified as high risk, the etiology of the risk, the nature of the treatment, and the personality structure and defenses of the pregnant woman (Kemp and Page 1987; Wolreich 1986).

In exploring the meaning, to women, of a medically complicated pregnancy, it is important to recognize that much of the self-esteem of women who choose motherhood may become entrenched in the successful completion of this task. The knowledge of carrying an "imperfect" pregnancy may affect a woman's self-esteem detrimentally and leave her with feelings of inadequacy and failure (Jones 1986; Raphael-Leff 1991). Indeed, Kemp and Page (1987) found that women carrying high-risk pregnancies scored lower than women with normal pregnancies on measures of self-esteem. More recently, Kemp and Hatmaker (1992) found that women with high-risk pregnancies also scored lower on a measure of self-actualization. If we subscribe to the view of pregnancy as an identification with the mother and the feminine ideal, then this low self-esteem and low self-actualization may even affect a woman's sense of herself as a woman.

## Psychologic Stages in High-Risk Pregnancy

Any event perceived as threatening by the mother may compromise her ability to master the various stages of pregnancy (Cohen 1979). In examining the impact of a designation of high risk on psychologic development in pregnancy, we have focused on the responses of the mother. The reactions of the partner and older children are also significant, however, and although beyond the scope of this chapter, must be considered in the care of the high-risk mother.

When the label of "high risk" is given, either before conception or very early on, the first psychologic task in pregnancy is more complex and at times paradoxical. These women must accept the pregnancy but concomitantly are faced with the threat to the survival of that pregnancy (Penticuff 1982). The normal ambivalence of early pregnancy may be prolonged and may persist for the duration of the pregnancy or until the perceived threat has subsided or resolved (Penticuff 1982).

In the next psychologic phase of pregnancy, one fundamental task is attachment to the fetus. Research examining this question in high-risk pregnancies is limited, and although earlier findings suggested that these mothers were no different from normal control subjects, clinical observation and more recent investigation suggest that the label of high risk may interfere with attachment. In two earlier studies, Kemp and Page (1986a, 1987) used fetal attachment measures to compare women carrying low- and high-risk pregnancies during their third trimester. They found no significant differences in degree of maternal attachment to the fetus. The authors speculated that a certain degree of denial regarding the severity, or even the presence, of the high risk designation may allow for attachment to proceed relatively normally. However, they also noted that the subjects were all beyond 28 weeks' gestation and may have become more optimistic because of the long duration of the pregnancy (Kemp and Page 1986a). Furthermore, because quickening usually occurs around 20 weeks' gestation, many may have actually begun the task of attachment to the fetus prior to receiving the diagnosis of high risk.

Therapists working with expectant parents with high-risk pregnancies have noted that this population holds off on developing feelings of attachment to the fetus for fear of disappointment (Moore 1983; Penticuff 1982). More recently, Kemp and Hatmaker (1992) looked at health-promoting and health-protective behaviors in pregnant women from a homogenous socioeconomic background. They found that women with high-risk pregnancies were less likely to engage in health-protective and health-promoting behaviors than were those with low-risk pregnancies. Although these findings run counter to what one might hope for in high-risk pregnancies, one can speculate that the absence of these behaviors may reflect an absent or diminished attachment to the fetus. In other words, attachment is negatively affected by the diagnosis of high risk; therefore, these women are less likely to demonstrate protective and nurturant behaviors toward their fetuses. Notably, unlike the earlier study on attachment, these women were polled between 20 and 41 weeks' gestation and thus some may have received their diagnoses before quickening, when attachment seems to begin. Although it seems likely that maternal attachment to the fetus is altered or delayed in high-risk pregnancies, more research is needed in this area to clarify how and when this occurs.

Separation issues, which also come to the fore once fetal movements are perceived, may also be affected by a high-risk pregnancy. Not only is the woman aware of fetal movements, but some of the interventions that she must undergo, either for her own health or for that of the fetus, help to underscore both their separateness as well as their merged status. The mother is acutely aware that medications she must take for her own health may pose risks to the developing fetus (Raphael-Leff 1991). Similarly, she may receive certain medications (for example, corticosteroids to mature fetal lungs) that are aimed at helping her fetus but may result in side effects for her. In the case of preexisting medical conditions, the pregnancy may jeopardize the mother's health or there may be a risk of passing on a genetic or infectious disorder to the infant. Finally, with the intrusion of medical intervention, the usual sense of being treated as a "pregnancy" may be exaggerated. The mother may feel overlooked—a vessel for the fetus toward whom all attention is being paid. Normal resentment toward the fetus at this time may be compounded and confused by feelings of guilt and responsibility.

The final weeks of pregnancy are notable for nesting behaviors as well as for a deepening dependency on social supports. With regard to nesting activity, Penticuff (1982) has suggested that preparatory behaviors are diminished or absent in high-risk pregnancies. For example, the couple may postpone preparing the nursery or selecting a name for the baby.

As described previously, dependency tends to increase throughout pregnancy and is greatest in the third trimester. The label of high risk has been thought to increase the normal dependency of pregnancy (Wolreich 1986). However, some controversy exists as to whether this increase is adaptive. Wolreich (1986) hypothesized that heightened dependency and the assumption of the "sick role" may make the frequency of visits and intensive testing more tolerable. In addition, the regression and passivity of pregnancy may allow for increased compliance with parental figures such as medical personnel. On the other hand, this increased dependency and tolerance of the "sick role" may mean that the mother anticipates a more negative outcome (Kemp and Page 1987). Such a belief may lead to a sense of learned helplessness, depression, and decreased compliance. In contrast, being treated as "sick" may be very difficult for some because these women often do not feel "ill" (Gupton et al. 1997; Gyves 1985). In such situations one might expect a more resistant or independent stance, which also results in decreased compliance with medical regimens.

In women who are hospitalized or are prescribed bed rest, regression and dependency may be further intensified by the enforced abandonment of usual activities, including work, and the provision of most aspects of daily care by others (Rogers 1989). Studies in recent years have looked at the effect of antepartum bed rest or hospitalization on psychologic functioning (Gupton et al. 1997; White and Ritchie 1984). Several issues have been found to create stress and anxiety in these women, such as concern about one's own health and that of the fetus, uncertainty and lack of control, feeling like a prisoner, feeling that one is missing out, concern about other children in the family, role reversals with the partner, and in the case of hospitalized patients, the separation from the usual supports of spouse and family (Gupton et al. 1997; White and Ritchie 1984). There is also financial stress if the expectant mother stops working or requires costly procedures, treatments, or services.

For many women with medically complicated pregnancies, the birth of a healthy baby signifies a resolution of the uncertainties experienced during pregnancy. Nevertheless, difficulties from earlier developmental periods may spill over into this next stage, leading to problems in the early mother–infant dyad and perhaps beyond (Bibring 1959; Penticuff 1982). In fact, Priel and Kantor (1988) found that women who had carried high-risk pregnancies not only perceived their newborn infants as more difficult than the "average" baby but also expected the "average" baby to be much "easier" than did mothers who had experienced normal pregnancies. Burger and colleagues (1993) found that at 4–8 years postpartum, mothers who had had complicated pregnancies viewed their children as vulnerable to illness almost twice as frequently as did women without pregnancy complications. This significant difference remained even when those infants who were in fact ill in the postpartum were removed from the analyses and only mothers with healthy newborns were included. Mothers with severe prenatal complications were also significantly more likely to report having had a postpartum depression. Viewing a child as more difficult or more vulnerable, as well as having postpartum depression, has serious implications for parent–child interactions. It would seem, then, that the psychologic difficulties that women with high-risk pregnancies may experience can have consequences that reach well into the postnatal period.

It should also be noted, however, that several studies examining pregnant women diagnosed as high risk have found that they manage fairly well. In a study examining the psychologic impact of the diagnosis of gestational diabetes, Spirito et al. (1989) found that most women coped well with this unanticipated development. Subjects were interviewed several weeks after the diagnosis was established, which may have allowed for a period of adjustment. Kemp and Page (1987) also found no significant difference in the anxiety levels of women carrying high-risk pregnancies and those carrying low-risk pregnancies. Again, this study looked at women in their third trimester who may also have had time to adjust and were therefore no longer anxious. As described previously, this study found no differences on measures of attachment; however, the authors did not look at the major tasks of this phase—that is, nesting behaviors and coping with increasing dependency needs. Thus, on certain measures of general adjustment, it is possible that for some women the diagnosis of high risk does not have a deleterious effect. However, when the specific psychologic tasks are examined at the appropriate developmental phase, a number of these women may be found to be struggling. Clearly, there is a paucity of well-designed studies examining these questions, and definitive conclusions are difficult to make at this time.

Women infected with HIV warrant special consideration. Some of their issues highlight difficulties pertinent to all medically ill women embarking on a pregnancy. Other issues differ distinctly. Sowell and Misener (1997) used focus groups to examine the reproductive choices of HIV-infected women. Participants who wanted children, once aware of their HIV status, saw childbearing as an opportunity to leave something behind when they were gone—an opportunity to feel complete. In a study of women having children after breast cancer, Dow (1994) also found women to report "feeling complete" as a rationale. Furthermore, for many breast cancer survivors, having children also meant getting well again, although they worried that they might not survive to see their children grow up. Regardless of whether this belief turned out to be accurate in the long run, getting well again has at least been a possibility for these women. For those infected with HIV, however, one of the struggles is knowing that they will probably succumb to their illness and leave their children behind. For some of the women in Sowell and Meisner's (1997) study, this knowledge influenced them to not have a baby.

Unique to HIV is the meaning of the disease in our culture and the stigmatization and shame that come with the diagnosis. De Ferrari et al. (1993a, 1993b) commented on some of the specific problems associated with HIV infection, such as discrimination, social isolation, poverty, grief, and in the case of pregnant women, guilt over potentially infecting an unborn child. Because a large proportion of HIV-infected pregnant women are substance abusers, their ongoing drug dependence makes them less able to be compliant with health care, thus compounding their sense of culpability and shame.

## Psychiatric Intervention

Working at the interface of psychiatry and obstetrics and gynecology can be both challenging and rewarding. Psychiatric involvement can be beneficial at every step of the process, from preconception through to the postpartum period. As noted by Bibring (1959), relatively simple interventions can result in significant change for the mother. Furthermore, the psychiatrist can play a role in helping others in the woman's immediate environment.

For some women the role of the psychiatrist may begin even before conception. In women with chronic diseases, prepregnancy counseling in conjunction with the obstetric team can be very helpful. Couples may need to feel that they have permission to *not* have a child or to explore options like surrogate pregnancy or adoption. Once the patient becomes pregnant, certain elements in her history may signal perinatal psychiatric difficulties, such as previous obstetric mishap, infertility, familial or congenital diseases, conflicts about separation from parents, and poor relationships with physicians (Cohen 1979; Nadelson 1978). Stewart and Lippert (1988) reviewed reasons for psychiatric referral during pregnancy and childbirth. They cited extreme ambivalence toward pregnancy, marital conflict related to the pregnancy, psychosocial problems, unstable environment, and prenatal anxiety as common reasons for referral. Another frequent referral question is to review the risk/benefit ratio of continuing psychotropic medications for a preexisting psychiatric disease during pregnancy or whether to initiate medications during the course of a pregnancy (see Chapter 5). Finally, psychiatric consultation is sometimes sought because of noncompliance with prenatal care. This typically occurs in pregnancies already considered high risk for medical or social reasons or because of substance abuse (Stewart and Lippert 1988). Once a patient is referred, the time-limited nature of pregnancy can be especially suited to short-term psychotherapeutic intervention aimed at improving adjustment and resolving conflicting feelings about the fetus (Bibring 1959; St-Andre 1993; Wolreich 1986).

Working with obstetric personnel can be challenging for the consultation-liaison psychiatrist. The medical team may have their own reactions to a jeopardized pregnancy that can interfere with providing optimal medical care and emotional support to the pregnant woman. Diplomatically helping the staff understand their responses can assist in modifying unhelpful, overinvolved, or even hostile behavior. Gyves (1985) noted stresses particular to the team working with high-risk pregnancies. First is the uncertainty of whether to label something as a problem and whether to inform the patient of it. Second, certain disorders have controversial treatments and dissent may exist within the team as to which direction to take. A further stress for the clinician can occur if the family chooses a course of action that differs from what is recommended. Finally, families often have very high expectations of the team, leaving little room for error in situations in which the outcomes can be devastating (Gyves 1985).

To be most effective, the psychiatrist working in this multifaceted area must have an understanding of the psychology of normal pregnancy, a familiarity with the medical and obstetric complications and management of high-risk pregnancy, and an appreciation of the psychologic reactions associated with high-risk status for the pregnant woman and her family. The impact of interventions at this time can be far-reaching, both for the new mother and for her baby.

# References

Benedek T: The psychobiology of pregnancy, in Parenthood: Its Psychology and Psychopathology. Edited by Anthony EJ, Benedek T. Boston, MA, Little, Brown, 1970, pp 137–151

Berk B: Body image and pregnancy: Bridging the mind–body connection. J Perinatol 13:300–304, 1993

Bibring GL: Some considerations of the psychological processes in pregnancy. Psychoanal Study Child 14:113–121, 1959

Bibring GL, Dwyer T, Huntington D, et al: A study of the psychological processes in pregnancy and the earliest mother-child relationship. Psychoanal Study Child 16:9–24, 1961

Biswas MK, Perloff DP: Cardiac, hemotalogic, pulmonary, renal, and urinary tract disorders in pregnancy, in Current Obstetric and Gynecologic Diagnosis and Treatment. Edited by Decherney AH, Pernoll ML. East Norwalk, CT, Appleton & Lange, 1994, pp 428–467

Bowers NA: The multiple birth explosion: implications for nursing practice. J Obstet Gynecol Neonatal Nurs 27:302–310, 1998

Burger J, Horwitz SM, Forsyth BW, et al: Psychological sequelae of medical complications during pregnancy. Pediatrics 91:566–571, 1993

Centers for Disease Control and Prevention: HIV testing among women aged 18–44 years: United States, 1991 and 1993. MMWR 45:733–737, 1996

Cohen RL: Maladaptation to Pregnancy. Semin Perinatol 3:15–24, 1979

De Ferrari E, Gegor CL, Summers L, et al: Nurse-midwifery management of women with human immunodeficiency virus disease. J Nurse Midwifery 38:86–96, 1993a

De Ferrari E, Paine LL, Gegor CL, et al: Midwifery care for women with human immunodeficiency virus disease in pregnancy: a demonstration project at the Johns Hopkins Hospital. J Nurse Midwifery 38:97–102, 1993b

Dow KH: Having children after breast cancer. Cancer Pract 2:407–413, 1994

Fleming AS, Ruble D, Krieger H, et al: Hormonal and experiential correlates of maternal responsiveness during pregnancy and the puerperium in human mothers. Horm Behav 31:145–158, 1997

Fowler MG, Melnick SL, Mathieson BJ: Women and HIV: epidemiology and global overview. Obstet Gynecol Clin North Am 24:705–729, 1997

Freud S: Femininity (1933), in The Standard Edition of the Complete Psychological Works of Sigmund Freud, Vol 22. Translated and Edited by Strachey J. London, England, Hogarth, 1964, pp 128.

Gabbe SG: Intrauterine growth retardation, in Obstetrics: Normal and Problem Pregnancies. Edited by Gabbe SG, Niebyl JR, Simpson JL. New York, Churchill Livingstone, 1986, pp 769–785

Gupton A, Heaman M, Ashcroft T: Bed rest from the perspective of the high-risk pregnant woman. J Obstet Gynecol Neonatal Nurs 26:423–430, 1997

Gyves MT: The psychosocial impact of high risk pregnancy. Adv Psychosom Med 12:71–80, 1985

Hofmeyr GJ, Marcos EF, Butchart AM: Pregnant women's perceptions of themselves: a survey. Birth 17:205–206, 1990

Hoyt L: HIV infection in women and children: special concerns in prevention and care. Postgrad Med 102:165–176, 1997

Jones MB: The high-risk pregnancy, in Nursing Assessment and Strategies for the Family at Risk, 2nd Edition. Edited by Johnson SH. Philadelphia, PA, JB Lippincott, 1986, pp 111–128.

Kemp VH, Hatmaker DD: Health practices and anxiety in low-income, high- and low-risk pregnant women. J Obstet Gynecol Neonatal Nurs 22:266–272, 1992

Kemp VH, Page CK: Maternal prenatal attachment in normal and high-risk pregnancies. J Obstet Gynecol Neonatal Nurs 15:179–184, 1986a

Kemp VH, Page CK: The psychosocial impact of a high-risk pregnancy on the family. J Obstet Gynecol Neonatal Nurs 15:232–236, 1986b

Kemp VH, Page CK: Maternal self-esteem and prenatal attachment in high-risk pregnancy. Matern Child Nurs J 16:195–206, 1987

Kestenberg JS: Regression and reintegration in pregnancy, in Female Psychology: Contemporary Psychoanalytic Views. Edited by Blum BL. New York, International Universities Press, 1977, pp 213–250.

Landon MB, Gabbe SG: Diabetes mellitus and pregnancy. Obstet Gynecol Clin North Am 19:633–651, 1992

Leifer M: Psychological changes accompanying pregnancy and motherhood. Genet Psychol Monogr 95:55–96, 1977

Lester EP, Notman MT: Pregnancy, developmental crisis, and object relations: psychoanalytic considerations. Int J Psychoanal 67:357–366, 1986

Mabie WC, Sibai BM: Hypertensive states of pregnancy, in Current Obstetric and Gynecologic Diagnosis and Treatment. Edited by Decherney AH, Pernoll ML. East Norwalk, CT, Appleton & Lange, 1994, pp 380–397

Mackey MC: Women's evaluation of their childbirth performance. Matern Child Nurs J 23:57–72, 1995

Marteau TM, Kidd J, Cook R, et al: Perceived risk, not actual risk, predicts uptake of amniocentesis. Br J Obstet Gynaecol 98:282–286, 1991

Minkoff H, Henderson C, Mendez H, et al: Pregnancy outcomes among mothers infected with human immunodeficiency virus and uninfected control subjects. Am J Obstet Gynecol 163:1598–1604, 1990

Moore ML: The high risk mother, in Realities in Childbearing, 2nd Edition. Edited by Moore ML. Philadelphia, PA, WB Saunders, 1983, pp 331–332

Morris MG: Psychoanalytic and literary perspectives on procreation conflicts in women. Psychoanal Rev 84:109–128, 1997

Nadelson CC: "Normal" and "special" aspects of pregnancy: a psychological approach, in The Woman Patient, Vol 1. Edited by Notman M, Nadelson C. New York, Plenum, 1978, pp 73–86.

Neuhaus W, Scharkus S, Hamm W, et al: Prenatal expectations and fears in pregnant women. J Perinatol Med 22:409–414, 1994

Nichols MR: Adjustment to new parenthood: attenders versus nonattenders at prenatal education classes. Birth 22:21–26, 1995

Palmer SM: Diabetes, in Current Obstetric and Gynecologic Diagnosis and Treatment. Edited by Decherney AH, Pernoll ML. East Norwalk, CT, Appleton & Lange, 1994, pp 368–379

Penticuff JH: Psychological implications in high-risk pregnancy. Nurs Clin North Am 17:69–78, 1982

Pernoll ML: Late pregnancy complications, in Current Obstetric and Gynecologic Diagnosis and Treatment. Edited by Decherney AH, Pernoll ML. East Norwalk, CT, Appleton & Lange, 1994a, pp 331–343

Pernoll ML: Third trimester hemorrhage, in Current Obstetric and Gynecologic Diagnosis and Treatment. Edited by Decherney AH, Pernoll ML. East Norwalk, CT, Appleton & Lange, 1994b, pp 398–409

Pernoll ML, Garmel SH: Early pregnancy risks, in Current Obstetric and Gynecologic Diagnosis and Treatment. Edited by Decherney AH, Pernoll ML. East Norwalk, CT, Appleton & Lange, 1994, pp 306–330

Pines D: Pregnancy and motherhood: interaction between fantasy and reality. Br J Med Psychol 45:333–343, 1972

Pines D: The relevance of early psychic development to pregnancy and abortion. Int J Psychoanal 63:311–319, 1982

Priel B, Kantor B: The influence of high-risk pregnancies and social support systems on maternal perceptions of the infant. Infant Mental Health Journal 9:235–244, 1988

Raphael-Leff J: Psychological Processes of Childbearing. London, England, Chapman and Hall, 1991, pp 48–102

Rogers MP: Psychological aspects of pregnancy in patients with rheumatic disease, in Rheumatic Disease Clinics of North America, Vol 15. Philadelphia, PA, WB Saunders, 1989, pp 361–374.

Rubin R: Cognitive style in pregnancy. Am J Nurs 70:502–508, 1970

Sandelowski M, Black PB: The epistemology of expectant parenthood. Western J Nurs Res 16:601–622, 1994

Schoenbaum EE, Webber MP: The underrecognition of HIV infection in women in an inner-city emergency room. Am J Public Health 83:363–368, 1993

Searle J: Fearing the worst: why do pregnant women feel "at risk"? Aust N Z J Obstet Gynaecol 36:279–286, 1996

Selwyn PA, Schoenbaum EE, Davenny K, et al: Prospective study of human immunodeficiency virus infection and pregnancy outcomes in intravenous drug users. JAMA 261:1289–1294, 1989

Sharp K, Brindle PM, Brown MW, et al: Memory loss during pregnancy. Br J Obstet Gynaecol 100:209–215, 1993

Sherwin BB: Estrogen and cognitive functioning in women. Proc Soc Exp Biol Med 217:17–21, 1998

Sherwin LN, Mele CN: Assessing and identifying the high-risk pregnancy: a holistic approach. Topics in Clinical Nursing 8:33–44, 1986

Sibai BM: Hypertension in pregnancy. Obstet Gynecol Clin North Am 19:615–631, 1992

Sokol RJ, Jones TB, Pernoll ML: Methods of assessment for pregnancy at risk, in Current Obstetric and Gynecologic Diagnosis and Treatment. Edited by Decherney AH, Pernoll ML. East Norwalk, CT, Appleton & Lange, 1994, pp 275–305.

Sowell RL, Misener TR: Decisions to have a baby by HIV-infected women. Western J Nurs Res 19:56–70, 1997

Spirito A, Williams C, Ruggiero L, et al: Psychological impact of the diagnosis of gestational diabetes. Obstet Gynecol 73:562–566, 1989

St-Andre M: Psychotherapy during opportunities and challenges. Am J Psychother 47:572–590, 1993

Stern DN: The Motherhood Constellation: A Unified View of Parent–Infant Psychotherapy. New York, Basic Books, 1995, pp 18–40

Stewart DE, Lippert GP: Psychiatric consultation-liaison services to an obstetrics and gynecology department. Can J Psychiatry 33:285–289, 1988

Trad P: Adaptation to developmental transformations during the various phases of motherhood. J Am Acad Psychoanal 19:403–421, 1991

White M, Ritchie J: Psychological stressors in antepartum hospitalization: reports from pregnant women. Matern Child Nurs J 13:47–56, 1984

Wolreich MM: Psychiatric aspects of high-risk pregnancy. Psychiatr Clin North Am 10:53–68, 1986

Zwelling E: Childbirth education in the 1990s and beyond. J Obstet Gynecol Neonatal Nurs 25:425–432, 1996

# Fetal Anomaly

GAIL ERLICK ROBINSON, M.D., D.PSYCH., F.R.C.P.C.
KATHERINE L. WISNER, M.D., M.S.

Fetal anomalies may be genetically programmed at conception by the transmission of defective genes or chromosomes or they may arise during pregnancy as a result of maternal illness or exposure to harmful substances. Prenatal genetic counseling and diagnostic techniques have made possible the in utero detection of a large number of these fetal defects. These technologic advances also bring psychologic stresses in the form of decisions about whether to have testing, anxieties related to the tests and the wait for results, and the possibility of having to choose whether to terminate a pregnancy.

This chapter discusses these reactions as well as the emotional consequences and management of elective genetic terminations or of giving birth to a child with a defect. The psychiatrist may have a role in direct counseling of patients who are adjusting to the emotional trauma of losing a wanted pregnancy or who are adapting to having a child with abnormalities. The psychiatrist may also be involved in supervising or assisting other members of the treatment team.

## Prepregnancy

### Risk of Hereditary Disorders

Geneticists and genetic counselors advise patients who are at risk for a hereditary disorder about the consequences of the disorder, the probability of developing the disease or transmitting the gene, and the ways in which this transmission may be prevented. Ideally, this information is given before pregnancy so the couple can make informed decisions about childbearing.

Counselors also provide general information on the risk of chromosome abnormalities for women of late maternal age. The risk of chromosomal abnormalities being detected at 16 weeks' gestation in a woman who is 35 years old is 1/250 for Down syndrome and 1/130 for all chromosome abnormalities. These risks increase until, in a woman who is 46 years of age, they are 1/15 and 1/10, respectively (Hook 1983). If a woman has previously given birth to an abnormal child, the geneticist uses clinical assessment of the affected infant, confirmation from medical records, and construction of a family genetic tree to make an accurate diagnosis and estimate the risk for future pregnancies.

Single gene or mendelian disorders have three inheritance patterns: autosomal dominant, autosomal recessive, and X-linked recessive or dominant genes. When one parent has an autosomal dominant disorder (such as tuberous sclerosis or Huntington's disease), there is a 50% probability that the offspring will be affected. Autosomal recessive disorders include the hemoglobinopathies and several progressive metabolic disorders such as Tay-Sachs disease. When both parents are carriers of an autosomal recessive condition the risk of transmission to children is 25%, and each child has a 50% risk of being a carrier. When the mother carries an X-linked recessive disorder (such as hemophilia or Duchenne dystrophy), there is a 50% risk that each son will be affected as well as a 50% probability that each daughter will be a carrier.

Most common birth defects, such as cleft lip, cleft palate, and neural tube defects, involve multifactorial inheritance. The recurrence risk of these disorders is rarely over 5% when only one parent is affected (Harper 1983). Chromosome disorders may involve numerical abnormalities caused by nondisjunction (e.g., Down syndrome due to trisomy 21) or structural abnormalities such as chromosome translocations (e.g., Down syndrome due to a translocation between chromosomes 14 and 21). The risk of nondisjunction after one occurrence is approximately 1%. With translocations, chromosomal material may be neither lost nor gained but merely out of place; in these cases, the translocation is said to be "balanced" and the individual will be a carrier (i.e., not symptomatic). Asymptomatic carriers of balanced translocations, however, have a 5%–20% risk of transmitting the unbalanced chromosome complement (i.e., too little or too much genetic material) to the child, who will, therefore, exhibit symptoms (Jackson 1980).

## Psychologic Reactions to Discovery of Risk Factors

The parents' perceived risk for any genetic disorder differs from the statistical risk (Swerts 1987). Five major factors influence perceived risk: 1) the potential degree of harm or lethality, 2) the degree to which the risk can be controlled through safety or rescue measures, 3) the number of people affected, 4) the degree of familiarity with the consequences and effects of the disorder, and 5) the degree to which the parents' exposure to the risk is voluntary.

Couples who have an increased risk for giving birth to a child with a genetic disorder are faced with the complications of a "natural" biologic process that is usually taken for granted. They may have a strong feeling of being defective. This presents a narcissistic threat to their self-esteem, to the extent that self-esteem is based on the expectation of creating a normal healthy child (Blumberg et al. 1975). A sense of guilt associated with being a carrier of a genetic disease may also be present. It is common for these couples to feel anger toward women who are enjoying normal pregnancies and to feel guilt because of difficulties with reproduction (G. E. Robinson and Stewart 1989). They may undergo a grieving process for the loss of their idealized family. Their sexual enjoyment may be affected by both their distress and by the realization that the procreative act can result in tragedy. Marital distress caused by this crisis complicates decisions about future pregnancies.

Genetic counseling and the possibility of detecting fetal defects prenatally play an important role in making decisions about further pregnancies (Boue et al. 1991). Over half of counseled families who have infants with Down syndrome and up to 80% of those who have a child with neural tube defects reported that they were positively influenced in their decision to have more children by the information received during counseling sessions. Preconception counseling may reduce the couples' guilt, their sense of defectiveness, and their grief.

## Pregnancy

## Indications for Prenatal Genetic Testing

The goals of prenatal diagnosis are detection of fetal genetic disorders, improvement of outcome, provision of information to prepare parents, and identification of severely affected pregnancies that parents can elect to terminate. Indications for prenatal testing include advanced maternal age (women over

35 years of age), a known balanced translocation in one of the parents, a previous child with a chromosome disorder or neural tube defect, a mother who is a carrier for an X-linked disease (to determine fetal gender and to provide molecular diagnosis, where applicable), and parents who are both carriers of recessively inherited metabolic disorders (Golbus et al. 1974). Some examples of the types of disorders that are common indications for prenatal diagnostic testing are shown in Table 3–1. This list is not exhaustive, as hundreds of conditions can now be diagnosed through prenatal testing.

The type of prenatal diagnostic test, the timing of testing, and the approximate waiting time for results are depicted in Table 3–2. Couples may not be willing to undergo prenatal diagnostic testing because of lack of information about the test, a perception of being at low risk for a fetal abnormality, concern about fetal injury or loss following the test, religious beliefs, or an unwillingness to consider elective termination as an option (Davies and Doran 1982; Dixson et al. 1981).

## Prenatal Diagnostic Tests

### Serum Screening

Alpha-fetoprotein (AFP) is a normal human fetal protein that is found in high concentrations in the fetal serum throughout gestation. Rising levels of AFP can be detected in the sera of pregnant women as early as 7 weeks' gestation, and levels increase steadily until at least 30 weeks' gestation (Burton 1988). Elevated levels of maternal serum AFP (MSAFP) can be used to detect 80%–85% of open neural tube defects and other malformations, including omphalocele or gastroschisis, intestinal atresias, congenital nephrosis, and Turner's syndrome. MSAFP levels are approximately 25% lower when the fetus has Down syndrome (Knight et al. 1988). The use of multiple markers (MSAFP, human gonadotropin, and unconjugated estriol) can detect 60%–85% of anomalies (Wenstrom et al. 1995).

MSAFP screening can be done with reasonable reliability between 15 and 21 weeks' gestation. About 4% of women will have an elevated MSAFP level on initial testing, and 30% of these women will have a normal result on repeat testing. For multiple marker screening, 8% of women will have a positive result on the initial test, but only 1%–2% of those will have an abnormal fetus (Carroll 1994). Patients who have abnormalities in the serum screening and are found through ultrasound and examination to have a single viable fetus at the anticipated gestational age may be advised to undergo amniocentesis.

TABLE 3–1. Indications for prenatal diagnostic testing

| Type of disorder | Example | Diagnostic ultrasound | MSAFP | CVS/Amniocentesis | | |
| --- | --- | --- | --- | --- | --- | --- |
| | | | | DNA analysis | Chromosome analysis | Enzyme analysis |
| Single-gene disorders, known or suspected | Cystic fibrosis | | | X | | |
| Multifactorial disorders, known or suspected | Neural tube disorders | X | X | | | |
| Chromosomal disorders in the consultand or a family member | Fragile X syndrome | | | X | X | |
| Abnormal trait or carrier state | Tay-Sachs disease | | | X | | X |
| Prenatal diagnosis for late maternal age or other causes | Down syndrome | X | X | | X | |
| Teratogen exposure | Fetal alcohol syndrome | X | | | | |

Note.   CVS = chorionic villus sampling; MSAFP = maternal serum alpha-fetoprotein.

TABLE 3–2.    Prenatal diagnostic testing

| Type of test | Time of testing (weeks of gestation) | Waiting time for results (weeks) |
| --- | --- | --- |
| Early amniocentesis | 10–14 | 2–3 |
| Chorionic villus sampling | 9–12 | 1–2 |
| Diagnostic ultrasound (routine screening) | 18–19 | Immediate |
| Midtrimester amniocentesis | 16–18 | 2–4 |
| Maternal serum screening | 15–21 | 1 |

Serum testing may create unnecessary maternal anxiety because some women will be falsely identified as having high-risk pregnancies (Evans et al. 1988). Patients undergoing genetic testing because of elevated MSAFP levels have been found to have a higher state of anxiety than those undergoing testing because of advanced maternal age. This anxiety only returns to normal levels after assurance of a definitively negative amniocentesis result (J. Robinson et al. 1984). Women who undergo serum screening have significantly lower anxiety levels in the third trimester of pregnancy than do women who have not been screened (Marteau et al. 1988).

### Ultrasound

Two main types of ultrasound are in common use: *continuous ultrasound* is used to detect moving structures such as the fetal heart, whereas *pulse ultrasound* is used to outline structures within the uterus. In obstetrics, ultrasound is used for the screening and diagnosis of fetal age, multiple pregnancy, intrauterine growth retardation, and fetal malformations including craniospinal defects such as anencephaly, cardiac defects, and musculoskeletal, gastrointestinal, and renal abnormalities. Diagnostic ultrasound has no known risks to the fetus or mother and produces little anxiety in low-risk women (Campbell et al. 1982). Women tend to view scans as benign procedures allowing them to confirm the baby is healthy (J. Green and Stratham 1996). Scans may promote maternal–fetal bonding (Campbell et al. 1982) and may lead to a decrease in behaviors such as smoking and drinking (Reading et al. 1982), especially in women who receive a high level of feedback during the ultrasound examination (Reading et al. 1988).

### Midtrimester Genetic Amniocentesis

Midtrimester genetic amniocentesis is carried out at approximately 16 weeks' gestation. After the exact positions of the placenta, fetus, and umbilical cord are determined by ultrasound, a needle is inserted through the abdomen into the amniotic sac. Amniotic fluid is withdrawn for AFP and karyotype testing.

In several studies, the rates of total fetal loss in the group receiving midtrimester amniocentesis (3.5%) and in nonrandomized control subjects (3.2%) were not significantly different. It is estimated that the risk of fetal loss because of midtrimester amniocentesis does not exceed 0.5% in experienced hands (Lowe et al. 1978). Serious fetal injury and bacterial infection within the uterus are extremely infrequent. The results are usually available 2–4 weeks later at approximately 20 weeks' gestation.

*Early Genetic Amniocentesis*

Early genetic amniocentesis can be performed between 10 and 14 weeks' gestation, although accuracy is greater at 12–14 weeks' gestation (Rooney et al. 1989). Preliminary reports suggested that early genetic amniocentesis was safer than chorionic villus sampling (CVS) (Godmilow et al. 1988) and as safe and accurate as midtrimester genetic amniocentesis (J. M. Johnson et al. 1996). Rates of procedure-related fetal loss have been reported to range between 3.3% and 6.6% (Hackett et al. 1991; Hanson et al. 1987), with an average loss of 2.7%. A recent multicenter study found that women who have early genetic amniocentesis have an increased risk of having children born with Talipes equinovarus (Canadian Early and Mid-trimester Amniocentesis Trial Group 1998).

*Chorionic Villus Sampling*

Chorionic villus sampling is another method of obtaining fetal cells for genetic analysis. Using ultrasound guidance, a catheter is inserted through the cervix or a needle is passed through the abdominal wall to aspirate chorionic tissue from the developing placenta. The material obtained is then sent for karyotype determination and other studies as indicated. In a multicenter, randomized clinical trial of CVS and midtrimester genetic amniocentesis, the difference between the rates of pregnancy loss with the two procedures was determined to be no greater than 2.8% for women 35 years of age and older (Canadian Collaborative CVS-Amniocentesis Clinical Trial Group 1989). The most likely risk is probably 1%–1.5%. Early reports about a possible association with fetal limb defects when CVS is performed at less than 10 weeks' gestation (Firth et al. 1991) have not been validated (Kuliev et al. 1996).

## Psychologic Consequences of Chorionic Villus Sampling, Midtrimester Genetic Amniocentesis, and Early Genetic Amniocentesis

Couples who undergo prenatal diagnostic testing may experience significant psychologic stress. Prior to testing, women worry the procedure will be painful, cause injury to the fetus, or result in miscarriage (J. Green and Stratham 1996; Marteau and Slack 1992). They may also be concerned about the results of the test (Evers-Kiebooms et al. 1988; Finley et al. 1977). Women with decreased social support have increased anxiety (J. Robinson et al. 1975). Beason and Golbus (1979) found increased anxiety in women who already had children with chromosomal disorders, but other investigators have not (Evers-Kiebooms et al. 1988; Tabor and Jonsson 1987). Women having the tests as a result of positive screening tests are particularly anxious (J. Green and Stratham 1996). No increase in anxiety has been found in women who have been adequately counseled, although counseling done immediately prior to the test was not found to be beneficial (Nielson 1981). Anxiety levels are also elevated in women prior to undergoing CVS (G. E. Robinson et al. 1988; Spencer and Cox 1987). A drop in anxiety immediately after testing has been noted for patients who underwent midtrimester genetic amniocentesis (Tabor and Jonsson 1987), early genetic amniocentesis (G. E. Robinson et al. 1998), or CVS (G. E. Robinson et al. 1988). Tabor and Jonsson (1987) found this to be especially true for younger women and women who perceive themselves to be at low risk for an abnormality. Older women remained anxious until the results were obtained. Beason and Golbus (1979) found an immediate drop in anxiety with a subsequent rise during the wait for a possible miscarriage and test results. Women receiving results earlier in the pregnancy experienced anxiety reduction much earlier than did the group receiving results after 17–18 weeks (G. E. Robinson et al. 1988, 1998). Even after obtaining the results, about 25% of women receiving midtrimester amniocentesis remained concerned about the outcome of the pregnancy (Dixson et al. 1981). McCormack et al. (1990) found that most patients had a better experience with CVS than with previous midtrimester genetic amniocentesis. Women who undergo CVS develop an increase in maternal–fetal bonding earlier than do those having midtrimester amniocentesis (Caccia et al. 1991).

## Pregnancy Loss After Testing

Women who have a miscarriage after a genetic procedure experience grief, guilt, and anger. Women who have CVS may perceive the procedure to be more risky and may feel additional guilt over having chosen it (G. E. Robinson et al. 1991). Also, because of the early timing of CVS, a miscarriage that would have spontaneously occurred may be falsely attributed to the procedure and create needless guilt. Even after genetic terminations or miscarriages, women tend to prefer earlier procedures (G. E. Robinson et al. 1988, 1998).

## Reactions to Detection of Fetal Anomaly

Detection of a fetal anomaly is always a disturbing event (J. Green and Stratham 1996). A pregnancy that has been desired and perhaps long sought may suddenly lose its value. The first reaction is one of shock and denial, either expressed openly or masked by an apparent calm acceptance of the diagnosis (Jackson 1980). It is often difficult for couples to absorb information during this period of shock. The second stage is characterized by anxiety as they try to come to terms with future plans and alternatives for care. Many individuals have problems grasping the meaning of probability figures and using them for decision-making (d'Ydewalle and Evers-Kiebooms 1987). Either parent may exhibit hostile and angry behavior directed at the partner, the physician, or the counselor. The parents may then enter a phase of depression as they deal with this difficult problem. These stages vary in length and severity and may fluctuate before the parents reach the stage of acceptance and equilibrium.

## Reactions to Genetic Termination

Reproductive loss for any reason is always distressing. In an elective termination because of genetic disorders (i.e., genetic termination), the couple must face not only the loss of a wanted pregnancy but the fact of making a conscious decision to end it (Leon 1995). Ideally, discussion about the actions to be taken if an abnormal result is discovered occurs during pretest counseling (Marteau 1995). If the disorder is incompatible with life, the decision may be reasonably straightforward. For many others, a clear identification of a problem with known consequences, such as Down syndrome, will allow them to make the choice despite ambivalence and pain. Problems in decision making increase with the identification of mosaicism or sex chromosomal disorders in which the outcome is not clearly a severe abnormality (Drugan et al. 1990). Acute grief reactions are experienced by 77%–92% of women and 82% of men following a genetic termination (Blumberg et al. 1975; Lloyd and

Lawrence 1985). This distress may last for many years after termination (White-van Mourik et al. 1992).

Couples often feel guilty about their decision to terminate a pregnancy. Couples who are at risk of having a child with an X-linked disorder and who terminate a pregnancy based only on knowledge of male gender must deal with the added guilt of knowing there is a 50% probability that the fetus would not have had the disorder (Blumberg et al. 1975). Couples may experience marital problems caused by projection of their anger onto each other or by isolation due to depression. The woman may have stronger feelings about the loss or may be more open about expressing her feelings. In an attempt to handle his own sadness as well as deal with his partner's grief, the man may suppress his own feelings.

The woman who has an induced abortion following genetic amniocentesis has probably experienced fetal movement, has usually been visibly pregnant, and has had to undergo delivery in order to terminate the pregnancy. It has been hypothesized that elective terminations following CVS may be less traumatic, but G. E. Robinson et al. (1991) found that women who had an elective termination following either method had equally elevated levels of depression.

Couples who terminate a pregnancy for genetic reasons experience a grief reaction and mourn for their unborn child (Magyari et al. 1987). Protocols for the management of neonatal death have been proposed (Langer and Ringler 1989; Magyari et al. 1987; Phipps 1981). In the protocol of Magyari et al. (1987), the finding of an abnormality is discussed immediately with the parents in the context of a nondirective planning meeting. The couple is given a factual description of the termination procedure. Mothers who choose termination are admitted to a private room on a nonmaternity ward where the spouses can remain together during the procedure. The psychologic management of pregnancy loss is discussed in more detail in Chapter 8.

## Selective Termination

Selective termination may be considered in multiple gestations in which one or more fetuses are severely abnormal or when continuation of the multiple pregnancy presents a risk to the mother or the pregnancy (Zaner et al. 1990). This problem is more common in infertile patients who achieve pregnancy after ovulation induction. Zaner et al. (1990) have argued that restricting selective termination to pregnancies of three or more fetuses provides the greatest chance of causing the least harm. They also advise early counseling for couples involved in ovulation induction to prepare them for the possibility of selective termination. McKinney et al. (1996) found that women who underwent selective reduction experienced guilt, ambivalence, and bereavement, but most felt they had made the right decision for themselves and their families.

## Fetal Gender Determination

Fetal gender determination can be done by ultrasound or chromosomal examination. In cases of X-linked recessive disorders, if the fetus is male and molecular analysis cannot detect whether it is affected, the couple may elect to terminate the pregnancy knowing that there is only a 50% chance it would be affected. Termination of fetuses of a particular gender merely for sociocultural reasons presents an ethical problem. Some physicians suggest that the gender of the fetus should be kept from the parents unless it is related to a genetic disorder. Others believe that caregivers do not have the right to withhold this information. Termination for the purpose of gender selection rarely occurs after midtrimester amniocentesis (S. R. Johnson and Elkins 1988).

## Psychologic Reactions to Perinatal Death

Stillbirth or neonatal death caused by genetic abnormalities elicits not only grief reactions but guilty feelings on the part of the parents for having produced a defective child. Waiting for the autopsy results to confirm or allay their fears of having passed on a chromosomal defect to their baby is painful. Carrying a chromosomal defect that may harm future children is emotionally distressing.

Children also react to the death of a sibling. The parents can assist by providing accurate information about the death, explaining that it was not the surviving child's fault, including the child in mourning ceremonies, and sharing parental grief (Leon 1990). Children's repetition of questions parallels the same phenomenon seen in parents' questioning of doctors. For a sibling who is free of a genetic illness, assurances that the fatality is not contagious and cannot happen to him or her can be helpful.

# Postpartum

## Psychologic Reactions to the Malformed Baby

The birth of a malformed baby constitutes an intense narcissistic injury for parents. Already coping with the psychophysiologic depletion that follows labor and delivery, these couples must also grieve the loss of the expected infant and accept the malformed child (Solnit and Stark 1961). They must attempt self-regulation in the face of chronic depression and rage when confronted with the disappointment inherent in producing a damaged child (Fajardo 1987). Couples may feel unable to accept the child because the narcissistic injury is intolerable, or alternatively, they may experience severe guilt leading to overinvolved parental dedication (Solnit and Stark 1961). Parents of children with problems such as congenital heart disease may have more problems accepting the child's condition because outwardly the child appears completely normal (Emery 1989). This stress intensifies any preexisting relationship difficulties. Men and women may handle the stress differently: women may be more preoccupied with hands-on care, whereas men may focus on trying to emotionally support the wife (Svavarsdottir and McCubbin 1996).

Mourning a malformed infant does not take place in the usual manner because the continuation of the child's life and the increased demands for physical care preoccupy most parents. Drotar et al. (1975) found that, despite reassurances, concern that the baby will die interferes with attachment to the child. Premature mourning for a child who subsequently recovers requires the parent to reverse psychologic energy and reintegrate the child into the family. Difficulty accomplishing this task can result in disturbed parent–child relationships and behavioral dysfunction in children (M. Green and Solnit 1964; Naylor 1982). The continuation of mourning into a persistent, depressed, self-reproachful state is more likely if the mother's mourning reaction is not understood and if the care and planning for the child are carried out without her active participation.

Parents of a malformed infant experience guilt and shame and frequently seek causal connections between the defect and prior thoughts, fantasies, wishes, or actions (Kessler et al. 1984). This guilt may or may not be realistic. Defenses against guilt include repression (behaviors such as substance abuse), intellectualization and rationalization, and isolation of affect. A common way for couples to handle the guilt is to decide against further reproduction.

Shame is frequently associated with responses to the anticipated or actual disapproval of others. Common defenses against shame include denial, reaction formation, compensation, or displacement, such as focusing on the deficiencies of the medical caregivers.

The parents must begin a lifelong reconciliation to the ongoing disappointments and special care required by the limitations of a child with a genetic defect. The child may be at risk of abuse, particularly if either parent has a history of child abuse, or of extreme social isolation from family and friends (Fost 1981).

Parents of children born with malformations may not remember the rational content of the first conversation with their doctor (Solnit and Stark 1961). They need repeated contact with their physician to accomplish the task of mourning. Parents also need assistance with decision structuring as they take responsibility for evaluative judgments and accept/reject decisions (Vlek 1987).

## Psychotherapy

In the initial stages of work with families in which a child is malformed, Solnit and Stark (1961) recommended support and clarification of the reality of the child's condition as the parents are able to discuss their questions and fears. Avoiding the interpretation of unconscious conflicts during mourning was recommended. Group support for parents of children with fatal genetic illnesses can decrease parental isolation, allow discussion of the parents' need for both closeness and distance from the infant, and calm their fears about events immediately preceding their child's death (Mack and Berman 1988). In such a group, the parents may be able to admire the lovable qualities about each other's children and share in each other's grief when the children die.

Zuskar (1987) advocated a short-term family crisis intervention model for managing the psychologic reactions to a baby born with genetic defects. This model includes multiple short meetings, initial work with the couple alone followed by placement into couples groups, an empathic and accepting therapeutic style to facilitate adaptation, provision of a supportive environment for emotional work, direct confrontation of beliefs about the fetus's impairment as causality, and attention to the marital relationship. Attention to biologic information and reproductive technology, the parents' psychologic capacities to receive information and use coping skills, and the parents' social milieu will allow the therapeutic team to develop a comprehensive treatment plan and achieve the most successful outcome.

## Acknowledgment

The authors wish to acknowledge the valuable assistance of Dr. Elaine Hutton in reviewing the information on genetics.

# References

Beason D, Golbus MS: Anxiety engendered by amniocentesis, in Risk, Communication, and Decision Making in Genetic Counseling. Edited by Epstein CJ, Curry CJ, Packman S, et al. (The National Foundation—March of Dimes Birth Defects Original Article Series). White Plains, NY, Alan R. Liss, 1979, pp 191–197

Blumberg BD, Golbus MS, Hanson, KH: The psychological sequelae of abortion performed for a genetic indication. Am J Obstet Gynecol 12:799–808, 1975

Boue J, Muller F, Simon-Bouy B, et al: Consequences of prenatal diagnosis of cystic fibrosis on the reproductive attitudes of parents of affected children. Prenat Diagn 11:209–214, 1991

Burton BK: Elevated maternal serum alpha-fetoprotein (MSAFP): interpretation and follow up. Clin Obstet Gynecol 31:293–305, 1988

Caccia N, Johnson JM, Robinson GE, et al: Impact of prenatal testing on maternal-fetal bonding: chorionic villus sampling versus amniocentesis. Am J Obstet Gynecol 165:1122–1125, 1991

Campbell S, Reading AE, Cox DN, et al: Ultrasound scanning in pregnancy: the short-term psychological effects of early real-time scans. J Psychosom Obstet Gynaecol 1:57–61, 1982

Canadian Collaborative CVS-Amniocentesis Clinical Trial Group: Multicentre randomized clinical trial of chorion villus sampling and amniocentesis. Lancet 1:1–6, 1989

Canadian Early and Mid-trimester Amniocentesis Trial (CEMAT) Group: Randomized trial to assess safety and fetal outcome of early and mid-trimester amniocentesis. Lancet 35:242–247, 1998

Carroll JC: Maternal serum screening. Can Fam Physician 40:1756–1764, 1994

Davies BL, Doran TA: Factors in a woman's decision to undergo genetic amniocentesis for advanced maternal age. Nurs Res 31:56–59, 1982

Dixson B, Richards T, Reinsch S, et al: Midtrimester amniocentesis: subjective maternal responses. J Reprod Med 26:10–16, 1981

Drotar D, Baskiewicz A, Irvin N, et al: The adaptation of parents to the birth of an infant with a congenital malformation: a hypothetical model. Pediatrics 56:710–717, 1975

Drugan A, Greb A, Johnson MP, et al: Determinants of parental decisions to abort for chromosome abnormalities. Prenat Diagn 10:483–490, 1990

d'Ydewalle G, Evers-Kiebooms G: Experiments on genetic risk perception and decision making: explorative studies. Birth Defects 23:209–225, 1987

Emery JL: Families with congenital heart disease. Arch Dis Child 64:150–154, 1989

Evans MI, Bottoms SF, Carlucci T, et al: Determinants of altered anxiety after abnormal maternal serum alpha-fetoprotein screening. Am J Obstet Gynecol 156:1501–1504, 1988

Evers-Kiebooms G, Swerts A, Van Den Berghe H: Psychological aspects of amniocentesis: anxiety feelings in three different risk groups. Clin Genet 33:196–206, 1988

Fajardo B: Parenting a damaged child: mourning, regression, and disappointment. Psychoanal Rev 74:19–43, 1987

Finley SC, Varner PD, Vinson PC, et al: Participants' reactions to amniocentesis and prenatal genetic studies. JAMA 238:2377–2379, 1977

Firth HV, Boyd PA, Chamberlain P, et al: Severe limb abnormalities after chorion villus sampling at 56–66 days gestation. Lancet 337:762–763, 1991

Fost N: Counseling families who have a child with a severe congenital anomaly. Pediatrics 67:321–324, 1981

Godmilow L, Weiner S, Dunn LK: Early genetic amniocentesis: experience with 600 consecutive procedures and comparison with chorionic villus sampling (abstract). Am J Hum Genet 43(suppl):A234, 1988

Golbus MS, Conte FA, Schneider EL, et al: Intrauterine diagnosis of genetic defects: results, problems and follow up of one hundred cases in a prenatal genetic detection centre. Am J Obstet Gynecol 118:897–905, 1974

Green J, Stratham H: Psychosocial aspects of prenatal screening and diagnosis, in The Troubled Helix: Social and Psychological Implications of the New Human Genetics. Edited by Marteau T, Richards M. Cambridge, England, Cambridge University Press, 1996, pp 140–163

Green M, Solnit A: Reactions to the threatened loss of a child: a vulnerable child syndrome. Pediatrics 34:58–66, 1964

Hackett GA, Smith JH, Rebello CTH: Early amniocentesis at 11–14 weeks gestation for the diagnosis of fetal chromosomal abnormality: a clinical evaluation. Prenat Diagn 11:35–40, 1991

Hanson FW, Zorn EM, Tennant FR, et al: Amniocentesis before 15 weeks' gestation: outcome, risks, and technical problems. Am J Obstet Gynecol 156:1524–1531, 1987

Harper PS: Genetic counseling and prenatal diagnosis. Br Med Bull 39:302–309, 1983

Hook EB: Chromosomal abnormality rates at amniocentesis and in live-born infants. JAMA 249:2034–2038, 1983

Jackson LG: Prenatal genetic counseling, in Psychosomatic Obstetrics and Gynecology. Edited by Youngs DD, Ehrhardt AA. New York, Appleton-Century-Crofts, 1980, pp 129–144

Johnson JM, Wilson RD, Winson EJT, et al: The early amniocentesis study: a randomized clinical trial of early amniocentesis versus midtrimester amniocentesis. Fetal Diagn Ther 11:85–93, 1996

Johnson SR, Elkins TE: Ethical issues in prenatal diagnosis. Clin Obstet Gynecol 31:408–420, 1988

Kessler S, Kessler H, Ward P: Psychological aspects of genetic counseling, III: management of guilt and shame. Am J Med Genet 17:673–697, 1984

Knight GJ, Palomaki GE, Haddow JE: Use of maternal serum alpha-fetoprotein measurements to screen for Down's syndrome. Clin Obstet Gynecol 31:306–327, 1988

Kuliev A, Jackson L, Froster U, et al: Chorionic villus sampling safety. Am J Obstet Gynecol 174:807–811, 1996

Langer M, Ringler M: Prospective counseling after prenatal diagnosis of fetal malformations and parental reactions. Acta Obstet Gynecol Scand 68:323–329, 1989

Leon IG: When a Baby Dies: Psychotherapy for Pregnancy and Newborn Loss. New Haven, CT, Yale University Press, 1990, pp 131–187

Leon IG: Pregnancy termination due to fetal anomaly: clinical considerations. Infant Mental Health Journal 16:112–126, 1995

Lloyd J, Lawrence KM: Sequelae and support after termination of pregnancy for fetal malformation. BMJ 290:907–909, 1985

Lowe CU, Alexander D, Bryla D, et al (eds): The NICHD Amniocentesis Registry: The Safety and Accuracy of Mid-Trimester Amniocentesis (DHEW Publication No. [NIH] 78-190) Bethesda, MD, Department of Health, Education, and Welfare, 1978

Mack SA, Berman LC: A group for parents of children with fatal genetic illnesses. Am J Orthopsychiatry 58:397–404, 1988

Magyari PA, Wedehase BA, Ifft RD, et al: A supportive intervention protocol for couples terminating a pregnancy for genetic reasons, in Strategies in Genetic Counseling (The National Foundation–March of Dimes Birth Defects Original Article Series, Vol 23). Edited by Paul NW, Travers H. White Plains, NY, Alan R. Liss, 1987, pp 75–83

Marteau TM: Toward informed decisions about prenatal testing: a review. Prenat Diagn 15:1215–1226, 1995

Marteau TM, Slack J: Psychological implications of prenatal diagnosis for patients and health professionals, in Prenatal Diagnosis and Screening. Edited by Brock DJH, Rodeck CH, Ferguson-Smith MA. London, England, Churchill Livingstone, 1992, pp 663–673

Marteau TM, Johnston M, Plenicar M, et al: Development of a self-administered questionnaire to measure women's knowledge of prenatal screening and diagnostic tests. J Psychosom Res 32:403–408, 1988

McCormack MJ, Rylance ME, MacKenzie WE, et al: Patients' attitudes following chorionic villus sampling. Prenat Diagn 10:253–255, 1990

McKinney, Tuber SB, Downey JI: Multifetal pregnancy reduction: psychodynamic implications. Psychiatry 59:393–407, 1996

Naylor A: Premature mourning and failure to mourn: their relationship to conflict between mothers and intellectually normal children. Am J Orthopsychiatry 52:679–687, 1982

Nielson CC: An encounter with modern medical technology: women's experiences with amniocentesis. Women Health 6:109–124, 1981

Phipps S: Mourning response and intervention in stillbirth: an alternative genetic counseling approach. Soc Biol 28:1–13, 1981

Reading AE, Campbell S, Cox DN, et al: Health beliefs and health care behaviour in pregnancy. Psychol Med 12:1–5, 1982

Reading AE, Cox DN, Campbell S: A controlled prospective evaluation of the acceptability of ultrasound in prenatal care. J Psychosom Obstet Gynaecol 8:191–198, 1988

Robinson GE, Garner DM, Olmsted M, et al: Anxiety reduction following chorionic villus sampling and genetic amniocentesis. Am J Obstet Gynecol 159:953–956, 1988

Robinson GE, Stewart DE: Motivation for motherhood and the experience of pregnancy. Can J Psychiatry 34:861–865, 1989

Robinson GE, Carr M, Olmsted MP, et al: Psychological reactions to pregnancy loss after prenatal diagnostic testing: preliminary results. J Psychosom Obstet Gynaecol 12:181–192, 1991

Robinson GE, Johnson JAM, Wilson RD, et al: Anxiety reduction after early and midtrimester prenatal diagnostic testing. Archives of Women's Mental Health 1:39–44, 1998

Robinson J, Tennes K, Robinson A: Amniocentesis: its impact on mothers and infants. A one-year follow-up study. Clin Genet 8:97–106, 1975

Robinson J, Hibbard BM, Lawrence KM: Anxiety during a crisis: emotional effects of screening for neural tube defects. J Psychosom Res 28:163–169, 1984

Rooney DE, MacLachlan N, Smith J, et al: Early amniocentesis: a cytogenetic evaluation. BMJ 299:25, 1989

Solnit AJ, Stark MH: Mourning and the birth of a defective child. Psychoanal Study Child 16:523–537, 1961

Spencer JW, Cox DN: Emotional responses of pregnant women to chorionic villi sampling or amniocentesis. Am J Obstet Gynecol 157:1155–1160, 1987

Svavarsdottir EK, McCubbin M: Parenthood transition for parents of an infant diagnosed with a congenital heart condition. J Pediatr Nurs 11:207–216, 1996

Swerts A: Impact of genetic counseling and prenatal diagnosis for Down syndrome and neural tube defects. Birth Defects 23:61–83, 1987

Tabor A, Jonsson MH: Psychological impact of amniocentesis on low risk women. Prenat Diagn 7:443–449, 1987

Vlek C: Risk assessment, risk perception, and decision making about courses of action involving genetic risk: an overview of concepts and methods, in Strategies in

Genetic Counseling (The National Foundation–March of Dimes Birth Defects Original Article Series, Vol 23). White Plains, NY, Alan R. Liss, 1987, pp 171–207

Wenstrom KD, Desai R, Owen J, et al: Comparison of multiple-marker screening with amniocentesis for the detection of fetal aneuploidy in women ≥ 35 years old. Am J Obstet Gynecol 173:1287–1292, 1995

White-van Mourik MCA, Connor JM, Ferguson-Smith MA: The psychosocial sequelae of a second-trimester termination of pregnancy for fetal abnormality. Prenat Diagn 12:189–204, 1992

Zaner RM, Boehm FH, Hill GA: Selective termination in multiple pregnancies: ethical considerations. Fertil Steril 54:203–205, 1990

Zuskar DM: The psychological impact of prenatal diagnosis of fetal abnormality: strategies for investigation and intervention. Women Health 12:91–103, 1987

# Psychiatric Disorders During Pregnancy

LAURA J. MILLER, M.D.

## Introduction

Pregnancy is a time of profound biologic, psychologic, and interpersonal change in the lives of many women. Although transient reactions of anxiety and sadness are common, most women navigate this transition without major psychopathology. However, for women who experience an episode of mental illness while pregnant, the effects on them, their offspring, and their families can be devastating. This chapter aims to summarize research and clinical findings that shed light on the interaction between pregnancy and psychiatric disorders and to suggest interventions that stem from these findings.

## Psychiatric Disorders Temporally Related to Pregnancy

### Schizophrenia and Related Psychotic Disorders

Changes brought about by deinstitutionalization and sociocultural factors have resulted in increased rates of pregnancy among women with schizophrenia (Miller 1997). Compared with demographically similar non–mentally ill women, women with schizophrenia have significantly fewer planned pregnancies and more unwanted pregnancies (McNeil et al. 1983; Miller and Finnerty 1996). Pregnancy among women with schizophrenia is often accompanied by risk factors such as substance abuse, poverty, homelessness, insufficient prenatal care, poor nutrition, poor social support, and being a victim of violence (McNeil et al. 1983; Miller and Finnerty 1996; Rudolph et al. 1990; Sacker et al. 1996; Stewart 1984). Risks are further increased by the direct effects of psychotic symptoms on behavior. For example, women with delusions about their pregnancies are significantly less likely to recognize labor than are mentally ill women without such delusions (Spielvogel and Wile 1992). Delusions related to pregnancy may also result in attempts at premature self-delivery, sometimes by self-injurious methods (Yoldas et al. 1996).

These risk factors result in increased morbidity for both pregnant women and their offspring. Most women with schizophrenia report a worsening of their mental status during pregnancy (McNeil et al. 1984). Many women lose assisted housing arrangements because they are pregnant (Bachrach 1988) and have difficulty finding facilities equipped to deliver needed mental health and prenatal care (Dolinar 1993). Offspring, in addition to inheriting a vulnerability to schizophrenia, suffer the consequences of increased obstetric complications (Sacker et al. 1996).

A central problem for many pregnant women with schizophrenia is the fear of losing custody of their babies. Anticipated custody loss may trigger exacerbations of psychosis and other grief-related reactions (Apfel and Handel 1993). Fear of custody loss often deters women from seeking intervention (Stewart 1984). Although symptoms of schizophrenia may affect parenting capability—for example, because of hallucinations and delusions about children, reduced ability to read and respond to nonverbal cues, interpersonal remoteness, and unpredictable behavior—many women with schizophrenia are capable of safe parenting. A comprehensive parenting assessment can serve as a basis for rational decisions about parenting capability. Such assessments use standardized tools to evaluate parenting behavior, mother–child attachment patterns, understanding of child development, and internal representations of the child (Jacobsen et al. 1997). The pattern and content of specific symptoms, insight into illness, acceptance of and response to treatment, comorbid risks, and social support are also assessed. Parenting rehabilitation strategies including parenting coaching, therapeutic nurseries, parenting support groups, and parenting classes can target specific parenting problems. Unfortunately, many mental health facilities are ill equipped to assess parenting capability and prepare women for custody determinations (Nicholson et al. 1993; Rudolph et al. 1990).

# Mood Disorders

## Major Depression

Mild to moderate symptoms of depression are relatively common during pregnancy, although episodes of major depression seem no more likely to occur during pregnancy than at other times in a woman's life (Affonso et al. 1991; Coble et al. 1994a; Kitamura et al. 1994; Kumar and Robson 1984; O'Hara 1986). Antenatal depressive symptoms are especially prevalent among adolescents, inner-city women, and women with past histories of major depression (Barnet et al. 1996; Coble et al. 1994a; Hobfoll et al. 1995). Psychosocial risk factors for depression during pregnancy include less social and spousal support, more previous children, early parental bereavement, and termination of a prior pregnancy (Affonso et al. 1991; Barnet et al. 1996; Demyttenaere et al. 1995; Hobfoll et al. 1995; Kitamura et al. 1994; Kumar and Robson 1984; O'Hara 1986).

Antenatal depression is significant not only because of its prevalence but also because of its consequences. Depression can impair the mother's nutritional intake and prenatal care, increase her likelihood of using potentially harmful addictive substances, and lead to suicide attempts (Coverdale et al. 1997; Pajer 1995). Untreated antenatal depression significantly increases the likelihood of postpartum depression (Barnet et al. 1996; Hobfoll et al. 1995), which in turn may affect the woman's long-term prognosis (Parry 1999) and parenting capability (Jacobsen 1999). A depressive outlook may also color women's decisions about pregnancy outcome and obstetric interventions (Coverdale et al. 1997). For example, some depressed women feel so inadequate that they cannot imagine raising a child and ask to terminate a pregnancy they might otherwise want to continue. Others may decline treatment for pregnancy complications because they believe a negative outcome is inevitable.

Diagnosing depression can be more difficult during pregnancy because insomnia, decreased energy, decreased concentration, and appetite changes are common to both pregnancy and depression. Screening instruments such as the Beck Depression Inventory may overdiagnose depression because of these overlapping somatic effects (Salamero et al. 1994), but these can be modified for use during pregnancy (O'Hara et al. 1984). More problematic, however, is underdiagnosis of depression during pregnancy. In clinics without screening measures, significant depression is often missed despite high levels of contact with health care professionals during pregnancy (Kumar and Robson 1984; Powers et al. 1993).

## Bipolar Mood Disorder

Because of the potential risks of prescribing mood-stabilizing medication during pregnancy (see Chapter 5), it is particularly important to understand the potential risks of untreated bipolar mood disorder during pregnancy. Although some women with bipolar disorder improve during pregnancy, sustaining euthymic baseline states without medication (Sharma and Persad 1995), others develop acute manic episodes if unmedicated. Untreated mania can decrease compliance with prenatal care, increase addictive drug use, increase high-risk sexual behavior that exposes both mother and fetus to sexually transmitted diseases including HIV infection, and increase the likelihood of the woman being a perpetrator or a victim of violence (Finnerty et al. 1996). When pregnancy complications develop, mania may interfere with obstetric treatment (e.g., making it impossible for a woman to maintain bed rest [Dickson et al. 1992] or comply with a diet for gestational diabetes mellitus [Finnerty et al. 1996]).

## Anxiety Disorders

### Panic Disorder

A subset of women experience a decrease in the frequency and severity of panic attacks during pregnancy (Villeponteaux et al. 1992), whereas other women experience new onset of panic disorder (Cowley and Roy-Byrne 1989) or worsening panic during pregnancy (Griez et al. 1995). Panic attacks occurring during pregnancy may be confused with preeclampsia (Benjamin and Benjamin 1993) or may contribute to complications like placental abruption, presumably by producing sympathetic nervous system arousal and transient hypertension (Cohen et al. 1989). Agoraphobia associated with panic disorder can compromise women's ability to visit a prenatal clinic (Olsen et al. 1992).

### Obsessive-Compulsive Disorder

Pregnancy is one of the most common triggers for the onset or exacerbation of obsessive-compulsive disorder (Neziroglu et al. 1992). When severe, compulsions may directly affect obstetric risk factors, such as when nutritious foods are avoided because of contamination fears or when time-consuming rituals preclude prenatal clinic visits. Obsessions sometimes include ego-dystonic thoughts of harming the fetus that women may be afraid to mention to others (Iancu et al. 1995). Occasionally, symptoms remit at the time of birth (Iancu et al. 1995), but this is not the norm.

## Posttraumatic Stress Disorder

Symptoms of posttraumatic stress disorder arising during pregnancy may be related to one of the following situations: 1) women with histories of sexual abuse whose traumatic memories are reactivated by the experience of pregnancy and childbirth; 2) women who develop posttraumatic stress disorder as a result of traumatic childbirth experiences; 3) women who develop both posttraumatic stress disorder and pregnancy because of a rape.

The experiences of pregnancy, childbirth, and obstetric interventions can reactivate memories of sexual abuse. Some women experience flashbacks and/or sensations analogous to forced intercourse and/or overwhelming feelings that their bodies are out of control, that they must depend on others in a way that frightens them (Rhodes and Hutchinson 1994). These feelings can result in difficulty collaborating with labor, so that there is a failure to progress. For example, a woman might tense her thigh and vaginal muscles rather than relax them to push, or might direct all of her pushing efforts into her arms, as if to "brake" the process of delivery. Other manifestations include dissociation during labor and regressive behavior, such as assuming a childlike voice, hiding under the covers, and assuming a fetal position (Rhodes and Hutchinson 1994). As a coping strategy, some women may attempt to control every aspect of delivery to the point at which they are seen as overcontrolling by obstetric staff. If the reasons for the behavior are not understood, obstetric personnel may come to regard the mother as an adversary who must be overcome in order to provide care to the baby (Josephs 1996). These patterns are especially common in pregnant adolescents because many pregnant teenagers have been sexually abused (Boyer and Fine 1992).

Even with no preexisting trauma history, childbirth itself is a sufficiently traumatic experience for some women that it produces symptoms of posttraumatic stress disorder (Ralph and Alexander 1994). Childbirth is sometimes inadvertently rendered more traumatic by prenatal classes that convey the impression that women who use analgesia during labor are failures (Stewart 1985). Although this feeling, in itself, is unlikely to cause posttraumatic stress disorder, it can be a contributory factor. Another vulnerable group is that of women who became pregnant as a result of rape. Many are unaware of the pregnancy for the first few months. Postrape counseling may help women recognize the possibility of pregnancy earlier as well as decrease the psychiatric sequelae.

## Sleep Disorders

It is normal for sleep patterns to be altered during pregnancy. The most common pattern consists of longer sleep and more naps in the first trimester, normal sleep in the second trimester, and numerous nighttime awakenings in the third trimester (Brunner et al. 1994; Coble et al. 1994b; Suzuki et al. 1993). Frequent awakenings toward the end of pregnancy are partly caused by increased urinary frequency, pain, fetal movements, and difficulty finding a comfortable position (Brunner et al. 1994; Suzuki et al. 1993). They may also be caused by qualitative changes in sleep architecture, perhaps hormonally induced (Brunner et al. 1994).

In some women, pregnancy is associated with new onset or recurrence of sleep disorders, including sleepwalking (Berlin 1988), night terrors (Snyder 1986), restless legs syndrome (O'Keeffe 1996), and obstructive sleep apnea (Littner and Brock 1996). Of these, the most common is restless legs syndrome, an unpleasant sensation in the legs that is relieved by movement and causes sleep disturbance because it usually occurs at night (O'Keeffe 1996). It occurs in up to 27% of pregnant women, especially in the second half of pregnancy. This disorder is associated with depression and is exacerbated by deficiencies of folate, vitamin $B_{12}$, and/or iron. The symptoms are also intensified by the use of caffeine, cigarette smoking, or alcohol, although the reasons for this are unknown. Treatment includes eliminating caffeine and alcohol ingestion; stopping smoking; supplementing with folate, $B_{12}$, and/or iron as indicated; and taking hot baths before bedtime. Severe cases can respond to psychopharmacology with L-dopa, bromocriptine, clonazepam, carbamazepine, clonidine, or oxycodone, but the risks of prescribing these agents during pregnancy must be taken into account (see Chapter 5).

Obstructive sleep apnea is rare during pregnancy but is important to detect because severe cases result in sufficient maternal hypoxemia to cause fetal intrauterine growth retardation. Noninvasive tests of fetal well-being, such as nonstress tests, serial ultrasound examinations, kick counts, and umbilical Doppler flow studies, can help determine whether the fetus is being affected by maternal sleep apnea (Littner and Brock 1996). In some cases, apnea is a result of sleeping in the supine position and can be remedied by instructing the woman to sleep on her side (Loube et al. 1996). In other cases, treatment measures such as continuous positive airway pressure, dental prostheses, tracheostomy, or overnight supplemental oxygen are necessary (Littner and Brock 1996).

## Factitious Disorders

In the context of pregnancy, factitious disorder is the feigning or intentional production of signs and symptoms of pregnancy complications. These can include vaginal bleeding, premature labor, premature rupture of membranes, vomiting, reduction in fetal movements, pyrexia, and seizures (Goodlin 1985; Jureidini 1993). Failure to detect the factitious nature of symptoms can result in misdiagnoses such as placenta previa, placental abruption, and fetal distress and can lead to premature delivery by cesarean section. Factitious disorder during pregnancy poses a risk for the later development of factitious disorder by proxy, which is the feigning or production by the mother of symptoms or illness in her child (Jureidini 1993), and of other forms of child abuse (Goodlin 1985).

Recognizing the factitious nature of symptoms is challenging but can be facilitated by 1) including factitious disorder in the differential diagnosis of pregnancy complications, 2) communicating with other health care providers for patients who seek care from multiple sites, and 3) eliciting a history of prior child custody loss. Management is usually best conducted by obstetricians in consultation with psychiatrists. Although patients rarely improve from direct interpretation of their behavior, an understanding of their motivations may be obtained through collateral historians and may guide intervention. Collaboration with child welfare agencies may offer protection for offspring as well as help motivate women to consider psychiatric intervention and parenting rehabilitation.

## Disorders Specific to Pregnancy

## Hyperemesis Gravidarum

Hyperemesis gravidarum is a condition of intractable vomiting during pregnancy that is of sufficient severity to result in electrolyte imbalance, weight loss, ketosis, acetonuria, and/or organ damage and is without a known organic cause other than pregnancy. Although mild nausea and vomiting are experienced in most normal pregnancies, hyperemesis gravidarum is relatively rare and occurs in approximately 0.5–10/1,000 pregnancies (Hod et al. 1994).

Endocrinologic explanations for the etiology of hyperemesis gravidarum have been postulated, although none have been clearly proven. The etiologic role of psychogenic factors has been controversial. Belief in such factors arose because vomiting ceased in some cases with placebo treatments, hospital admission alone, or psychosocial interventions. Psychodynamic explanations initially centered on vomiting as an unconscious attempt to get rid of the fetus (O'Brien and Newton 1991).

Empirical studies have suffered from methodologic difficulties, including a lack of adequate control subjects and a failure to differentiate the psychologic causes of hyperemesis from its effects. One well-controlled follow-up study found no evidence of significant differences in long-term psychopathology between women with hyperemesis and control subjects, although acute psychiatric disturbance could not be excluded (Majerus et al. 1960). Other studies have found hyperemesis to be associated with factors such as hysterical personality, below-average intelligence, poor mother–daughter relationships, unplanned and/or undesired pregnancies, susceptibility to hypnosis, and eating disorders (Apfel et al. 1986; Fairweather 1968; Fitzgerald 1984). Hyperemesis has also been conceptualized as a learned behavior in response to psychosocial "triggers" that vary from woman to woman. In some cases, it is postulated that the "trigger" is an extreme anxiety response to "normal" nausea and vomiting of pregnancy, which in turn worsens the nausea and vomiting, creating a "vicious circle" (Deuchar 1995).

Overall, available data suggest a spectrum of psychophysiologic causation, with some cases heavily influenced by psychopathology, others apparently unrelated to psychologic disturbance, and some having both emotional and somatic determinants. A logical clinical approach begins with screening for the presence of a personality disorder, current interpersonal conflict, eating disorder, ambivalence about the pregnancy, extreme anxiety, and/or specific psychosocial "triggers" of vomiting. Noting apparent connections between the factors and the symptoms can guide effective treatment.

## Denial of Pregnancy

Difficulties with recognizing and accepting pregnancy fall on a continuum from disavowal of the emotional reality of pregnancy through suppression of awareness of pregnancy to psychotic denial of pregnancy. Emotional denial occurs in women who acknowledge that they are pregnant yet do little or nothing to alter their lives accordingly. For example, they do not change diet, wardrobe, exercise regimen, or future plans. They do not fantasize about the baby, think of names for the baby, or prepare a nursery. This type of denial is often seen in women who have lost a prior baby, such as through stillbirth. In these cases, working through unresolved grief may help mothers bond with their new babies and allow those babies to have identities separate from those of their lost siblings. This pattern is also seen in many women who use addictive drugs and feel guilty about potential consequences (Spielvogel and Hohener 1995).

More extreme denial may be seen in women who suppress awareness of pregnancy through all or most of gestation. Typically, such women gain little or no weight; those who do gain weight attribute it simply to "getting fat." Many have episodes of bleeding throughout the pregnancy; those who do not may attribute amenorrhea to menopause or to irregular periods. Few experience typical pregnancy-related symptoms such as nausea; those who do experience such symptoms attribute them to other causes. Symptoms and signs of labor are misinterpreted; for example, contractions may be experienced as the urge to defecate and ruptured membranes as urination. During labor and delivery, these women often show signs of dissociation. In most cases, significant others do not know that the women are pregnant. In part, this is because the women conceal signs of pregnancy, but in many cases it seems to reflect a profound interpersonal isolation and lack of intimacy with significant others. Pregnancy is usually discovered during labor or after the birth of the baby but is occasionally discovered earlier by accident—for example, by viewing fetal bones on X-rays that the mother receives for unrelated complaints ( Brezinka et al. 1994; Brozovsky and Falit 1971; Finnegan et al. 1982).

Women who deny pregnancy in this way are a heterogeneous group. Risk factors for this form of denial include 1) young age (most reported cases are in adolescents); 2) passivity (e.g., women who do not refuse unwanted sex and/or do not insist on contraception, then become pregnant and do not seek abortions even if they want them); 3) family and/or cultural taboos (e.g., families or subcultures in which it is "unthinkable" to become pregnant while unmarried or families in which a woman believes dire consequences will result from pregnancy—"If you ever got pregnant, your father would have a heart attack!"); 4) history of sexual abuse, leading women to deny pregnancy in order to stave off traumatic memories; 5) limited intelligence or paucity of knowledge about reproductive anatomy and physiology; 6) relevant life stressors, such as separation from the father of the child; and 7) social isolation (Brezinka et al. 1994; Finnegan et al. 1982; Resnick 1970; Saunders 1989; Spielvogel and Hohener 1995).

Certain obstetric and gynecologic conditions also enhance the likelihood of pregnancy denial. These include breech presentation, which causes body habitus to be less recognizable as pregnant, and irregular menses, which make pregnancy-related amenorrhea less noticeable (Brezinka et al. 1994).

The consequences of extreme pregnancy denial can include failure to receive prenatal care; inadequate nutrition during pregnancy; failure to avoid pregnancy-related risks such as radiologic procedures or teratogenic drugs; failure to notice warning signs of premature labor, premature rupture of membranes, or other pregnancy complications; unassisted delivery, sometimes accompanied by complications such as excessive bleeding or infection; neonaticide, occurring either actively (e.g., the mother is overwhelmed by fear and rage after the sudden breakdown of defensive denial and kills the baby) or passively (e.g., the baby drowns in the toilet because of being mistaken for a bowel movement); and loss of custody of the child (Brezinka et al. 1994; Resnick 1970; Saunders 1989; Spielvogel and Hohener 1995).

Psychotic denial of pregnancy usually occurs in women with preexisting psychotic disorders, most commonly schizophrenia. It consists of maintaining the belief that one is not pregnant despite experiencing the physical changes of pregnancy and experiencing positive pregnancy tests, ultrasound examinations, fetal heart tones, and even the baby after birth. In many cases, the denial comes and goes and is intensified by stress. Psychotic denial is more common in women who have lost custody of a baby and/or anticipate losing custody, suggesting that it is a defense against overwhelming feelings of loss (Miller 1990).

Denial and its resultant risks can be minimized by screening for pregnancy in high-risk populations (e.g., adolescents and women with schizophrenia or drug addiction), discussing sexuality and reproduction in a nonjudgmental manner, and screening for past sexual abuse and past fetal/neonatal loss. Emotional denial often responds to brief, focused psychotherapy. Extreme, nonpsychotic denial usually collapses in the face of external validation of pregnancy, but supportive psychotherapeutic and family interventions may be necessary depending on the sources of denial and the consequences of acknowledging the pregnancy. Psychotic denial may respond to pharmacotherapy and supportive psychotherapy; if persistent, however, hospitalization may be required in order to to avoid precipitous, unassisted delivery and/or harm to the fetus or neonate (Miller 1990; Spielvogel and Hohener 1995).

## General Principles of Intervention During Pregnancy

The increased contact with health care professionals afforded by prenatal care allows for early detection of psychiatric disorders during pregnancy. Early detection, in turn, allows prompt intervention and prevention of exacerbations later in pregnancy or postpartum. This may decrease the need for medication during pregnancy, decrease obstetric complications, and promote optimal parenting.

Early detection can be promoted by the use of screening tools designed for this purpose (Powers et al. 1993). Mental health screening questions can be incorporated into general prenatal intake histories in the form of self-administered questionnaires (on paper or computer) or as semistructured interviews. In addition to instruments that screen for general psychiatric symptoms, instruments are available that have been developed specifically for use with pregnant women in prenatal care settings. These include the Maternal Attitudes to Pregnancy Instrument (MAPI; Blau et al. 1964), the Life Events Scale for Obstetric Groups (Barnett et al. 1983), the Maternal Adjustment and Maternal Attitudes scale (MAMA; Kumar et al. 1984), and the Pregnancy Psychologic Attitudes Test (PPAT; Mamelle et al. 1989).

When psychiatric symptoms are present, a comprehensive psychiatric evaluation can assist in making a diagnosis and guiding interventions. For certain symptoms, specific forms of psychotherapy may be particularly effective: for example, cognitive-behavioral therapy for depression, obsessive-compulsive disorder, and panic disorder; relaxation techniques and hypnosis for hyperemesis gravidarum; or interpersonal psychotherapy for depression. In cases of severe psychiatric disorders, the risks of active symptoms may outweigh potential risks of pharmacotherapy or electroconvulsive therapy during pregnancy (see Chapter 5). Decisions about somatic treatment during pregnancy must take into account not only the risks of treatment and of untreated symptoms but also the patient's insight into her illness, her ability to recognize early symptoms, her social supports, and her therapeutic alliance. Involving the family members and self-help support networks of pregnant women may be helpful, given the high levels of psychosocial stress associated with many antenatal psychiatric conditions.

When presenting mentally ill pregnant women with decisions about obstetric interventions, it is important to evaluate whether and how psychiatric symptoms are affecting the decision-making process. For women with prior histories of psychiatric disorder who become pregnant, health care directives stating treatment preferences can be written in anticipation of possible relapse (Coverdale et al. 1997). For women with extreme anxiety about obstetric interventions (e.g., in cases of posttraumatic stress disorder), helping them gain and maintain a sense of control is helpful. This can be facilitated, for example, by avoiding unnecessary vaginal examinations, preparing them emotionally for necessary examinations, getting explicit permission to touch them before doing so, and maintaining their active involvement in decision making throughout the pregnancy (Rhodes and Hutchinson 1994). After difficult labors, postnatal debriefing either individually or in a group may prevent the later development of anxiety symptoms (Ralph and Alexander 1994).

For patients who require psychiatric hospitalization during pregnancy, setting up collaborative links between mental health, obstetric, and pediatric staff can facilitate optimal care (Miller 1992; Muqtadir et al. 1986). In some cases, hospitalization can be avoided with prenatal home visits by case managers and nurse midwives, such as for women with agoraphobia.

Major mental illness during pregnancy raises questions about a woman's ability to care for her baby after birth. Assessment of parenting capability (Jacobsen et al. 1997), followed by provision of extra social support and parenting rehabilitation when needed, may decrease the possibility of custody loss and may improve the future course of the lives of the mother, the baby, and the rest of the family.

# References

Affonso D, Lovett S, Paul S, et al: Predictors of depression symptoms during pregnancy and postpartum. J Psychosom Obstet Gynaecol 12:255–271, 1991

Apfel R, Handel MH: Madness and the Loss of Motherhood: Sexuality, Reproduction, and Long-Term Mental Illness. Washington, DC, American Psychiatric Press, 1993

Apfel R, Kelley S, Frankel F: The role of hypnotizability in the pathogenesis and treatment of hyperemesis gravidarum. J Psychosom Obstet Gynaecol 5:179–186, 1986

Bachrach LL: Chronically mentally ill women: an overview of service delivery issues, in Treating Chronically Mentally Ill Women. Edited by Bachrach LL, Nadelson CC. Washington, DC, American Psychiatric Press, 1988, pp 1–17

Barnet B, Joffe A, Duggan AK, et al: Depressive symptoms, stress, and social support in pregnant and postpartum adolescents. Arch Pediatr Adolesc Med 150:64–69, 1996

Barnett BE, Hanna B, Parker G: Life event scales for obstetric groups. J Psychosom Res 27:313–320, 1983

Benjamin J, Benjamin M: Panic disorder masquerading as pre-eclampsia. Eur J Obstet Gynecol Reprod Biol 51:81–82, 1993

Berlin RM: Sleepwalking disorder during pregnancy: a case report. Sleep 11:298–300, 1988

Blau A, Welkowitz J, Cohen J: Maternal attitude to pregnancy instrument. Arch Gen Psychiatry 10:324–331, 1964

Boyer D, Fine D: Sexual abuse as a factor in adolescent pregnancy and child maltreatment. Fam Plann Perspect 24:4–12, 1992

Brezinka C, Huter O, Biehl W, et al: Denial of pregnancy: obstetrical aspects. J Psychosom Obstet Gynaecol 15:1–8, 1994

Brozovsky M, Falit H: Neonaticide: clinical and psychodynamic considerations. J Am Acad Child Psychiatry 10:673–683, 1971

Brunner DP, Munch M, Biedermann K et al: Changes in sleep and sleep electroencephalogram during pregnancy. Sleep 17:576–582, 1994

Coble PA, Reynolds CF, Kupfer DJ, et al: Childbearing in women with and without a history of affective disorder, I: psychiatric symptomatology. Compr Psychiatry 35:205–214, 1994a

Coble PA, Reynolds CF, Kupfer DJ, et al: Childbearing in women with and without a history of affective disorder, II: electroencephalographic sleep. Compr Psychiatry 35:215–224, 1994b

Cohen LS, Rosenbaum JF, Heller VL: Panic attack–associated placental abruption: a case report. J Clin Psychiatry 50:266–267, 1989

Coverdale JH, McCullough LB, Chervenak FA, et al: Clinical implications of respect for autonomy in the psychiatric treatment of pregnant patients with depression. Psychiatr Serv 48:209–212, 1997

Cowley DS, Roy-Byrne PP: Panic disorder during pregnancy. J Psychosom Obstet Gynaecol 10:193–210, 1989

Demyttenaere K, Lenaerts H, Nijs P, et al: Individual coping style and psychological attitudes during pregnancy predict depression levels during pregnancy and during postpartum. Acta Psychiatr Scand 91:95–102, 1995

Deuchar N: Nausea and vomiting in pregnancy: a review of the problem with particular regard to psychological and social aspects. Br J Obstet Gynecol 102:6–8, 1995

Dickson LR, Miller WH, Hyatt MC: Pregnancy complicated by acute mania and preeclampsia. Psychosomatics 33:221–224, 1992

Dolinar LJ: Obstacles to the care of patients with medical-psychiatric illness on general hospital psychiatry units. Gen Hosp Psychiatry 15:14–20, 1993

Fairweather DVI: Nausea and vomiting in pregnancy. Am J Obstet Gynecol 102:135–175, 1968

Finnegan P, McKinstry E, Robinson GE: Denial of pregnancy and childbirth. Can J Psychiatry 27:672–674, 1982

Finnerty M, Levin Z, Miller LJ: Acute manic episodes in pregnancy. Am J Psychiatry 153:261–263, 1996

Fitzgerald CM: Nausea and vomiting in pregnancy. Br J Med Psychol 57:159–165, 1984

Goodlin RC: Pregnant women with Munchausen syndrome. Am J Obstet Gynecol 153:207–210, 1985

Griez EJL, Hauzer R, Meijer J: Pregnancy and estrogen-induced panic (letter). Am J Psychiatry 152:1688, 1995

Hobfoll SE, Ritter C, Lavin J, et al: Depression prevalence and incidence among inner-city pregnant and postpartum women. J Consult Clin Psychol 63:445–453, 1995

Hod M, Orvieto R, Kaplan et al: Hyperemesis gravidarum: a review. J Reprod Med 39:605–612, 1994

Iancu J, Lepkifker J, Dannon P, et al: Obsessive-compulsive disorder limited to pregnancy. Psychother Psychosom 64:109–112, 1995

Jacobsen T: Effects of postpartum disorders on parenting and on offspring, in Postpartum Mood Disorders. Edited by Miller LJ. Washington, DC, American Psychiatric Press, 1999, pp 119–139

Jacobsen T, Miller LJ, Kirkwood KP: Assessing parenting competency in individuals with serious mental illness: a comprehensive service. J Ment Health Adm 24:189–199, 1997

Josephs L: Women and trauma: a contemporary psychodynamic approach to traumatization for patients in the Ob/Gyn psychological consultation clinic. Bull Menn Clin 60:22–38, 1996

Jureidini J: Obstetric factitious disorder and Munchausen syndrome by proxy. J Nerv Ment Dis 181:135–137, 1993

Kitamura T, Toda MA, Shima S, et al: Early loss of parents and early rearing experiences among women with antenatal depression. J Psychosom Obstet Gynaecol 15:133–139, 1994

Kumar R, Robson KM: A prospective study of emotional disorders in childbearing women. Br J Psychiatry 144:35–47, 1984

Kumar R, Robson KM, Smith AMR: Development of a self-administered questionnaire to measure maternal adjustment and maternal attitudes during pregnancy and after delivery. J Psychosom Res 28:43–51, 1984

Littner MR, Brock BJ: Snoring in pregnancy: disease or not? Chest 109:859–861, 1996

Loube DI, Poceta JS, Morales MC, et al: Self-reported snoring in pregnancy: association with fetal outcome. Chest 109:885–889, 1996

Majerus PW, Guze SB, Delong WB, et al: Psychologic factors and psychiatric disease in hyperemesis gravidarum: a follow-up study of 69 vomiters and 66 controls. Am J Psychiatry 117:421–428, 1960

Mamelle N, Measson A, Munoz F, et al: Development and use of a self-administered questionnaire for assessment of psychologic attitudes toward pregnancy and their relation to a subsequent premature birth. Am J Epidemiol 130:989–998, 1989

McNeil TF, Kaij L, Malmquist-Larsson A: Pregnant women with nonorganic psychosis: life situation and experience of pregnancy. Acta Psychiatr Scand 68:445–457, 1983

McNeil TF, Kaij L, Malmquist-Larsson A: Women with nonorganic psychosis: pregnancy's effect on mental health during pregnancy. Acta Psychiatr Scand 70:140–148, 1984

Miller LJ: Psychotic denial of pregnancy: phenomenology and clinical management. Hospital and Community Psychiatry 41:1233–1237, 1990

Miller LJ: Comprehensive care of pregnant mentally ill women. J Ment Health Admin 19:170–177, 1992

Miller LJ: Sexuality, reproduction, and family planning in women with schizophrenia. Schizophr Bull 23:623–635, 1997

Miller LJ, Finnerty M: Sexuality, pregnancy, and childrearing among women with schizophrenia spectrum disorders. Psychiatr Serv 47:502–506, 1996

Muqtadir S, Hamann MW, Molnar G: Management of psychotic pregnant patients in a medical-psychiatric unit. Psychosomatics 27:31–33, 1986

Neziroglu F, Anemone R, Yaryura-Tobias JA: Onset of obsessive-compulsive disorder in pregnancy. Am J Psychiatry 149:947–950, 1992

Nicholson J, Geller JL, Fisher WH, et al: State policies and programs that address the needs of mentally ill mothers in the public sector. Hospital and Community Psychiatry 44:484–489, 1993

O'Brien B, Newton N: Psyche versus soma: historical evolution of beliefs about nausea and vomiting during pregnancy. J Psychosom Obstet Gynaecol 12:91–120, 1991

O'Hara MW: Social support, life events, and depression during pregnancy and the puerperium. Arch Gen Psychiatry 43:569–573, 1986

O'Hara MW, Neunaber DJ, Zekoski EM: Prospective study of postpartum depression: prevalence, course, and predictive factors. J Abnorm Psychol 93:158–171, 1984

O'Keeffe ST: Restless legs syndrome: a review. Arch Intern Med 156:243–248, 1996

Olsen ME, Toeppen-Sprigg B, Krell MA: Prenatal care and delivery in an agoraphobic woman: a case report. J Reprod Med 37:466–468, 1992

Pajer K: New strategies in the treatment of depression in women. J Clin Psychiatry 56(suppl 2):30–37, 1995

Parry B: Postpartum depression in relation to other reproductive cycle mood changes, in Postpartum Mood Disorders. Edited by Miller LJ. Washington, DC, American Psychiatric Press, 1999, pp 21–45

Powers ZL, Zahorik P, Morrow B: An evaluation of residents' recognition of depressive symptoms in obstetrical patients. J Tenn Med Assoc 86:147–149, 1993

Ralph K, Alexander J: Borne under stress. Nurs Times 90:28–30, 1994

Resnick PJ: Murder of the newborn: a psychiatric review of neonaticide. Am J Psychiatry 126:1414–1420, 1970

Rhodes N, Hutchinson S: Labor experiences of childhood sexual abuse survivors. Birth 21:213–220, 1994

Rudolph B, Larson GL, Sweeny S, et al: Hospitalized pregnant psychotic women: characteristics and treatment issues. Hospital and Community Psychiatry 41:159–163, 1990

Sacker A, Done DJ, Crow TJ: Obstetric complications in children born to parents with schizophrenia: a meta-analysis of case-control studies. Psychol Med 26:279–287, 1996

Salamero M, Marcos T, Gutierrez F, et al: Factorial study of the BDI in pregnant women. Psychol Med 24:1031–1035, 1994

Saunders E: Neonaticides following "secret" pregnancies: seven case reports. Public Health Rep 104:368–372, 1989

Sharma V, Persad E: Effect of pregnancy on three patients with bipolar disorder. Ann Clin Psychiatry 7:39–42, 1995

Snyder S: Unusual case of sleep terror in a pregnant patient (letter). Am J Psychiatry 143:391, 1986

Spielvogel A, Hohener HC: Denial of pregnancy: a review and case reports. Birth 22:220–226, 1995

Spielvogel A, Wile J: Treatment and outcomes of psychotic patients during pregnancy and childbirth. Birth 19:131–137, 1992

Stewart D: Pregnancy and schizophrenia. Can Fam Physician 30:1537–1542, 1984

Stewart D: Possible relationship of postpartum psychiatric symptoms to childbirth education programmes. J Psychosom Obstet Gynaecol 4:295–301, 1985

Suzuki S, Dennerstein L, Greenwood KM, et al: Melatonin and hormonal changes in disturbed sleep during late pregnancy. J Pineal Res 15:191–198, 1993

Villeponteaux VA, Lydiard RB, Laraia MT, et al: The effects of pregnancy on preexisting panic disorder. J Clin Psychiatry 53:201–203, 1992

Yoldas Z, Iscan A, Yoldas T et al: A woman who did her own caesarean section. Lancet 348:135, 1996

# Psychotropic Drugs and Electroconvulsive Therapy During Pregnancy and Lactation

DONNA E. STEWART, M.D., D.PSYCH., F.R.C.P.C.
GAIL ERLICK ROBINSON, M.D., D.PSYCH., F.R.C.P.C.

Any discussion on the effects of psychotropic drugs in pregnancy and lactation must start by stating the limits to our knowledge. Many studies have failed to consider confounding variables such as diagnosis; maternal age; use of alcohol, tobacco, or street drugs; gravidity; socioeconomic status; previous pregnancy loss; genetic history; use of multiple drugs; timing of drug exposure; and dosage. Few prospective controlled studies of the treatment of psychiatric disorders in pregnant women are available (Altshuler et al. 1996). Moreover, drugs that consistently produce defects in other animals may not have similar effects in humans (Elia et al. 1987). It is wise to remember that the U.S. Food and Drug Administration (1979) has not approved any psychotropic drugs for administration during pregnancy and urges caution in their use. A multidisciplinary task force is developing new guideline documents (Center for Drug Evaluation and Research 1997). During the 1990s, patterns of psychotropic drug exposure in pregnancy changed. Selective serotonin reuptake inhibitors are now the most commonly prescribed antidepressant drugs, and a host of new antianxiety and psychotropic drugs have been approved for clinical use.

# Effects of Pregnancy on Drug Metabolism, Action, and Side Effects

Pregnant women may receive psychotropic drugs for several reasons. Some may be undergoing treatment with antidepressants, antipsychotics, mood stabilizers, or minor tranquilizers, either for an acute psychiatric illness or for maintenance therapy, when they become pregnant. Other women may develop a psychiatric illness that requires treatment during pregnancy or lactation (Robinson et al. 1986).

The potential benefits of pharmacotherapy in the pregnant or lactating woman must be carefully weighed against the possible risks to the woman and her developing fetus or infant. The risk side of the risk/benefit equation includes the risks of maternal and newborn toxicity, side effects and withdrawal, and fetal physical or behavioral teratogenicity (Cohen et al. 1989). Although the benefits of psychotropic drugs for the severely psychotic, depressed, or suicidal pregnant woman may outweigh the risks to the infant, a careful appraisal of current knowledge in this area is essential before a rational clinical decision can be reached (Robinson et al. 1986). This chapter contains current information on the use of antipsychotics, antidepressants, mood stabilizers, and anxiolytics during pregnancy and lactation. Use of electroconvulsive therapy (ECT) in pregnancy is also discussed.

Despite public education, drug use in pregnancy is still commonplace. Because more than 50% of pregnancies are unplanned, many drug exposures will occur before the pregnancy is even diagnosed. Rayburn et al. (1982) showed that 90% or more of all pregnant women take one or more drugs in addition to dietary supplements during pregnancy. In a North American study, Heinonen et al. (1977) reported that 36% of pregnant women took sedatives, tranquilizers, or antidepressants at some time during their pregnancies.

Several physiologic changes in pregnancy alter the effects of drugs. Data on drug metabolism rates, dosages, and side effects in nonpregnant women may not apply to pregnant women. The significant increases in total body water content that occur during pregnancy may result in lower drug serum concentrations than are found in nonpregnant women. Total protein is also reduced in pregnancy, thereby altering drug binding. A physiologic drop in blood pressure in the second trimester of pregnancy may result in orthostatic hypotension, causing significant problems in pregnant women treated with some antipsychotic and tricyclic antidepressant drugs. The emptying rate of the gastrointestinal tract is decreased by 30%–50%, and gastric acid is decreased, thus altering drug absorption. Constipation, a common condition in pregnancy, may be worsened by medications with anticholinergic side effects. Glomerular filtration rates are increased in pregnancy, causing some drugs such as lithium to be excreted more quickly and thereby requiring higher doses to achieve therapeutic serum levels. Hepatic hydroxylases involved in drug metabolism may be inhibited during pregnancy (Mortola 1989; Wisner and Perel 1988).

The physiologic changes of pregnancy necessitate careful monitoring of a woman's drug response, side effects, and toxicity throughout the pregnancy and early postpartum period (Wisner and Perel 1988). Higher doses are sometimes required in pregnancy to achieve therapeutic serum levels. After delivery, the doses may need to be decreased to prevent maternal toxicity (Koplan 1983; Stewart 1988).

All psychotropic drugs cross the placenta and enter the fetal circulation to some degree. The penetration to the fetal compartment is influenced by the characteristics of the drug, the dosage, and the stage of pregnancy (Mirkin 1976). When repeated doses of a psychotropic drug are administered to sustain plasma concentrations, the drug is usually distributed equally to mother and fetus (G.H. Levy 1981). Both the placenta and the fetus have enzyme systems involved in drug metabolism, but many details are as yet incompletely understood (Chao and Juchau 1983). It is also known that some enzyme systems are not mature at birth, impairing the ability of the newborn's liver to conjugate the metabolites of common drugs such as diazepam (Kanto 1982). Thus, fetal physiology must also be considered in prescribing psychotropic drugs in pregnancy.

## General Effects on the Fetus and Neonate

### Morphologic Teratogenicity

During the first several cell divisions, the developing embryo is thought to be protected against the effects of drugs administered to the mother because the placenta has not yet formed. This period of protection is between conception (approximately day 14) and the first missed period (approximately day 28 of a 28-day cycle). After the first missed period, however, the placenta is sufficiently developed to transfer drugs in the maternal circulation to the developing fetus (Cohen 1989).

It is impossible to guarantee that any psychotropic drug is not teratogenic and able to cause fetal deformity because the baseline rate of birth defects in the Western World is approximately 3%, and the cause of most birth defects remains unknown (Beeley 1986). Although the incidence of birth defects caused by drugs is probably low, low levels of teratogenicity caused by drugs are extremely difficult to distinguish from the spontaneous occurrence of anomalies and require large exposure samples (American Medical Association 1983).

Several factors, however, are known to increase the teratogenic risks of a drug: 1) exposure to the drug during organogenesis (central nervous system, gestational days 10–25; limb development, days 24–26; cardiovascular system development, days 20–40); 2) dosage and regularity of use (lack of maternal toxicity does not indicate lack of fetal toxicity); 3) interaction with other environmental factors, such as other drugs, alcohol, tobacco, and other toxins; and 4) the genetic constitution of the mother and fetus. It is hypothesized that the continuum of abnormal development ranges from fetal death (resulting in miscarriage or stillbirth) to physical malformation, growth retardation, or functional deficits (behavioral teratogenicity) (J. G. Wilson 1977).

## Behavioral Teratogenicity

The rapidly developing field of behavioral teratogenicity includes functional deficits such as delayed behavioral maturation, abnormal activity, and impaired problem solving and learning, all of which may develop following fetal exposure to teratogens (Vorhees and Butcher 1982). Research in animals has shown that most drugs that act on the central nervous system have a low potential for physical teratogenicity but a higher potential as behavioral teratogens, which probably arises from less-severe damage (Vorhees and Butcher 1982). Many behavioral teratogenic agents may not yet have been identified in humans because they are unaccompanied by physical malformation. Few studies on the long-term follow-up of children exposed to psychotropic drugs in utero are available. (See specific information on major tranquilizers, antidepressants, and lithium in the section on "Known Effects of Specific Psychotropic Drug Groups" in this chapter.) Other investigators have criticized the available studies for their small sample sizes, lack of data on dosage and timing, circumscribed inquiry, lack of standardized psychometric instruments, and inadequate follow-up period (Edlund and Craig 1984). It is therefore unwise to assume that any psychotropic agent is "safe" in pregnancy (Wisner and Perel 1988), although the use may be appropriate in many clinical situations. Use of psychotropic drugs during pregnancy and lactation should include thoughtful weighing of risks of prenatal exposure versus risks of maternal mental illness or relapse following drug discontinuation (Altshuler et al. 1996).

## Effects of Psychotropic Drugs During Second and Third Trimester and Labor

Psychotropic drugs appear to be safer during the second and third trimester of pregnancy. Major malformations are not produced during the second and third trimesters, but drugs can affect the growth and functional development of the fetus. In particular, the central nervous system continues to develop throughout pregnancy and the neonatal period, and damage after the first trimester can produce microcephaly, mental retardation (Beeley 1986), and behavioral teratogenicity. Some clinicians recommend that the drug doses be lowered or discontinued approximately 2 weeks prior to the expected date of delivery to reduce the possibility of side effects, toxicity, and withdrawal in the newborn (Kerns 1986; Robinson et al. 1986; Wisner and Perel 1988), whereas other experts do not discontinue psychotropic drugs before labor in order to reduce the risk of in vitro fetal withdrawal or maternal relapse of psychiatric illness (Altshuler et al. 1996).

Both the major and the minor tranquilizers have been used by obstetricians during labor to reduce anxiety, increase relaxation, or decrease nausea. Long-acting benzodiazepines, however, should be avoided in the third trimester because they adversely affect the neonate (Mandrelli et al. 1975). If benzodiazepines are required they should be used in the lowest effective dose for the shortest period of time necessary to minimize fetal exposure (Altshuler et al. 1996).

## Effects on the Neonate

Antipsychotics, tricyclic antidepressants, and benzodiazepines are lipid soluble and largely protein bound and are slowly eliminated from the newborn. The neonate may be more susceptible to these drugs because liver enzymes are not fully developed; plasma protein concentrates are lower, leading to increased free drug available to act on the brain; the blood-brain barrier is incomplete; and the immature central nervous system may be more sensitive to these drugs (Altshuler et al. 1996; Nahas and Goujard 1978).

## Effects During Lactation

Psychotropic drugs, like most medications, are excreted to some degree in breast milk. The concentration of the drug in breast milk depends on its solubility, protein binding, and drug pH compared with plasma (Robinson et al. 1986). There are wide variations among drugs, and concentrations may vary in breast milk samples taken at different times of the day.

The American Academy of Pediatrics Committee on Drugs (1994) has classified major and minor tranquilizers and antidepressants under the category of "drugs whose effects on nursing infants is unknown but may be of concern." Various case reports of toxic effects, drowsiness, impaired temperature regulation, and no ill effects have been described in breastfed infants of mothers receiving psychotropic or mood-stabilizing drugs (Gelenberg 1987). The effects of these drugs on the immature neurotransmitter system are unknown (Mortola 1989; Robinson et al. 1986).

Wisner et al. (1996) reviewed the use of antidepressants during lactation, and although they found limited findings to be reassuring, they recommended an expanded database of mother–baby serum levels, behavioral assessments of babies during nursing and longitudinal development, and evaluation of nurslings.

# Known Effects of Specific Psychotropic Drug Groups

## Antipsychotic Agents

### Teratogenicity

Numerous reports in the literature describe individual or short series of cases in which the use of neuroleptics in the first trimester has coincided with the occurrence of congenital anomalies (Table 5–1). Results of larger studies are conflicting.

The French National Institute of Health and Medical Research conducted a retrospective study involving 12,764 births (Rumeau-Rouquette et al. 1977). Infants in the control group demonstrated congenital malformation not considered to be related to chromosomal abnormalities in 1.6% of cases. Of the 315 women who received phenothiazines during the first trimester, 3.5% gave birth to malformed infants. This was considered a statistically sig-

**TABLE 5–1.** Psychotropic drugs in pregnancy and lactation

| Drugs | Teratogenicity | Effects on the neonate | Lactation |
|---|---|---|---|
| **Antipsychotics** | | | |
| Phenothiazines (especially aliphatics) | Congenital anomalies increased if used weeks 6–10. Cardiovascular anomalies increased. Use with caution in first trimester. Appears to be fairly safe. | Third trimester use of neuroleptics may cause extrapyramidal symptoms in infant: excessive crying, motion, hypertonia, hyperreflexia, respiratory distress, vasomotor instability, and slow early learning tasks. Jaundice possible, especially in prematures. | Excreted in breast milk. No serious side effects reported as yet; increased drowsiness. Use with caution. |
| Butyrophenones | No evidence at present for teratogenicity. | | Haloperidol toxic in animal studies. Use with caution. |
| Clozapine, olanzapine; respiradone, quetiapine | Unknown. | Effects unknown. | Effects unknown. |
| **Antidepressants** | | | |
| Tricyclics and heterocyclics | No link with fetal deformity or limb dysgenesis. Use with caution in first trimester. Appears to be fairly safe. | Withdrawal symptoms in infant may include heart failure, tachycardia, myoclonus, seizures, respiratory distress, urinary retention, cyanosis, irritability, feeding difficulty. | Excreted in breast milk. No effects shown for amitriptyline, nortriptyline, desipramine, clomipramine, or dothiapin. |
| Serotonin reuptake inhibitors | Caution in first trimester. Data on fluoxetine, paroxetine, sertraline, and fluvoxamine show no evidence of malformation. Appear fairly safe. | Fluoxetine-exposed infants show no difference up to school age compared with control subjects. Other drugs unknown. | Small amounts in breast milk. Early data show no serious effects for sertraline, fluoxetine, or paroxetine. |
| Monoamine oxidase inhibitors | Phenelzine teratogenic in animals. Avoid in first trimester. | Effects unknown. | Effects unknown. |

**TABLE 5–1.** Psychotropic drugs in pregnancy and lactation (continued)

| Drugs | Teratogenicity | Effects on the neonate | Lactation |
|---|---|---|---|
| **Mood stabilizers** | | | |
| Lithium carbonate | Increased cardiovascular anomalies. Use with caution in first trimester. Give in small divided doses if necessary. Refer for fetal ultrasonography. | Third trimester use may cause hypotonia, lethargy, cyanosis, poor sucking, shallow respiration, low Apgar score, arrhythmias, hypotension. | Excreted in breast milk. Severe toxic reactions. Contraindicated while breastfeeding. |
| Valproic acid | Spina bifida reported (1%–5%). | Effects unknown. | Limited data compatible with breastfeeding. (American Academy of Pediatrics) |
| Carbamazepine | Craniofacial defects and spina bifida reported. | Effects unknown. | Limited data compatible with breast feeding (American Academy of Pediatrics) |
| **Anxiolytics** | | | |
| Benzodiazepines | Safety in first trimester not established. Incidence of cleft lip/palate may be increased. | With chronic use in pregnancy, withdrawal symptoms include tremor, hypertonia, and hyperreflexia. High doses prior to delivery result in low Apgar scores, hypothermia, and neurologic depression. Floppy infant syndrome, decreased sucking rate, and jaundice possible. | Excreted in breast milk. Lethargy, jaundice, poor temperature regulation possible. Long half life drugs contraindicated while breastfeeding. |
| Meprobamates | Cleft lip/palate, and other severe congenital anomalies possible. Do not use. | | |

**TABLE 5–1.** Psychotropic drugs in pregnancy and lactation (*continued*)

| Drugs | Teratogenicity | Effects on the neonate | Lactation |
|---|---|---|---|
| Barbiturates | Associated with dose-related growth retardation, facial dysmorphism, oral clefts, and skeletal anomalies when used in first trimester. | Chronic use in pregnancy associated with withdrawal in infant 10–14 days after birth; increased tone, tremor, and irritability. | Long-term effects unknown. |
| Hydroxyzine | Teratogenic in animals. | Jitteriness, myoclonic jerks, and hypotonia possible after large doses prior to delivery. | |
| Antiparkinsonian agents | No studies. Usually given with neuroleptic. Amantadine teratogenic in animals. Cardiovascular malformation? | Effects unknown. | Effects unknown. |

nificant increase in malformations (especially following the use of aliphatic phenothiazines), but it is not clear whether confounding variables such as dosage, concurrent drugs, and maternal health and age were taken into account.

Slone et al. (1977) reported the results of the Collaborative Perinatal Project of 5,282 gravidas and their children, including 1,309 cases of prenatal exposure to phenothiazines. The authors found no significant increase in the incidence of congenital malformations related to exposure in the first trimester except for a questionable association with cardiovascular malformations. Perinatal mortality rate, birth weight, and IQ at age 4 were all found to be normal in this group.

The California Child Health and Development Project, which studied over 19,000 births, originally showed no increase in congenital anomalies following phenothiazine use in pregnancy (Milkovich and van den Berg 1976). On reanalyzing the data, Edlund and Craig (1984) demonstrated a trend toward increased congenital anomalies when the drugs were given after 4 weeks, the most critical period being from 6–10 weeks' gestation. The exposed samples yielded an incidence of congenital anomalies of 5.4% versus 3.2% in the control subjects.

Studies to date have not revealed a significant increase in fetal abnormalities for pregnant women receiving thioridazine, perphenazine, trifluoperazine, fluphenazine, or haloperidol (Ananth 1975; Goldberg and DiMascio 1978). No evidence has been found of teratogenicity for the dibenzoxazepines, thioxanthenes, or diphenylbutylpiperidines; their safety in pregnancy, however, has not been established.

Caution must be exercised in drawing conclusions from these studies. Edlund and Craig (1984) and others have pointed out numerous confounding methodologic errors. Many studies may have minimized potential effects by looking at nonpsychotic populations using small amounts of drugs as antiemetics or anxiolytics rather than the dosages typically used to treat psychoses. There is also some evidence that children of psychotic women have a higher risk of fetal damage independent of drug exposure (Stewart 1984; Wrede et al. 1980). On the basis of available data it appears that psychotic illness per se may confer the greatest increase in risk of poor fetal outcome. Perinatal exposure to low-potency phenothiazines may confer an additional risk of poor outcome in 4/1,000 patients (0.4%) (Altshuler et al. 1996). In general, the higher-potency drugs such as haloperidol appear to be safer; however, little data are yet available on clozapine, olanzapine, respiradone, or quetiapine.

## Effects on the Neonate

The use of neuroleptics in the last trimester has been reported to cause extrapyramidal symptoms in the neonate, sometimes lasting up to 6 months (W. Levy and Wisniewski 1974). Infants regularly exposed to neuroleptics in the third trimester may be especially difficult to care for because they may suffer from excessive motion, crying and sucking, hypertonicity, hyperreflexia, and vasomotor instability. Brazelton (1970) found effects on neonatal weight, response to nursing, and early learning tasks, but these seemed to occur only in the immediate postnatal period.

## Effects on Breastfeeding Infants

The quantity of major tranquilizers excreted in breast milk is usually less than 30% of the maternal plasma concentration (Ananth 1978). An exception may be haloperidol excretion, which was reported in one case study to be approximately 60% (Whalley et al. 1981). Aside from some drowsiness with chlorpromazine and some galactorrhea with chlorpromazine and thioridazine, no significant human neonatal side effects have been reported despite several large studies (Ananth 1978). Some studies in animals, however, have shown behavioral abnormalities in offspring following administration of haloperidol during lactation (Ananth 1978). Infants who are breastfed while their mothers are receiving major tranquilizers should be carefully clinically monitored. Serum levels in the infant may be helpful in assessing risk and drowsiness.

## Long-Term Effects on Children Exposed in Utero

Slone et al. (1977) studied 4-year-old children whose mothers had received phenothiazines during pregnancy and found their IQ scores to be the same as those of a control population. Kris (1965) followed-up a small sample of children who had been exposed to 50–150 mg chlorpromazine in utero and found the children to be "healthy" with "normal behavior." The flaws of these studies are described in the "Behavioral Teratogenicity" section earlier in this chapter.

# Antidepressants

## Teratogenicity

Crombie et al. (1975) reviewed 10,000 pregnancies in England and Wales, and Kuenssberg and Knox (1972) reviewed another 15,000 pregnancies in

Scotland. The Finnish Register of Congenital Malformations for 1964–1972 was used by Idanpaan-Heikkila and Saxen (1973) to analyze 2,784 cases of birth defects and an equal number of matched control births. No link was found between fetal deformities, including limb dysgenesis, and the use of tricyclic antidepressants in pregnancy in these studies. The Collaborative Perinatal Project (Heinonen et al. 1977) prospectively examined the relationship of tricyclic antidepressants to pregnancy outcome but the numbers were too small to justify generalizations. The European Network of the Teratology Information Services has prospectively collected and evaluated data on 689 pregnancies exposed to tricyclic and nontricyclic antidepressants. The incidence of spontaneous abortion and late fetal/neonatal deaths was within normal limits. Two-thirds of mothers were receiving multiple drugs and 95% were exposed in the first trimester. Of infants without malformations, 31 had neonatal problems associated with chronic multidrug use, especially near term. Evaluated after the first few weeks of postnatal life, 97% of live-born babies were morphologically normal and there was no increase in particular malformations or patterns of defects (McElhatton et al. 1996).

A prospective study from a drug exposure in pregnancy registry was unable to demonstrate any teratogenicity following first-trimester exposure to fluoxetine (Pastuszak et al. 1993). A study of infants exposed to fluoxetine in utero showed no increased rate of major birth defects but found higher rates of minor abnormalities, preterm births, low birth weights, and admissions to special nurseries (Chambers et al. 1996). However, this study did not control for depression effects, was randomized, and the women receiving fluoxetine were older than control mothers. A well-designed study of infants exposed to tricyclic drugs or fluoxetine in utero was unable to demonstrate any teratogenic, birth weight, Apgar score, language development, IQ, or social development changes in exposed infants followed-up to school entry compared with unexposed control infants (Nulman et al. 1997). A recent meta-analysis of epidemiologic studies showed no association between first-trimester fluoxetine use and human teratogenic effects (Addis and Koren 2000). In another study, no congenital anomalies were found in 63 infants exposed to paroxetine in the first trimester (Inman et al. 1993). A recent study of exposure to sertraline (147 women), paroxetine (97 women), and fluvoxamine (26 women) showed no increase of infant teratogenicity at birth (Kulin et al. 1998).

Inadequate data are available to evaluate new antidepressants such as bupropion, trazodone, buspirone, nefazadone, mirtazapine, or venlafaxine. Monoamine oxidase inhibitors have been shown to have teratogenic properties (Heinonen et al. 1977; Poulson and Robson 1964). Although the numbers in these studies are small, it is probably wise to use other antidepressants in pregnancy.

Stimulants such as methylphenidate or amphetamines are also used to treat depression. Unfortunately, most case reports of their use in pregnancy are from women who abused these drugs. In large doses these drugs are associated with fetal growth retardation, premature delivery, irritability, jerkiness, shrill cries, lassitude, and apnea (Briggs et al. 1994; Oro and Dixon 1987). One study found medical use of amphetamines to be associated with fetal oral clefs (Milkovich and van den Berg 1977).

## Effects on the Neonate

Withdrawal symptoms, irritability, and convulsions in the neonate have been reported following the use of desipramine, imipramine, and nortriptyline during pregnancy (Shearer et al. 1972; Webster 1973). There have been case reports of infants born with heart failure, tachycardia, bowel obstruction, respiratory distress, and urinary retention. Signs of toxicity in the infants of mothers taking large amounts of these medications just before delivery may include breathlessness, cyanosis, tachypnea, irritability, seizures, and feeding difficulties (Ananth 1976; Eggermont et al. 1972). More admissions to special care nurseries were reported in infants exposed to fluoxetine in utero (Chambers et al. 1996).

## Effects on Breastfeeding Infants

Controversy exists concerning the effects of antidepressants on breastfeeding infants. Sovner and Orsulak (1979) suggested that amounts of imipramine and desipramine in breast milk samples are similar to those found in plasma and recommended that women not breastfeed while receiving antidepressants because of concern about subtle effects on the neurologic or behavioral maturation of the infant.

Wisner et al. (1996, 1999) critically reviewed the literature on antidepressants during lactation and reported that amitriptyline, nortriptyline, desipramine, clomipramine, dothiapin, and sertraline were not found in quantifiable amounts in nurslings and no adverse effects were reported. The authors felt these were the drugs of choice for breastfeeding women. Adverse effects were reported in some young infants whose mothers has been treated with doxepin or fluoxetine during breastfeeding; however, they found that infants older than 10 weeks showed no accumulation of drugs and were at low risk for adverse effects. Moreover, Chambers et al. (1999) found lower weight gain in 26 breastfed infants whose mothers were receiving fluoxetine. However, Stowe et al. (2000) found only low concentrations of paroxetine in infants' serum and a lack of any observable adverse effects after maternal use while breastfeeding.

Current information, therefore, does not warrant an absolute recommendation on the use of antidepressant drugs in women who are breastfeeding, because the risk/benefit ratio must be assessed on an individual basis. Infants who are breastfed while their mothers are receiving antidepressants should be carefully clinically monitored, and infant serum levels of antidepressants should be measured in cases of extended drug exposure (Birnbaum et al. 1999). The American Academy of Pediatrics (1994) does not believe that maternal antidepressant use precludes breastfeeding, but it classifies antidepressants as "drugs whose effects on nursing infants are unknown but may be of concern."

## Lithium, Carbamazepine, and Valproic Acid

### Teratogenicity

Weinstein (1980) reviewed the records of The International Register of Lithium Babies and found an 11% rate of malformation in 225 exposed infants. Of these malformations, 8% were Ebstein's anomaly or other major cardiovascular malformations. Ebstein's anomaly is a rare condition that occurs in 1 infant per 20,000 live births. Subsequent investigators (Kallen and Tandberg 1983) also reported that exposure to lithium is linked to cardiovascular anomalies, resulting in a contraindication for lithium in the first trimester. Two more-recent studies (Jacobson et al. 1992; Zalzstein et al. 1990), however, suggested that the link to Ebstein's anomaly is much weaker than previously reported.

A pooled overview of studies suggests the risk of Ebstein's anomaly following first trimester lithium exposure is 10–20 times as common as in the general population (0.1%) (Altshuler et al. 1996). Therefore, in women with unstable bipolar disorder or a recent severe affective illness, it may be reasonable to continue lithium and screen for cardiovascular effects with a targeted ultrasound at week 18 of gestation. The use of lithium in the second and third trimesters may infrequently cause a large fetal goiter that may necessitate a cesarean section (Nars and Girard 1977) or may cause cardiac arrhythmias (Llewellyn et al. 1998).

Carbamazepine, previously considered safe in pregnancy, has now been associated with fetal craniofacial defects, developmental delay, nail hypoplasia (Jones et al. 1989), and spina bifida (Rosa 1991). Caution should be exercised until further data are available.

Valproic acid, another mood stabilizer used in bipolar affective disorder, has been associated with spina bifida in 1%–5% of the offspring of mothers treated during the first trimester. The risks of valproic acid are even greater than those of lithium for teratogenic potential, and its use is probably contraindicated in pregnancy.

Several other malformations, including ear rotation, short nose, depressed nasal bridge, elongated upper lip, and fingernail hypoplasia, have been described in infants with in utero exposure to anticonvulsants (Gaily and Granstrom 1992; Scolnik et al. 1994).

## Effects on the Neonate

Life-threatening toxicity from lithium has been noted in some newborns of mothers receiving lithium in the third trimester, particularly when maternal lithium levels exceed therapeutic levels (Morrell et al. 1983). Affected babies may show hypotonia, lethargy, cyanosis, depressed Apgar scores, hypotension, cardiac arrythmias, poor sucking reflex, and shallow respiration (Ananth 1976; Llewellyn et al. 1998; N. Wilson et al. 1983). Lithium levels may remain high for more than a week; the serum half-life in infants has been estimated at 96 hours (MacKay et al. 1976).

## Effects on Breastfeeding Infants

Levels of lithium in breast milk average 40%–50% of those in maternal serum, and levels in infant serum are approximately equal to those in breast milk (Schou and Amdisen 1973). Lithium in breast milk has been associated with cyanotic episodes, lethargy, hypothermia, and hypotonia in the neonate (Tunnessen and Hertz 1972). Because the long-term effects of lithium on neonates are unknown, mothers receiving lithium are advised not to breastfeed (Ananth 1978; Robinson et al. 1986; Wisner and Perel 1988). Use of lithium during lactation is considered contraindicated by the American Academy of Pediatrics (1994). Valproic acid and carbamazepine are considered compatible with breastfeeding by the American Academy of Pediatricians (1994), but the available data are very limited.

## Long-Term Effects on Children Exposed in Utero

Schou (1976) discovered no significant differences in physical or mental anomalies at age 5 between children exposed to lithium in utero and their unexposed siblings. This study was too poorly designed, however, to draw definitive conclusions.

## Anxiolytics

### Teratogenicity

Several studies have yielded conflicting evidence about the relationship between the use of benzodiazepines during pregnancy and the occurrence of fetal malformations, especially cleft lip with or without cleft palate. In a pooled overview of studies (Aarskog 1975; Laegreid et al. 1990; Rosenberg et al. 1983; Safra and Oakley 1975; Saxen and Saxen 1975; St. Clair and Schirmer 1992), use of benzodiazepines in first trimester increased the odds of having oral clefts. Because the subjects were heterogeneous, several benzodiazepines were studied, and the anomalies were reported in different drugs, the final answer to the oral cleft question remains uncertain and caution should be exercised. The literature on in utero benzodiazepine exposure and behavioral teratogenicity in humans is limited, but some studies suggest that benzodiazepine exposure may cause developmental delays (Viggedal et al. 1993).

### Effects on the Neonate

Benzodiazepines that are lipid soluble and have a low molecular weight can easily cross the placenta, especially late in pregnancy (Kanto 1982). The long half-lives of these drugs may result in marked accumulation in the mother and the fetus when regularly administered (Mirkin 1976). Chronic use of diazepam throughout pregnancy has been reported to lead to withdrawal symptoms including tremor, hypertonia, and hyperreflexia lasting up to 8 weeks in the neonate (Volpe 1981). These irritable infants are difficult to care for. Mandrelli et al. (1975) reported hypotonia, low Apgar scores, hypothermia, impaired response to cold, and neurologic depression in infants whose mothers had received high doses of diazepam prior to delivery. The muscular hypotonia sometimes found in these infants has been labeled *floppy infant syndrome* (Gillberg 1977). Use of injectable diazepam at delivery has been linked to kernicterus because of competition between bilirubin and the preservative sodium benzoate (Schiff et al. 1971). Long-acting benzodiazepines should be avoided in the third trimester because they may inhibit newborn respiration and diminish responsiveness immediately after birth. Moreover, the immature liver has difficulty metabolizing these drugs (Kanto 1982). Larger doses of diazepam may result in low Apgar scores at birth, apneic spells, hypotonia, and poor sucking (Cree et al. 1973). All sedative drugs have been associated with decreased newborn sucking rates (Kanto 1982).

Chronic use of barbiturates prior to delivery can lead to withdrawal symptoms in the newborn that may not occur until 10–14 days after birth. Symptoms may include tremulousness, crying, irritability, hyperphagia, and increased tone (Hill and Stern 1979).

### Effects on Breastfeeding Infants

Benzodiazepines constitute a risk to nursing newborns because they produce lethargy and impaired temperature regulation. They are not metabolized in the fetal liver or gut, and from days 1–4 the infant is unable to conjugate them with glucuronic acid, which may result in newborn jaundice (Kanto 1982). If a mother needs benzodiazepines on a prolonged basis, breastfeeding is contraindicated because of the possibility of accumulation and lack of data on the effects of long-term exposure through breast milk (Mortola 1989; Robinson et al. 1986). When given to the nursing mother in therapeutic doses, phenobarbital appears to have little or no demonstrable effect on the infant, but long-term effects are unknown (Ananth 1978).

## Agents Used to Treat the Extrapyramidal Side Effects of Neuroleptics

Few studies are available on the specific teratogenicity of agents used to treat the extrapyramidal side effects of neuroleptics in the first trimester because these agents are coadministered with neuroleptics. Some reports link diphenhydramine to congenital anomalies (Heinonen et al. 1977), and cardiovascular malformation has been reported in an infant exposed to amantadine during the first trimester (Nora et al. 1975).

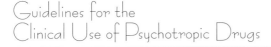

## Guidelines for the Clinical Use of Psychotropic Drugs

The goals for treating psychiatric disorders in pregnancy may be altered to achieve control of symptoms rather than complete remission. Nonpharmacologic strategies, such as cognitive-behavioral therapy, interpersonal therapy, dynamic psychotherapy, family therapy, marital therapy, light therapy, ECT, environmental support, and sometimes hospitalization, may be preferable to the use of drugs in first trimester (Mortola 1989; Nurnberg and Prudic 1984; Wisner et al. 1999). Despite these strategies, psychotropic drugs are sometimes required, particularly if the woman is so severely depressed or psychotic that her well-being or that of her fetus is in jeopardy (Altshuler et al. 1996). A severely ill woman may fail to eat properly, may not attend appointments for prenatal care, and may respond to command hallucinations to harm herself or her fetus. The American Medical Association (1983) recommends the following guidelines for physicians when prescribing drugs to women of childbearing age or those who are already pregnant: 1) avoid unnecessary exposure to drugs and select those drugs with the most favorable risk/benefit ratios; 2) inform patients of the implications of drug exposures in pregnancy; 3) when drugs are necessary, advise patients of the need for contraceptive measures when indicated; and 4) identify and report any birth defects.

In general, psychotropic drugs should be used in pregnancy only when they are clearly indicated for the prophylaxis or treatment of psychiatric illness and then only in the lowest effective doses for the shortest period of time necessary. An individual risk/benefit appraisal is required. Because of altered pharmacokinetics and metabolism during pregnancy, higher doses may be required than are used in nonpregnant women. It is generally believed that divided maternal doses have less effect on the fetus than once-daily dosing schedules. New drugs should be avoided until safety and side effects have been well established through use in nonpregnant women (Wisner and Perel 1988).

## Antipsychotics

Few data support the choice of one antipsychotic over another during pregnancy. Halogenated phenothiazines, however, appear to slightly increase teratogenicity (Rumeau-Rouquette et al. 1977). We favor high-potency agents because they usually cause fewer autonomic, anticholinergic, hypotensive, sedative, and cardiovascular side effects. We currently prescribe haloperidol during pregnancy and lactation in the lowest effective divided dose and try to avoid its use in the first trimester when possible.

## Antidepressants

Because the dose–response curves and therapeutic efficacy of any antidepressant have not yet been established in pregnancy, the choice of which of these drugs to use is primarily based on side effects and safety. We tend to favor nortriptyline, desipramine, or fluoxetine during pregnancy and lactation because of their reduced side effects (including hypotension), better published evidence for safety, and the correlation between serum levels and therapeutic effect. Tricyclic antidepressants and fluoxetine have the most robust published, long-term, neurobehavioral data on exposed infants (Nulman et al. 1997). We administer the lowest effective dose and try to avoid first-trimester exposure when possible. We avoid maprotilene because maternal seizures have been reported (Edwards 1979) and monoamine oxidase inhibitors because they may be teratogenic (Heinonen et al. 1977). Data evaluating some of the newer serotonin reuptake inhibitors or reversible monoamine oxidase inhibitors in pregnancy are still insufficient.

## Lithium and Carbamazepine

General recommendations for use of lithium in women of childbearing age include the following: 1) the drug should be given for unequivocal indications; 2) patients should be warned of the possible teratogenic and toxic effects on the fetus; 3) effective contraception should be encouraged; 4) the drug should be gradually withdrawn in first trimester in cases of unexpected pregnancy (except in severe or unstable bipolar illness); and 5) referral for a targeted ultrasound examination to detect fetal cardiovascular malformations should be considered (Gelenberg 1983; Llewellyn et al. 1998; Weinstein 1980).

A recent study showed that recurrence risks for bipolar disorder rose sharply in the postpartum period when lithium was discontinued during pregnancy (Viguera et al. 2000). Recurrence risk was greater after rapid discontinuation than after gradual discontinuation. We reserve lithium in pregnancy and lactation for patients with unstable or severe bipolar disorder and usually taper the dose by 30% the week before the expected due date to reduce the risk of toxicity. Recent studies suggest that lithium may be less teratogenic than previously thought (see earlier discussion). Patients maintained on lithium should be closely monitored and targeted ultrasound should be performed at gestational week 18 to examine for cardiovascular malformation. Weinstein (1980) has suggested that when lithium is used in pregnancy, sodium-depleting diuretics and low-salt diets should be avoided, serum lithium levels should be closely monitored (at least once per month in early pregnancy and weekly toward the end), care should be taken to distinguish the nausea and vomiting of pregnancy from those associated with lithium toxicity, serum levels should be kept at the lowest effective level, and lithium should be given in three to five equal doses not exceeding 300 mg/dose. Lithium levels should be carefully monitored after delivery to avoid toxicity because physiologic fluid shifts occur.

We reserve carbamazepine and valproate for women who have lithium-resistant unstable bipolar disorder. We augment with folate, 4 mg/day in the hope that this may reduce the risk of neural tube defect. An ultrasound is performed at gestational weeks 10–19 to rule out neural tube defect and other congenital anomalies.

## Anxiolytics

Nonpharmacologic interventions should be the main strategy for the management of most anxiety or insomnia during pregnancy and lactation. These interventions include relaxation, cognitive-behavioral therapy, psychotherapy, and environmental change and support. No anxiolytic can be regarded as completely safe in pregnancy or lactation, but if circumstances dictate (such as in panic disorder), lorazepam may be a reasonable choice because of its lack of active metabolites and its glucuronide metabolism, high potency, and good absorption (Wisner and Perel 1988). The drug should be given at the lowest effective dosage for the briefest possible time and avoided, if possible, in the first trimester and near term. It is prudent to bear in mind that sleep disturbance and anxiety are common in late pregnancy and that risk/benefit considerations seldom warrant hypnotics or anxiolytics at this time except for the treatment of severe anxiety and panic disorder. Use of antidepressants to control panic disorder should also be considered.

## Electroconvulsive Therapy in Pregnancy

### Indications

Electroconvulsive therapy is generally regarded as a safe and effective treatment for specific psychiatric diagnoses in pregnancy and the puerperium (National Institute of Health Consensus Conference 1985) and is underused in treating pregnant women with psychiatric illnesses. It is primarily useful for severe depression, psychosis with affective features, and catatonia. ECT may be prescribed in the following situations: 1) on an emergency basis when the psychiatric status of the mother presents a hazard to herself or the fetus, 2) as a back-up for failure of other treatments in severe psychiatric conditions, and 3) to avoid the risk of exposure to potential teratogens in first trimester (Fink

1981). It may also be used in pregnant patients who have a history of successful ECT treatment. ECT is an effective treatment for postpartum psychosis that allows continuation of breastfeeding if desired.

## Clinical Considerations

Remick and Maurice (1978) and Wise et al. (1984) have commented on the lack of conclusive data on ECT in pregnancy and have suggested the following guidelines:

1. Thorough physical examination
2. Involvement of an obstetrician
3. Consideration of high-risk pregnancy as a relative contraindication
4. External fetal monitoring for several hours before and after ECT
5. Endotracheal intubation
6. Low-voltage, nondominant ECT with electroencephalographic monitoring
7. Electrocardiographic monitoring of the mother
8. Oxygen pretreatment and assisted ventilation until the return of spontaneous respiration in the mother
9. Evaluation of maternal arterial blood gases during or after ECT
10. Doppler ultrasonography of fetal heart rate
11. Tacodynamometer recording of uterine tone
12. Glycopyrrolate as anticholinergic of choice
13. Screening for pseudocholinesterase deficiency if using succinylcholine
14. Weekly non-stress tests of fetal well-being
15. Careful monitoring and control of maternal blood pressure

The patient should be placed in the left lateral position with a wedge under the right hip to ensure that the gravid uterus does not obstruct blood flow through the inferior vena cava. These very cautious considerations are for general information only, and the advice of an obstetrician and anesthesiologist should be obtained for the individual patient.

## Conclusions

The clinician presented with a psychiatrically ill pregnant or lactating patient must make important clinical decisions about psychotropic drugs and ECT in the face of considerable uncertainty (Kuller et al. 1996). Careful attention to the most recent and reliable information available and consideration of the unique features of each patient's circumstances will assist in weighing the risk/ benefit ratio and determining the best clinical strategy. Written documentation of the factors considered, the patient's informed consent, and careful, ongoing monitoring are vital in the optimal management of this difficult clinical dilemma.

# References

Aarskog D: Association between maternal intake of diazepam and oral clefts (letter). Lancet 2:921, 1975

Addis A, Koren G: Safety of fluoxetine during the first trimester of pregnancy: a meta-analytical review of epidemiological studies. Psychol Med 30:89–94, 2000

Altshuler LL, Cohen L, Szuba, MP, et al: Pharmacologic management of psychiatric illness during pregnancy: dilemmas and guidelines. Am J Psychiatry 153:592–606, 1996

American Academy of Pediatrics Committee on Drugs: The transfer of drugs and other chemicals into human milk. Pediatrics 84:924–936, 1989

American Academy of Pediatrics Committee on Drugs: The transfer of drugs and other chemicals into human milk. Pediatrics 93:137–150, 1994

American Medical Association: Drug interactions and adverse drug reaction, in American Medical Association Drug Evaluations. Chicago, AMA, 1983, pp 31–44

Ananth J: Congenital malformations with psychopharmacologic agents. Compr Psychiatry 16:437–445, 1975

Ananth J: Side effects on fetus and infant of psychotropic drug use during pregnancy. Int Pharmacopsychiatry 11:246–260, 1976

Ananth J: Side effects in the neonate from psychotropic agents excreted through breast-feeding. Am J Psychiatry 135:801–805, 1978

Beeley L: Adverse effects of drugs in the first trimester of pregnancy. Clin Obstet Gynecol 13:177–195, 1986

Birnbaum CS, Cohen LS, Bailey JW, et al: Serum concentrations of antidepressants and benzodiazepines in nursing infants: a case series (abstract). Pediatrics 104:e11, 1999

Brazelton TB: Effect of prenatal drugs on the behavior of the neonate. Am J Psychiatry 126:1261–1266, 1970

Briggs G, Freeman R, Yaffe S: Drugs in Pregnancy and Lactation. Baltimore, MD, Williams & Wilkins, 1994

Center for Drug Evaluation and Research: Notice of part 15 hearings: prescription drugs and biological products labeling. Federal Register 20247, 1997

Chambers CD, Johnson KA, Dick LN, et al: Birth outcomes in pregnant women taking fluoxetine. N Engl J Med 335:1010–1015, 1996

Chambers CD, Anderson PO, Thomas RG, et al: Weight gain in infants breastfed by mothers who take fluoxetine (abstract). Pediatrics 104:e61, 1999

Chao ST, Juchau MR: Placental drug metabolism, in Teratogenesis and Reproductive Toxicology. Edited by Johnson EM, Kochhar DM. New York, Springer-Verlag, 1983, pp 31–48

Cohen LS, Heller VL, Rosenbaum JF: Treatment guidelines for psychotropic drug use in pregnancy. Psychosomatics 30:25–33, 1989

Cree JE, Meyer J, Hailey DM: Diazepam in labour: its metabolism and effect on the clinical condition and thermogenesis of the newborn. BMJ 4:251–255, 1973

Crombie DL, Pinsent RJ, Fleming DM, et al: Fetal effects of tranquilizers in pregnancy. N Engl J Med 293:198–199, 1975

Edlund MJ, Craig TJ: Antipsychotic drug use and birth defects: an epidemiologic reassessment. Compr Psychiatry 25:32–37, 1984

Edwards JG: Antidepressants and convulsions. Lancet 2:1368–1369, 1979

Eggermont E, Raveschot J, Deneve V, et al: The adverse influence of imipramine on the adaptation of the newborn infant to extrauterine life. Acta Paediatr Belg 26:197–204, 1972

Elia J, Katz IR, Simpson GM: Teratogenicity of psychotherapeutic medications. Psychopharmacol Bull 23:531–586, 1987

Fink M: Convulsive and drug therapies in depression. Annu Rev Med 32:405–412, 1981

Gaily E, Granstrom ML: Minor abnormalities in children of mothers with epilepsy. Neurology 42(suppl):128–131, 1992

Gelenberg AJ: When a woman taking lithium wants to have a baby. Biological Therapies in Psychiatry 6:19–20, 1983

Gelenberg AJ: Antidepressants in milk. Biological Therapies in Psychiatry 10:1, 1987

Gillberg C: "Floppy infant syndrome" and maternal diazepam. Lancet 2:244, 1977

Goldberg HL, DiMascio A: Psychotropic drugs in pregnancy, in Psychopharmacology: A Generation of Progress. Edited by Lipton MA, DiMascio A, Killam KF. New York, Raven Press, 1978, pp 1047–1055

Heinonen OP, Slone D, Shapiro S: Birth Defects and Drugs in Pregnancy. Littleton, MA, Publishing Sciences Group, 1977

Hill RM, Stern L: Drugs in pregnancy: effects on the fetus and newborn. Drugs 17:182–197, 1979

Idanpaan-Heikkila J, Saxen L: Possible teratogenicity of imipramine-chloropyramine. Lancet 2:282–284, 1973

Inman W, Kubota K, Pearce G: Prescription event monitoring of paroxetine. Prescription Event Monitoring Reports 1993, pp 1–44

Jacobson SJ, Jones K, Johnson K, et al: Prospective multicentre study of pregnancy outcome after lithium exposure during first trimester. Lancet 339:530–533, 1992

Jones KL, Lacro RV, Johnson KA, et al: Pattern of malformations in the children of women treated with carbamazepine during pregnancy. N Engl J Med 320:1661–1666, 1989

Kallen B, Tandberg A: Lithium and pregnancy: a cohort study on manic depressive women. Acta Psychiatr Scand 68:134–139, 1983

Kanto JH: Use of benzodiazepines during pregnancy, labour, and lactation with particular reference to pharmacokinetic considerations. Drugs 23:354–380, 1982

Kerns LL: Treatment of mental disorders in pregnancy. J Nerv Ment Dis 174:652–659, 1986

Koplan CR: The use of psychotropic drugs during pregnancy and nursing, in Practitioner Guide to Psychiatric Drugs, 2nd Edition. Edited by Bassuk EL, Schoonover SC, Gelenberg AJ. New York, Plenum, 1983, pp 353–372

Kris EB: Children of mothers maintained on pharmacotherapy during pregnancy and postpartum. Curr Ther Res Clin Exp 7:785–789, 1965

Kuenssberg EV, Knox JD: Imipramine in pregnancy. BMJ 2:292, 1972

Kulin N, Pastuszak A, Sage SR, et al: Pregnancy outcome following maternal use of the new selective seratonin reuptake inhibitors. JAMA 279:609–610, 1998

Kuller JA, Bashford RA, Wells SR, et al: Pharmacologic treatment of psychiatric disease in pregnancy and lactation: fetal and neonatal effects. Obstet Gynecol 87:789–794, 1996

Laegreid L, Olegard R, Conradi N, et al: Congenital malformations and maternal consumption of benzodiazepines: a case-control study. Dev Med Child Neurol 32:432–441, 1990

Llewellyn A, Stowe ZN, Strader JR: The use of lithium and management of women with bipolar disorder during pregnancy and lactation. J Clin Psychiatry 59(suppl):57–64, 1998

Levy GH: Pharmacokinetics of fetal and neonatal exposure to drugs. Obstet Gynecol 58(suppl):95–165, 1981

Levy W, Wisniewski K: Chlorpromazine causing extrapyramidal dysfunction in newborn infants of psychotic mothers. NY State J Medicine 74:684–685, 1974

MacKay AV, Loose R, Glen AI: Labour on lithium. BMJ 1:878, 1976

Mandelli M, Morselli P, Nordic S, et al: Placental transfer of diazepam and its deposition in the newborn. Clin Pharmacol Ther 17:564–572, 1975

McElhatton PR, Hanneke MG, Elefant E, et al: The outcome of pregnancy in 689 women exposed to therapeutic doses of antidepressants: a collaborative study of the European Network of Teratology Information Services. Reprod Toxicol 10:285–294, 1996

Milkovich L, van den Berg BJ: An evaluation of the teratogenicity of certain antinauseant drugs. Am J Obstet Gynecol 125:244–248, 1976

Milkovich L, van den Berg BJ: Effects of antenatal exposure to anorectic drugs. Am J Obstet Gynecol 129:637–642, 1977

Mirkin BL: Drug disposition and therapy in the developing human being. Pediatr Ann 5:542–557, 1976

Morrell P, Sutherland GR, Buamah PK, et al: Lithium toxicity in a neonate. Arch Dis Childhood 58:538–539, 1983

Mortola JF: The use of psychotropic agents in pregnancy and lactation. Psychiatr Clin North Am 12:69–87, 1989

Nahas C, Goujard J: Phenothiazines, benzodiazepines, and the fetus, in Reviews in Perinatal Medicine. Edited by Scarpelli EM, Cosini EV. New York, Raven Press, 1978, pp 243–280

Nars PW, Girard J: Lithium carbonate intake during pregnancy leading to large goitre in a premature infant. Am J Dis Child 131:924–925, 1977

National Institute of Health Consensus Conference: Electroconvulsive therapy. JAMA 254:2103–2108, 1985

Nora JJ, Nora AH, Way GL: Cardiovascular maldevelopment associated with maternal exposure to amantadine. Lancet 2:607, 1975

Nulman I, Rovet J, Stewart DE, et al: Neurodevelopment of children exposed in utero to antidepressant drugs. N Engl J Med 4:258–262, 1997

Nurnberg GH, Prudic J: Guidelines for treatment of psychosis during pregnancy. Hospital and Community Psychiatry 35:67–71, 1984

Oro AS, Dixon SD: Perinatal cocaine and methamphetamine exposure: maternal and neonatal correlates. J Pediatr 111:571–578, 1987

Pastuszak A, Schick-Boschetto B, Zuber C, et al: Pregnancy outcome following first trimester exposure to fluoxetine (Prozac). JAMA 269:2246–2248, 1993

Poulson E, Robson JM: Effect of phenelzine and some related compounds on pregnancy. J Endocrinol 30:205–215, 1964

Rayburn W, Wible-Kant J, Bledsoe J: Changing trends in drug use during pregnancy. J Reprod Med 27:569–575, 1982

Remick RA, Maurice WL: ECT in pregnancy. Am J Psychiatry 135:761–762, 1978

Robinson GE, Stewart DE, Flak E: The rational use of psychotropic drugs in pregnancy and postpartum. Can J Psychiatry 31:183–190, 1986

Rosa F: Spina bifida in infants of women treated with carbamazepine during pregnancy. N Engl J Med 324:674–677, 1991

Rosenberg L, Mitchell AA, Parsells JL, et al: Lack of relation of oral clefts to diazepam use during pregnancy. N Engl J Med 309:1282–1285, 1983

Rumeau-Rouquette C, Goujard J, Huel C: Possible teratogenic effects of phenothiazines in human beings. Teratology 15:57–64, 1977

Safra MD, Oakley GP: Association between cleft lip with or without cleft palate and prenatal exposure to diazepam. Lancet 2:478–540, 1975

Saxen I, Saxen L: Letter: association between maternal intake of diazepam and oral clefts. Lancet 2:498, 1975

Schiff D, Chan G, Stern L: Fixed drug combinations and the displacement of bilirubin from albumin. Pediatrics 8:139–141, 1971

Schou M: What happened later to the lithium babies? Follow-up study of children born without malformations. Acta Psychiatr Scand 54:193–197, 1976

Schou M, Amdisen A: Lithium and pregnancy: lithium ingestion by children breastfed by women on lithium treatment. BMJ 2:138, 1973

Scolnik D, Nulman I, Rovet J, et al: Neurodevelopment of children exposed in utero to phenytoin and carbamazepine monotherapy. JAMA 271:767–770, 1994

Shearer WT, Schreiner RL, Marshall RE: Urinary retention in a neonate secondary to maternal ingestion of nortriptyline. J Pediatr 81:570–572, 1972

Slone D, Suskind V, Heinonen OP, et al: Antenatal exposure to the phenothiazines in relation to congenital malformations, perinatal mortality, birth weight and intelligence quotient score. Am J Obstet Gynecol 128:486–488, 1977

Sovner R, Orsulak PJ: Excretion of imipramine and desipramine in human breast milk. Am J Psychiatry 136:451–452, 1979

St. Clair SM, Schirmer RG: First trimester exposure to alprazolam. Obstet Gynecol 80:843–846, 1992

Stewart DE: Schizophrenia and pregnancy. Can Fam Physician 30:1537–1542, 1984

Stewart DE: Prophylactic lithium in postpartum affective psychosis. J Nerv Ment Dis 176:485–489, 1988

Stowe ZN, Cohen LS, Hostetter A, et al: Paroxetine in human breast milk and nursing infants. Am J Psychiatry 157:85–189, 2000

Tunnessen WW Jr, Hertz CG: Toxic effects of lithium in newborn infants: a commentary. J Pediatr 81:804–807, 1972

U.S. Food and Drug Administration: Drug Bulletin. Washington, DC, U.S. Food and Drug Administration, September 1979, pp 22–23

Viggedal G, Hagberg BS, Laegreid L, et al: Mental development in late infancy after prenatal exposure to benzodiazepines: a prospective study. J Child Psychol Psychiatry 34:295–305, 1993

Viguera AC, Nonacs R, Cohen LS, et al: Risk of reucrrence of bipolar disorder in pregnant and nonpregnant women after discontinuing lithium maintenance. Am J Psychiatry 157:179–184, 2000

Volpe JJ: Teratogenic effects of drugs and passive addiction, in Neurology of the Newborn. Edited by Volpe JJ. Philadelphia, PA, WB Saunders, 1981, pp 601–635

Vorhees CV, Butcher RE: Behavioral teratogenicity, in Developmental Toxicology. Edited by Snell K. New York, Praeger, 1982, pp 249–298

Webster PAC: Withdrawal symptoms in neonates associated with maternal antidepressant therapy. Lancet 2:318–319, 1973

Weinstein MR: Lithium treatment of women during pregnancy and in the post-delivery period, in Handbook of Lithium Therapy. Edited by Johnson FN. Lancaster, England, MTP Press, 1980, pp 421–429

Whalley LJ, Blain PG, Prime JK: Haloperidol secreted in breast milk. BMJ 282:1746–1747, 1981

Wilson JG: Current status of teratology: general principles and mechanisms derived from animal studies, in Handbook of Teratology: General Principles and Etiology, Vol 1. Edited by Wilson JG, Fraser FC. New York, Plenum, 1977, pp 47–74

Wilson N, Forfar JC, Godman MJ: Atrial flutter in the newborn resulting from maternal lithium ingestion. Arch Dis Childhood 58:538–539, 1983

Wise MG, Ward SC, Townsend-Parchman W, et al: Case report of ECT during high-risk pregnancy. Am J Psychiatry 141:99–101, 1984

Wisner KL, Findling RL, Perel JM: Antidepressant treatment during breastfeeding. Am J Psychiatry 153:1132–1137, 1996

Wisner KL, Gelenberg AJ, Leonard H, et al: Pharmacologic treatment of depression during pregnancy. JAMA 282:1264–1269, 1999

Wrede G, Mednick SA, Huttenen MO, et al: Pregnancy and delivery complications in the births of an unselected series of Finnish children with schizophrenic mothers. Acta Psychiatr Scand 62:369–381, 1980

Zalzstein E, Koren G, Einarson T, et al: A case-control study on the association between first trimester exposure to lithium and Ebstein's anomaly. Am J Cardiol 65:817–818, 1990

# Adolescent Pregnancy

DIANA L. DELL, M.D., F.A.C.O.G.

## Scope of the Issue

Each year in the United States about 10% of all adolescent women between the ages of 15 and 19 become pregnant. Of these, only about 13% consciously planned their pregnancies; approximately 33% will abort their pregnancies; 14% will miscarry; and 52% will bear children. Of the 500,000 adolescent women who give birth each year, more than 175,000 are 17 years of age or younger. Of these 500,000 births, only 75% are first births and 72% are out of wedlock (Maynard 1997).

The United States has far higher rates of pregnancy, childbirth, and abortion among adolescents than other Western industrialized nations (e.g., Canada, England, Wales, France, Sweden, and the Netherlands). The adolescent abortion rate in the United States is often higher than the entire pregnancy rate (abortion plus childbearing) seen in the other nations even though access to abortion services is much easier in other countries. Rates of unintended or mistimed pregnancy do not appear to be a function of higher rates of sexual activity among teenagers in the United States, because rates of sexual activity are about the same in all of the nations compared. The bottom line is that American teens do not practice contraception as often or as effectively as teens in other nations (Zabin and Hayward 1993).

Unfortunately, the largest differences in birth rates are usually seen at the youngest ages: for example, the birth rate for 14-year-old women in the United States is 5/1,000, which is four times higher than that of second-ranking Canada. Among American women aged 18 years or younger, there are fewer births in affluent areas and much higher rates for birth and abortion concentrated in the most economically deprived areas. These economically deprived areas are the same areas that have the highest rates for infant mortality, violent deaths among youths, violent crime, illicit drug use, and homicide (Zabin and Hayward 1993)

The question of why adolescents do not use contraception more effectively has been the object of intensive research. In a recent survey of 200 consecutively enrolled patients aged 13–18 years in an adolescent-oriented maternity program, more than 40% of the respondents had positive attitudes toward childbearing. Interviewed during the third trimester, 20% of respondents said that they did not mind getting pregnant, 17.5% said "I wanted to get pregnant," and 5% said that their boyfriend wanted them to get pregnant. Only 12% of participants attributed their pregnancies to contraceptive failure. Even smaller percentages cited a fear or dislike of contraceptive side effects (5%) or a fear of parental discovery and/or disapproval (5%) as the reason for not using contraception. The authors concluded that a positive attitude toward pregnancy rather than a negative attitude toward contraceptive technologies was most likely to predict whether adolescents used contraception (Stevens-Simon et al. 1996b).

## Normal Adolescent Development

Attempting to understand the phenomenon of adolescent pregnancy and to provide adequate care for pregnant adolescents requires an understanding of the cognitive and psychosocial development of adolescents. Although age ranges are often assigned to the developmental tasks for early, middle, and late adolescence, the chronologic age does not always correspond to the level of maturity. Additionally, an individual adolescent may be functioning at one level cognitively and at another level psychosocially (Drake 1996).

In the terms used by Piaget (see Singer and Revenson 1978), cognitive development moves from the concrete operations of children to the formal operations that begin in adolescence. During the stage of concrete operations, children can manipulate concrete objects but can function only in the present, with no capacity to conceptualize the future. With the emergence of formal operations at about 11 years of age, adolescents learn to evaluate the environment in less concrete ways. They develop increasing capacities to think logically, work with abstract ideas, predict consequences of behavior, and speculate about future events (Drake 1996). Normal psychosocial development is often divided into three stages, each of which spans about 3 years.

Some authors have further defined stages of psychosexual development that roughly correspond to the same chronologic time spans.

Early adolescence is characterized by turmoil stemming from the physical changes of puberty, loss of body control, and an intense preoccupation with physical appearance (Drake 1996). Adjusting to their new body image makes early adolescents self-conscious and raises their concerns about being normal and appearing acceptable. Psychosexual development may correspond with undifferentiated exploratory sexual behavior with members of the same or opposite sex (Stevens-Simon and Reichert 1994). Very early adolescents seldom seek sexual activity but may be an especially vulnerable group for sexual advances from others (Drake 1996).

Middle adolescence focuses on self-identification and self-realization. Girls show more interest in developing intense, loving relationships with boys. Boys are more interested in the pleasure of sexual activity than in the maintenance of loving relationships (Drake 1996). Both genders exhibit behavior that is more defiant, narcissistic, and self-reliant. With narcissism comes a sense of personal omnipotence and what Elkind describes as "personal fables," which are stories about one's own uniqueness and invulnerability. For boys, this may be a sense of immortality that fosters risk-taking behavior; for girls, it may be a belief that she cannot become pregnant so she does not need to use contraception (Lewis and Volkmar 1990, p. 218). Middle adolescents often loosen their emotional ties to the family of origin and begin to engage in a series of experimental, monogamous, heterosexual relationships (Stevens-Simon and Reichert 1994).

In late adolescence, there is a progression away from the narcissistic sense of personal omnipotence toward a more integrated, solid sense of oneself and how that self copes with and integrates into the adult world. Psychosexually, the move is toward developing stable, mutually intimate relationships (Drake 1996; Stevens-Simon and Reichert 1994).

The developmental stage at which an adolescent woman becomes sexually active is extremely critical. Her level of cognitive and psychosocial development will predict not only how well she protects herself from pregnancy but how she responds to the event of pregnancy if she fails to adequately practice contraception.

Because early adolescents are still very present oriented, self-centered, and less capable of abstract thinking, they have difficulty accepting the reality of a pregnancy. They often deny that they are pregnant, even in the presence of an enlarging abdomen or positive pregnancy test. They are secretive and when possible will often conceal pregnancy until an advanced stage of gestation. They seldom have more than a casual relationship with the father of the fetus. They anticipate and often receive very negative reactions when family members become aware of the pregnancy. Unless directed by parents or other adults, they tend to seek prenatal care late or not at all. Once enrolled in prenatal care, they have difficulty focusing on threats to their own health or the health of the fetus. They are not emotionally ready to assume a parenting role and require adult guidance and assistance with the responsibility for infant care (Drake 1996).

Middle adolescent women often have begun some form of sexual experimentation. They move from a stage of exploratory behavior toward a stage of developing intense, loving relationships. If pregnancy occurs at this stage, the woman often has a deeper emotional attachment to the father of the fetus. She may have consciously or unconsciously chosen to become pregnant as a means of confirming her feminine identity, as a means of securing a closer relationship with the father of the fetus, or as a means of gaining adult status. Some adolescent women, especially those who are doing poorly in school or do not have opportunities for advanced education and career training, will choose pregnancy during this time as a career choice of motherhood over education/employment (Drake 1996).

Depending on the circumstances surrounding the decision to seek pregnancy or the more ambivalent posture of just not using contraception, middle adolescents still tend to seek prenatal care later in pregnancy than do more mature groups. However, middle adolescents are more capable than early adolescents of making the needs of the fetus a priority and of assuming responsibility for parenting, although assistance with child care is needed to allow completion of educational goals (Drake 1996).

Late adolescents have a much stronger sense of themselves and a stronger relationship with the father of the fetus. They are more like adult women in most categories: they seek prenatal care earlier, are motivated to do what is best for a healthy pregnancy, and can usually assume the task of parenting on their own (Drake 1996).

## Abnormal Adolescent Development

Sexual victimization in childhood can adversely affect normal adolescent psychosexual development in addition to being independently associated with a broad spectrum of physical, emotional, and behavioral problems. The association between prior sexual abuse and adolescent pregnancy is very strong.

Numerous studies have demonstrated that former victims of sexual abuse are overrepresented in adolescent prenatal programs, with some groups appearing more at risk than others (Stevens-Simon and Reichert 1994). In one sample of 535 pregnant adolescents, 66.2% had some history of sexual victimization; Of these, 70% of the white adolescents had been abused prior to conception compared with 42% of black adolescents and 37% of Hispanic adolescents (Boyer and Fine 1992).

Rainey et al. (1995) prospectively queried 202 consecutive nonpregnant, sexually active, nulliparous adolescent women aged 13–19 who sought routine medical care at two teen centers. In this group, 20% reported prior sexual abuse. Sexually abused and nonabused girls reported similar ages at menarche; similar rates of miscarriages, abortions, and sexually transmitted disease; similar ages for initiation of consensual sexual intercourse; similar frequencies of intercourse; and similar rates of contraceptive use. Sexually abused adolescents were three times more likely than their nonabused peers to state that they were seeking pregnancy (34.2% vs. 11.3%, $P < 0.001$). Abused patients expressed more concerns about their ability to conceive, were more likely to report previous pregnancy testing, were twice as likely to report feeling that something was wrong with them and that they could not conceive, and were more likely to have older boyfriends who encouraged them to get pregnant. The authors postulated that infertility concerns could be another expression of the low self-esteem commonly seen in adolescents with prior sexual abuse (Rainey et al. 1995).

In the same study it was noted that sexually abused girls were more likely to report socially deviant behaviors: smoking cigarettes, frequent alcohol use, other illicit drug use, and involvement with the police or juvenile court system within the preceding 6 months. The authors speculated that adolescent pregnancy may be another manifestation of self-destructive and socially deviant behavior attributable to prior sexual victimization (Rainey et al. 1995).

Ongoing violent behavior and sexual victimization are also related to adolescent pregnancy. Current estimates suggest that up to 30% of college-age women have had at least one violent incident in a dating relationship. In one large urban sampling, 32% of pregnant adolescents reported having been physically or sexually abused during the prior year and 22% were being abused during the current pregnancy. Abused women tended to enter prenatal care later: 24% of the abused adolescents in this sample entered prenatal care during the third trimester compared with 9% of those who were not abused (Parker 1993).

In abusive relationships, both male and female partners tended to express more negative feelings toward the pregnancy: 51% of abused women reported negative feelings about the pregnancy compared with 31% of non-abused women, and 29% of the abusing partners reported negative feelings about the pregnancy compared with 13% of the nonabusing partners (Parker 1993).

## Process of Pregnancy Resolution

### Late Diagnosis

For reasons that are not always clear, adolescent women often prolong the interval between suspecting and confirming that they are pregnant. This delay accounts for complications associated with late entry into prenatal care and higher rates of elective second trimester abortion. Bluestein and Rutledge (1992) reviewed the literature that has been generated to explain this delay and found that this phenomenon was not adequately explained by socio-demographic attributes (including age, race, education, or ability to pay for pregnancy testing) or by clinical attributes (including parity, contraceptive practices, menstrual regularity, and presence of pregnancy symptoms). They surveyed 123 pregnant adolescents aged 14–19 years, 54% of whom carried their pregnancies and 46% of whom aborted their pregnancies. The mean duration of delay in seeking a pregnancy test was 4.35 weeks. In this sample, only difficulty in acknowledging the pregnancy exerted a significant net effect on delayed testing ($P < 0.05$). Interestingly, difficulty acknowledging the pregnancy was also associated with depressive symptoms ($P < 0.01$), problems talking with partners ($P < 0.05$), and an initial negative reaction to the pregnancy ($P < 0.01$) (Bluestein and Rutledge 1992).

Difficulty acknowledging a pregnancy may be a manifestation of denial that reflects cognitive immaturity. For other adolescents it may represent psychosocial immaturity, with ambivalence or feelings of guilt about sexual activity. Whatever the reasons, during this period of delay pregnant adolescents may be alone as they face difficult decisions concerning their pregnancy (Bluestein and Rutledge 1992).

### Counseling

Although unwanted or mistimed pregnancy can create a crisis in the life of a woman at any age, adolescent women are at special risk because of their own developmental issues. Early and middle adolescents, for example, have not completed individuation and are ill-equipped for making autonomous decisions; older adolescents may have more decision-making ability but are unaccustomed to making decisions of this magnitude. Counseling for pregnancy resolution must explore all available options: abortion, adoption, and keeping the baby. It should include the family whenever possible, must be free of counselor bias, and must be provided in very practical terms that will facilitate appropriate decision making (J. H. Gold 1991).

## Keeping the Pregnancy

Farber (1991) conducted in-depth interviews with 28 unmarried adolescent mothers from six subgroups, identified as black and white teens from middle-class, working-class, and lower-class families. In her sample, the process of recognizing the pregnancy took many forms, ranging from immediate acknowledgment to a long period of denial. Fears about the anticipated response of the parents was a consistent finding, both before and especially after confirmation of the pregnancy. Nonetheless, the young women, with only one exception, looked immediately to their families for direction and generally were advised to keep the child. Only one subject even referred to the father of the fetus in the decision-making process (Farber 1991).

All adolescent women in this study bore their pregnancy and kept their child. This decision was seldom based simply on the desire to be a mother. The pregnant adolescent was not acting as an isolated individual able to calculate the best outcome for her own self-interest and proceed toward a decision consistent with her level of self-esteem, career aspirations, or cultural load. Parents and extended family members often exerted direct influence on the parenting decision, and the final choice of pregnancy resolution included concerns about obedience to parents and grandparents, a belief in the sanctity of life, acceptance of the consequences of their actions, and the perceived best interests of the child (Farber 1991).

One case illustrates how final resolution can be a complex and difficult process that ultimately may be based on identifying the least harmful alternative. One black middle-class teen who had planned to go to medical school did not acknowledge her pregnancy until her preferred choice of safe abortion was no longer an option. She had to choose among hurting her beloved grandmother who opposed adoption, maintaining the support of her mother who favored adoption, and guarding against endangering her career aspirations through early motherhood. She ultimately kept her child, to be raised with assistance from her mother (Farber 1991).

Although the sample size of Farber's study was small, some trends were evident. One consistent pattern was the overwhelmingly negative reaction of the families of black middle-class teenagers, with reactions ranging from disappointed shock to fury. Black middle-class and working-class families expressed marked disappointment about their daughters' futures. Among white middle-class and working-class families, the first expression of concern was about potential complications of being pregnant at such a young age. The families of black lower-class teens were also hurt, disappointed, and angry, but the black lower-class teens themselves expressed either positive or neutral feelings about the pregnancy, and with one exception did not report fearing the parents' reaction. Lower-class teens and their parents, especially the mothers, quickly accepted as inevitable that the young woman would keep and raise her child (Farber 1991).

## Abortion

Although abortion has been legal in the United States since 1973, the availability and accessibility of abortion services to adolescent women has been changing dramatically over the past few years. Decreased public funding, decreased provider availability, and parental consent laws have had a disproportionate effect on adolescent and economically deprived women.

For the adolescent woman to make decisions about her pregnancy, she needs information about what specific alternatives are available to her, including the abortion options specific to her stage of gestation as well as community resources that are available for either abortion or prenatal care. If she chooses abortion, she has a much greater need than does an older woman for intensive education about female physiology and specific characteristics of the abortion procedure that will be used. Accurate information about the sensations she will experience can markedly diminish immediate and longer-term negative responses (Zakus and Wilday 1987).

Despite politically motivated reports to the contrary, abortion is followed by relatively few psychologic sequelae. Most women experience some anticipatory grieving during the decision-making process; after the abortion procedure, the resolution of that grief response is relatively rapid, with most women reporting a sense of relief and a rapid return to their previous level of functioning (J. H. Gold 1991; Zakus and Wilday 1987).

Several categories of women have been identified who may be at special risk for emotional difficulties in the months or years after an abortion:

- Women who feel they are not free to make their own choice about terminating a pregnancy. Adolescents are particularly vulnerable to feeling that parents or partners "coerced" them into having an abortion (Zakus and Wilday 1987). Unfortunately, the same may also be true for an adolescent woman who carries a pregnancy to term against her wishes; she will experience the same regret, guilt, and anger as the woman coerced into having an abortion (J. H. Gold 1991).

- Women with a history of sexual abuse. Not only are previously abused adolescent women at greater risk for pregnancy, they appear at greater risk for experiencing gynecologic examinations and the abortion procedure itself as an additional trauma (Zakus and Wilday 1987).
- Women with other unresolved grief reactions. For adolescents, it is very common for the crisis of pregnancy to result in dissolution of the relationship with the father of the fetus. Grieving the loss of that relationship may compound the transient abortion-related grief reaction (Zakus and Wilday 1987).
- Women with preexisting psychiatric disorders (Zakus and Wilday 1987).

Adolescent women who appear at special risk for emotional difficulties in the wake of pregnancy resolution decisions should be identified in the initial counseling—whether they decide to carry or abort their pregnancies. These women often benefit from crisis intervention strategies that address the current life situation and the patient's own coping skills (Zakus and Wilday 1987).

## Adoption

A generation ago, adoption was the most popular option for out-of-wedlock pregnancy, especially among white adolescents and families. Currently, less than 5% of adolescents who give birth choose adoption as the preferred resolution of their pregnancy. In an effort to understand this dramatic shift, Custer (1993) conducted in-depth interviews of 21 unmarried white adolescents carrying an unplanned pregnancy. The subjects, their significant others, and people they identified as being influential in helping to make decisions about the future were interviewed during the last trimester of pregnancy and again at 6–8 weeks postpartum. The most important phenomenon noted was the absence of societal sanctions against adolescent parenthood, concurrent with reciprocal sanctions against relinquishing a child for adoption. The culture was now saying that it is acceptable to be a single adolescent mother but definitely *not* acceptable to give away a baby (Custer 1993).

Societal sanction appeared to be primarily centered on the idea of adoption not being good for the child. Numerous subjects voiced concern that the child would suffer, that it would not be loved and would therefore hate the birth mother. There was also an element of societal disapproval related to the perception that adolescents should assume responsibility for their actions: "It's your responsibility to take care of the situations you get yourself into. If you don't want the kid, why were you messing around?" (Custer 1993).

The apparent lack of accurate knowledge among adolescents about adoption was startling. Only limited information was provided to the patients by the health care professionals who provided prenatal care. Only three of the subjects had any degree of accurate knowledge about adoption, only eight re-called being asked if they were considering adoption, and only two remem-bered actually receiving any adoption information or counseling at any time during the pregnancy (Custer 1993). Custer concluded that anticipation of psychologic distress is the most powerful immediate barrier to adolescents giving up their infants for adoption. The combination of general societal sanctions, low levels of knowledge, and absence of professional intervention served to confirm the adolescents' beliefs that severe, intolerable, and ongo-ing psychologic distress would accompany giving up an infant for adoption (Custer 1993). This conclusion gains additional strength when considered in the context of psychosocial development—middle adolescents conform to so-cietal standards to avoid censure by authority figures, whereas late adoles-cents conform to maintain the respect of impartial observers and avoid self-condemnation (Drake 1996).

## General Health Care for Adolescent Women

Confidentiality is a major issue in dealing with adolescent patients. Adoles-cents are more likely to give an accurate history if assured that whatever in-formation they provide is not shared with others unless safety is an issue, as in suspected abuse/neglect or suicidal ideation. Conveying this information to both patients and parents at the initial visit is helpful (Brown-Jones and Orr 1993). Even with this assurance, adolescents may have difficulty communi-cating information about sexuality to adults who resemble parental authority figures.

### Sexual Activity

Physical maturation profoundly influences the onset of sexual activity and the subsequent risk for adolescent pregnancy. Hormone production in girls usually begins between 7 and 9 years of age, with rapid escalation from age

9 until the onset of menstruation. The age of menarche in girls from Western industrialized nations has been steadily declining for the past 100 years, with the average age now cited as 12.6 years. Earlier physical maturation means that the variance between physical maturation and psychosocial maturation is probably greater than that found in previous generations. This disparity may place peripubertal girls at greater risk for pregnancy and the acquisition of sexually transmitted diseases before they have the cognitive and psychosocial skills to manage a sexual life (Zabin and Hayward 1993).

Menarche can be considered a marker for the initiation of sexual behavior, with age of first intercourse for girls usually occurring within 2–3 years after menarche. The impact is most evident at the youngest ages; by age 13, almost 40% of those girls whose menarche occurred at 11 years or younger are sexually active; 20% of girls with menarche at age 13–14 are sexually active at or before menarche; and only 10% of those with menarche after age 14 are sexually active at or before menarche (Brown-Jones and Orr 1993; Zabin and Hayward 1993).

Half of all first pregnancies in adolescents occur within the first 6 months of sexual activity, with about 20% occurring in the first month. Early adolescents are less likely than older adolescents to use contraception or to use it effectively; they also have longer delays between initiation of sexual activity and seeking contraceptive services: 23.5 months for women age 15 or younger versus 10.6 months for women ages 16–19. Because this activity is occurring in a phase in which the adolescent is relating increasingly to peers and less to parents, the presence of a sexually active and/or noncontracepting peer group may have a much greater impact on younger adolescents than it would have at a later age (Zabin and Hayward 1993).

## Sexually Transmissible Disease

Three million adolescents acquire a sexually transmissible disease every year. They are at greater risk than adults for several reasons: they are more likely to have multiple sex partners, more likely to have high-risk partners, and less likely to use barrier protection for intercourse. For adolescent women there is the additional issue of having an immature cervix, which does not provide the same barrier to infection that a more mature cervix provides and is more likely to be injured by sexually transmissible organisms. In fact, many of the serious health consequences of sexually transmissible diseases that appear in adults, such as cancer and infertility, are the result of infections acquired during adolescence (Donovan 1997).

All adolescent women should be encouraged to use both a reliable method of female birth control and condoms. This process is facilitated both by empowering young women to take charge of their bodies and by demonstrating the correct use of condoms on a mannequin in the office setting. Many adolescent women have never seen or touched a condom and the office demonstration dramatically reduces anxiety, which may facilitate increased use (Brown-Jones and Orr 1993).

Unfortunately, evidence indicates that physicians do not always provide adequate information or screening services for sexually transmitted disease. Mahler (1997) screened 1,217 California physicians who were board certified in either family medicine, internal medicine, obstetrics and gynecology, or pediatrics regarding the routine services they provided to adolescents. Only 47% said that they asked all patients aged 15–18 whether they were sexually active and 3% said that they never asked; only 31% furnished all teenaged patients with information about sexually transmitted disease, including HIV.

Once an adolescent has demonstrated sexual activity by presenting for pregnancy testing, it is important to do immediate screening for sexually transmitted disease. Matson et al. (1993) followed-up 168 pregnant adolescents from low socioeconomic backgrounds from their original pregnancy diagnosis to their first prenatal visit. Of those patients who had screening pelvic examinations at the time of pregnancy testing, 29% were positive for gonorrhea, chlamydia, or both. This study design would not detect syphilis, HIV, or other blood-borne infections. The average delay from pregnancy diagnosis to first prenatal visit (at which routine evaluations for sexually transmitted diseases are normally done) was 35.7 days, with 40% of patients seen more than a month after pregnancy diagnosis and an additional 25% seen more than 46 days later.

The implications generated by these data are important for both the mother and the fetus. Adolescents are an increasing percentage of the HIV-positive population, with theoretic concerns that their future risk is enormous (D'Angelo et al. 1994). Because recent data show a marked decrease in transplacental transmission of the virus when HIV pregnant women are treated with antiviral agents during pregnancy, finding ways to ensure early screening and treatment of all HIV-positive women is a public health imperative.

## Emergency Contraception

Emergency contraception is used after unprotected intercourse to prevent pregnancy, but is used so infrequently that it has been called "the best-kept contraceptive secret in America" (M. A. Gold et al. 1997). The most common method used is the "Yuzpe" method: two oral contraceptive pills, each containing 50 μg of ethinyl estradiol, are taken within 72 hours of unprotected intercourse, followed by two additional 50-μg pills 12 hours later. Some women experience nausea from this estrogen dose, so an antiemetic may be helpful; if vomiting occurs, the dose should be repeated.

In Great Britain, where all contraceptive pills can be purchased over the counter, a pill that is packaged and marketed specifically for postcoital use is also available (M. A. Gold et al. 1997). In the United States, the Food and Drug Administration has approved the use of oral contraceptives in this manner, but information about the method has been slow to disseminate.

Emergency contraception may be especially suited for use in the adolescent population, in which first intercourse is usually unplanned and unprotected. The Yuzpe method reduces the risk of pregnancy after unprotected intercourse by 75% and could decrease the abortion rate by 50%. Nonetheless, when college students were screened in one women's health clinic, 85% of students who had previously had an abortion did not know anything about emergency contraception (M. A. Gold et al. 1997).

Other agents, including mefipristone or antiprogesterone preparations, may also be suited for postcoital use. Further research about long-term effects of postcoital contraception and increased education about this method for primary care physicians who treat adolescents are sorely needed.

## Prenatal Care for Adolescent Women

Adolescents appear to have increased risks for certain potentially serious conditions during pregnancy, including pregnancy-induced hypertension, anemia, preterm labor, preterm delivery, and having low-birth-weight infants. Whether these increased risks are primarily a function of age or secondary to other variables (Scholl et al. 1994) is an ongoing research issue. The real challenge is to find ways that help pregnant adolescents achieve the best possible outcomes for themselves and their infants.

When an adolescent woman becomes pregnant, her level of cognitive development and her level of psychosocial development will predict how she behaves with regard to herself and her pregnancy. Not only does she face the usual developmental tasks for her stage of adolescence, but she now has the added developmental tasks superimposed by the pregnancy (Drake 1996). The field of maternal–child nursing has had a longstanding appreciation for these principles and has contributed much of the information in this important area.

A recent publication by Drake (1996) provided an especially useful summation of these principles. Table 6–1 outlines the developmental tasks of adolescence as they are experienced by pregnant adolescent in the early, middle, and late stages of cognitive and psychosocial development. Table 6–2 outlines the developmental tasks of pregnancy as they are experienced by early, middle, and late adolescents.

# Special Populations of Pregnant Adolescents

## Substance Abuse

Use of psychoactive substances during pregnancy has become an area of growing concern over the past two decades. This concern is fueled by statistics showing that new drug use occurs among women at a rate twice that among men. In one study from Maryland, baseline statistics showed that 16% of all newborns in 1986 were designated as high risk based on maternal drug use. Four years later, the number had increased almost threefold, to 46%. Although it was unclear whether the apparent increase in drug-exposed infants was secondary to increased surveillance or higher rates of drug use, the authors felt certain that no reduction had occurred in the proportion of women using drugs during pregnancy (Marques and McKnight 1991).

A prominent finding in the Maryland study was that white pregnant teens were much more likely to fall into the two highest-risk groups for drug abuse compared with only 12% of black pregnant teens. The authors contrasted their findings with another public health population in Florida in which black adolescents were 10 times more likely to be tested and thus appeared to have higher rates of substance abuse (Marques and McKnight 1991).

Similar findings were noted in another study that examined prenatal alcohol use in adolescents. Significantly more white adolescents were among the moderate/heavy drinkers than black adolescents. Drinking is common during adolescence and adolescents have different patterns of drinking than adults. One national survey reported that more than 27% of female high school seniors reported at least one occasion in the 2 weeks prior to questioning when they had consumed five or more drinks. When compared with a cohort of pregnant adults, pregnant adolescents of both races had higher rates

TABLE 6–1. Achievement of developmental tasks of adolescence by the pregnant adolescent

| Developmental tasks of adolescence* | Early pregnant adolescents | Middle pregnant adolescents | Late pregnant adolescents |
|---|---|---|---|
| Achievement of a stable identity | Weakly developed sense of self. Much difficulty in adapting to the demands of pregnancy. Too much turmoil and confusion for identity formation. Responsibilities of parenthood may be thrust on them. | A developing sense of self. May still be developing ideas of what they want to do, how they want to behave. Pregnancy may have been desired to confirm feminine identity. | A strong sense of self. Have developed feminine identities and are able to adapt to pregnant and parenting roles like adult mothers. |
| Body image | Body in stage of rapid growth. Awkward and self-conscious about being different. May conceal the pregnancy. | Body reaching maturity. Usually react negatively to body image changes imposed by pregnancy. | Comfortable with mature body and maternal appearance. |
| Sexuality | Prefer same-gender peers. Usually have only casual relationship with the father of the fetus. | May have entered relationship with father of the fetus but relationship lacks depth and closeness. May have desired the pregnancy to strengthen the relationship with the father. | Able to form close relationships with both genders. Have a stable relationship with the father of the fetus. |
| Personal value system | Premoral or preconventional (Kohlberg 1964). Obey to avoid punishment. Conform to obtain rewards, have favors returned (Mercer 1990). Need concrete incentives to comply with recommendations for healthy prenatal behaviors. | Role conformity or conventional (Kohlberg 1964). Maintain good relationships for others' approval. Conform to avoid censure by authorities and resultant guilt (Mercer 1990). Do what is suggested for prenatal care to avoid reproach by parents or health care providers. | Self-accepted moral principles (Kohlberg 1964). Conform to maintain respect of impartial observer and to avoid self-condemnation (Mercer 1990). Self-motivated to do what is best for a healthy pregnancy. |

**TABLE 6–1.**  Achievement of developmental tasks of adolescence by the pregnant adolescent *(continued)*

| Developmental tasks of adolescence* | Early pregnant adolescents | Middle pregnant adolescents | Late pregnant adolescents |
|---|---|---|---|
| Vocation/career | In the sixth to ninth grade. Not able to be future oriented or concerned about career choices. Also are not able to have motherhood as a role without support. | In the tenth to twelfth grade. If doing poorly in school and not encouraged to have educational and employment goals, motherhood may be primary role. | May have completed high school. Are able to define career choices and goals. May combine choices and goals. May combine employment or education with motherhood. |
| Independence from parents | Dependent on parents or other adults. Need much assistance with parenting resposibilities. | Usually still dependent on parents or another adult. Share parenting responsibility with adult family members. | May be independent if gainful employment is available for them or their partners. Can take primary responsibility for parenting with the father of the fetus. |

* As identified by Mercer (1990).

*Source.*  Drake P: "Addressing Developmental Needs of Pregnant Adolescents." *J Obstet Gynecol Neonatal Nurs* 25:518–524, 1996. Reprinted with permission of Association of Women's Health, Obstetric, and Neonatal Nurses (AWHONN).

TABLE 6–2. Achievement of developmental tasks of pregnancy by adolescents

| Developmental tasks of pregnancy* | Early adolescents | Middle adolescents | Late adolescents |
|---|---|---|---|
| Seeking safe passage | Hampered by denial of pregnancy. Not able to clearly state questions and concerns. Seek prenatal care late or not at all. | May not be assertive in expressing concerns. Late prenatal care is common. | Actively seek information about pregnancy, birth, and infants. Usually start prenatal care in the middle trimester. |
| Acceptance of the pregnancy by self and others | High levels of secrecy and denial of pregnancy may occur. Usually strong negative reaction by families. | May have chosen the mothering role to gain mature status. Families' reaction usually negative: shock, anger, guilt, and sadness (Johnson 1995). | Mixed reaction of adolescents, partners, and families. More acceptance if adolescents are financially independent. |
| Acceptance of the reality of the unborn child | Have difficulty focusing on the fetus because they are present-oriented, self-centered, and concrete thinkers. | May be willing to make the needs of the fetus first priority. Influenced by developing feminine identities and the significance of the mothering role. | Able to focus on the fetus. Can understand the consequences of behavior on fetal growth and development. |
| Acceptance of the reality of parenthood | Not emotionally ready to assume a parenting role. Require adult guidance and assistance to share responsibility for infant care. | May be able to take on some responsibility for parenting. To continue own education, assistance with child care from adults is necessary. | Can get prepared and assume the tasks of parenting competently. |

* As identified by Rubin (1984).

*Source.* Drake P: "Addressing Developmental Needs of Pregnant Adolescents." *J Obstet Gynecol Neonatal Nurs* 25:518–524, 1996. Reprinted with permission of Association of Women's Health, Obstetric, and Neonatal Nurses (AWHONN).

of binge drinking during the first trimester, and adolescent binge drinking did not decrease until after the first trimester. Heavy drinking was a risk factor for later recognition of pregnancy in both adult and adolescent cohorts, which has important implications for prevention of fetal alcohol syndrome (Cornelius et al. 1994).

In the same study, the use of marijuana and crack/cocaine decreased during pregnancy for both adolescents and adults. Tobacco use, on the other hand, decreased in the adult cohort but actually increased in the adolescent cohort. The proportion of tobacco smokers in the adolescent sample increased from 52% to 64% during pregnancy; black adolescent women were less likely to use tobacco than white adolescent women; and by the third trimester, 92% of the white adolescents were smoking (Cornelius et al. 1994).

Berenson et al. (1992) surveyed 342 pregnant adolescents from diverse ethnic origins to explore the relationship between violence and substance abuse. They reported that adolescent women with a history of combined physical and sexual assault were seven times more likely to use psychoactive substances than were adolescents without a history of assault. Substance abuse was five times more likely for those who had been sexually victimized and three times more likely for those who had been physically assaulted. Drug use was most strongly associated with assault by a mate, whereas alcohol and tobacco were more commonly associated with assault by a member of the victim's family of origin.

Scafidi et al. (1997) evaluated psychosocial stress in 104 adolescent mothers between the ages of 13 and 21 years. Drug-abusing adolescent mothers experienced more psychosocial stressors than did adolescent mothers who were not substance abusers. Drug-abusing adolescent mothers also reported poorer physical health, poorer mental health, lower vocational and educational status, more family and peer relations problems, less constructive use of leisure time, and poorer social skills than the comparable group. Overall, poor mental health was the most significant factor associated with drug abuse in this cohort of adolescent mothers.

## Mental Illness

Kovacs et al. (1994) noted that the investigations prospectively examining mental illness in children as a predictor of adolescent pregnancy were limited. The authors used existing longitudinal data from a psychiatric clinic sample of 83 girls who were aged 8–13 years at study entry. They followed-up with the girls over time and identified 25 girls who had had their first pregnancies at age 18 or younger. The authors had postulated that girls with depressive disorders should be at greater risk for adolescent pregnancy, but the data did not support this theory. In the final multivariant analysis, only conduct disorders appeared to have a major role. Among girls with conduct disorders, 54.8% had teen pregnancies versus 12% of girls with other diagnoses.

In a subsequent study by Zoccolillo et al. (1997), the role for conduct disorder as a predictor of greater risk for adolescent pregnancy was also acknowledged; 9 of 25 pregnant adolescent women studied had that diagnosis. In addition, conduct disorder was also a major risk factor for polysubstance use, with 67% of the subjects in this study also meeting diagnostic criterion for substance abuse or dependence. The authors suggested that screening for conduct disorder may be an efficient way to identify girls at especially high risk for early pregnancy; screening is relatively easy, most adolescents will not meet the criterion, and intensive pregnancy prevention efforts could be directed toward those who do.

A common explanation for poor contraception and unwanted pregnancy in past years has been an assumption that these behaviors were a reflection of poor self-esteem. Matsuhashi and Felice (1991) found just the opposite in the first reported study assessing body perceptions in pregnant adolescents. They assessed 43 primiparous pregnant adolescents, aged 14–18 years, during the third trimester of pregnancy. In comparison with a never-pregnant control group matched for age, race, Tanner stage of pubertal development, and socioeconomic status, the pregnant girls reported higher overall self-esteem, a more positive body image, a surer self-identity, and feelings of being more productive as family members. The authors suggested that some adolescent girls may actually be developing their own sexual identity through a pregnancy.

That principle may apply to repeat pregnancy rates as well. Stevens-Simon et al. (1996a) assessed attitudes toward childbearing in a racially diverse group of 200 consecutively enrolled, poor, pregnant adolescents aged 13–18 years in an adolescent-oriented maternity program. During the first postpartum year, the repeat pregnancy rate was 11.5%. Those adolescents who became pregnant again were more likely to have expressed positive attitudes toward childbearing during the index pregnancy (60.9% vs. 39.6%; $P = 0.05$). Interestingly, they were also more likely to have reported a miscarriage prior to the index pregnancy (30% vs. 9%; $P = 0.04$), and those with miscarriage prior to the index pregnancy conceived more quickly after the index pregnancy. Those who conceived again within 1 year were more likely to have dropped out of school before high school graduation ($P = 0.004$), more often admitted to the use of illicit drugs ($P = 0.05$), had more frequently moved away from their parental home ($P = 0.006$), and were more likely to have rated their families as unsupportive during the index pregnancy ($P = 0.009$). They were not significantly different with regard to age, race, Medicaid use, or depression scores, but they were less likely to have planned postpartum levonorgestrel (Norplant) use during the index pregnancy (22% vs. 49%; $P = 0.02$).

## Planning for the Future

As we look for conclusions about the complex issue of adolescent pregnancy, the only thing that is perfectly clear is that it is multifactorial and does not have any simple or easy solutions. It is imperative that we begin finding solutions, because our population is in a phase that will produce an accelerated number of middle and late adolescents during this decade. McElroy and Moore (1997) estimated that between the years 1990 and 2000, the number of women ages 15–19 would increase by 1 million. Unless significant reductions are achieved in the adolescent birth rate, we can anticipate a substantial increase in the number of births in this group.

## References

Berenson AB, San Miguel VV, Wilkinson GS: Violence and its relationship to substance abuse in adolescent pregnancy. J Adolesc Health 13:470–474, 1992

Bluestein D, Rutledge CM: Determinants of delayed pregnancy testing among adolescents. J Fam Pract 35:406–410, 1992

Boyer D, Fine D: Sexual abuse as a factor in adolescent pregnancy and child maltreatment. Fam Plann Perspect 24:4–11, 19, 1992

Brown-Jones L, Orr DP: Health care for the adolescent female. Compr Ther 19:291–299, 1993

Cornelius MD, Richardson GA, Day NL, et al: A comparison of prenatal drinking in two recent samples of adolescents and adults. J Stud Alcohol 55:412–419, 1994

Custer M: Adoption as an option for unmarried pregnant teens. Adolescence 28:891–902, 1993

D'Angelo LJ, Brown R, English A, et al: HIV infection and AIDS in adolescents: a position paper of the Society for Adolescent Medicine. J Adolesc Health 15:427–434, 1994

Donovan P: Confronting a hidden epidemic: the Institute of Medicine's report on sexually transmitted diseases. Fam Plann Perspect 29:87–89, 1997

Drake P: Addressing developmental needs of pregnant adolescents. J Obstet Gynecol Neonatal Nurs 25:518–524, 1996

Farber NB: The process of pregnancy resolution among adolescent mothers. Adolescence 26:697–716, 1991

Gold JH: Adolescents and abortion, in Psychiatric Aspects of Abortion. Edited by Stotland NL. American Psychiatric Press, Washington, DC, 1991

Gold MA, Schein A, Coupey SM: Emergency contraception: a national survey of adolescent health experts. Fam Plann Perspect 29:15–19, 1997

Kohlberg L: Development of moral character and moral ideology, in Review of Child Development Research. Edited by Hoffman ML, Hoffman W. New York, Russell Sage Foundation, 1964, pp 383–431

Kovacs M, Krol RSM, Voti L: Early onset pathology and the risk for teenage pregnancy among clinically referred girls. J Am Acad Child Adolesc Psychiatry 33:106–113, 1994

Johnson PA: Adolescent sexuality, pregnancy, and parenthood, in Maternity Nursing. Edited by Bobak IM, Lowdermilk DL, Jensen MD. St. Louis, MO, Mosby, 1995, pp 722–747

Lewis M, Volkmar FR: Clinical Aspects of Child and Adolescent Development. Media, PA, Williams and Wilkins, 1990, pp 212–247

Mahler K: Physicians often omit sexual health services from adolescents' care. Fam Plann Perspect 29:91–92, 1997

Marques PR, McKnight AJ: Drug abuse risk among pregnant adolescents attending public health clinics. Am J Drug Alcohol Abuse 17:399–413, 1991

Matson SC, Pomeranz AJ, Kamps KA: Early detection and treatment of sexually transmitted disease in pregnant adolescents of low socioeconomic status. Clin Pediatr 32:609–612, 1993

Matsuhashi Y, Felice ME: Adolescent body image during pregnancy. J Adolesc Health 12:313–315, 1991

Maynard RA: The study, the context, and the findings in brief, in Kids Having Kids: Economic Costs and Social Consequences of Teen Pregnancy. Edited by Maynard RA. Washington, DC, Urban Institute Press, 1997

McElroy AW, Moore KA: Trends over time in teenage pregnancy and childbearing: the critical changes, in Kids Having Kids: Economic Costs and Social Consequences of Teen Pregnancy. Edited by Maynard RA. Washington, DC, Urban Institute Press, 1997

Mercer R: Parents at Risk. New York, Springer, 1990

Parker B: Abuse of adolescents: what can we learn from pregnant teenagers? AWHONNS Clin Issues Perinat Womens Health Nurs 4:363–370, 1993

Rainey DY, Stevens-Simon C, Kaplan DW: Are adolescents who report prior sexual abuse at higher risk for pregnancy? Child Abuse Negl 19:1283–1288, 1995

Rubin R: Maternal Identity and the Maternal Experience. New York, Springer, 1984

Scafidi FA, Field T, Prodromidis M, et al: Psychosocial stressors of drug-abusing disadvantaged adolescent mothers. Adolescence 32:93–100, 1997

Scholl TO, Hediger ML, Belsky DH: Prenatal care and maternal health during adolescent pregnancy: a review and meta-analysis. J Adolesc Health 15:444–456, 1994

Singer DG, Revenson TA: A Piaget Primer: How a Child Thinks. New York, New American Library, 1978

Stevens-Simon C, Reichert S: Sexual abuse, adolescent pregnancy, and child abuse. Arch Pediatr Adolesc Med 148:23–27, 1994

Stevens-Simon C, Kelly L, Singer D: Absence of negative attitudes toward childbearing among pregnant teenagers. Arch Pediatr Adolesc Med 150:1037–1043, 1996a

Stevens-Simon C, Kelly L, Singer D, et al: Why pregnant adolescents say they did not use contraceptives prior to conception. J Adolesc Health 19:48–53, 1996b

Zabin LS, Hayward SC: Adolescent Sexual Behavior and Childbearing. Newbury Park, CA, Sage, 1993

Zakus G, Wilday S: Adolescent abortion option. Soc Work Health Care 12:77–91, 1987

Zoccolillo M, Meyers J, Assiter S: Conduct disorder, substance dependence, and adolescent motherhood. Am J Orthopsychiatry 67:152–157, 1997

# Postpartum Disorders

GAIL ERLICK ROBINSON, M.D., D.PSYCH., F.R.C.P.C.
DONNA E. STEWART, M.D., D.PSYCH., F.R.C.P.C.

Mental disturbance following childbirth was first mentioned by Hippocrates, but the first good clinical description of postpartum psychosis was written by a French psychiatrist, Louis Marcé, in 1858. There was little interest in this disorder until Paffenberger (1961) showed that admission to mental hospitals was enormously increased during the first month postpartum and Hamilton (1962) argued that puerperal psychosis was a distinct disorder. Psychologic disturbances can occur in the postpartum period in the form of maternity ("baby") blues, postnatal depression, or psychosis. Although any psychiatric disorder may present or recur in the postpartum period, it is clear that affective disorders are most common. Not uncommonly seen after delivery, however, are adjustment, attachment, obsessive-compulsive, and anxiety disorders as well as schizophrenia.

## Postpartum Adaptation

The postpartum period involves numerous physiologic, psychologic, and sociocultural changes. All of the following have been investigated as possible etiologic factors in postpartum disorders.

### Biologic Factors

Dramatic changes in hormone and electrolyte balance and fluid volume level occur during labor and the postpartum period. After birth, progesterone and estriol rapidly fall, returning to prepregnancy levels by 3 days after delivery. When estrogen falls after birth, prolactin, which has risen during pregnancy, is no longer blocked and lactation is initiated. Suckling by the infant stimulates the secretion of oxytoxin. The usual cyclic variation of androgens is absent during both pregnancy and lactation. Plasma corticosteroids reach a peak during labor and decrease significantly within 4 hours postpartum. Thyroid function returns to prepregnancy levels approximately 4 weeks after delivery. Beta-endorphins rise during labor, reach a peak immediately before delivery, and decline after parturition. Plasma renin falls after childbirth. Sodium excretion rises and calcium excretion falls. Several days after birth, a rapid weight loss occurs. Testosterone is associated with greater reported mood disturbances after delivery (Buckwalter et al. 1999).

Several methodologic problems have hampered studies on the biologic basis of postpartum disorders. Early researchers could not accurately assay hormones, particularly free, unbound plasma concentrations. Psychologic rating scales used in various studies differed; some, confounded by the normal physical symptoms of the puerperium, were obviously inappropriate measures of maternal mental states. Blood sampling often took place at inappropriate times, ignoring activities such as breastfeeding that can alter hormone levels. Seasonal variations in hormones and circadian rhythmicity were often overlooked. Studies that examined one hormone in isolation were inadequate because of complex endocrine interrelationships.

## Psychosocial Factors

Transition to parenthood has a significant impact on both men and women, their relationship as a couple, and their work and social activities. New conflicts may arise and old ones resurface. Problems in the relationship between the woman and her own mother may increase her difficulties in the development of her new maternal identity. She must also come to terms with her own femininity.

A woman's postpartum adaptation is intimately linked to the quality of the relationship with her partner (Zelkowitz and Milet 1996). A supportive relationship with the child's father can help mitigate the stresses of being a new mother. In many cases, the family system must be reorganized, and many couples adopt more traditional roles. Couples with reasonably egalitarian relationships often have more difficulty adjusting to new parenthood because, regardless of previous philosophies, it is usually the mother who accepts the major share of parenting tasks. The parents must decide how their new roles will affect their previous work patterns and implement the necessary changes. With the added burden of child care, the relationship between the partners often suffers, and there is less time for socializing. Groups of other new parents can be very supportive in helping the couple work through these normal adjustments. Age, parity, culture, expectations, financial problems, and housing difficulties may all affect normal postpartum reactions and the developing relationship between the mother and her new baby.

## Infant Feeding

It is generally agreed that breastfeeding is best for young infants, for both nutritional and other health reasons. It may also facilitate mother–child bonding. Although 65% of North American mothers begin breastfeeding, only 25% continue for 4 months. Although they are aware of the benefits of breastfeeding, many mothers prefer bottle feeding for various reasons (Wollett 1987), including modesty, discomfort, an unsupportive environment, difficulties in breastfeeding, a wish to share feeding responsibilities with others, or uncertainty about the amount of breast milk provided. The father's attitude toward breastfeeding often plays a vital role. Either partner's beliefs about the effect of breastfeeding on contraception or breast size and shape can also influence its acceptance. In addition, women who are returning to the workplace shortly after the birth may find it impossible to continue breastfeeding, whereas women on a demand schedule may feel overburdened by the responsibility of being available every few hours. Some women think their husbands will become more involved if they choose bottle-feeding. A woman's attitude toward breastfeeding is greatly improved with support from her physician, hospital staff, and other health care providers. Information and support about breastfeeding is valuable in helping women weather the difficult first few weeks after birth. It is vital, however, that the woman not be made to feel guilty, whatever her informed choice.

## Maternity Blues

Maternity blues is a common, benign, transitory condition occurring in the first 10 days postpartum. Its incidence ranges from 28%–80% (Harris 1980; Lanczick et al. 1992).

## Clinical Presentation

Maternity blues typically begin 3–4 days after delivery (Stein 1982) and peak on days 4–5. The most frequently reported symptom is weeping. In the first few hours after delivery, crying may be accompanied by happy feelings. Handley et al. (1980) felt that depressed mood is characteristic of maternity blues, whereas Kennerley and Gath (1986) found that although women described themselves as "low spirited" they did not consider themselves to be depressed. Emotional lability seems to be a characteristic feature. Elation ("postpartum pinks") may also occur and may be mild or predict more serious mood disturbance.

Researchers have also described irritability, lack of affection for the baby, hostility toward the husband, sleep disturbance, headaches, feelings of unreality, depersonalization, exhaustion, and restlessness in women suffering from maternity blues. Although many mothers describe themselves as being absentminded, distracted, and lacking in concentration, psychologic tests have produced no evidence that cognitive impairments are common (Kennerley and Gath 1986).

## Etiology

### Psychosocial Factors

No clear correlations have been established between maternity blues and various psychosocial factors. Maternity blues have been reported in all social classes (Ballinger et al. 1979; Stein 1980) and in many different cultures (Davidson 1972; Harris 1980). The condition is unrelated to marital status (Davidson 1972), although associations have been reported with poor marital relationships (Ballinger et al. 1979; Cutrona 1984). No positive association has been reported between the blues and other external stressors (Paykel et al. 1980; Pitt 1973). Hospital delivery does not appear to be a causal factor, because there is an equal incidence in home deliveries (Yalom et al. 1968).

Contradictory findings have been reported for the association of maternity blues with personality factors (Nott et al. 1976; Pitt 1973), the primiparous state (Ballinger et al. 1979; Nott et al. 1976; Stein 1980), ambivalent attitudes toward pregnancy (Nilsson and Almgren 1970), fear of labor (Ballinger et al. 1979; Kennerley and Gath 1986), and anxiety and depression during pregnancy (Davidson 1972; Handley et al. 1980). O'Hara et al. (1991) reported a history of personal and family depression, more problems with social adjustment, and stressful life events in women who get postnatal blues compared with women who do not.

## Biologic Factors

The high incidence, typical onset at 3 days postpartum, fluctuating course, and lack of clear psychosocial causation of maternity blues have led many researchers to suspect a biologic cause. However, no consistent correlations have been found between maternity blues and prolactin, cortisol, thyroid hormones, beta-endorphins, norepinephrine, 5-hydroxytryptamine, cyclic adenosine monophosphate, electrolytes, or pyridoxine (George and Sandler 1988). O'Hara et al. (1991) reported higher levels of free and total estriol before and after delivery in women who develop blues compared with those who do not. Harris et al. (1994) found a relationship between severity of the blues and the high levels and steep rate of rise of progesterone antenatally as well as a steep drop postnatally.

## Obstetric and Gynecologic Factors

Yalom et al. (1968) noted a higher incidence of obstetric anomalies or subjective discomfort during pregnancy in women with maternity blues, whereas Pitt (1973) and Ballinger et al. (1979) did not. No link was found among maternity blues and physiologic monitoring during pregnancy (Blumberg 1980), cesarean section (Kendell et al. 1981), or breastfeeding compared with bottle-feeding (Ballinger et al. 1979; Cox et al. 1982). Researchers have reported that women who experience maternity blues were of a younger age at menarche (Yalom et al. 1968), have a shorter menstrual flow (Yalom et al. 1968), experience more menstrual irregularities (Handley et al. 1980), and have a history of premenstrual tension (Ballinger et al. 1979) compared with those who do not experience this condition. Davidson and Robertson (1985), however, failed to find any association with previous menstrual difficulties.

## Treatment

Women with maternity blues benefit from reassurance that the symptoms are common and will disappear quickly. Emotional support and instruction on newborn care may also be helpful. Women should be advised to seek help if symptoms are severe or persist for more than 2 weeks.

## Prognosis

Most women completely recover from maternity blues in a few days to 2 weeks. In a small number, however, the symptoms escalate into more serious psychiatric conditions. Many women experience maternity blues after each pregnancy.

# Disorders of the Mother–Infant Relationship

Disorders of the mother–infant relationship range from delayed attachment to infanticide. Studies of these disorders are limited by problems in methodology, including the difficulty of measuring maternal–infant attachment.

## Incidence

Delayed attachment is reported in approximately 10% of mothers. Absolute rejection of the infant and obsessive, hostile thoughts about the baby are seen in 1% of mothers. Estimates of child abuse vary greatly and depend on the criteria used and cultural norms. Infanticide occurs in 1/50,000 births in the United Kingdom (Brockington and Cox-Roper 1988).

## Clinical Presentations

Approximately 40% of primiparous women experience mild detachment or negative feelings toward their infants in the immediate postnatal period, with a gradual increase in the strength of maternal feelings over the ensuing few weeks (Robson and Powell 1982). In more severe, persistent disorders of attachment, the mother expresses disinterest, neglect, and failure to protect, nurture, or interact with the infant. Delayed attachment can be primary or can occur secondary to another psychiatric disorder, such as an adjustment disorder, depression, mania, psychosis, anxiety, obsessive-compulsive disorder, or personality disorders. Margison (1982) has described infant rejection in which the mother shows persistent hostility, often wishes the child had never been born, and is determined to avoid the maternal role. Other women may feel normally loving toward their infants but may be afraid of contact because of obsessional, intrusive, and distressing thoughts about their babies, including impulses to harm them (Brockington and Cox-Roper 1988).

## Etiology

Cultural factors and social class influence the way a woman first relates to her child (Robson and Powell 1982). The role of maternal personality factors in facilitating or interfering with attachment is still being studied. Women who have had disrupted or inadequate mothering themselves (Frommer and O'Shea 1973) and single teenage mothers without social supports should be considered at special risk for attachment disorder. Painful and difficult childbirth experiences have also been linked to early maternal detachment (Robson and Kumar 1980). Congenital defects or prematurity in the infant may result in a lack of attachment or rejection because of fear of subsequent loss. Problems with obsessional hostile feelings toward the newborn may be a manifestation of obsessive-compulsive illness or depression (Beck 1995). Socioeconomic or environmental stresses tend to exacerbate difficulties in attachment. Persistent rejection of the newborn is found most frequently in unwanted pregnancies (Resnick 1970).

## Management

Most delays in attachment resolve spontaneously within the first few days or weeks postpartum. Education about delayed attachment may alleviate the mother's guilt. Although it has not been clearly established that brief separation leads to attachment disorders, it is important to maintain close contact if either the mother or the baby requires hospitalization. Mothers who suffer from continued bonding problems may benefit from practical advice and support concerning infant care, psychotherapy to explore the determinants of the problem, behavioral approaches designed to decrease anxiety when coping with the baby, and occasionally joint admission to a mother–infant unit. Severe disturbances of attachment, in which the infant is at serious risk of abuse or neglect, may require protective custody, joint treatment, or enforced supervision where available. Obsessional thoughts of hostility toward the baby may respond to psychotherapy, often combined with pharmacotherapy with an antidepressant such as clomipramine or a selective serotonin reuptake inhibitor. Women with attachment difficulties secondary to other psychiatric disorders should be reassessed after the primary disorder has been treated.

## Effects on the Neonate

Delayed attachment or early temporary separation from the mother has not been proven to have significant long-term effects on the baby (Robson and Powell 1982). Children who suffer from ongoing lack of bonding, however, may show failure to thrive, stunted emotional and cognitive development, and difficulty in developing peer relationships. These infants are also at more risk of being abused and rejected. A comprehensive review of infanticide (Resnick 1970) found that the victims of neonaticide (murder of the newborn within 24 hours of its birth) were most commonly unwanted babies of mothers who were young, unmarried, and without evidence of psychosis or depression. Many of the women were denied or failed to seek an abortion for an unwanted pregnancy they were afraid to reveal to their families.

# Postnatal Depression

Postnatal depression is an affective disorder lasting more than 2 weeks, the severity of which meets criteria for DSM-IV affective disorder (American Psychiatric Association 1994). Carefully designed research has cast doubt on the existence of postnatal depression as a distinct entity (O'Hara and Zekoski 1988). In a group of pregnant women and matched, nonpregnant control women, rates of depression were 10.6% for postpartum women during the first 9 weeks after delivery and 10.0% for control subjects. O'Hara and Zekoski (1988) concluded that there was no evidence that postpartum subjects were at greater risk for depression than control subjects. However, hospitalization rates to psychiatric hospitals are higher in the 30 days after delivery than at any other time in a woman's life (Paffenberger 1961). Regardless of whether postpartum depression is a distinct illness, the subsequent negative consequences to the mother, her marital relationship, and her child make postnatal depression an important condition to diagnose and treat.

## Prevalence and Epidemiology

A meta-analysis of numerous studies found the average prevalence rate of postnatal depression to be 13% (O'Hara and Swain 1996). Lower occupational status of the mother and lower family income were found to be small but significant predictors of depression, whereas maternal age, marital status, education, parity, and length of relationship with partner all failed to significantly predict postnatal depression (O'Hara and Swain 1996; O'Hara and Zekoski 1988).

## Clinical Presentation

Postnatal depression usually begins within 1–6 months after delivery. In some women, maternity blues simply continue and become more severe. In others, a period of well-being is followed by gradual onset of depression, characterized by tearfulness, despondency, emotional lability, guilty feelings, anorexia, and sleep disturbances as well as feelings of being inadequate to cope with the infant, poor concentration and memory, fatigue, and irritability (Robinson and Stewart 1986). Some women may worry excessively about the baby's health or feeding habits and see themselves as "bad," inadequate, or unloving mothers.

## Etiology

### Psychosocial Factors

Studies of postnatal depression have been handicapped by methodologic errors and the inability to identify it as a distinct disorder. A relationship has been reported, however, between measurable anxiety during pregnancy and the level of postpartum depressive symptoms (Hayworth et al. 1980; Watson et al. 1984). Kumar and Robson (1984) found no increase in previous psychiatric diagnoses in women with postpartum depression, in contrast with the findings of O'Hara (1986) and O'Hara et al. (1983). O'Hara (1986) also found that a higher percentage of depressed subjects (66.7%) had a family history of depression than did nondepressed women (20.7%).

Several well-designed studies (Braverman and Roux 1978; Kumar and Robson 1984) have reported an increased risk of postpartum depression in women who experience marital problems during pregnancy. Hopkins et al. (1986), however, failed to confirm this finding. Women with postnatal depression perceived their husbands to be less supportive than did women who were not depressed, but these differences were apparent only postpartum, not during pregnancy (O'Hara 1986; O'Hara et al. 1983). Cutrona (1984) found that the availability of companionship and a feeling of belonging to a group were more important predictors of good adjustment than was intimacy with the husband. Only a few studies (Hopkins et al. 1986) found no association between measures of social support and the occurrence of postnatal depression. No relationship has been demonstrated between various obstetric variables and postnatal depression.

Contradictory findings have been reported concerning the contribution of a poor relationship between the woman and her mother to postnatal depression (Kumar and Robson 1984; Nilsson and Almgren 1970; Paykel et al. 1980; Watson et al. 1984). Although O'Hara et al. (1984) and Cutrona (1984) found a relationship between external stressors and higher levels of postpartum depressive symptoms, Hopkins et al. (1986) found a relationship only with having a baby who is difficult to care for or a baby with neonatal complications. Similarly, Kumar and Robson (1984) found no association between stressful life events and postnatal depression.

## Biologic Factors

Although it has been suggested that postnatal depression is caused by low levels of progesterone or estrogen or high levels of prolactin, no significant relationships have been found (Harris 1994; Hendrick et al. 1998). Some women may be especially vulnerable to normal hormonal changes that may trigger depression (Hendrick et al. 1998; Stewart and Boydell 1993). Alder and Cox (1983) found that women who were breastfeeding their infants and taking oral contraceptives postpartum had a higher risk of depression at 3–5 months postnatally than did women who were breastfeeding exclusively but not taking oral contraceptives. No conclusive evidence relating the various neurotransmitter systems, free or total tryptophan levels, or cortisol levels and postnatal depressive symptoms has been demonstrated (Llewellyn et al. 1997). However, Harris (1996) showed a minor association of postnatal depression and thyroid dysfunction in thyroid antibody–positive women.

## Summary of Etiologic Factors

The most relevant etiologic factors for postnatal depression are those found in association with depression in general: personal or family psychiatric history of depression; lack of support, especially from the spouse; and occurrence of a number of negative life events around the time of delivery (O'Hara and Swain 1996; Stowe and Nemeroff 1995).

## Treatment

Postnatal depression is treated on both a psychosocial and a biologic basis. Identification and acknowledgment of the depression itself may be a helpful feature, dispelling the woman's fears of physical disease and personal inadequacy. Individual or group psychotherapy may help the woman resolve conflicts about mothering or her new role. Joint counseling is indicated if there are conflicts with or a lack of support from her partner. Information about newborn care, social assistance, and practical supports such as homemaking may also be beneficial. Medication, such as nortriptyline, 75–100 mg/day; desipramine, 150–300 mg/day; fluoxetine, 20–60 mg/day; paroxetine, 20–60 mg/day; or sertraline, 50–150 mg/day, is helpful for many depression and anxiety disorders. The use of minor tranquilizers to reduce anxiety should be limited to brief or adjunctive therapy to reduce the risk of dependency. Estradiol has been reported as a useful treatment in two small studies and requires further investigation (Ahokas et al. 2000; Gregoire et al. 1996). Chapter 5 discusses the use of drugs in the breastfeeding mother.

## Prevention

Discussion of postpartum mood disorders during prenatal classes is likely to improve early detection and presentation for treatment. Gordon and Gordon (1960) found that patients with a postnatal depression who received active social intervention as well as dynamic psychotherapy required shorter treatment and were less likely to require hospitalization. The women attending these groups, especially those accompanied by their husbands, experienced fewer emotional problems than did those in the control group. Halonen and Passman (1985), Shereshefsky and Lockman (1973), and Broussard (1976) found that either prenatal counseling or relaxation training could decrease the level of the woman's distress and improve the marital relationship postpartum. In a study of 15 women, Wisner and Wheeler (1994) found that starting antidepressants within the first 24 hours after birth in women with a history of postnatal depression decreased the expected recurrence rate. Oral estrogen has been proposed as prophylaxis for women with histories of affective disorders occurring only in the puerperium, but studies remain limited (Sichel et al. 1995).

## Prognosis

Postnatal depression usually lasts several months if not treated (Kumar and Robson 1984; Watson et al. 1984). Women may have difficulties in bonding with their infants and may express feelings of rejection, dislike, or indifference (Margison 1982; Teti et al. 1995). Women with postnatal depression are also more likely to experience future episodes of depression (Caplan et al. 1989). Although the occurrence of a postnatal depression does not guarantee behavioral, cognitive, or social problems in the toddler or young child, exposure to maternal depression in the early postpartum months may have an enduring influence on the child's psychological adjustment (Murray et al. 1999). Subsequent depression in these women has been associated with poor adjustment of the child at 4 years of age (Caplan et al. 1989; Phillips and O'Hara 1991).

Puerperal Psychoses

Puerperal psychoses are psychotic disorders arising after childbirth. Contro-versy exists over the specificity and timing of these disorders because early research suffered from confounding variables such as differences in case def-initions and the time period allowed for the occurrence of such disorders (Brockington et al. 1982). Consequently, some authors consider these disor-ders to be distinct entities with specific etiologies, clinical presentations, and prognoses (Brockington et al. 1982; Hamilton 1962), whereas most believe that they are simply episodes of psychotic illness triggered by the stresses of pregnancy and delivery (Kendell et al. 1987). Although women with schizo-phrenia frequently suffer from psychotic relapses within weeks after delivery, most authorities now agree that most postpartum psychoses are affective dis-orders (Kendell et al. 1987).

Brockington et al. (1982) found that early postpartum psychosis could be blindly differentiated from nonpuerperal psychosis. McNeil (1986) found that manic postpartum disturbances were characterized by more confusion and disorganized speech than were nonpuerperal episodes, and postpartum psychoses were generally characterized by more disorganized behavior. Oth-er distinctive characteristics included a symptom-free phase between delivery and onset of psychosis, marked confusion, changeability, unpredictability in clinical features, and distinguishing psychologic characteristics related to con-cerns about motherhood (Hamilton 1982). Clouding of consciousness (Pro-theroe 1969) and an excess of Schneiderian symptoms (Kadrmas et al. 1979) are also characteristic features.

## Incidence and Prevalence

The incidence of psychiatric admission for postpartum psychosis is 1–2 per 1,000 postpartum women. The relative risk of admission for psychosis within the first 30 days following childbirth is 21.7, decreasing to 12.7 in the first 90 days. Despite this decrease over time, the relative risk remains elevated for 2 years following delivery. Women with a history of bipolar affective disorder appear to be particularly vulnerable (Kendell et al. 1987).

## Epidemiology

Primiparous women appear to have a higher risk for postpartum psychosis; in Edinburgh, 62% of cases occurred in primiparous women versus 47% in the general population (Kendall et al. 1981). No significant relationship to maternal age (Kendell et al. 1987), class, or culture has been found. Although Kendell et al. (1987) found an increased number of admissions in single women, this finding may be related to a lack of spousal support (Paffenberger 1964).

## Early Versus Late Onset

McNeil (1986, 1987, 1988a, 1988b) found a number of significant differences between women who had early onset (within 3 weeks of delivery) and those with late onset postpartum illness. Women with early onset psychoses tended to have affective illnesses, to be primiparous, younger, and to have suffered emotional disturbance during pregnancy. Women with late onset illnesses tended to have schizophreniform illnesses; were older, of lower socioeconomic class, and single; and had suffered premorbid mental problems and more emotional disturbances before pregnancy but fewer during pregnancy.

## Clinical Presentation

Most postpartum psychoses begin within the first 3 weeks after delivery. There is nearly always an asymptomatic period of 2–3 days after delivery. Prodromal symptoms include sleep disturbances, fatigue, depression, irritability, and emotional lability. The mother often has difficulty caring for her infant. Characteristically, she feels confused, perplexed, bewildered, and dreamy and may complain of poor memory, although performance on formal mental tests is often normal (Brockington et al. 1982). Clinical presentation may be an atypical or brief reactive psychosis, major affective disorder, schizophreniform disorder, or an organic brain syndrome.

The most common presentation of puerperal psychosis is an affective disorder. In psychotic depression, the woman is tearful; has psychomotor retardation, sleep, and appetite disturbances; and is preoccupied with feelings of guilt and worthlessness. She may have delusions about the infant's being dead or defective. She may deny having given birth or have hallucinations commanding her to harm the baby. These typical depressive features are often accompanied by a sense of confusion.

In postpartum mania, the woman is excited, euphoric, grandiose, irritable, and hyperactive. She requires little sleep, and her appetite may be markedly reduced or exaggerated. She may have grandiose delusions about her baby. Insight is usually lacking.

In a schizophreniform presentation, the woman demonstrates thought disorder, delusions, inappropriate affect, hallucinations, agitation, motor retardation, bizarre delusional ideas about herself or her child, and lack of insight.

Women who present with an "organic brain syndrome" have prominent symptoms of confusion, bewilderment, and memory loss. This syndrome may be caused by medical conditions such as encephalitis, autoimmune disorders, endocrine disturbance, electrolyte imbalance, or sepsis but can occur in the absence of any recognizable medical disorder (Robinson and Stewart 1986; Welner 1982) and may be an atypical presentation of bipolar affective disorder.

## Etiology

Researchers have been unable to confirm a link between puerperal psychosis and levels of prolactin, thyroxine, estrogen, progesterone, adrenocortcoids, follicle stimulating hormone, or beta-endorphins (Brockington et al. 1982; Steiner 1979; Stewart et al. 1988). A 2.5-fold increased incidence of puerperal psychosis is seen after cesarean compared with vaginal delivery (Kendell et al. 1981). Other obstetric variables have not been found to increase risk.

Studies by Protheroe (1969) and Winokur et al. (1978) suggested that although an inherited predisposition to psychotic illness exists, a specific inherited predisposition to puerperal illness does not. However, a strong link has been found between bipolar disorder and puerperal psychosis with affective symptoms: women with a history of bipolar affective disorder have a 50% chance of developing postpartum psychosis (McNeil 1987). Women with a history of manic episodes are especially at risk for developing postpartum psychosis (Brockington et al. 1982). Moreover, the severity of past psychiatric illness appears to be significantly related to the occurrence of postpartum psychosis (McNeil 1987). First-degree relatives of women with bipolar disorders also have an increased incidence (20%) of postpartum psychosis (Uddenberg and Englesson 1978). Women with a history of schizophrenia have a 24% chance of developing postpartum psychosis (McNeil 1986).

## Treatment

Treatment of puerperal psychosis usually requires admission to a hospital, particularly if the mother is at risk of harming herself or her child through neglect, abuse, or acting on delusions or hallucinations. Mothers may be admitted independently or (preferably) together with their infants, if feasible. The woman's partner should be involved in the treatment from the beginning. Puerperal psychosis requires both pharmacologic and psychosocial therapy.

Specific drug treatments vary with the presentation. For depressive psychosis, an antidepressant such as nortriptyline, desipramine, or a serotonin reuptake inhibitor combined with a major tranquilizer such as haloperidol, 1–10 mg/day, or olanzapine, 5–15 mg/day, usually controls the psychotic symptoms as well as the depression. If the patient does not respond to these medications, electroconvulsive therapy is often effective, usually providing complete remission after six to eight treatments.

Hypomanic or manic presentations are treated with lithium carbonate in daily doses of 600–1,200 mg until a therapeutic serum level of 0.8–1.2 mg/L is reached. Patients who are unresponsive to lithium carbonate may be treated with other mood stabilizers such as carbamazepine or valproic acid. A major tranquilizer may be necessary to control acute symptoms until an adequate serum level of lithium or another mood stabilizer is obtained.

Women who present with a schizophreniform disorder should be treated with a major tranquilizer such as haloperidol, 4–10 mg/day or olanzapine, 5–15 mg/day. Those who do not respond adequately sometimes benefit from a trial of electroconvulsive therapy, particularly if affective or catatonic symptoms are present.

Conflicts about mothering, career, marital problems, issues relating to the woman's own mother, and concerns about femininity may require attention after the psychotic symptoms remit. Idealistic expectations of parenthood often need to be explored. The woman requires both practical and emotional support from her spouse, family, and friends, sometimes including education about child care. Individual or marital therapy may be indicated. Community social services may be extremely helpful for the mother and infant after discharge.

## Prognosis

Prior to the development of psychotropic drugs, untreated puerperal psychosis required an average of 5–8 months of hospitalization, with many women continuing to have symptoms for many years (Brockington et al. 1982). Current treatments have substantially shortened the psychotic episodes: 95% of adequately treated women improve within 2–3 months.

Reviewing the results of several studies, Brockington et al. (1982) found that 31% of women suffered a further puerperal episode and that psychosis complicated 21% of future pregnancies. They estimated the risk for each succeeding pregnancy to be 20% and postulated that the risk was higher in women with more severe psychosis and multiple risk factors. Prophylactic lithium given immediately after delivery to women with a history of postpartum affective psychosis appears to reduce the recurrence risk to 10% (Stewart et al. 1991). Careful follow-up is indicated after subsequent deliveries, both for support and early case identification and treatment.

Schopf et al. (1984) found that 65% of women studied had at least one nonpuerperal relapse and only 25% remained free of later psychopathology. Of those who had nonpuerperal relapses, 43% had been diagnosed as suffering from affective psychosis, 38% from schizoaffective psychosis, and only 19% from schizophrenia. They found that nonpuerperal relapses were strongly related to a family history of psychosis and the occurrence of a psychotic episode before the index episode. Davidson and Robertson (1985) looked specifically at women in whom the puerperal illness was the first onset of illness. Overall, 56% had at least one recurrent illness during follow-up. Of those women diagnosed as having unipolar depression, 40% had a nonpuerperal illness, whereas 30% had another puerperal disorder. Those diagnosed as having bipolar affective disorders had a 66% recurrence of nonpuerperal disorders and a 50% occurrence of subsequent puerperal psychosis. All of the women who had schizophrenia developed a chronic illness with frequent exacerbations.

## Effect on the Mother–Child Relationship

Evidence on the long-term effects on children of mothers with puerperal psychosis is conflicting. The psychiatric history, premorbid personality, nature and timing of the puerperal psychosis, current marital and environmental circumstances, degree of life stress, access to support, and health and temperament of the baby may all play a role. In the United Kingdom, many women are admitted to hospitals with their babies, either to a specialized mother–infant unit or to a general psychiatric ward. Although it is difficult to do randomized, controlled studies of the effectiveness of mother–infant admissions, a beneficial effect on the parent–child relationship and on parenting competence is apparent when measured 2 years later (Stewart 1989).

It is difficult to predict which infants may be at risk of harm from their mothers. Most women who commit neonaticide are not psychotic at the time (Resnick 1970). Filicide (the murder of a child by its parent more than 24 hours after birth), however, is most often associated with mental illness as part of a suicide attempt, as a response to hallucinations or delusions, as a delusional attempt to prevent the child from suffering, or as an accidental result of a violent outburst. Women with manic, depressed, or schizophrenic illnesses may also place their children at risk through neglect and lack of judgment, and careful supervision is required while the mother is ill and recovering.

# Postpartum Anxiety Disorders

Anxiety disorder with or without panic attacks may develop de novo in the postpartum period (Metz et al. 1988) or a previous anxiety disorder may be exacerbated at this time (Cowley and Roy-Byrne 1989). Panic attacks are typical in nature and respond to the usual pharmacologic treatments. The extent to which pregravid anxiety disorder predicts the occurrence of postpartum anxiety is unknown (Cohen et al. 1994). Postpartum worsening of panic attacks is hypothesized to be caused by the rapidly changing concentrations of reproductive hormones on monoaminergic binding sites (Charney et al. 1990) or to the relationship between falling progesterone levels during the postpartum period and resulting rises in blood $PCO_2$ (Villeponteaux et al. 1992). The presence of even mild symptoms of panic disorder during pregnancy may indicate the possibility of a postpartum anxiety disorder and the need for treatment with antidepressant medication, such as imipramine 150–300 mg/day, fluoxetine 10–40 mg/day, or sertraline 25–100 mg/day, with or without cognitive behavior therapy (Cohen et al. 1994).

## Postpartum Obsessive-Compulsive Disorders

Development of obsessive-compulsive disorders and obsessive-compulsive symptoms is not uncommon in the early postpartum period. Women with these disorders usually experience unwanted intrusive thoughts about harming their babies and may avoid situations in which they feel they are at risk of acting on their thoughts (e.g., bathing or sleeping with the infants, preparing food with sharp knives). Not infrequently, women with postpartum depression may also develop obsessive-compulsive symptoms. These women usually recover promptly when treated with serotonin reuptake inhibitor antidepressants or clomipramine combined with supportive psychotherapy. However, some postpartum women appear to have a pure obsessive-compulsive disorder without affective changes (Williams and Koran 1997). These women are often more treatment resistant, although success has been experienced using higher doses of serotonin reuptake inhibitor antidepressants (e.g., fluoxetine 80 mg/day) with cognitive-behavioral therapy over a period of several months.

## Conclusions

Postpartum psychiatric disorders have a major impact on women, their children, and their families. It is important for physicians to be aware of the possibility that a woman will develop an emotional disorder in the postpartum. Frequently, women are discharged home within 24 hours of birth, isolated, and do not see a health care provider again until their 6-week postpartum follow-up visit, when it may be discovered that they have been ill for many weeks. Women may hesitate to admit feeling depressed or unattached to the baby. Health care providers may dismiss their signs and symptoms as normal reactions to new motherhood. Women who may be particularly vulnerable to developing a postpartum disorder include those who have a history of psychiatric disorders, especially a bipolar affective disorder; are anxious or depressed during pregnancy; are younger mothers; lack a support network; have had difficult deliveries; or are under other current stresses. All women, however, should be considered to be at increased risk and a strong case can be made for screening for psychosocial risk factors during prenatal and postpartum care (Evins et al. 2000; Reid et al. 1998). There is a great need for physicians and community-based groups to provide information, support, and reassurance to new mothers and to participate in detecting and treating postpartum illness at an early stage.

## References

Ahokas A, Aito M, Rimon R: Positive treatment effect of estradiol in postpartum psychosis: a pilot study. J Clin Psychiatry 61:166–169, 2000

Alder EM, Cox JL: Breast feeding and postnatal depression. J Psychosom Res 27:139–144, 1983

American Psychiatric Association: Diagnostic and Statistical Manual of Mental Disorders, 4th Edition. Washington, DC, American Psychiatric Association, 1994

Ballinger CB, Buckley DE, Naylor GJ, et al: Emotional disturbance following child-birth: clinical findings and urinary excretion of cyclic AMP. Psychol Med 9:293–300, 1979

Beck CT: The effects of postpartum depression on maternal–infant interaction: a meta-analysis. Nurs Res 44: 298–304, 1995

Blumberg N: Effects of neonatal risk, maternal attitude, and cognitive style on early postpartum adjustment. J Abnorm Psychol 89:139–150, 1980

Braverman J, Roux JF: Screening for the patient at risk for postpartum depression. Obstet Gynecol 52:731–736, 1978

Brockington IF, Cox-Roper A: The nosology of puerperal mental illness, in Motherhood and Mental Illness, Vol 2: Causes and Consequences. Edited by Kumar R, Brockington IF. London, Wright, 1988, pp 1–16

Brockington IF, Winokur G, Dean C: Puerperal psychosis, in Motherhood and Mental Illness, Vol 1. Edited by Kumar R, Brockington IF. London, Academic Press, 1982, pp 37–70

Broussard ER: Evaluation of televised anticipatory guidance to primiparae. Community Ment Health J 12:203–210, 1976

Buckwalter JG, Stanczyk FZ, McCleary CA, et al: Pregnancy, the postpartum, and steroid hormones: effects on cognition and mood. Psychoneuroendocrinology 24:69–84, 1999

Caplan HL, Cogill SR, Alexandra H, et al: Maternal depression and the emotional development of the child. Br J Psychiatry 154:818–822, 1989

Charney DS, Woods SW, Nagy LM, et al: Noradrenergic functions in panic disorder. J Clin Psychiatry 51:5–11, 1990

Cohen LS, Sichel DA, Dimmock JA, et al: Postpartum course in women with pre-existing panic disorder. J Clin Psychiatry 55:289–292, 1994

Cowley DS, Roy-Byrne PP: Panic disorders during pregnancy. J Psychosom Obstet Gynaecol 10:193–210, 1989

Cox JL, Connor Y, Kendell RE: Prospective study of the psychiatric disorders of childbirth. Br J Psychiatry 140:111–117, 1982

Cutrona CE: Causal attributions and perinatal depression. J Abnorm Psychol 92:161–172, 1983

Cutrona CE: Social support and stress in the transition of parenthood. J Abnorm Psychol 93:378–390, 1984

Davidson JR: Postpartum change in Jamaican Women: a description and discussion on its significance. Br J Psychiatry 121:659–663, 1972

Davidson J, Robertson E: A follow-up study of postpartum illness 1946–1978. Acta Psychiatr Scand 71:451–459, 1985

Evins GG, Theofrastous JP, Galvin SL: Postpartum depression: a comparison of screening and routine clinical examination. Am J Obstet Gynecol 182:1080–1082, 2000

Frommer EA, O'Shea G: Antenatal identification of women liable to have problems in managing their infants. Br J Psychiatry 123:149–156, 1973

George A, Sandler M: Endocrine and biochemical studies in puerperal mental disorders, in Motherhood and Mental Illness, Vol 2: Causes and Consequences. Edited by Kumar R, Brockington IF, London, Wright, 1988, pp 78–112

Gordon RE, Gordon KK: Social factors in the prevention of postpartum emotional problems. Obstet Gynecol 15:433–438, 1960

Gregoire AJP, Kumar R, Everitt B et al: Transdermal oestrogen for treatment of severe postnatal depression. Lancet 347:930–933, 1996

Halonen JS, Passman RH: Relaxation training and expectation in the treatment of postpartum distress. J Consult Clin Psychol 53:839–845, 1985

Hamilton JA: Postpartum Psychiatric Problems. St. Louis, MO, CV Mosby, 1962

Hamilton JA: The identity of postpartum psychosis, in Motherhood and Mental Illness, Vol 1. Edited by Brockington IF, Kumar R. London, Academic Press, 1982, pp 1–20

Handley SL, Dunn TL, Waldron G, et al: Tryptophan, cortisol, and puerperal mood. Br J Psychiatry 136:498–508, 1980

Harris B: Maternity blues. Br J Psychiatry 136:520–521, 1980

Harris B: Biological and hormonal aspects of postpartum depressed mood. Br J Psychiatry 164:288–292, 1994

Harris B: Hormonal aspects of postnatal depression. International Review of Psychiatry 8:27–36, 1996

Harris B, Lovett L, Newcombe RL, et al: Cardiff puerperal mood and hormone study paper 2: maternity blues and major endocrine changes: the progesterone factor. BMJ 308:949–953, 1994

Hayworth J, Little BC, Carter SB, et al: A predictive study of postpartum depression: some predisposing characteristics. Br J Med Psychol 53:161–167, 1980

Hendrick V, Altshuler LL, Suri R: Hormal changes in the postpartum and implications for postpartum depression. Psychosomatics 39:93–101, 1998

Hopkins J, Campbell SB, Marcus M: The role of infant-related stressors in postpartum depression. J Abnorm Psychol 96:237–241, 1986

Kadrmas A, Winokur G, Crowe R: Postpartum mania. Br J Psychiatry 135:551–554, 1979

Kendell RE, Rennie D, Clarke JA, et al: The social and obstetrics correlates of psychiatric admission in the puerperium. Psychol Med 11:341–350, 1981

Kendell RE, Chalmers JC, Platz C: Epidemiology of puerperal psychoses. Br J Psychiatry 150:662–673, 1987

Kennerley H, Gath D: Maternity blues reassessed. Psychiatr Dev 1:1–17, 1986

Kumar R, Robson KM: A prospective study of emotional disorders in childbearing women. Br J Psychiatry 144:35–47, 1984

Lanczick M, Spingler H, Heidrich A et al: Postpartum blues: depressive disease or pseudoneurasthenic syndrome. J Affect Disord 25:47–52, 1992

Llewellyn AM, Stowe ZN, Nemeroff CB: Depression during pregnancy and puerperium. J Clin Psychiatry 58:26–32, 1997

Marcé LV: Traite de la Folie des Femmes Enceintes, des Nouvelles Accouchees et des Nourrices. Paris, France, Balliere, 1858

Margison F: The pathology of the mother–child relationship, in Motherhood and Mental Illness, Vol 1. Edited by Brockington IF, Kumar R. London, Academic Press, 1982, pp 191–232

McNeil TF: A prospective study of postpartum psychoses in a high risk group, I: clinical characteristics of the current postpartum episodes. Acta Psychiatr Scand 74:205–216, 1986

McNeil TF: A prospective study of postpartum psychoses in a high risk group, II: relationships to demographic and psychiatric history characteristics. Acta Psychiatr Scand 75:35–43, 1987

McNeil TF: A prospective study of postpartum psychoses in a high risk group, III: relationship to mental health characteristics during pregnancy. Acta Psychiatr Scand 77:604–610, 1988a

McNeil TF: A prospective study of postpartum psychoses in a high risk group, IV: relationship to life situation and experience of pregnancy. Acta Psychiatr Scand 77:645–653, 1988b

Metz A, Sichel DA, Goff DC: Postpartum panic disorder. J Clin Psychiatry 49:278–279, 1988

Murray L, Sinclair D, Cooper P, et al: The socioemotional development of 5-year-old children of postnatally depressed mothers. J Child Psychol Psychiatry 40:1259–1271, 1999

Nilsson A, Almgren P: Perinatal emotional adjustment: a prospective investigation of 165 women. Acta Psychiatr Scand Suppl 220:65–141, 1970

Nott, PN, Franklin M, Armitage C, et al: Hormonal changes and mood in the puerperium. Br J Psychiatry 128:379–383, 1976

O'Hara MW: Social support, life events and depression during pregnancy and the puerperium. Arch Gen Psychiatry 43:569–573, 1986

O'Hara MW, Swain AM: Rates and risk of postpartum depression: a meta-analysis. International Review of Psychiatry 8:37–54, 1996

O'Hara MW, Zekoski EM: Postpartum depression: a comprehensive review, in Motherhood and Mental Illness, Vol 2: Causes and Consequences. Edited by Kumar R, Brockington IF. London, Wright, 1988, pp 17–63

O'Hara MW, Rehm LP, Campbell SB: Postpartum depression: a role for social network and life stress variables. J Nerv Ment Dis 171:336–341, 1983

O'Hara MW, Neunaber DJ, Zekoski EM: A prospective study of postpartum depression: prevalence, course and predictive factors. J Abnorm Psychol 93:158–171, 1984

O'Hara MW, Schlechte JA, Lewis DA, et al: Prospective study of postpartum blues: biologic and psychosocial factors. Arch Gen Psychiatry 48:801–806, 1991

Paffenberger RS: The picture puzzle of postpartum psychosis. J Chronic Dis 13:161–173, 1961

Paffenberger RS: Epidemiological aspects of postpartum mental illness. Br J Prevent Soc Med 18:189–195, 1964

Paykel ES, Emms EM, Fletcher J, et al: Life events and social support in puerperal depression. Br J Psychiatry 136:339–346, 1980

Phillips LHC, O'Hara MW: Prospective study of postpartum depression: 4½ year follow-up of women and children. J Abnorm Psychol 2: 151–155, 1991

Pitt B: Maternity blues. Br J Psychiatry 122:431–435, 1973

Protheroe C: Puerperal psychoses: a long term study 1927–1961. Br J Psychiatry 115:9–30, 1969

Reid AJ, Biringer A, Carroll JD, et al: Using the ALPHA form in practice to assess antenatal psychosocial health. Can Med Assoc J 159:677–684, 1998

Resnick PJ: Murder of the newborn: a psychiatric review of neonaticide. Am J Psychiatry 126:1414–1420, 1970

Robinson GE, Stewart DE: Postpartum psychiatric disorders. CMAJ 134:31–37, 1986

Robson KM, Kumar R: Delayed onset of maternal affection after childbirth. Br J Psychiatry 136:347–353, 1980

Robson KM, Powell E: Early maternal attachment, in Motherhood and Mental Illness, Vol 1. Edited by Brockington IF, Kumar R. London, Academic Press, 1982, pp 155–190

Schopf J, Bryois C, Jonquiere M, et al: On the nosology of severe psychiatric postpartum disorders. Eur Arch Psychiatry Neurol Sci 234:54–63, 1984

Shereshefsky PM, Lockman RF: Comparison of counselled and non-counselled groups, in Psychological Aspects of a First Pregnancy. Edited by Shereshefsky PM, Yarrow LJ. New York, Raven, 1973, pp 151–163

Sichel DA, Cohen LS, Robertson LM, et al: Prophylactic estrogen in recurrent postpartum affective disorder. Biol Psychiatry 38:814–818, 1995

Stein GS: The pattern of mental change and body weight change in the first postpartum week. J Psychosom Res 24:165–171, 1980

Stein GS: The maternity blues, in Motherhood and Mental Illness, Vol 1. Edited by Brockington IF, Kumar R. London, Academic Press, 1982, pp 119–154

Steiner M: Psychobiology of mental disorders associated with childbearing: an overview. Acta Psychiatr Scand 60:449–464, 1979

Stewart DE: Psychiatric admission of mentally ill mothers with their infants. Can J Psychiatry 34:34–38, 1989

Stewart DE, Boydell KM: Psychologic distress during menopause: associations across the reproductive life cycle. Int J Psychiatry Med 23:157–162, 1993

Stewart DE, Addison AM, Robinson GE, et al: Thyroid function in psychosis following childbirth. Am J Psychiatry 145:1579–1581, 1988

Stewart DE, Klompenhouwer JL, Kendell RE, et al: Prophylactic lithium in postpartum affective psychosis: 3 centres' experience. Br J Psychiatry 158:393–397, 1991

Stowe ZN, Nemeroff CB: Women at risk for postpartum-onset major depression. Am J Obstet Gynecol 173:639–645, 1995

Teti DM, Messinger DS, Gelfand DM, et al: Maternal depression and the quality of early attachment: an examination of infants, pre-schoolers and their mothers. Dev Psychol 31:364–376, 1995

Uddenberg N, Englesson I: Prognosis of postpartum disturbance. Acta Psychiatr Scand 58:201–212, 1978

Villeponteaux VA, Lydiard RB, Laraia MT, et al: The effects of pregnancy on pre-existing panic disorder. J Clin Psychiatry 53:201–203, 1992

Watson JP, Elliott SA, Rugg AJ, et al: Psychiatric disorder in pregnancy and the first postnatal year. Br J Psychiatry 144:453–462, 1984

Welner A: Childbirth-related psychiatric illness. Compr Psychiatry 23:143–154, 1982

Williams KE, Koran LM: Obsessive-compulsive disorder in pregnancy, the puerperium and the premenstruum. J Clin Psychiatry 58:330–334, 1997

Winokur G, Behar D, Vanvalkenburg C, et al: Is a familial definition of depression both feasible and valid? J Nerv Ment Dis 166:764–768, 1978

Wisner KL, Wheeler RN: Prevention of recurrent postpartum major depression. Hospital and Community Psychiatry 45:1191–1196, 1994

Wollett A: Who breastfeeds? The family and cultural context. J Reprod Infant Psychol 5:127–131, 1987

Yalom I, Lunde DT, Moos RH, et al: Postpartum blues syndrome: a description and related variables. Arch Gen Psychiatry 18:16–27, 1968

Zelkowitz P, Milet TH: Postpartum psychiatric disorders: their relationship to psychological adjustment and marital satisfaction in the spouses. J Abnormal Psychol 105: 281–285, 1996

# Perinatal Loss

IRVING G. LEON, PH.D.

Grief following perinatal loss has been discovered relatively recently by the medical profession. Thirty years ago perinatal death was considered a nonevent by medical caregivers (Bourne 1968)—perhaps a disappointment, but certainly not a significant loss. Medical practice, accordingly, was oriented toward suppressing emotional reactions to the loss: parental contact with the dead baby was virtually unthinkable. Tranquilizers were dispensed to dull parental, especially maternal, distress. Parents were advised to forget what had happened and women were advised to try to become pregnant again as soon as they physically recovered. Today, the standard of care by medical caregivers is exactly the opposite: parents are now encouraged to see, touch, hold, name, and bury their stillborn or dead infant to make that child's life and death more real. Tranquilizers are avoided; instead, parents are encouraged to grieve together. They are usually urged to wait until this loss has been sufficiently grieved before embarking on another pregnancy.

Recent longitudinal, prospective studies indicate that at 6 months after pregnancy loss, women report significantly greater distress—anxiety, physical complaints, and especially depression—than do their counterparts delivering healthy babies; these differences tend to wane by 1 year (Beutel et al. 1995; Janssen et al. 1996; Neugebauer et al. 1997; Vance et al. 1995). This finding confirms the consensus held by most researchers and clinicians that over the course of the year following perinatal loss most women are able to resume preloss functioning, accompanied by a lingering, transient "shadow grief" (Peppers and Knapp 1980) often triggered by important anniversaries and reminders of the loss. However, about 25% of women experiencing pregnancy loss may be expected to have more serious and often enduring psychiatric difficulties following this loss (Zeanah 1989). This chapter explores why pregnancy and newborn demise is such a difficult loss to endure, identifies the many ways this loss affects family members, and suggests medical and psychiatric approaches that may deter the development of psychiatric difficulty and effectively address those problems when they arise.

# Epidemiology and Etiology

*Perinatal loss* is typically defined as fetal demise beyond 20 weeks' gestation through infant death 1 month postpartum and occurs in approximately 1.2% of all pregnancies in the United States (Cunningham et al. 1997). Although this rate is less than half the perinatal mortality rate in the United States in 1950, it is still significantly higher than other industrialized countries with wide differences among different groups in our country. There are half as many perinatal deaths in Japan than in the United States and the perinatal mortality rate for blacks in America is almost twice that of whites (Herz 1993). In short, we can do better.

About 15%–25% of all recognized pregnancies result in miscarriage. The actual rate of spontaneous abortions may be twice as high, because a subclinical early pregnancy loss is more likely to be viewed as a "late period" than a miscarriage (DeLuca and Leslie 1996). Ectopic pregnancies, increasing more than threefold between 1970 and 1986, now occur in almost 2% of all pregnancies (Stone 1995).

It is beyond the scope of this chapter to review medical aspects of pregnancy loss, but a few basic points are worth noting. Although most miscarriages are caused by major genetic abnormalities in the embryo or fetus that are not likely to recur, perinatal loss is usually the result of maternal factors leading to preterm delivery of a nonviable fetus. Many maternal factors, such as cervical incompetence, hypertension, and diabetes, are now successfully treated. The increasing incidence of ectopic pregnancies is due to the higher incidence of pelvic inflammatory disease and complications resulting from the use of intrauterine devices and from surgeries leading to tubal damage (Stone 1995).

Most of the psychologic investigation and the resulting changes in medical practice have focused on the relatively infrequent late-term perinatal loss, especially stillbirth. Furthermore, although with wider application of existing medical technology it is possible to reduce the rate of perinatal loss even further, the greater frequency of pregnancy among older women will increase their rate of miscarriages. Although there was a greater appreciation (and study) of the impact of miscarriages through the 1990s, there continues to be virtually no investigation of the specific psychologic repercussions of ectopic pregnancy losses.

This chapter more broadly considers miscarriages and ectopic pregnancies as well as perinatal death, noting the relevant differences among these losses. Related losses such as infertility (see Chapter 10) and pregnancy termination for fetal anomaly (See Chapter 3) will not be discussed in detail, although both are usually profound losses that complicate and magnify subsequent pregnancy losses. Because sudden infant death syndrome (SIDS) or "crib death" does not entail the unique aspects of a loss around pregnancy and also involves the death of an older infant, its repercussions are usually different and are not discussed here. Finally, elective abortion, when chosen without pressure from others during an unwanted pregnancy, usually does not result in the extended grief reaction of other pregnancy losses (Blumenthal 1991; Dagg 1991) and therefore is not discussed.

## Historical and Cross-Cultural Considerations

### Historical Review

Before the 1970s, the lack of awareness among medical and psychologic caregivers that perinatal loss generally evokes intense grief mirrored society's minimization or ignorance of this loss. As a logical outgrowth of their pioneering work on the development of parental attachment to the newborn, consolidated in "bonding," Kennell et al. (1970) were among the first to recognize the pattern of grieving following the death of a baby. Mounting appreciation during the 1970s of the usually profound grief following perinatal loss culminated in the first major study of this death by Peppers and Knapp in 1980 (*Motherhood and Mourning: Perinatal Death*) followed by more than a dozen handbooks over the next 15 years directed toward bereaved parents. In seeking to describe the normative pattern of grieving perinatal loss, clinical investigators during the 1970s demonstrated, ironically, how *individualized* the reactions to this loss were, thus providing richly textured and highly personal accounts (Grubb 1976; E. Lewis 1976).

Throughout the 1980s, quantitative investigations reported that perinatal loss in the Western industrialized world was a major loss of a family member (see reviews by Leon [1990, 1992b] and Zeanah [1989] for more detail). However, methodologic flaws such as failing to develop measures specific to perinatal loss or to track the course of this grief made it difficult to appreciate what is unique about this death at the inception of life as well as to identify early risk factors leading to later psychologic difficulties.

Hospital practice, however, dramatically improved during the 1980s. This decade marked the increasingly routine use of protocols embedded in perinatal bereavement programs helping parents to grieve. Kellner et al. (1981) pioneered perhaps the earliest multidisciplinary, hospital-based perinatal mortality counseling program, integrating effective delivery of services with data collection for research. RTS Bereavement Services (formerly Resolve Through Sharing) offered specialized training to hundreds of hospitals (especially obstetric nurses confronting perinatal losses in their patients) throughout the country (Limbo and Wheeler 1986). Finally, pastoral and lay caregivers—many of whom were dismayed by their own perinatal losses being ignored by medical professionals—played a crucial role in developing self-help groups and materials emphasizing the vital importance of social support and increasing recognition of this previously overlooked loss. Under the leadership of Sister Jane Marie (Lamb 1986) for over a decade, SHARE (founded in 1977) provided a model for over 400 community-based self-help groups oriented to pregnancy loss throughout the world. Ilse's (1990) work, *Empty Arms*, is perhaps the brochure most frequently distributed to parents following a perinatal loss to help them normalize powerful reactions and encourage them to construct memories to facilitate grieving.

During the late 1980s and early 1990s, more sophisticated self-report measures of perinatal loss were developed and increasingly used, thus helping to track longitudinally the course of perinatal bereavement as well as to understand better the different dimensions of this loss. Using their Perinatal Bereavement Scale, Theut et al. (1989, 1990) reported that recovery from pregnancy loss was often facilitated by a successful subsequent pregnancy. Using the Perinatal Grief Scale, a 33-item questionnaire increasingly becoming the standard in the field, Toedter et al. (1988) distinguished three distinct factors (i.e., active grieving, difficulty coping, and despair) that make up perinatal loss. They reported that it was not the intensity of initial grief but rather prepregnancy mental health that appeared to have the greatest impact on difficulties in coping and depression for couples 2 years postloss (Lasker and Toedter 1991). These important studies challenged some of the prevailing "clinical wisdom" and results of earlier, poorer research. For example, it had been believed (and recommended) that the bereaved couple should complete grieving before beginning the next pregnancy and that a more intense, early grief reaction predicted prolonged difficulties.

## Cross-Cultural Reactions to Pregnancy Loss

Because societal beliefs in part structure the boundaries of life and death in which perinatal loss is experienced, cultural attribution is a crucial ingredient in understanding the impact of pregnancy losses. Aside from a few general (Lawson 1990; Layne 1990) and anecdotal (T. H. Lewis 1975; Mammen 1995) accounts, culture has been largely ignored. Although quantitative studies have usually found sociodemographic variables to be poor predictors of psychologic and behavioral responses to perinatal loss (Kellner et al. 1984; Lasker and Toedter 1991; Nicol et al. 1986), qualitative examination of how different subgroups within our culture respond to perinatal loss continues to be lacking.

A recent volume edited by Cecil (1996a), *The Anthropology of Pregnancy Loss,* begins to correct the omission of cross-cultural investigation by providing ethnographic descriptions of pregnancy loss in rural India, Jamaica, New Guinea, Tanzania, and Cameroon as well as historical accounts of pregnancy loss in eighteenth-century England and early-twentieth-century Ireland.

The experience of pregnancy and its demise becomes part of the very fabric of a culture's beliefs and identity. In particular, pregnancy loss is commonly attributed to the woman being estranged from her spiritual and social world. Whether viewed as a target of evil spirits in India (Jeffery and Jeffery 1996) and Cameroon (Savage 1996) or as a victim of sorcery in Jamaica (Sobo 1996) and New Guinea (Winkvist 1996), the woman is still commonly viewed as ultimately responsible for reproductive outcome. In many of these cultures, pregnancy loss is considered a punishment for actual misdeeds (Wembah-Rashid 1996), for negative emotions such as anger, envy, or jealousy (Savage 1996), or for breaking societal taboos (Winkvist 1996). Physical explanations coexist with social/spiritual perspectives, allowing for the possibility of less condemning and more sympathetic responses (Chalmers 1996; Wembah-Rashid 1996; Winkvist 1996). Notably absent in virtually all of these cultural accounts is the grief reaction now almost ubiquitously reported in Western studies. Because many of these unborn children were regarded as not fully human (Savage 1996; Wembah-Rashid 1996; Winkvist 1996) or as the product of some transgression, mourning was often actively discouraged. Pregnancy loss simply did not signify the death of a valued, potential member of society. Importantly, many of these cultures believe pregnancy begins during the second trimester, often at quickening (Jeffery and Jeffery 1996; Sobo 1996; Wembah-Rashid 1996), thereby making the most common pregnancy loss, early miscarriage, a true nonevent.

Depending on the societal definition of pregnancy and the causal explanations for these losses, grieving is not an inevitable or even appropriate response for all or most members of a community. We also need to respect the nonmedical, seemingly irrational ideas of many women who experience these losses. Many Western women describe feelings of being punished for misdeeds ("What did I do to deserve this?") or attribution of pseudomedical explanations (e.g., eating certain foods, having intercourse during pregnancy, exercising), suggesting that we in the West share a need with non-Western cultures to create more social, personal, and spiritual understandings of these losses beyond what science can tell us. Indeed, not only medically sound explanations (Dunn et al. 1991) but even inaccurate, self-blaming beliefs may provide some reason for these losses, some sense of control and efficacy against their recurrence (Affleck et al. 1985; Tennen et al. 1986).

Although data are limited, it may be surmised that grief reactions to pregnancy loss were significantly less intense and common in the early twentieth century in the West. Several investigators have suggested that the more common occurrence of perinatal and infant loss in undeveloped countries today (Scheper-Hughes 1991) and in the West many years ago (Cecil 1996c) may have led to the view that such a loss was "just one of those things" (Cecil 1996c, p. 190), an almost expected disappointment but not a tragedy. Again, when infant mortality was high, babies were often not recognized as fully human and not worthy of much grief; the development of maternal attachment during pregnancy may have only gradually become a cultural norm, consolidating as the odds for survival increased (Cecil 1996b; Scheper-Hughes 1991). Today, a woman who becomes pregnant again after a perinatal loss may take a task-oriented, unenthusiastic approach to the pregnancy, thus avoiding the usual attachment to the unborn child until a healthy baby is born (Phipps 1985). Finally, historical accounts indicate that not much more than a century ago in the United States, children were still viewed as economic assets rather than as solely objects of love and caregiving (Mason 1994; Zelizer 1985). The medical discovery of perinatal grief in the past quarter-century perhaps naturally followed how increasingly normative that grief became in the preceding 50 years.

## Impact of Perinatal Loss on the Mother

There are many aspects to the psychologic repercussions of pregnancy loss. The unique nature of this loss is critically important and often missed by studies that compare or evaluate this loss with other family losses (such as death of a spouse or older child). The following areas can be used as a clinical guide for assessing maternal responses and risk factors. This discussion includes clinical issues faced by mental health workers, whether as part of a multidisciplinary team in the hospital at the time of loss (Kellner et al. 1981) or as a therapist working with the client sometime after the loss.

## Mourning the Death of a Baby

By the last trimester of pregnancy, both of the expectant parents, but especially the mother, develop an intense attachment to their unborn child as a unique, separate person (Condon 1985; Lumley 1982; Stainton 1990). Parental images of the unborn child are so powerfully consolidated by this time that a statistically significant degree of continuity exists in parental perception of the baby's temperament (e.g., activity, rhythmicity, adaptability, mood) in utero and postpartum (Zeanah et al. 1985).

Based on this attachment, parents grieve the death of their unborn child, already a beloved family member before birth. The usual pattern of grieving has been recognized for over 50 years (Lindemann 1944). After the initial shock and numbness on learning of the death (especially if it was unexpected), a period of intense confusion usually follows, with lapses in memory, anxiety, restlessness, irritability, and somatic distress. As the reality of the death gradually "sinks in," the bereaved parents yearn for the return of the deceased. Inconsolable sadness, preoccupation with memories of the deceased, and intensely painful periods of loneliness, guilt, anger, and hopelessness wash over the bereaved. Over the next year, the parents gradually become reconciled to this permanent loss; everyday activities are resumed, vigor in other relationships and the world in general is renewed, and capacity to feel pleasure is restored.

It usually takes more work to make perinatal loss feel real. Because so much of the image of the unborn child is imbued with fantasies during pregnancy (Deutsch 1945; Pines 1972), it comes as no surprise that couples after perinatal loss often struggle with whether a pregnancy actually occurred (Helmrath and Steinitz 1978; Lovell 1983). The raw material of memories fueling the grieving process is scarce or absent following perinatal loss. For this reason, virtually all researchers and clinicians working in this area recommend giving parents as many opportunities as possible to get to know their baby—seeing and holding their child and going home with mementoes and pictures testifying to their baby's existence. Much of perinatal loss involves grieving the loss of the future—relinquishing the wishes, hopes, and fantasies about one who could have been. It may be accurate to say that most grieving involves retrospective mourning (i.e., detaching oneself from the relationship that once was), whereas perinatal loss demands prospective mourning (i.e., detaching oneself from the relationship that was to be) (Leon 1990). Recent studies of bereavement in general (Klass et al. 1996) and of the death of a child (Knapp 1986; Rubin 1985) or that of a child's parent (Altschul 1988; Harris 1995) in particular suggest that it is normal for an intermittent, usually attenuated, grief to recur throughout one's life following major losses. This may occur after perinatal loss when the lost child-to-be would have reached the age at which cherished wishes for him or her would have occurred.

A critical determinant of the magnitude and quality of grief following perinatal loss is how much and in what way the child was wanted and loved. The common research finding of more profound grief following a later-term pregnancy loss (Cuisinier et al. 1993; Goldbach et al. 1991; Janssen et al. 1997; Kirkley-Best and Kellner 1982; Theut et al. 1989; Toedter et al. 1988) is logical based on the deepening attachment usually formed toward the child-to-be as the pregnancy progresses. Similarly, the generally muted, limited, or even absent grief following uncoerced decisions to surrender unwanted pregnancies or children—such as by elective abortion (Blumenthal 1991; Dagg 1991), relinquishing a child for adoption (Cushman et al. 1993; McLaughlin et al. 1988), or surrogacy (Fischer and Gillman 1991; Hanafin 1987; Schmulker and Aigen 1989)—provides powerful testimony that the woman's attachment to her baby is a variable, psychologic process rather than a biological, instinctive inevitability. These same losses usually provoke much more intense grief when the babies are in fact wanted—such as when the pregnancy is terminated because of fetal anomaly (Leon 1995; Zeanah et al. 1993) or when the loss is an essentially involuntary decision (e.g., studies of extended birthmother grief when adoption was only feasible choice available, prior to the legal availability of abortions or societal acceptability of unmarried parenthood [Deykin et al. 1984; Rynearson 1982].

To understand grief following pregnancy loss, clinicians should remember that along with the commonly felt loss of a very real baby may be the just as powerful evocation of a prior loss. Images of the child-to-be are a conglomeration of current and earlier object ties (Bibring 1959), a kind of projective screen of salient relationships among which incompletely mourned people may figure quite prominently. Not infrequently, an intractable, more chronic grief following perinatal loss may involve the unconscious resurfacing of an earlier loss, especially the death of a parent while the woman was still in childhood (Leon 1987, 1990).

Clinicians must recognize that grieving is a highly individual and variable process (Parkes 1985; Zizook and DeVaul 1985), not one that can be readily put on a schedule or compartmentalized into stages. Studies of grief in general (Wortman and Silver 1989) and perinatal loss in particular (Lin and Lasker 1996) indicate that most people do not, in fact, follow the stepwise pattern and diminuition of grief so frequently assumed.

## Repairing Narcissistic Losses

Reproduction fulfills many cherished wishes and ambitions that have little to do with parenting a child and everything to do with enhancing self-esteem. Pregnancy promotes self-worth and enriches feminine identity by fostering a sense of omnipotence, both in the act of creation and in becoming a parent (who is imbued with so much power in the mind of the young child); affirming gender identity through reproduction; and defusing death anxiety by ensuring a biologic continuity in projecting oneself into the next generation (Leon 1990, 1992b).

Pregnancy loss, therefore, causes multiple blows to self-worth and self-image. The growing intimation of omnipotence is shattered by this loss. The woman is unable to experience even the usual sense of control over her body. She faces the harsh finality of death when she least expects it, in the very act of creating life. Her own mortality is awakened, as she sometimes fears she will die as well. Pride in her femininity is transformed into shame and humiliation. Ultimately, she feels she has failed. Many of the usual reactions to pregnancy loss—persisting worthlessness, intense guilt, rage at the unfairness of it all, feelings of emptiness and fragmentation, and psychosomatic symptoms (Furman 1978; Kohut 1971; Lasker and Toedter 1991; Peppers and Knapp 1980)—may be better understood as resulting from the profound deprivation of normal narcissistic motives of pregnancy rather than the usual pattern of grieving the death of one's baby (i.e., object loss) (Leon 1990, 1992b).

Such profound narcissistic damage helps explain why many women experience a significant improvement in well-being when they are able to achieve a successful pregnancy following pregnancy loss (Hunfeld et al. 1997; Murray and Callan 1988; Theut et al. 1990). This enables them not only to parent but to repair a damaged self.

Narcissistic rage directed at medical caregivers may originate in the intense disappointment and hurt of the loss but is invariably compounded when caregivers are unable to appreciate the magnitude of this loss. Empathic communication that enables the woman to feel understood is vital in reducing narcissistic damage and healing self-esteem (Leon 1990). Quantitative studies indicate that after pregnancy loss, parents expressed significantly higher self-esteem when they were satisfied with the support they received from hospital caregivers (Murray and Callan 1988); the degree of parent satisfaction with care was directly related to the attentiveness and sensitivity of health care professionals rather than the total number of interventions they received (Lasker and Toedter 1994; Radestad et al. 1996b). In the words of Furman (1978), "For the professional person to tell the parents just to bear it is not enough; to be with them and to extend oneself in bearing it can do much more" (p. 216).

Women who suffer miscarriage or ectopic pregnancy may experience additional narcissistic damage because of its occurrence in the early part of pregnancy when there is usually much less separation between fetus and self and also because of the bodily damage to the fallopian tubes often accompanying ectopics. Furthermore, because most psychologic interventions are designed to grieve the loss of a baby, these early losses are often minimized, neglected, or ignored, resulting in patients reporting greater dissatisfaction in their care than those suffering later perinatal losses (Cuisinier et al. 1993; Lasker and Toedter 1994; Radestad et al. 1996a).

## Surmounting Developmental Interference

Pregnancy ushers in a new stage of development—parenthood (Leifer 1977; Shectman 1980)—that profoundly changes self-perception, perception of the meaning and purpose of life, and the value of family and relationships. As with any other developmental advance, turmoil in one's inner world is heightened, often leading to confusion, anxiety, and insecurity. This process of inner disorganization facilitates reintegration and further development of the personality, optimally increasing adaptation (Benedek 1959; Bibring 1959).

Pregnancy loss is a crisis within a crisis. Instead of progression to the next developmental stage, developmental interference occurs. Studies demonstrate that having had children previously reduces the depressive consequences of pregnancy loss (Graham et al. 1987; Janssen et al. 1997; Neugebauer et al. 1992b, 1997; Toedter et al. 1988). Women who have lost a pregnancy often talk of not getting on with their life goals, plans, and dreams. They feel stuck, off track, as if running in place.

Interpersonal isolation compounds the sense of internal stagnation. The woman may feel profoundly estranged and lonely, cut off from family and friends who are moving on with their lives and having families of their own. Soon after a pregnancy loss, it is often too painful to go to places frequented by young families. Many of the usual responses to perinatal loss, such as visualizing or hearing a baby, wishing to have another baby as soon as possible, and feeling intense pain and envy when exposed to other babies, may come from the frustration of not being able to parent.

Pregnancy losses near the beginning and end of a woman's reproductive life may also complicate developmental issues. For the teenager, pregnancy may be less a wish to parent than to feel like an adult or, regressively, seek to feel loved by (i.e., be taken care of by) a baby (Mishne 1986; Rosenthal 1993). When such a pregnancy is lost, the young woman must contend with the thwarted needs both to grow up and to satisfy early childhood longings, often quickly prompting another pregnancy. For women who have delayed parenthood into their 30s or later, the perceived danger of never becoming a biologic parent looms over this loss.

## Reviving Psychologic Conflicts

In their extensive review of the perinatal loss literature, Bourne and Lewis (1992) note a relative absence of psychoanalytic work in the area of revived psychologic conflicts. This absence may be the result of an unspoken allegiance to some traditional but now outdated psychoanalytic belief that unconscious psychologic conflicts cause perinatal loss (Leon 1996b).

Earlier conflicts and relationship paradigms may be activated by and interwoven with a perinatal loss. Clinical accounts (Condon 1986; Leon 1987, 1990, 1996a) and quantitative studies (Hunfeld et al. 1997; Lasker and Toedter 1991; Toedter et al. 1988) indicate that earlier psychologic problems, especially prior depression (Beutel et al. 1995; Janssen et al. 1997; Neugebauer et al. 1997), can interfere with the successful resolution of perinatal loss. Although complicated grief following perinatal loss can often be treated with short-term psychotherapy (Leon 1987, 1990, 1996a), serious, ongoing character problems may require more extended therapy to prevent further regression and to address aspects of grief (especially rage and guilt) intensified by the personality disorder.

## Mastering Exacerbating Circumstances of the Loss

The circumstances and causes of a loss typically are crucial factors influencing the course and outcome of bereavement (Bowlby 1980; Raphael 1983).

Clinical (Parkes 1980; Volkan 1970) and quantitative (Lundin 1984; Prigerson et al. 1997) studies indicate that a sudden, unexpected loss—trauma complicating grief—significantly interferes with adaptive resolution of grief, often resulting in higher psychiatric and physical morbidity. The ability to gradually digest and process a major loss before the actual death—anticipatory mourning—usually facilitates grief resolution, clearly documented in the significantly greater likelihood of parents to adaptively mourn the loss of an older child from a terminal illness as opposed to a sudden death (Knapp 1986; Leon 1990; Rando 1983).

Pregnancy loss is typically an unexpected death, often resulting in some traumatic aftermath. Flashbacks of the hospital experience, intense anxiety on returning to the hospital, and initial numbness soon after the loss are all tell-tale signs that the trauma needs to be processed before and while the death is grieved.

Other circumstances complicating the loss also need to be considered. Loss of a baby who survived some time after birth, thus leading to increased maternal attachment, often results in more extended grief. Medical threats to the mother's life concurrent with pregnancy loss (such as ectopic pregnancy and preeclampsia/eclampsia) may provoke an additional degree of trauma. When mothers engage in behavior contributing to fetal death (e.g., substance abuse) or demonstrably substandard medical care is provided, the intensity of guilt or rage may complicate coping with the loss. Skillful clinical acumen and tact will be necessary to determine and communicate how much the understandable preoccupation with this aspect of the loss is an adaptive catharsis of trauma or a barrier to dealing with other critical issues (e.g., grieving the baby's death). Only by encouraging a detailed telling of the story will it be possible to assess the degree of trauma as well as to begin to resolve that trauma.

## Other Important Factors

### Infertility Compounding Perinatal Loss

Clinical experience (Leon 1990, 1996a) indicates that infertility profoundly complicates pregnancy loss. Infertility usually heightens the developmental interference with realizing parenthood. The grief over a pregnancy loss following infertility may be exacerbated by how precious and long overdue this pregnancy has been—a psychic gestation measured often in years rather than months. Infertility may interfere with grief resolution by denying the opportunity for closure and reparation during the subsequent pregnancy and birth of a healthy child (Kirkley-Best and Kellner 1982; Peppers and Knapp 1980; Theut et al. 1989). The stigma associated with infertility (Griel 1991; Menning 1988) and the ensuing feelings of shame, failure, and worthlessness create additional obstacles to obtaining psychologic help (Leon 1990, 1996a), thus demanding clinical sensitivity in normalizing the psychologic repercussions. That some members of the psychiatric, especially psychoanalytic, community continue to believe that unconscious conflicts cause perinatal loss (e.g., Pines 1990) and infertility (e.g., Bydlowski and Dayan-Lintzer 1988) provides a haunting reminder of how much women, in one way or another, are held responsible for reproductive outcome in our culture (and many others) and how much psychiatric thinking has served that social ideology.

## Social Support Mediating Aftermath

Perhaps more than any other single variable, the availability or absence of social support may influence both the process and outcome of pregnancy loss. When couples are able to mutually understand and support each other (Forrest et al. 1982; Janssen et al. 1997; LaRoche et al. 1984; Nicol et al. 1986; Toedter et al. 1988; Tudehope et al. 1986) and medical caregivers are felt to be sensitively responsive to the loss (Harmon et al. 1984; Murray and Callan 1988; Smith and Borgers 1988), grief is reportedly more tolerable and the outcome more benign. Social support essentially means providing empathy, engendering a feeling of being understood, appreciated, and respected. One's pain is taken seriously and compassionately. It is defined less by what is said and how many things are done than by how these things are said and done (Furman 1978; Leon 1992a; Swanson-Kauffman 1986).

## Job Stress or Relief

Often-overlooked factors influencing the aftermath of pregnancy loss are the demands and satisfactions of work. Most women will still be grieving on returning to work. A fulfilling job can be extremely therapeutic in reducing narcissistic injury by promoting a feeling of competence again and by offering a welcome distraction from the continuous pain of grief. Other aspects of the work environment may make grieving more difficult or even intolerable. Total indifference by coworkers may be especially disorienting and painful. Some corporate or professional work climates may not tolerate even a muted grief. For health care workers, a "macho" medical ethos may permit compassion for one's patients while expecting immediate recovery for oneself. Medical, especially obstetric, caregivers need to be reminded that returning to a job so closely related to their loss may require that reentry be gradual and that their anxiety, sadness, and numbing while on the job is valid and normal.

## Putting Religious Faith to the Test

Almost universally, the meanings and causality of pregnancy loss are sought beyond the answers of science. Not how, but *why* did this happen to me? Religious beliefs may ease or intensify distress. Believing in the child's continued existence in heaven and an eventual reunion there following one's own death may be comforting and may relieve some of the pain of separation. Even if one does not claim to know God's purpose, believing that a God or gods exists (in whatever form one's religion describes) and that such a death is not without meaning can be reassuring. For others, religious beliefs become a source of increased guilt, a feeling of being punished. For those whose belief in God is based on a sense of fairness and justice, this loss may severely challenge their faith, leading to a bitter or cynical retreat from God or an eventual modification and reaffirmation of that faith. Clerical counselors may be most prepared to discuss religious matters, but all clinicians should inquire about and be ready to address these concerns. One need not (maybe cannot) have the answers in order to be enormously helpful by facilitating the processes of searching, questioning, challenging, abandoning, changing, and finding religious faith.

# Family Reactions

## Mothers and Fathers: Grieving Apart and Together

Although fathers clearly grieve for their unborn, stillborn, and newborn children who die, their grief tends to be significantly less intense and shorter than that of their mates (Benfield et al. 1978; Helmrath and Steinitz 1978; Smith and Borgers 1988; Theut et al. 1989; Vance et al. 1991, 1995; Zeanah et al. 1995). Peppers and Knapp (1980) attributed this pattern of incongruent grieving to the significantly earlier and more intense attachment by the expectant mother to the unborn child within her body compared with that of the prospective father. Although attempting to be supportive, husbands often betray impatience and irritation over their wives' seemingly endless grieving. Husbands fear their wives will never "get over it," and often want to "get back to normal" before their wives are ready.

The texture of grief often differs between mothers and fathers. Because the child-to-be is more a part of the woman's physical and psychologic self and felt to be more under her control, maternal guilt and diminished self-esteem tend to be more important ingredients of grief among women than among men (Leon 1990). For a man, relief over his wife's physical recovery may also eclipse grief over what has been lost.

Cultural gender roles that discourage masculine expression of intense feelings in general and of sadness in particular often magnify the different expressions of perinatal loss by fathers and mothers (Gilbert and Smart 1992). Men believe that they should be "strong." Social norms reinforce these role expectations—husbands are often asked how their wives are doing, with little concern about how they themselves are faring. They may feel ashamed and fear losing control of their intense emotions. They may grieve alone, crying in the car on the way to work, or their frustration and disappointment may be channeled into a more acceptably masculine emotion—anger.

Men are often assigned and assume the responsibility of taking care of their wives and managing concrete tasks, such as funeral arrangements, thus reinforcing the masculine preference to act rather than to feel. The sense of helplessness may propel them to work overtime to combat depressed feelings, to avoid being with a depressed wife, and to find some sense of accomplishment on the job. They may seek out distractions in sports or, more problematically, retreat into substance abuse. A husband may feel it is his duty to cheer his wife up rather than share his grief with her, increasing his wife's isolation and estrangement from him. Although his wife may crave physical affection and cuddling in order to feel loved, he is more likely to press for sexual intercourse as a way of feeling close to her, leading each to feel disappointed by the other.

These are general patterns. Some men experience a deeper loss of their child than do their wives following pregnancy loss. Notwithstanding these normative differences, most couples successfully weather the storm, eventually reporting increased closeness and a stronger marital bond (Gilbert and Smart 1992; Harmon et al. 1984; Helmrath and Steinitz 1978; Peppers and Knapp 1980). No evidence of increased incidence of divorce following perinatal loss has been found.

Couples' work can be an especially timely and appropriate intervention after pregnancy loss. It may provide a bridge to appreciate and empathize with the partner's experience—modeled by the clinician when appropriate—that is enriched by exploration of salient individual issues.

## Effects on Siblings: The Invisible Loss

Perinatal sibling loss has been called the "invisible loss" because the dead baby usually is not seen, little is heard about the loss, and often the sibling's many questions, confusions, and feelings go unacknowledged (Leon 1986b). This has significantly improved over the past 15 years. Siblings are increasingly allowed or encouraged to see the baby as they participate in opportunities for the whole family to grieve. However, the professional blindspot in this area continues, with virtually no quantitative research on the impact of perinatal loss on siblings and the most effective ways of helping them cope with this loss.

As early as age 2 or 3 years, a child can begin to grasp the essential concept of death as the permanent cessation of all functioning (Bowlby 1980; Furman 1974). Preschoolers, however, dramatically distort causality. "Magical thinking" and egocentrism dominate their interpretation of events. Thus, a child's jealousy toward the new baby during pregnancy may, after perinatal loss, become a conviction that he or she caused the death. At the same time, sibling rivalry should not be the only lens through which perinatal sibling loss is viewed. If permitted, young children (especially beyond toddlerhood) often powerfully and poignantly grieve their sibling's death. Ultimately, the child's developmental level, individual dynamics (including reactions to this pregnancy), and family style of grieving will decisively influence the child's reactions to this loss.

Clinicians can play a valuable role in helping parents understand and cope with their children's reactions to perinatal loss. The range of normal reactions should be reviewed with parents. Anxiety is common ("Will someone else die too?"). Depressed feelings may be based on many factors, including guilt ("Was I to blame?"), lowered self-worth due to neglect ("Nobody pays attention to me anymore"), and grief over the loss. These feelings may take the form of tired, bored, or angry behavior or of somatic complaints. It is normal for children to become preoccupied with death for a while, staging mock funerals or asking many questions about what happens to the body. A child's reluctance to show any interest may be based on the family's overt or unspoken rules about avoiding that topic. Children may also respond nurturantly toward their parents' grief ("What can I do to make the pain go away, Mommy?"). Perinatal sibling loss may foster a child's empathy.

Attending the funeral usually helps even young children by making the death concrete and providing social support. The child needs to be prepared for what he will see and hear and have a trusted adult nearby to answer any questions that arise. *It is crucial that parents explain what happened and how the baby died in clear, simple, concrete terms using words the child can understand.* This should be done when pregnancy loss occurs early (e.g., miscarriage or ectopic) as well as late; parents often deny a child's knowledge about the pregnancy or believe such a discussion creates an unnecessary burden, overlooking how the sometimes devastating impact of miscarriage (Beutel et al. 1995; Herz 1984; Neugebauer et al. 1992a, 1997) will be more confusing and troubling to children if not put into some understandable context. Drawing pictures can be a useful aid. Having the child repeat the explanation in his or her own words may tell the parent what has been understood or confused. It may be necessary to clarify for a younger child that the death was not caused by anything he or she felt or did but rather by a baby disease that cannot happen to anyone older in the family. Children may also need to hear that the parents' sadness over the death of the baby does not mean that they love their living children any less, although it may be hard for them to be as attentive when they are so sad. It helps parents to talk about the death, sad as they may be, and helps them feel better about themselves as parents when they are able to help their children cope with the loss and answer any questions.

A mental health consultation with a clinician familiar with childhood grief may be warranted when sibling distress becomes chronic. As with adult responses, unresolved perinatal sibling loss is often associated with earlier problems predating the loss. Clinical studies (Leon 1986a, 1986b, 1990) strongly suggest that children's disturbed reactions to perinatal sibling loss were strongly linked to a failure by parents to provide accurate and clear information about the loss and to support their child's feelings; to parental unresolved grief usually leading to an extended disruption in parenting; or to parents engaging the child in destructive patterns of family interaction, including scapegoating, extreme overprotectiveness, or using a subsequent child as a replacement for the dead baby.

## Caregiver and Community Responses

### How Caregivers Respond

Early work exploring the reactions of caregivers to perinatal loss focused on their tendency to resort to psychologic defenses to protect themselves against the intense feelings aroused by these losses (Bourne 1968; Klaus and Jnell 1982; Peppers and Knapp 1980; Stack 1982). This temporary relief of their own distress was bought, however, at the high price of failing to engage with their bereaved patients as well as blocking more effective coping. Among obstetricians, widespread knowledge of parental grief following perinatal loss (Kirkley-Best et al. 1985) has enabled them to be more helpful to their patients.

Medical training that dictates that it is unprofessional to have strong feelings because of the danger of becoming "emotionally involved" with one's patients must be challenged. Such thinking is bad for patients and caregivers. It is natural for medical caregivers who have participated in a pregnancy to feel loss, sometimes profound, at its demise. It is just as natural for caregivers to feel sad when they are with people who are grieving, helping them feel they are not alone and that their pain is shared by others. Bereaved parents need to see that their caregivers care.

Medical caregivers frequently feel guilty, inadequate, and helpless after a pregnancy loss, even when they know they did nothing wrong. They may fail to recognize the enormous importance of their emotional response to their vulnerable patients. What medical caregivers say and do at the critical time of this loss is not forgotten. Heartfelt, comforting words or touches can become lifelong sustaining memories that promote healing, just as seeming indifference can leave painful scars, irreparably damaging the patient–doctor relationship.

Overwhelming helplessness in the wake of pregnancy loss may cause trauma among medical caregivers: unforgettable memories returning as flashbacks or dissociative detachment masking as indifference. The cumulative strains on caregivers who regularly deal with these losses can be debilitating. Measures for resolving the occupational grief and trauma that affect medical caregivers need to be devised at individual, group, and institutional levels (Gilliland and James 1993).

## How Friends and Extended Family React

Until recently, there was little communal recognition of and compassion for perinatal loss. Talk about the baby was often replaced with a deafening silence that seemed to say, contrary to parents' grief, that nothing had happened and no one had died (Helmrath and Steinitz 1978; Peppers and Knapp 1980). Well-meaning advice intended to comfort and distract the bereaved was more likely to impede grieving by encouraging suppression ("Just try not to think about it and you'll feel better"), reinforcing maternal guilt ("It was meant to be"), and denying the loss ("You can always have another child").

Many people still recoil from the tragedy of pregnancy loss. Fearing they will say the wrong thing, they will often say nothing. It is also common to expect bereaved parents to return to "normal" and become their "old selves" within weeks or a few months at most.

It may be especially difficult for grandparents to tolerate their children's grieving. Grandparents often avoid talking about the baby for fear they will "upset" their children, which in turn leads bereaved parents to feel more isolated and misunderstood. Although adult siblings can be an important source of support, if siblings are pregnant or have young children, envy felt by the bereaved parents may be intolerable, increasing estrangement from extended family.

The most beneficial source of community support and understanding for perinatal loss has been self-help groups in which bereaved parents reaffirm for one another the normalcy of grieving by providing a place where those feelings may be freely expressed (Klauss and Jnell 1982; Peppers and Knapp 1980; Wilson and Soule 1981). For those whose grief has abated, these groups may provide a valuable channel for supporting others, transforming self-preoccupation into altruism (Videka-Sherman 1982). However, only a small percentage of the bereaved ever attend a self-help group; this resource is rarely used by minorities or the most socially isolated. Recommending a support group should never substitute for a caregiver's listening and responding to perinatal grief.

## Psychologic Management of Pregnancy Loss

### Hospital Practice

Klaus and Jnell (1982) provided the basic model of preventive intervention following perinatal loss. Doctors empathically but honestly keep parents fully informed of the baby's condition when problems emerge. Immediately after the death, the doctor meets with parents to give the tragic news, offer comfort and support, and answer any medical questions they may have. Parents are encouraged to validate their loss by having contact with their baby as well as taking home pictures and mementoes of the baby (e.g., footprints, baby bracelet, receiving blanket, and lock of hair). Dulling grief with sedation is avoided. Instead, the normalcy of the intense grief that can be anticipated (including rage, irrational guilt, and somatic symptoms) is explained. Because the parents are often in a state of shock at the time of death, a second meeting is scheduled for a few days later to discuss many of the same concerns, continuing to provide support and empathy for their feelings. The importance of sharing their grief is emphasized, as is the fact that no one is to blame. Parents are usually encouraged not to attempt another pregnancy until they have grieved this loss (at least 6 months). At 3 to 6 months after the loss, a third meeting is scheduled to review the autopsy findings, address any new issues, and determine whether additional follow-up meetings or mental health referral is needed.

With minor variations this basic approach has become the standard of care for all pregnancy losses, including outpatient obstetric practice (Leppert and Pahlka 1984). Many hospitals have created their own multidisciplinary grief support teams (Brown 1992; Kellner et al. 1981; Lake et al. 1983). An alternative approach is training all obstetric caregivers—often with the aid of protocols—in the hospital management of perinatal loss (Carr and Knupp 1985; Hutti 1988). A danger exists that sole reliance on grief specialists ("let them do it") will devalue the importance of all medical caregivers developing skills in responding to these losses.

However caregiving is delivered, it needs to be individualized (Leon 1992a). Too great a reliance on specific instructions will deplete the genuine interaction with bereaved parents that is the essence of good care. As important as contact with the dead baby is for most parents in order to make the loss real and to help them grieve their loss, such contact is not equivalent to mourning. Quantitative studies have not yet conclusively demonstrated that such contact facilitates grieving or is indispensable. Caregivers need to guard against exercising undue pressure on parents to view their baby. Caregivers will never go wrong when they allow themselves to empathize with their patients. By listening carefully, caregivers may be able to sense to what extent the loss is experienced as the death of a child, a profound blow to self-worth, the revival of an earlier loss or trauma, and/or an obstacle to becoming a parent. Finally, because these losses so often leave parents traumatized in the wake of feeling profoundly helpless, empowering them by offering options rather than dictating care is usually therapeutic. For example, instructing parents to wait at least 6 months before attempting another pregnancy is less effective than discussing the pros and cons about timing future pregnancies, allowing the parents to decide what is best for them (Davis et al. 1989).

Although models of follow-up care are available (Ewton 1993; Ilse and Furrh 1988; Maguire and Skoolicas 1988), insufficient follow-up after the family leaves the hospital is a serious deficiency in the management of pregnancy loss. In addition to facilitating continued grieving, follow-up care may provide the needed support for the next emotionally difficult pregnancy, fraught with anniversary revivals of anxiety and grief (Bourne and Lewis 1984; Phipps 1985). Research has repeatedly emphasized both the value of follow-up contact and how often it is overlooked. A single 15- to 40-minute phone call within 10 days of a neonatal death significantly reduced loneliness, depression, and guilt 2–6 months postloss (Schreiner et al. 1979). Even research interviews at 6 weeks and 6 months after a miscarriage appeared to have unintended therapeutic effects (Neugebauer et al. 1992b). Other investigations (Clyman et al. 1979; Helstrom and Victor 1987; Kellner et al. 1984) have indicated that up to 75% of parents who experienced a pregnancy loss wanted to discuss the details of the death or come in for a follow-up appointment 2–4 months after the loss. A recent national maternal health survey reported that over 50% of the sample experiencing perinatal loss wanted more information (Covington and Theut 1993).

## Mental Health Considerations

Mental health professionals play a crucial role in the continuum of caregiving for pregnancy loss. They can make diagnostic differentiations, such as distinguishing intense, immediate grief reactions from frankly psychotic episodes or appreciating the impact of earlier characterologic disturbance, such as borderline personality. They may serve valuable educational and supervisory roles. Accustomed to equating care with overt procedures, medical caregivers often need to learn that empathic listening and responding to a parent's intense grief is not "doing nothing," but is in fact beneficial. Outside the hospital as therapists, mental health professionals may mitigate the potentially destructive and chronic consequences of unresolved grief.

Thanatologists typically distinguish more-or-less normal grief from the range of pathologic or complicated grief reactions, including chronic, delayed, inhibited, or distorted mourning (Bowlby 1980; Horowitz et al. 1997; Jacobs 1993; Worden 1982). Treatment recommendations are similarly divided between supportive counseling oriented toward facilitating resolution of normal grief and interpretive psychotherapy directed toward defusing pathologic reactions (Worden 1982).

Although distinguishing self-remitting grief reactions from disturbed responses requiring psychologic intervention certainly has both heuristic and practical value, my clinical experience suggests these distinctions are best viewed as two poles on a continuum. That is, many if not most bereavements possess aspects of normal and disturbed grief; treatments, similarly, blend aspects of counseling and psychotherapy. Many responses viewed as symptomatic of distorted grief (e.g., furious hostility, depersonalization, loss of patterns of social interaction, and agitated depression) (Lindemann 1944) are not unusual reactions in the months following perinatal loss. It has been notoriously difficult to predict accurately the individuals at risk for later psychologic problems (Kellner et al. 1984; LaRoche et al. 1984; Leon 1990; Zeanah 1989). Too many quantitative studies continue to view marked distress and depressive symptoms in the weeks and first months following pregnancy loss as psychiatric disturbance (e.g., Friedman and Gath 1989; Neugebauer et al. 1997) rather than intense grief. Patterns of grieving in general (Klass et al. 1996; Wortman and Silver 1989) and perinatal loss in particular (Brown 1993; Lin and Lasker 1996) do not fit the dichotomy of normal versus pathologic grieving. Those labeled as having uncomplicated grief may be discouraged from seeking the help they could use, whereas those burdened with the idea of being "sick" may be too frightened to obtain the help they need. Many women who seek psychotherapy after perinatal loss describe significant unresolved childhood loss, disappointment, or emotional deprivation, especially with their own mothers, that has indirectly been awakened by this loss (Leon 1990).

During the year following pregnancy loss, psychologic help may prevent the development of further disturbance by facilitating grief and addressing maladaptive reactions based on prior emotional difficulties and/or inadequate social support—especially between the partners—two of the factors most convincingly associated with later emotional problems in quantitative studies (Lasker and Toedter 1991; Zeanah 1989). Substance abuse, the development of severe psychosomatic problems, suicidal behavior, or serious intent (not solely the thoughts or wishes of dying that are common) require immediate attention. When grief, depression, impaired job performance and interpersonal functioning, or any other emotional or behavioral difficulties do not begin to subside over the second half of the first year, treatment may be indicated. In subsequent years, psychotherapy may effectively address emotional difficulties based on earlier unresolved pregnancy loss that have become entwined with a prior unresolved loss or other latent conflicts and/or deficits (Condon 1986; Leon 1987, 1990; Turco 1981).

If the bereaved parent is able to form an effective therapeutic alliance, antidepressants usually are not necessary, because considerable symptomatic relief is generally achieved with short-term psychotherapy. In the presence of immobilizing depression or suicidal risk, antidepressants may be needed. With the increased use of selective serotonin reuptake inhibitors (e.g., fluoxetine, sertraline, and paroxetine) causing fewer side effects, antidepressants are increasingly being prescribed for depressive reactions associated with bereavement. Antidepressants without regular psychotherapy are not the appropriate treatment for maladaptive grief reactions.

## Treating Pregnancy Loss

Whatever the setting, a consultation sets the stage for treating pregnancy loss. Flexibility is crucial both in the number of sessions needed (usually three to six) and whether the partner is included, which is initially based on a client's wish. Consultation balances the tasks of crisis intervention, counseling, and assessment. The first session usually involves the patient telling the story of what happened (not, I would emphasize, a psychiatric interview with history-taking designed to obtain a DSM diagnosis). This approach fosters the therapeutic alliance, facilitates grieving and processing trauma by making the events real for the client and clinician, and highlights what is unique about this loss. The therapist counsels by providing direction as needed (e.g., the importance of sharing feelings with one's partner and explaining the appropriate details to one's children) and almost always by offering reassurance about the normalcy of intense grief (i.e., "you're not going crazy"). Psychological evaluation clarifies the multiple factors that make this loss so difficult, provides a history, and develops a diagnosis as the consultation progresses.

Flexibly structured short-term psychotherapy is usually the optimal intervention for recent perinatal loss (Leon 1987, 1990, 1996a). Even if long-term intensive psychotherapy appears warranted based on significant prior disturbance, clients rarely are prepared to accept that recommendation: they are not seeking characterologic change at this time, are inclined to experience such a recommendation as another narcissistic blow, and need the prospect of short-term relief. Clients are empowered by deciding when they are ready to stop rather than having to submit, helplessly, to a prescribed number of sessions, whether by theoretical design (Mann 1973) or according to the limits of managed care. Usually, one can be optimistic about significant improvement within 3–4 months following the consultation. By the end of the consultation, it can be valuable to distinguish—to the degree they can be heard—the longer-term issues that will not be the focus of these sessions, thereby setting realistic expectations for the treatment.

A cardinal principle in treating pregnancy loss is flexibility. All modalities should be considered and a multimodal approach used when appropriate. Although individual work may focus on complicated intrapsychic dynamics, marital work may be crucial in clarifying the different responses to this loss, and family work may promote a safe family atmosphere to grieve. Therapists need to be careful not to usurp the parental role in addressing this loss with children. Having a preferred orientation does not prevent using other approaches when warranted. Cognitive-behavioral techniques may be quite effective with specific symptoms (e.g., encouraging systematic desensitization with phobic reactions related to avoiding grief-evoking stimuli). A flexible approach to the frequency of meetings is also helpful. Weekly meetings are the norm, although more frequent sessions on short notice during more emotionally intense times (e.g., anniversaries) are effective, as are less-frequent meetings, especially in tracking the extended stresses of infertility treatments or a future pregnancy.

The positive therapeutic relationship is not the means but the essence of this work. If a solid alliance cannot be established, the prospects for effective short-term therapy are poor. Grieving is understood not solely as an intrapsychic process but also as an interpersonal transaction. In a sense this is an adaptive form of projective identification (Hinshelwood 1991) in which the bereaved, overwhelmed by the sadness of her loss, is assisted in expressing and getting through the pain of her grief by its being shared and felt by another. This process demands stable object relatedness in the bereaved (i.e., having basic trust in others) and a willingness by the therapist to participate in a subdued fashion in the grieving. Maintaining an empathic connection is more important than getting it right (i.e., interpretation of unconscious conflicts). Past dynamics are explored only as they influence current loss issues. Transference expression is not encouraged and interpreted only when necessary (i.e., when threatening the alliance).

Taking account of subcultural attitudes and religious beliefs, not as stereotypes but as normative contexts from which individual differences emerge, is another important facet of what the loss means to the parent. Challenging the stigmatization associated with some of these losses (e.g., infertility, pregnancy termination for fetal anomaly, adoption counseling) promotes a recognition of the social forces that help shape their impact.

Depending on the situation and timing, the therapist may gently encourage or advise against certain actions (e.g., it usually does couples no good to exacerbate intense grief by attending baby showers before they are ready or by celebrating major holidays when they feel they have nothing to celebrate). This is not telling them what to do but rather giving them permission to do what they already know is right for them.

Terminations vary. Even when the help has been deeply appreciated, endings tend to be more brief and less intense in this work than in more traditional therapies. The therapist will usually have an intuitive sense of a premature, unexpected, avoidant "bolting" as opposed to a readiness to end soon because the work is drawing to a close. Ironically, although the essence of this work is grieving multiple losses, the loss of the therapist is usually not grieved by the patient but is instead relinquished without much fanfare, as a transitional object loses its significance for the young child—once indispensable to her sense of security and well-being, but now expendable (Winnicott 1953).

## Conclusions

Although major advances have been made in the understanding and management of pregnancy loss, more work is needed, especially in appreciating the individual experience of this loss. More case clinical studies are needed to design interventions—studies that involve families, fathers, and children as well as mothers. Quantitative measures assessing the multiple dimensions of this loss (such as the Perinatal Grief Scale [Toedter et al. 1988]) are vital in tracking the course and outcome of reactions beyond a uniform model of grieving (Lin and Lasker 1996). Nonclinical studies must go into greater depth than the self-reports found in anecdotal handbooks. All of these approaches broaden our understanding of normal and maladaptive reactions to pregnancy loss, enabling a more individualized approach in hospital and psychologic practice than currently exists. Finally, integrating the impact of subcultural, ethnic, and religious influences on the individual phenomenology of these losses will provide a much needed anchor in the social realm.

## References

Affleck G, McGrade B, Allen B, et al: Mothers' beliefs about behavioral causes for their developmentally disabled infant's condition: what do they signify? J Pediatr Psychol 10:293–303, 1985

Altschul S (ed): Childhood Bereavement and its Aftermath. Madison, CT, International Universities Press, 1988

Benedek T: Parenthood as a developmental phase. J Am Psychoanal Assoc 7:389–417, 1959

Benfield DG, Leib SA, Vollman J: Grief response of parents to neonatal death and parent participation in deciding care. Pediatrics 62:171–177, 1978

Beutel M, Deckardt R, von Rad M, et al: Grief and depression after miscarriage: their separation, antecedents and course. Psychosom Med 57:517–526, 1995

Bibring G: Some consideration of the psychological processes in pregnancy. Psychoanal Study Child 14:113–121, 1959

Blumenthal SJ: Psychiatric consequences of abortion: overview of research findings, in Psychiatric Aspects of Abortion. Edited by Stotland NL. Washington, DC, American Psychiatric Press, 1991, pp 17–37

Bourne S: The psychological effects of stillbirths on women and their doctors. J R Coll Gen Pract 16:103–112, 1968

Bourne S, Lewis E: Delayed psychological effects of perinatal deaths: the next pregnancy and the next generation. BMJ 289:209–210, 1984

Bourne S, Lewis E: Psychological Aspects of Stillbirth and Neonatal Death, An Annotated Bibliography. London, England, Tavistock Clinic, 1992

Bowlby J: Attachment and Loss, Vol 3: Loss. New York, Basic Books, 1980

Brown Y: The crisis of pregnancy loss: a team approach to support. Birth 19:82–89, 1992

Brown Y: Perinatal loss: a framework for practice. Health Care Women Int 14:469–479, 1993

Bydlowski M, Dayan-Lintzer M: A psychomedical approach to infertility: "suffering from sterility." J Psychosom Obstet Gynaecol 9:139–151, 1988

Carr D, Knupp S: Grief and perinatal loss: a community hospital approach to support. J Obstet Gynecol Neonatal Nurs 14:130–139, 1985

Cecil R (ed): The Anthropology of Pregnancy Loss. Oxford, England, Berg, 1996a

Cecil R: Introduction: an insignificant event? Literary and anthropological perspectives on pregnancy loss, in The Anthropology of Pregnancy Loss. Edited by Cecil R. Oxford, England, Berg, 1996b, pp 1–14

Cecil R: Memories of pregnancy loss: recollections of elderly women in northern Ireland, in The Anthropology of Pregnancy Loss. Edited by Cecil R. Oxford, England, Berg, 1996c, pp 179–196

Chalmers B: Cultural variations in South African women's experiences of miscarriage: implications for clinical care, in The Anthropology of Pregnancy Loss. Edited by Cecil R. Oxford, England, Berg, 1996, pp 153–177

Clyman R, Green C, Mikkelsen C, et al: Do parents utilize physician follow-up after the death of their newborn? Pediatrics 64:665–667, 1979

Condon JT: The parental-foetal relationship: a comparison of male and female expectant parents. J Psychosom Obstet Gynaecol 4:271–284, 1985

Condon JT: Management of established pathological grief reaction after stillbirth. Am J Psychiatry 143:987–992, 1986

Covington SN, Theut SK: Reactions to perinatal loss: a qualitative analysis of the national maternal and infant health survey. Am J Orthopsychiatry 63:215–222, 1993

Cuisinier MCJ, Kuijpers JC, Hoogduin CAL, et al: Miscarriage and stillbirth: time since the loss, grief intensity, and satisfaction with care. Eur J Obstet Gynecol Reprod Biol 52:163–168, 1993

Cunningham FG, MacDonald PC, Grant NF, et al: Williams' Obstetrics, 20th Edition. Stamford, CT, Appleton & Lange, 1997

Cushman LF, Kalmuss K, Namerow PB: Placing an infant for adoption: the experience of young birthmothers. Soc Work 38:264–272, 1993

Dagg PKB: The psychological sequelae of therapeutic abortion: denied and completed. Am J Psychiatry 148:578–585, 1991

Davis DL, Stewart M, Harmon RJ: Postponing pregnancy after perinatal death: perspectives on doctor advice. J Am Acad Child Adolesc Psychiatry 28:481–487, 1989

DeLuca MA, Leslie PW: Variation in risk of pregnancy loss, in The Anthropology of Pregnancy Loss. Edited by Cecil R. Oxford, England, Berg, 1996, pp 113–130

Deutsch H: The Psychology of Women, Vol 2: Motherhood. New York, Grune & Stratton, 1945

Deykin E, Campbell L, Patti P: The postadoptive experience of surrendering parents. Am J Orthopsychiatry 54:271–280, 1984

Dunn DS, Goldbach KR, Lasker JN, et al: Explaining pregnancy loss: parents' and physicians' attributions. Omega 23:13–23, 1991

Ewton DS: A perinatal loss follow-up guide for primary care. Nurse Pract 18:30–36, 1993

Fischer S, Gillman I: Surrogate motherhood: attachment, attitudes, and social support. Psychiatry 54:13–20, 1991

Forrest G, Standish E, Baum J: Support after perinatal death: a study of support and counseling after perinatal bereavement. BMJ 285:1475–1479, 1982

Friedman T, Gath D: The psychiatric consequences of spontaneous abortion. Br J Psychiatry 155:810–813, 1989

Furman E: A Child's Parent Dies. New Haven, CT, Yale University Press, 1974

Furman E: The death of the newborn: care of the parents. Birth and Family Journal 5:214–218, 1978

Gilbert KR, Smart LS: Coping with Infant or Fetal Loss: The Couple's Healing Process. New York, Brunner/Mazel, 1992

Gilliland BE, James RK: Crisis Intervention Strategies, 2nd Edition. Pacific Grove, CA, Brooks/Cole Publishing, 1993

Goldbach KR, Dunn DS, Toedter LS, et al: The effects of gestational age and gender on grief after pregnancy loss. Am J Orthopsychiatry 61:461–467, 1991

Graham MA, Thompson SC, Estrada M, et al: Factors affecting psychological adjustment to fetal death. Am J Obstet Gynecol 157:254–257, 1987

Griel AL: Not Yet Pregnant: Infertile Couples in Contemporary America. New Brunswick, NJ, Rutgers University Press, 1991

Grubb C: Body image concerns of a multipara in the situation of intrauterine fetal death. Matern Child Nurs J 5:93–116, 1976

Hanafin H: Surrogate parenting: reassessing human bonding. Presented at the annual meeting of the American Psychological Association, New York, August 28, 1987

Harmon R, Glicken A, Siegel R: Neonatal loss in the intensive care nursery: effects of maternal grieving and a program for intervention. J Am Acad Child Psychiatry 23:68–71, 1984

Harris M: The Loss That is Forever: The Lifelong Impact of the Early Death of a Mother or Father. New York, Dutton, 1995

Helmrath T, Steinitz E: Death of an infant: parental grieving and the failure of social support. J Fam Pract 6:785–790, 1978

Helstrom L, Victor A: Information and emotional support for women after miscarriage. J Psychosom Obstet Gynaecol 7:93–98, 1987

Herz E: Psychological repercussions of pregnancy loss. Psychiatr Ann 14:454–457, 1984

Herz E: Perinatal loss, in Psychological Aspects of Women's Health Care. Edited by Stewart DE, Stotland NL. Washington DC, American Psychiatric Press, 1993, pp 139–161

Hinshelwood RD: A Dictionary of Kleinian Thought, 2nd Edition. Northvale, NJ, Jason Aronson, 1991

Horowitz, MJ, Siegel B, Holen A, et al: Diagnostic criteria for complicated grief disorder. Am J Psychiatry 154:904–910, 1997

Hunfeld JAM, Wladimiroff JW, Passchier J: Prediction and course of grief four years after perinatal loss due to congenital anomalies: a follow-up study. Br J Med Psychol 70:85–91, 1997

Hutti MH: A quick reference table of interventions to assist families to cope with pregnancy loss or neonatal death. Birth 15:33–35, 1988

Ilse S: Empty Arms: Coping after Miscarriage, Stillborn, and Infant Death, 2nd Edition. Maple Plains, MN, Wintergreen Press, 1990

Ilse S, Furrh CB: Development of a comprehensive follow-up care program after perinatal and neonatal loss. J Perinat Neonatal Nurs 2:23–33, 1988

Jacobs S: Pathologic Grief: Maladaptation to Loss. Washington DC, American Psychiatric Press, 1993

Janssen HJEM, Cuisinier MCJ, Hoogduin KAL, et al: Controlled prospective study on the mental health of women following pregnancy loss. Am J Psychiatry 153:226–230, 1996

Janssen HJEM, Cuisinier MCJ, de Graauw PHM, et al: A prospective study of risk factors predicting grief intensity following pregnancy loss. Arch Gen Psychiatry 54:56–61, 1997

Jeffery P, Jeffery R: Delayed periods and falling babies: the ethnophysiology and politics of pregnancy loss in rural north India, in The Anthropology of Pregnancy Loss. Edited by Cecil R. Oxford, England, Berg, 1996, pp 17–37

Kellner K, Kirkley-Best E, Chesborough S, et al: Perinatal mortality counseling program for families who experience a stillbirth. Death Education 5:29–35, 1981

Kellner K, Donnelly W, Gould S: Parental behavior after perinatal death: lack of predictive demographic and obstetric variables. Obstet Gynecol 63:809–814, 1984

Kennell J, Slyter, H, Klaus M: The mourning response of parents to the death of a newborn infant. N Engl J Med 283:344–349, 1970

Kirkley-Best E, Kellner K: The forgotten grief: a review of the psychology of stillbirth. Am J Orthopsychiatry 52:420–429, 1982

Kirkley-Best E, Kellner K, LaDue T: Attitudes towards stillbirth and death threat level in a sample of obstetricians. Omega 15:317–327, 1985

Klass D, Silverman PR, Nickman SL (eds): Continuing Bonds/ New Understandings of Grief. Bristol, PA, Taylor and Francis, 1996

Klaus M, Jnell J: Parent-Infant Bonding, 2nd Edition, St. Louis, MO, C.V. Mosby, 1982

Knapp R: Beyond Endurance: When a Child Dies. New York, Schocken Books, 1986

Kohut H: The Analysis of the Self. New York, International Universities Press, 1971

Lake M, Knuppel RA, Murphy J, et al: The role of a grief support team following stillbirth. Am J Obstet Gynecol 146:877–881, 1983

Lamb JM: SHARE, in Parental Loss of a Child. Edited by Rando T. Champaign, IL, Research Press, 1986, pp 499–507

LaRoche C, Lalinec-Michaud M, Engelsmann F, et al: Grief reactions to perinatal death: a follow-up study. Can J Psychiatry 29:14–19, 1984

Lasker JN, Toedter LJ: Acute versus chronic grief: the case of pregnancy loss. Am J Orthopsychiatry 61:510–522, 1991

Lasker JN, Toedter LJ: Satisfaction with hospital care and interventions after pregnancy loss. Death Studies 18:41–64, 1994

Lawson LV: Culturally sensitive support for grieving parents. Am J Matern Child Nurs 15:76–79, 1990

Layne LL: Motherhood lost: cultural dimensions of miscarriage and stillbirth in America. Women Health 16:69–98, 1990

Leifer M: Psychological changes accompanying pregnancy and motherhood. Genet Psychol Monogr 95:55–96, 1977

Leon IG: Intrapsychic and family dynamics in perinatal sibling loss. Infant Mental Health Journal 7:200–213, 1986a

Leon IG: The invisible loss: the impact of perinatal loss on siblings. J Psychosom Obstet Gynaecol 5:1–14, 1986b

Leon IG: Short-term psychotherapy for perinatal loss. Psychotherapy 24:186–195, 1987

Leon IG: When a Baby Dies: Psychotherapy for Pregnancy and Newborn Loss. New Haven, CT, Yale University Press, 1990

Leon IG: Perinatal loss: a critique of current practices. Clin Pediatr 31:366–374, 1992a

Leon IG: The psychoanalytic conceptualization of perinatal loss: a multidimensional model. Am J Psychiatry 149:1464–1472, 1992b

Leon IG: Pregnancy termination after fetal anomaly: clinical considerations. Infant Ment Health J 16:112–126, 1995

Leon IG: Reproductive loss: barriers to psychoanalytic treatment. J Am Acad Psychoanal 24:341–352, 1996a

Leon IG: Revising psychoanalytic understandings of perinatal loss. Psychoanal Psychol 13:161–176, 1996b

Leppert PC, Pahlka BS: Grieving characteristics after spontaneous abortion: a management approach. Obstet Gynecol 64:119–122, 1984

Lewis E: The management of stillbirth: coping with an unreality. Lancet 2:619–620, 1976

Lewis TH: A culturally patterned depression in a mother after loss of a child. Psychiatry 38:92–95, 1975

Limbo RK, Wheeler SR: When a Baby Dies: A Handbook for Healing and Helping. La Crosse, WI, Resolve Through Sharing, 1986

Lin SX, Lasker JN: Patterns of grief reaction after pregnancy loss. Am J Orthopsychiatry 66:262–271, 1996

Lindemann E: Symptomatology and management of acute grief. Am J Psychiatry 101:141–148, 1944

Lovell A: Some questions of identity: late miscarriage, stillbirth, and perinatal loss. Soc Sci Med 17:755–761, 1983

Lumley J: Attitudes to the fetus among primigravidae. Aus Paediatric J 18:106–109, 1982

Lundin T: Morbidity following sudden and unexpected bereavement. Br J Psychiatry 144:84–88, 1984

Maguire D, Skoolicas S: Developing a bereavement follow-up program. J Perinat Neonatal Nurs 2:67–77, 1988

Mammen OK: Women's reaction to perinatal loss in India: an exploratory, descriptive study. Infant Ment Health J 16:96–101, 1995

Mann J: Time-Limited Psychotherapy. Cambridge, MA, Harvard University Press, 1973

Mason MA: From Father's Property to Children's Rights: The History of Child Custody in the United States. New York, Columbia University Press, 1994

McLaughlin SD, Pearce SD, Manninen DL, et al: To parent or relinquish: consequences for adolescent mothers. Soc Work 33:320–324, 1988

Menning BE: Infertility: A Guide for the Childless Couple, 2nd Edition. New York, Prentice Hall, 1988

Mishne JM: Clinical Work with Adolescents. New York, Free Press, 1986

Murray J, Callan VJ: Predicting adjustment to perinatal death. Br J Med Psychol 61:237–244, 1988

Neugebauer R, Kline J, O'Connor P, et al: Depressive symptoms in women in the six months after miscarriage. Am J Obstet Gynecol 166:104–109, 1992a

Neugebauer R, Kline J, O'Connor P, et al: Determinants of depressive symptoms in the early weeks after miscarriage. Am J Public Health 82:1332–1339, 1992b

Neugebauer R, Kline J, Shrout P, et al: Major depressive disorder in the 6 months after miscarriage. JAMA 277:383–388, 1997

Nicol MT, Tompkins JR, Campbell NA, et al: Maternal grieving response after perinatal death. Med J Aust 144:287–295, 1986

Parkes CM: Bereavement counseling: does it work? BMJ 281:3–6, 1980

Parkes CM: Bereavement. Br J Psychiatry 146:11–17, 1985

Peppers L, Knapp R: Motherhood and Mourning: Perinatal Death. New York, Praeger, 1980

Phipps S: The subsequent pregnancy after stillbirth: anticipatory parenthood in the face of uncertainty. Int J Psychiatry Med 15:243–264, 1985

Pines D: Pregnancy and motherhood: interaction between fantasy and reality. Br J Med Psychol 45:333–343, 1972

Pines D: Pregnancy, miscarriage and abortion: a psychoanalytic perspective. Int J Psychoanal 71:301–307, 1990

Prigerson HG, Bierhals AJ, Kasl SV, et al: Traumatic grief as a risk factor for mental and physical morbidity. Am J Psychiatry 154:616–623, 1997

Radestad I, Nordin C, Steineck G, et al: Stillbirth is no longer managed as a nonevent: a nationwide study in Sweden. Birth 23:209–215, 1996a

Radestad I, Steineck G, Nordin C, et al: Psychic and social consequences of women in relation to memories of a stillborn child: a pilot study. Gynecol Obstet Invest 41:194–198, 1996b

Rando T: An investigation of grief and adaptation in parents whose children have died of cancer. J Pediatric Psychol 8:3–20, 1983

Raphael B: The Anatomy of Bereavement. New York, Basic Books, 1983

Rosenthal M: Adolescent pregnancy, in Psychological Aspects of Women's Health Care. Edited by Stewart DE, Stotland NL. Washington DC, American Psychiatric Press, 1993, pp 97–114

Rubin S: Maternal attachment and child death: on adjustment, relationship, and resolution. Omega 15:347–352, 1985

Rynearson E: Relinquishment and its maternal complications: a preliminary study. Am J Psychiatry 139:338–340, 1982

Savage OMN: "Children of the rope" and other aspects of pregnancy loss in Cameroon, in The Anthropology of Pregnancy Loss. Edited by Cecil R. Oxford, England, Berg, 1996, pp 95–109

Scheper-Hughes N: Social indifference to child death. Lancet 337:1144–1147, 1991

Schmulker I, Aigen BP: The terror of surrogate motherhood: fantasies, realities, and viable legislation, in Gender in Transition: A New Frontier. Edited by Offerman-Zuckerberg J. New York, Plenum, 1989, pp 235–248

Schreiner R, Gresham E, Green M: Physician's responsibility to parents after death of an infant. Am J Dis Child 133:723–726, 1979

Shectman KW: Motherhood as an adult developmental phase. Am J Psychoanal 40:273–281, 1980

Smith A, Borgers S: Parental grief response to perinatal death. Omega 19:203–214, 1988

Sobo EJ: Cultural explanations for pregnancy loss in rural Jamaica, in The Anthropology of Pregnancy Loss. Edited by Cecil R. Oxford, England, Berg, 1996, pp 39–58

Stack J: Reproductive casualties. Perinatal Press 6:31–36, 1982

Stainton MC: Parents' awareness of their unborn infant in the third trimester. Birth 17:92–96, 1990

Stone LR: Pregnancy losses, in Primary Care of Women. Edited by Lemcke D, Pattison J, Marshall L. Norwalk, CT, Appleton & Lange, 1995, pp 531–539

Swanson-Kauffman K: Caring in the instance of unexpected early pregnancy losses. Top Clin Nurs 8:37–46, 1986

Tennen H, Affleck G, Gershman K: Self-blame among parents of infants with perinatal complications: the role of self-protective motives. J Pers Soc Psychol 50:690–696, 1986

Theut SK, Pedersen FA, Zaslow MJ, et al: Perinatal loss and parental bereavement. Am J Psychiatry 146:635–639, 1989

Theut SK, Zaslow MJ, Rabinovich B, et al: Resolution of parental bereavement after a perinatal loss. J Am Acad Child Adolesc Psychiatry 29:521–525, 1990

Toedter, LJ, Lasker JN, Alhadeff JM: The Perinatal Grief Scale: development and initial validation. Am J Orthopsychiatry 58:435–449, 1988

Tudehope DI, Iredell J, Rodgers D, et al: Neonatal death: grieving families. Med J Aust 144:290–292, 1986

Turco R: The treatment of unresolved grief following loss of an infant. Am J Obstet Gynecol 141:503–507, 1981

Vance JC, Foster WJ, Najman JM, et al: Early parental responses to sudden infant death, stillbirth or neonatal death. Med J Aust 155:292–297, 1991

Vance JC, Najman JM, Thearle MJ, et al: Psychological changes in parents eight months after the loss of an infant from stillbirth, neonatal death, or sudden infant death syndrome: a longitudinal study. Pediatrics 96:933–938, 1995

Videka-Sherman L: Coping with the death of a child. Am J Orthopsychiatry 52:688–698, 1982

Volkan V: Typical findings in pathological grief. Psychiatr Q 44:231–250, 1970

Wembah-Rashid JAR: Explaining pregnancy loss in matrilineal southeast Tanzania, in The Anthropology of Pregnancy Loss. Edited by Cecil R. Oxford, England, Berg, 1996, pp 75–93

Wilson A, Soule D: The role of a self-help group in working with parents of a stillborn baby. Death Education 5:175–186, 1981

Winkvist A: Water spirits, medicine men, and witches: avenues to successful reproduction among the Abelam, Papua New Guinea, in The Anthropology of Pregnancy Loss. Edited by Cecil R. Oxford, England, Berg, 1996, pp 59–74

Winnicott DW: Transitional objects and transitional phenomena. Int J Psychoanal 34:89–97, 1953

Worden JW: Grief Counseling and Grief Therapy: A Handbook for the Mental Health Practitioner. New York, Springer, 1982

Wortman C, Silver R: The myths of coping with loss. J Consult Clin Psychol 57:349–357, 1989

Zeanah CH: Adaptation following perinatal loss: a critical review. J Am Acad Child Adolesc Psychiatry 28:467–480, 1989

Zeanah CH, Keener M, Stewart L, et al: Prenatal perception of infant personality: a preliminary investigation. J Am Acad Child Psychiatry 24:204–210, 1985

Zeanah CH, Dailey J, Rosenblatt M, et al: Do women grieve after terminating pregnancies because of fetal anomalies? A controlled investigation. Obstet Gynecol 82:270–275, 1993

Zeanah CH, Danis B, Hirshberg L, et al: Initial adaptation in mothers and fathers following perinatal loss. Infant Ment Health J 16:80–93, 1995

Zelizer VA: Pricing the Priceless Child: The Changing Social Value of Children. New York, Basic Books, 1985

Zizook S, DeVaul R: Unresolved grief. Am J Psychoanal 45:370–379, 1985

# Gynecology

# Psychological Aspects of the Menstrual Cycle

MARGARET F. JENSVOLD, M.D.
CORINNA E. DAN, R.N., B.S.N.

Biomedical researchers have commonly viewed the menstrual cycle as a confounding factor in research rather than as a legitimate subject of scientific study. This view has contributed to the exclusion of women of reproductive age from much health research (Kinney et al. 1981). At the same time a plethora of media articles have conveyed primarily negative images of the menstrual cycle and of premenstrual syndrome, along with conflicting diagnostic and treatment information and jokes (Chrisler and Levy 1990). If women and their health care providers are confused about the menstrual cycle, there is good reason.

Nevertheless, we do have some knowledge. Research during the past couple of decades has helped clarify what the questions are and has pointed to directions for future research. This chapter is intended not to be entirely comprehensive, citing all research findings, but rather to present current research findings and illustrative points to provide a framework for clinicians, researchers, and health care consumers for conceptualizing the role of the menstrual cycle in psychiatry.

Many, if not most, physiologic parameters vary in a circadian manner (e.g., body temperature, cortisol level, thyrotropin-releasing hormone level, sleep-wake), usually without causing symptoms and often with the person not even aware that the changes are occurring. Likewise, many physiologic parameters vary over the course of the normal menstrual cycle, not causing symptoms and often with the woman being unaware of the change. Cultural factors are well documented to have a significant influence on expectations and perceptions related to the menstrual cycle. With both physiologic and cultural factors contributing to changes over the menstrual cycle, how is one to make sense of pathology related to this cycle? This chapter addresses the physiology, cultural considerations, and diagnosis and treatment related to the menstrual cycle with attention to methodologic and political concerns.

# Physiology

## Normal Menstrual Cycle

The core events of the normal menstrual cycle are an integrally interconnected neuroendocrine feedback loop: the hypothalamic–pituitary–ovarian axis.[1] Readers are referred elsewhere for detailed accounts of the endocrine events of the normal menstrual cycle (Severino and Moline 1989; Speroff et al. 1982). The menstrual cycle can be thought of as consisting of two phases, the follicular phase and the luteal phase, with cyclicity occurring in a number of organs and tissues (Figures 9–1 and 9–2). What is happening suprahypothalamically over the course of the menstrual cycle is less known to us, but animal research shows that neurotransmitters cycle catamenially[2] in various parts of the brain (McEwen 1988). The uterus is not a core player in the normal menstrual cycle, but rather is a target organ for hormonal action. Its regular, recurrent menstrual flow is an external indicator to the woman that yet another menstrual cycle has been completed and that a new one is beginning.

What constitutes the endogenous time clock of the menstrual cycle is relatively unknown at present. The suprachiasmatic nucleus and associated structures are suspected (Kawakami et al. 1980). Circadian cycling is thought to be driven by the suprachiasmatic nucleus, with light input through the retinohypothalamic tract serving as a zeitgeber, or entraining factor, that affects the cycle length but not the presence or absence of the circadian cycle altogether. In the absence of light–dark cues the circadian time clock freeruns, still cycling in a regular circadian manner but with a slightly longer cycle length on average (27 hours free running compared with 24 hours day–night entrained). Whether ovarian input to the brain serves as a zeitgeber—simply entraining the timing of a catamenial cycle that would freerun without ovari-

[1]A hypothalamic–pituitary–gonadal axis exists in men as well, of course: the hypothalamus–pituitary–testicular axis. That it has no external indicator of its timing does not in itself mean that it does not have an endogenous timing mechanism.

[2] *Catamenial* means of or related to menses or the menstrual cycle.

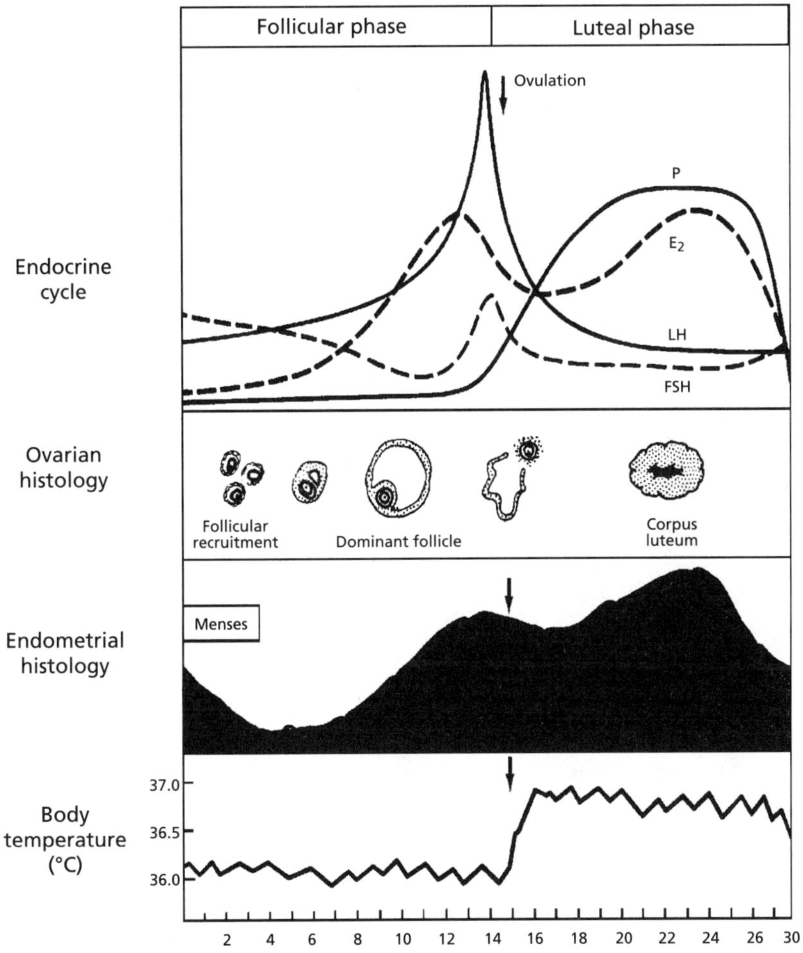

**FIGURE 9–1.** The normal menstrual cycle. Hormonal, ovarian, endometrial, and basal body temperature changes and their relationships throughout the normal menstrual cycle are shown. E2 = estradiol; FSH = follicle stimulating hormone; LH = luteinizing hormone; P = progesterone.

*Source.* Reprinted from Carr BR, Wilson JD: "Disorders of the Ovary and Female Reproductive Tract," in *Harrison's Principles of Internal Medicine*, 11th Edition. Edited by Braunwald E, Isselbacher KJ, Petersdorf RG, et al. New York, McGraw-Hill, 1987, p. 1823. Copyright 1987, The McGraw-Hill Companies. Used with permission.

an input—or whether ovarian input is integral to the continued catamenial cycling of the brain is not entirely known. There is some evidence in each direction. Gonadotropin-releasing hormone (GnRH) agonist treatment evi-

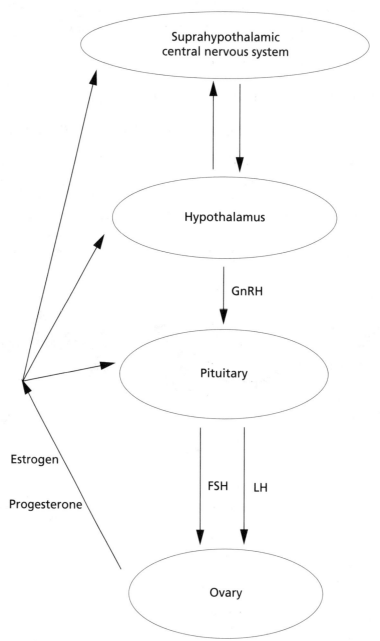

**FIGURE 9-2.** Hypothalamic–pituitary–ovarian axis. The pathways of endogenous and exogenous hormones are shown. FSH = follicle-stimulating hormone; GnRH = gonadotropin-releasing hormone; LH = luteinizing hormone.

dence indicates that when ovarian input is removed, catamenial cycling of central nervous system symptoms stops (Hammarback and Backstrom 1988). On the other hand, a study of patients with premenstrual syndrome using a progesterone antagonist, RU-486, showed that when the normal hormonal milieu of the latter quarter of the menstrual cycle is removed, thus displacing the timing of menstrual flow, menstrually related mood symptoms still occur at the usual time in some patients (Schmidt et al. 1991). This indicates either that endocrine events earlier in the cycle ordain the timing of the cyclic mood symptoms or that central nervous system cycling continues independently of the peripheral hormonal milieu, at least for a time.

An exogenous factor affecting the menstrual cycle that has been studied is the presence of other cycling females. The tendency toward synchrony of cycles among females who spend an extended time together is mediated by pheromones produced by the women themselves that expedite or delay the onset of the ovarian cycle (McClintock 1984).

## Variability in the Normal Menstrual Cycle

An occasional anovulatory cycle or shortened luteal phase is not uncommon. However, certain groups are more prone to menstrual irregularities, including heavy exercisers, anorexics, and women taking neuroleptic medications (Sullivan and Lukoff 1990) or abusing substances. At least for heavy exercisers, anovulatory cycles appear to be associated with increased bone loss.

## Cultural Aspects

Evidence for a strong cultural influence on our view of the menstrual cycle comes from several fronts. Menstrual taboos have existed across cultures and across time, including today. Deutsch (1944) discussed the psychologic meaning of menstruation, pointing out the reasons why women deny and hide it and also pointing out the tendency to prefer to view the menstrual cycle as a "biologic function" rather than as having great psychologic significance for the woman. The words we use to describe the menstrual cycle convey our tendency to view it negatively, rather than positively (Martin 1987). Premenstrual syndrome seems to be to the twentieth century what neurasthenia was to the nineteenth century—a nebulous disorder primarily of women that involves the menstrual cycle, has numerous symptoms, etiologies, and treatments proposed, and conveys a negative view of women (King 1989).

Premenstrual syndrome meets the criteria for a culture-bound syndrome. It constitutes a "negotiated reality"—that is, its reality is "that negotiated between those who treat it and those who suffer it" (Morokoff 1991). Premenstrual syndrome is unique in the extent to which the societal negotiation process has been overt and public—with research, debates, protests, letters back and forth, and papers supporting various points of view. The tentative compromise solution placed late luteal phase dysphoric disorder (LLP-DD) in the appendix to DSM-III-R (American Psychiatric Association 1987), highlighting its negotiated and controversial status. In DSM-IV (American Psychiatric Association 1994), premenstrual dysphoric disorder (PMDD) is listed as an affective disorder, with recognition of this entry as a "criteria set and axes provided for further study." This latest placement is being debated by researchers and clinicians who are concerned about categorizing this cohort of women as depressed (Severino 1996). In general, the inclusion of PMDD in the main body of DSM-IV is seen as a step forward in improving the diagnosis and treatment of this disorder (Steiner 1997).

Symbolic analysis of culture-bound syndromes provides an understanding not afforded by the biomedical approach alone (Morokoff 1991; Severino 1996). Johnson (1987) argued that premenstrual syndrome addresses the traditional concepts of women and work, reinforcing the cultural double-bind of the imperative for women to be both productive and reproductive. Although women with premenstrual syndrome may be unable to work for a limited period of time, they must still relate to others in a manner that is pleasing (as is culturally mandated) most of the time. Formal evaluations of cognitive functioning in women with premenstrual syndrome indicate no reduction in cognitive performance even though the women reported increased feelings of inadequacy (Morgan et al. 1996). What is new is not the negative view of women as being weak, emotional, and unable to work, which in premenstrual syndrome is captured in the premenstrual phase, but rather the positive view of women as strong, powerful, and capable, which is captured in the nonpremenstrual phases of the menstrual cycle.

Interpreted literally, premenstrual syndrome allows women access to power most of the time, while invalidating them and their experience part of the time. However, a regularly disabled woman is not seen as a capable woman, and the woman with premenstrual syndrome may be angry or assertive premenstrually and submissive the rest of the time, whether or not appropriate to the circumstances (including oppression). Morokoff (1991) argued that premenstrual syndrome captures our cultural ambiguity regarding women and conception, with symptoms occurring at the time of greatest ambiguity about whether the woman *has* conceived and, more important, whether the woman *should* conceive. Premenstrual syndrome appears to constitute a transitional compromise for a culture in which women's roles have changed and men's roles have not.

Studies show that women report more negative symptoms when they believe they are premenstrual than when they are led to believe that they are not premenstrual. A study analyzing women's perception of perimenstrual impairment found that with positive reframing of changes that occur perimenstrually, impairment decreased (Morse 1997). Studies also indicate that women report more premenstrual symptoms when they are aware of the focus of the study than when they are not (Hamilton et al. 1989). These findings substantiate an expectancy component to symptom reporting. This psychosomatic aspect of symptom occurrence may complicate research findings (Mortola 1998).

## Pathology and the Menstrual Cycle

Does a unique disorder of primarily psychologic symptoms occurring only premenstrually exist? If so, what is the relationship of it to other psychiatric and medical disorders? Do other psychiatric and medical disorders themselves vary with the menstrual cycle?

A brief history of the term *premenstrual syndrome* is necessary to put into context our modern conceptualization of these questions. When Frank coined the term *premenstrual tension* in 1931, he distinguished between what he considered to be three different groups of women. The first group had mild symptoms premenstrually, such as fatigue, that he considered to be normal. The second group included women with systemic illnesses that varied with the menstrual cycle; he cited two examples, a patient with catamenial asthma and one with catamenial epilepsy. The third group was a small minority of women who experienced what he called "premenstrual tension," a disorder of severe emotional symptoms occurring premenstrually, including suicidality, a "personality change," and/or reckless behavior for which they later had remorse. Relief of these symptoms occurred with onset of menses. Subsequent writers from the 1930s to the 1950s added progressively more and more symptoms to the list of possible premenstrual tension symptoms, such that by the 1950s it was recommended that any and all symptoms that vary with the menstrual cycle be considered as falling under the rubric of premenstrual tension, including asthma attacks and seizures. Dalton first used *premen-*

*strual syndrome* in medical literature in 1953, a change that emphasized the wide variety of possible symptoms, both physical and psychologic. As all symptoms related to the menstrual cycle became lumped together, a great deal of confusion followed and it became necessary to ask certain questions: Is there really a single premenstrual syndrome, or many? Is progesterone the drug of choice for all cases of premenstrual syndrome, as claimed by Dalton (1964)? Frank's (1931) original delineation of a severe syndrome with primarily psychologic symptoms, distinct from either systemic illnesses varying with the menstrual cycle or normal, mild symptoms, was lost in the confusion. In recent years research has started bring us out of the confusion, and, in the process, has pointed us back toward Frank's forward-looking original impressions.

## Disorders Varying with the Menstrual Cycle

### Dysmenorrhea

*Dysmenorrhea* is defined as recurrent, catamenial pelvic pain. *Primary dysmenorrhea* occurs in the absence of discrete pathophysiology and *secondary dysmenorrhea* occurs in the presence of discrete pathophysiology, including uterine fibromyomas and endometriosis. Now that primary dysmenorrhea is known to be caused by an excess of prostaglandins in the endometrial tissue and is treatable with prostaglandin synthetase inhibitors, it should no longer be considered a manifestation of neurosis or dismissed as "just part of being a woman" or just a symptom of premenstrual syndrome.

### Medical Disorders

The frequency or intensity of symptoms of a number of medical disorders vary by menstrual cycle phase, including lupus erythematosus, acute intermittent porphyria, herpes genitalis, pneumothorax, and others (M. Jensvold and G. V. Foster, unpublished manuscript, 1984). Among women with migraines, 10%–70% have migraines occurring regularly during or just before menses (Digre and Damasio 1987; Lokken et al. 1997). In a study of asthma, 35% of reproductive-age women with asthma reported that their asthma symptoms worsened just before or at the time of menses. Daily spirometry only confirmed significant deterioration in airway resistance at the time of menses in the group who reported an association of symptoms to the menstrual cycle (Hanley 1981).

## Psychiatric Disorders

What evidence indicates that psychiatric disorders vary with the menstrual cycle? A few studies have begun to address this question.

Bulimia.    In two prospective studies of bingeing behavior in bulimic women, one study found a modest but statistically significant premenstrual exacerbation of binge eating, without an increase in depression (Gladis and Walsh 1987). One prospective study found a significantly increased frequency of binge episodes in the luteal phase (Price et al. 1987). A third study analyzing the clinical similarities of PMDD and bulimia found a comorbidity of 16.6% for PMDD and bulimia and only a 2.3% comorbidity for women not affected by PMDD. The researchers also found a common personality dimension, harm avoidance, to be more frequent in women with PMDD and bulimia suggesting that similarities exist between the two disorders (Verri et al. 1997). A report of two patients contrasted one whose bulimic bingeing increased regularly premenstrually and one whose bulimic bingeing showed no association to the menstrual cycle (McDaniel 1989).

Panic disorder.    In three studies of panic disorder, 40%–90% of the women studied retrospectively reported worsening of panic or anxiety premenstrually. Using prospective ratings, two of the studies found no evidence of menstrual cycle–related changes in panic (Cook et al. 1990; Stein et al. 1989), but the third found significant worsening in intensity of full situation panic attacks, with other parameters not showing significant variation. The authors concluded that actual fluctuations in anxiety symptoms across the menstrual cycle were rather small (Cameron et al. 1988). Yonkers's (1997a) analysis of PMDD and panic concluded that women with premenstrual syndrome experienced increased occurrence of panic attacks and "that biological mechanisms or vulnerabilities are shared in women with panic and women with PMDD" (p. 62)

Affective disorders.    A great deal of evidence links affective symptoms and the menstrual cycle. Overlap exists among symptoms reported by women with PMDD and those reported by women with other affective disorders (Yonkers 1997b). Prevalence rates for premenstrual depression were found to be 65% by several groups examining prevalence in patients with current or lifetime diagnoses of affective disorder. In patients complaining of premenstrual depression, 39% exhibited depression through daily ratings and 36% showed intermittent depression throughout the cycle (McMillan and Pihl

1987). Patients who pursued treatment for premenstrual depression were found to be at high risk for suicide attempts because of the increased severity and intensity of symptoms (Stout et al. 1986). Additionally, one recent study of 113 women found a correlation between premenstrual suicide attempts and a history of previous psychiatric illness (Baca et al. 1998). Lifetime diagnoses of major depressive disorder were found to have prevalence rates of 57%–100% among women in five different samples who suffered from premenstrual depression. Complaints of premenstrual depression have been found to have predictive value in terms of future depression (Graze et al. 1990). Halbreich (1997) has suggested that premenstrual syndrome symptoms constitute "an expression of vulnerability traits" (p. 20) that may also indicate traits for depression or anxiety.

Data suggest a susceptibility to psychopathologic cycling among women. Most people with rapid cycling bipolar disorder are women (Wehr et al. 1988). The same is true of those with seasonal affective disorder. However, the mood disorders of only a few of these women cycle in relation to the menstrual cycle (Conrad and Hamilton 1986; Kukopulos et al. 1985; Wehr et al. 1988). The reasons for women's increased susceptibility to cyclic disorders are not known, and the mechanisms of the interrelationships between mood and cycling are not well understood.

**Posttraumatic stress disorder and dissociative disorders.** Some evidence exists of a menstrual cycle–related pattern in posttraumatic symptoms and dissociative disorders in some women who present complaining of premenstrual syndrome (Jensvold et al. 1989).

## Premenstrual Syndrome and Premenstrual Dysphoric Disorder

Two definitions of premenstrual syndrome are currently in use in the research and clinical literature, a "common" definition and PMDD. A third definition, LLPDD, was briefly in use while the disorder was listed in the appendix to DSM-III-R. For the purposes of this chapter, we will indicate the name used in the cited report with an understanding that LLPDD and PMDD are very similar—the definition of PMDD includes one more symptom than that of LLPDD, a subjective sense of being overwhelmed or out of control (Severino 1996). The "common" definition mentioned above requires a combination of common psychologic and physical symptoms that occur premenstrually and are absent during the follicular phase. Commonly cited psychologic symptoms include sadness, irritability, and tension or anxiety, and commonly cited physical symptoms include bloating and breast tenderness. PMDD, in contrast, has been used to date only in some of the most recent mental health literature, as would be expected, because it is a recently available diagnosis. It emphasizes psychologic symptoms (physical symptoms are optional), includes a severity criterion, and requires confirmation on daily prospective ratings (see Figure 9–3).

| | | Daily ratings (DR) | |
|---|---|---|---|
| | | + | − |
| Self-report (SR) | + | Concordant<br><br>Positive | Discordant<br><br>False-positive SR<br>or<br>False-negative DR |
| | − | Discordant<br><br>False-negative SR<br>or<br>False-positive DR | Concordant<br><br>Positive |

FIGURE 9–3. Meeting diagnostic criteria by self-report and daily ratings.

Is there a unique disorder, PMDD, that can be distinguished from other disorders? Women can be identified who report severe symptoms, including occupational or social impairment, that occur only premenstrually; who are confirmed to fulfill PMDD criteria on prospective ratings; and who do not seem to have another current psychiatric illness (Steiner 1997). Recent placement of PMDD in the main body of DSM-IV indicates its reliability and validity as a diagnostic category. Based on phenomenology and course, studies support classification as a depressive mood disorder. Whether PMDD, as conceptualized, is the optimal taxonomy continues to be explored (Halbreich et al. 1983; Hamilton and Gallant 1990; Spitzer et al. 1989). Certainly, rigor is needed in our categorizations so that research and treatment may be most appropriately directed.

What is the relationship of PMDD to other psychiatric disorders? One of the diagnostic criteria for PMDD is that the symptoms are not attributable to another psychiatric disorder. However, in the presence of another psychiatric disorder, it is hard to know whether the premenstrual symptoms are attributable to that psychiatric disorder. Categorization of PMDD as a mood disorder in DSM-IV is supported by study findings of low serotonin and melatonin metabolism as well as numerous studies reporting symptom improvement with selective serotonin reuptake inhibitors (Parry 1997). In one comparison of PMDD and depression, PMDD is suggested to be an expression of traits indicating vulnerability to depression (Halbreich 1997), whereas another study suggests that biologic cognitive studies and treatment response factors help to differentiate PMDD from other mood disorders (Yonkers 1997B). The true nature of the relationship between concurrent PMDD and other psychiatric disorders remains to be elucidated.

## Findings in Premenstrual Syndrome Research

**Prevalence of symptoms.**   Several studies have shown at least 75% of women reporting at least one symptom occurring premenstrually. However, the number of women who report that symptoms are severe or bothersome enough to warrant treatment is much lower. Psychologic symptoms are often reported to be the most distressing. Positive changes also occur premenstrually (Stewart 1989) but are often overlooked. Two studies have examined the prevalence of women who fulfill diagnostic criteria for LLPDD. One study, a community-based survey with prospective ratings, found that 3.4% of reproductive-age women reported severe symptoms (R. F. Haskett, unpublished data, May 1987). In the other study, 4.6% of college-age women reported severe symptoms (Rivera-Tovar and Frank 1990), suggesting that 3%–5% of women of reproductive age may meet criteria for LLPDD. A more recent study of women with PMDD also endorsed the 3%–5% figure (Gehlert and Hartlage 1997).

**Prevalence of Axis I and Axis II disorders.**   Only one study has examined lifetime prevalence of both Axis I and Axis II disorders in women meeting criteria for LLPDD. Depression was found to be more prevalent in women with LLPDD in this study than in those in the community-based Epidemiologic Catchment Area study, although the prevalence of other psychiatric disorders was similar in both studies. Of women meeting LLPDD criteria, 78% had a lifetime history of Axis I disorder, with prior depression being most prevalent; 10% met criteria for Axis II disorders, with avoidant personality being most prevalent; and 20% had current psychiatric disorders despite attempts to exclude women with current psychiatric disorders (Pearlstein et al. 1990). In a study in which data were pooled from five institutions (Hurt et al. 1992), 670 women who sought treatment for premenstrual syndrome were examined, of whom 39% were found to have only past psychiatric disorders, 27% had a current psychiatric disorder, and 33% had no psychiatric history. The authors concluded that LLPDD was not synonymous with another psychiatric disorder and that past psychiatric history increased the risk of LLPDD. Present psychiatric disorder was not shown to increase the risk of LLPDD over that observed in women with no psychiatric history. The prevalence of LLPDD varied substantially as a function of the four methods of analyzing daily ratings data (Hurt et al. 1992).

**Hormone studies.** Numerous studies have been conducted but have shown no consistent abnormalities in peripheral hormone levels in women with premenstrual syndrome (Rubinow et al. 1988). Some evidence exists of a hormone axis instability (Roy-Byrne et al. 1987), and several studies have now shown abnormalities in serotonin metabolism (Ashby et al. 1990), whereas others have linked fluctuating serotonin-receptor concentrations with changes in estrogen and progesterone levels (Biegon et al. 1980). Circadian phase shifts may be implicated in some patients (Parry and Wehr 1987; Parry et al. 1997). The concept of "multiple cyclic change . . . occurring as a diversified, dynamic, time-related process" (Halbreich et al. 1988, p.183) is probably more accurate than any hypothesis of unitary abnormalities in accounting for the diversity of symptoms reported with premenstrual syndrome. One recent study found hypothalamic and pituitary hormone differences between women with premenstrual syndrome and control subjects that suggested neurobiologic vulnerability in women who experience premenstrual syndrome symptoms (Rosenstein et al. 1996). A second study found a decrease in premenstrual syndrome symptoms with ovarian suppression, indicating that women with premenstrual syndrome may be experiencing atypical sensitivity to normal hormonal changes (Schmidt et al. 1998). In a recent analysis of existing hormonal studies and treatment modalities, Mortola (1998) suggested that premenstrual syndrome is "the result of a complex interaction between ovarian steroids and neurotransmitters" (p. 256).

## Methodologic and Political Issues in Premenstrual Syndrome Research

**Prospective ratings.** The method used to analyze daily ratings greatly affects the percentage of women meeting the diagnostic criteria. Currently, daily ratings are seen as the standard for diagnosis, with negative prospective ratings automatically taking precedence over the woman's positive self-report. Cases with discordant retrospective self-report and prospective ratings should be examined more closely for the presence of any of a number of factors contributing to the discordance. Reasons to trust prospective ratings over self-report are the evidence of misattributions and negative expectancies. However, several reasons exist for not assuming that prospective ratings are necessarily the ultimate conveyor of truth, including the possibility of inadvertently creating false-positives or false-negatives by setting cutoffs too low or too high; intercycle variability; and evidence that as many men as women fulfill diagnostic criteria for premenstrual syndrome on the basis of prospective ratings (Gallant 1991). Approaches to discordant cases should be individualized; for example, if a psychiatric disorder is present in the follicular phase, treatment of that disorder is indicated.

Some evidence indicates that more severe cases show greater concordance in self-report and daily ratings and less severe cases show greater discordance. In one well-designed study, retrospective reports of premenstrual syndrome were predictive of future major depression even in women without a past history of depression and without a family history of depression. Retrospective reports were a better predictor in this study than daily ratings (Graze et al. 1990).

**Diagnostic options.** Official psychiatric diagnostic nomenclature has denoted a unique disorder of primarily psychologic symptoms premenstrually: PMDD. Alternatives to the current denotation are still being debated among clinicians and practitioners. These include a psychiatric disorder with a menstrually related or catamenial pattern (similar to the seasonal pattern denotation in DSM-IV) or a category of hormone-related disorders in which male disorders related to hormones could also be denoted.

**Chasm between research and practice.** Current research practices automatically exclude from most premenstrual syndrome research women whose self-report and daily ratings are discordant and women who choose not to comply with 2 months of daily ratings. The diagnosis of PMDD, as currently specified, diagnoses moderate cases—women who have impairment premenstrually but who can tolerate and are willing to complete 2 months of ratings prior to treatment. However, clinicians are presented with cases that run the full spectrum of severity. Thus a chasm exists between research (which needs rigorously defined homogeneous patient populations) and clinical needs (with the mandate to help all women who present for help).

**Political issues.** Stotland (unpublished paper, 1991) has pointed out two main categories of risks to women from an LLPDD/PMDD diagnosis. The first of these is the risk to all women if common, menstrually related experiences are pathologized. The second risk is that of "the impact of a narrowly defined LLPDD on the majority of women who now present for treatment of PMS who would be excluded." To say either that all women who have menstrual cycles have a disorder or that no women who have menstrual cycles have a menstrually related disorder is to minimize the subject and to fail to listen to women's experience.

Symptoms are not synonymous with syndromes and must be distinguished. The media often portray as mild or moderate premenstrual syndrome what researchers would call normal (Chrisler and Levy 1990). Concern that women with normal menstrual cycles and minimal or no symptoms will be declared to have disorders is not lessened by the fact that some symptom rating scales still used in the field classify all women as having varying severities of premenstrual syndrome and provide no way of classifying a woman as not having premenstrual syndrome.

No other diagnosis requires prospective ratings to confirm the patient's self-report. Mandatory compliance with daily ratings of patients with other disorders has not been studied (Stotland 1991). The assumptions that prospective ratings are always correct and that discordance between prospective ratings and the woman's retrospective self-report automatically invalidates that self-report may be discriminatory. Hormones contribute to disorders or symptoms in men, such as aggressivity, but do not receive attention as such.

**Law.** Use of premenstrual syndrome as a legal defense has succeeded in Canada and England, but this defense has been controversial and generally unsuccessful in the United States and barriers to its successful use seem to be formidable (Severino and Moline 1989). Concern has been expressed that, with its use, all women will be on trial. Numerous questions remain about the implications if premenstrual syndrome is successfully used as a defense. For example, what should be done with the premenstrual syndrome offender who fails or refuses to obtain court-ordered treatment? Is there clear evidence treatment will succeed in light of the enigmatic pathophysiology?

Treatment and the Menstrual Cycle

## Chronotherapy

*Chronobiology* has been described as

> the broad spectrum of interacting and interdigitating rhythms that all togeth-
> er comprise the *time structure* of a living organism . . . [By learning the patterns
> of] biological variations we can compare, correlate, and finally predict their
> course. This development makes it necessary and possible for physicians to
> concentrate more closely on the individual needs of their patients through
> *patient-monitoring* and *time-specified medications.* (Haen 1988, p. 7)

Studies of the timing of melatonin release in women with PMDD have revealed that nocturnal melatonin concentrations are lower in women with
PMDD compared with those in control subjects (Parry 1997). Parry (1997)
suggests that changing sleep cycles and using light therapy can alter melatonin circadian rhythms, thus effecting mood changes.

The issue of chronotherapy, or timing therapy, has received much less
attention in psychiatry than it deserves. The question arises that if symptoms
occur during certain menstrual cycle phases for a particular woman, when
should treatment be administered? Should it be administered constantly
(throughout the menstrual cycle), periodically (recurrently, e.g., premenstrually only), or at varying times (e.g., with increased dosages premenstrually)?
The question also arises whether fluctuations in symptoms are caused by
physiologic variables (which would occur in any woman with a normal menstrual cycle), pathologic variables (which would occur only in persons with
the disorder), or as an interactive process between the two. If the latter, what
is the nature of this interaction?

Lithium treatment illustrates these concepts well. Individual cases document that for some women with bipolar illness, mood symptoms and lithium
levels vary according to menstrual cycle phase. One woman's bipolar illness
was in good control when she was receiving a constant dose of lithium except
for a premenstrual recurrence of symptoms, at which time her serum lithium
levels dropped premenstrually. When her lithium dosage was increased premenstrually, her serum levels remained constant with good control of symptoms (Conrad and Hamilton 1986). In another case, a woman with bipolar
illness had regular recurrence of hypomania earlier in the cycle, depression
later in the cycle, and symptomatic relief with onset of menses. Her lithium
levels were lowest when she was hypomanic, highest when she was de-

pressed, and intermediate with euthymic mood (Kukopulos et al. 1985).

Do physiologic factors account for these changes in lithium levels? A study of lithium levels in regularly menstruating women found that serum lithium levels following administration of a single dose of lithium were identical regardless of the phase of the menstrual cycle and regardless of whether the women were receiving oral contraceptive medication (Chamberlain et al. 1990). This finding indicates that physiologic factors in the normal menstrual cycle do not account for menstrual cycle–related changes in lithium levels and that these changes are probably more related to changes in pathology (i.e., manic or depressive, rather than luteal or follicular). In a study of 54 persons with rapid cycling bipolar illness, 92% were women, but none was found to switch moods in relation to the menstrual cycle, highlighting the fact that not all women with bipolar illness cycle in relation to the menstrual cycle (Wehr et al. 1988). Also, Hatotani et al. (1983) found an association between mood and the menstrual cycle in bipolar patients but found that mood was sometimes slightly out of synchronization with the menstrual cycle. This raises the question of how mood and the menstrual cycle are really associated. Why does bipolar illness entrain to the menstrual cycle in some regularly menstruating women but not all? What accounts for cycling that moves in and out of synchronization with the menstrual cycle? What is the role of oral contraceptive medication in entraining pathology to the menstrual cycle or in freeing it from entrainment? The data raise as many questions as they answer.

## Interaction Between Endogenous Hormones and Psychotropic Medications

Women take more medications, including more psychotropic medications, than do men, but even when corrected for the number of medications taken, women have more adverse effects to medications than do men. Almost certainly one of the contributing factors to this is a lack of attention to the menstrual cycle. By not taking the menstrual cycle into account, the clinician risks either overtreating or undertreating the patient. If the phase of the menstrual cycle is not considered, cycle-dependent symptoms may be misinterpreted as side effects or ineffectiveness of the medication.

Clinically significant side effects in relation to gender or hormone levels are known for mood stabilizers (lithium), antidopaminergic and antipsychotic drugs, anticonvulsants (e.g., phenytoin), some benzodiazepines (e.g., diazepam), propranolol, and alcohol (Hamilton 1991). One patient's premenstrual depression was documented to require a varying dose of antidepressant medication throughout the cycle. She tolerated a constant low dose of tricyclic antidepressant well but this dose was only partially effective. A constant higher dose was effective for premenstrual symptoms, but was not tolerated in the follicular phase. Finally, a varying dosage of tricyclic antidepressant, with higher dosage premenstrually, was both effective and well tolerated (Jensvold et al. 1992). One study of the effects of benzodiazepines over the menstrual cycle in women with premenstrual syndrome found a decreased sensitivity at the γ-aminobutyric acid/benzodiazepine-receptor complex, indicating a decreased treatment effectiveness that was especially marked during the third week of the menstrual cycle (Sundstrom et al. 1997). Women with catamenial epilepsy had a marked decrease in phenytoin during menses compared with control subjects and with women with noncatamenial epilepsy. Recurrent premenstrual failure of migraine prophylaxis was associated with lower steady-state serum levels of propranolol during menses. Some drugs do not show clearly significant menstrual cycle effects, including salicylates, aminopyrine, nitrazepam, and paracetamol. Without systematic monitoring of drug–hormone interactions, the drug differences that have come to our attention can be considered to be the "tip of the iceberg." Future studies will find that some drugs do not show any substantial menstrual cycle–related effects, but we do not yet know which drugs those are.

When menstrual cycle–related effects have been found, they often occur in subgroups of women (e.g., those receiving lithium or phenytoin), with reported effects generally tending toward increased clearance premenstrually (Hamilton 1991). Sex steroid hormones can have differential effects on partial pathways for various metabolites. Competition between drugs and hormones for the same metabolic sites may account for some of the differences in metabolic rates (Hamilton 1991) in women as compared with men or over time. Interindividual differences in the use of alternative metabolic pathways or in the levels of or sensitivity to endogenous sex steroid hormones may explain why only some women experience menstrual cycle–related effects (Hamilton 1991).

## Interaction Between Exogenous Hormones and Psychotropic Medications

### Oral Contraceptives

In a review of interactions between oral contraceptives and other medications, Teichmann (1990) concluded that medications showing clinically significant interactions included antidepressant medications, antihypertensives, insulin, synthetic glucocorticoids, theophylline, and caffeine. The *Medical Drug Reference* (Ellsworth et al. 1997) lists clinically significant interactions between oral contraceptives or estrogens and 16 medication classifications. Oral contraceptives tend to increase clearance of drugs metabolized by glucuronidation (e.g., some benzodiazepines) and decrease clearance of drugs metabolized by oxidative pathways, including the P450 cytochrome oxidase system (e.g., imipramine, diazepam, caffeine, and chlordiazepoxide).

Of women of reproductive age in the United States, 27% receive oral contraceptive medication, which means that a number of women presenting to psychiatrists are using or will use chemical contraceptive agents (Hatcher et al. 1994). Psychiatric side effects of oral contraceptives were more frequent in older, higher-dosage preparations, but mood effects have been observed in the lower-dose preparations and we have observed these low-dose oral contraceptive mood effects to be responsive to antidepressant medication. Oral contraceptives may entrain psychopathology to the menstrual cycle in some cases or free symptoms from entrainment to the menstrual cycle in others. In one large study, 276 oral contraceptive users were compared with 276 nonusers. Research indicated that oral contraceptive users experienced longer patterns of perimenstrual negative mood than did nonusers (Bancroft and Rennie 1993). In some cases, a woman may need to stop hormonal therapy in order to know what role the oral contraceptive is playing in her symptoms, whether exacerbating them, ameliorating them, or having no effect at all.

Contraceptive medications now available to women in the United States include combination medication (estrogen and progestogen for 21 days followed by a hormone-free week, the most commonly used preparations); sequential medication, including triphasic pills (varying dosages of hormone sequentially, also commonly used); mini-dose progesterone (daily oral micronized progesterone, which has fewer side effects but is less commonly used because of its slightly decreased effectiveness as a contraceptive agent); long-acting subcutaneous progesterone injection (DepoProvera); and long-acting subcutaneous progesterone implant (Norplant). Other long-acting progesterone derivatives and chemical contraceptive agents are being tested and used in Europe, Scandinavia, and elsewhere (Hatcher et al. 1994).

## Postmenopausal Hormone Replacement Therapy

In a survey study, 32% of postmenopausal women were found to use hormone replacement therapy (HRT) (Harris et al. 1990). HRT differs from oral contraceptives in that it uses natural conjugated estrogens that do not affect the cytochrome P450 oxidase system, whereas oral contraceptives use synthetic estrogens (e.g., ethinyl estradiol) that do affect that system. Also, the dosages of hormones are about 1.1–2.5 times higher in oral contraceptives than in HRT.

Hormone replacement therapy can cause mood effects, with progesterone thought to be responsible for recurrent dysphoric moods associated with HRT (Magos et al. 1986); however, estrogen has been shown to trigger rapid mood cycling in vulnerable women (Oppenheim 1984). Consequently, women with histories of affective disorders should be monitored closely for mood effects when HRT is started.

Postmenopausal hormone therapy is known to cause symptoms similar to those of premenstrual syndrome in some women (Magos et al. 1986), in effect, an iatrogenic premenstrual syndrome. This leads some women to present to psychiatrists for treatment of new-onset or recurrent premenstrual-like symptoms or mood symptoms. We have found that symptoms can be minimized by decreasing the hormone dose or changing the timing, for example, changing the 10-day interval of progestogen from once monthly to once every 3 months. If these interventions do not provide sufficient relief, then stopping HRT or adding a psychotropic agent should be considered.

## Gonadotropin-Releasing Hormone Agonists

Potent agonists bind powerfully to GnRH receptors at the level of the pituitary, thus blocking the pulsatile action of GnRH. After transiently increasing release of luteinizing hormone and follicle-stimulating hormone from the pituitary, GnRH agonists then paradoxically block the pituitary's normal response to GnRH, thus effecting a "chemical oophorectomy." This therapy must be used with extreme caution. Use of GnRH for endometriosis and other conditions is growing. Three forms of GnRH agonists are now available: intramuscular, intranasal, and depot GnRH. The forms vary with respect to ease of administration and in how much control one has over the administered dose. Estrogen deficiency–related symptoms, including hot flashes and osteoporosis, are considerations.

GnRH agonists have been reported to help severe premenstrual symptoms, although some women experience transient worsening during the first month of treatment. One woman's first hypomanic episode was precipitated by GnRH; some women's mood disorders, previously linked to the menstrual cycle, have become unlinked from cycle on GnRH. A recent study at the National Institute of Mental Health concluded that GnRH administration successfully improved the symptoms of premenstrual syndrome. Symptoms recurred with administration of estradiol and progesterone, indicating that the interruption of the body's natural hormonal changes can improve premenstrual syndrome symptoms (Schmidt et al. 1998).

## Gynecologic versus Psychotropic Medications for the Treatment of Premenstrual Symptoms

Because the hypothalamic–pituitary–ovarian axis is an interconnected feedback loop, interventions at different levels of the feedback loop may, at least theoretically, affect a particular targeted menstrually related symptom.

### Gynecologic Treatments

Several methods that prevent ovulation have been tried for the relief of premenstrual syndrome. Surgical ovariectomy (Casson et al. 1990) and chemical ovariectomy using GnRH (Hammarback and Backstrom 1988; Schmidt et al. 1998) appear to provide lasting relief of severe premenstrual psychologic and physical symptoms, although their use is inappropriate for most patients with premenstrual syndrome and requires psychiatric screening and long-term follow-up studies. Hysterectomy without ovariectomy provides more variable results, as would be expected, because it removes menses—the external time cue—but the hormonal cycle remains intact. Danazol, an androgenic agent, inhibits ovulation and provides relief for some premenstrual symptoms, particularly mastalgia, but appears to cause or exacerbate depression and irritability in some patients. Oral contraceptives appear to worsen premenstrual syndrome in some women, have no effect on others, and perhaps ameliorate symptoms in others.

Progesterone as a treatment for premenstrual syndrome is now essentially disproven; numerous double-blind, controlled studies have failed to show its superiority over placebo (Hurt et al. 1992) and a progesterone antagonist study disproved the hypothesis that luteal-phase progesterone plays a role in causing catamenial mood symptoms (Schmidt et al. 1991).

### Psychotropic Agents

A study of fluoxetine treatment for LLPDD found that premenstrual physical symptoms as well as psychologic symptoms were helped by fluoxetine (Stone et al. 1991). Further studies of serotonin reuptake inhibitors such as fluoxetine and sertraline have indicated that both symptomatic and functional impairment decrease with treatment (Yonkers et al. 1997). Other studies have shown efficacy of both alprazolam and desipramine treatment over placebo for LLPDD/PMDD.

## Nonbiologic Treatments of Menstrually Related Symptoms

Dynamic issues regarding the menstrual cycle and what it means to the individual woman are important in some cases. Menstrual cyclicity can have an indirect impact on psychotherapy as well, with some psychotherapeutic work being more possible, more necessary, or more or less effective during certain phases. One example is the woman with state-dependent, recurrent premenstrual flashbacks of earlier trauma (Jensvold et al. 1989). If expectancies or misattributions are thought to play a significant role with a particular patient, then cognitive therapy techniques, interpersonal therapy, or feminist therapy, which examines the woman in her environmental context (including societal influences) rather than narrowly focusing on intrapsychic factors, may be helpful. Support groups may also play a useful role in treatment because group members recognize dysfunctional behavioral or emotional patterns or expectancies and develop increased insight and confidence and improved coping.

## Conclusion

It seems now that Frank was forward looking in 1931 in distinguishing among women with a unique psychologic disorder occurring premenstrually, women with mild symptoms, and women whose systemic illnesses varied with the menstrual cycle. Excessive lumping together of disorders over subsequent decades has caused confusion among researchers, clinicians, patients, and the public. State-of-the-art research is now sorting out various threads and addressing questions implied by Frank's clinical observation: Is there validity to a single diagnostic category describing psychologic symptoms occurring only premenstrually? Do other psychiatric disorders vary with the menstrual cycle? How can one address real problems without stigmatizing women and without playing into the already excessively negative views of the menstrual cycle and of women? What are the roles of gynecologic agents and of psychotropic agents in treating psychiatric disorders related to the menstrual cycle? Psychiatric symptoms and the menstrual cycle represent a confluence in which mind–body issues can be addressed in interesting and important ways, with the potential for much to be learned about chronobiology, brain–endocrine interactions, and cultural overlay as well as the promise of improving the health of women patients.

# References

American Psychiatric Association: Diagnostic and Statistical Manual of Mental Disorders, 3rd Edition Revised. Washington, DC, American Psychiatric Association, 1987

American Psychiatric Association: Diagnostic and Statistical Manual of Mental Disorders, 4th Edition. Washington, DC, American Psychiatric Association, 1994

Ashby C, Carr L, Cook C, et al: Alteration of 5-HT uptake by plasma fractions in the premenstrual syndrome. J Neural Transm Gen Sect 79:41–50, 1990

Baca G, Sanchez A, Gonzalez P, et al: Menstrual cycle and profiles of suicidal behaviour. Acta Psychiatr Scand 97:32–35, 1998

Bancroft J, Rennie D: The impact of oral contraceptives on the experience of perimenstrual mood, clumsiness, food craving and other symptoms. J Psychosom Res 37:195–202, 1993

Biegon A, Bercovitz H, Samuel D: Serotonin receptor concentration during the estrous cycle in the rat. Brain Res 187:221–225, 1980

Cameron O, Kuttesch D, McPhee K, et al: Menstrual fluctuation in the symptoms of panic anxiety. J Affect Disord 15:169–174, 1988

Casson P, Hahn P, Vugt D, et al: Lasting response to ovariectomy in severe intractable premenstrual syndrome. Am J Obstet Gynecol 162:99–105, 1990

Chamberlain S, Hahn P, Casson P, et al: Effect of menstrual cycle phase and oral contraceptive use on serum lithium levels after a loading dose of lithium in normal women. Am J Psychiatry 147:907–909, 1990

Chrisler J, Levy K: The media construct a menstrual monster: a content analysis of PMS articles in the popular press. Women Health 16:89–104, 1990

Conrad C, Hamilton J: Recurrent premenstrual decline in serum lithium concentration: clinical correlates and treatment implications. J Am Acad Clin Psychiatry 26:852–853, 1986

Cook B, Noyes R, Garvey M, et al: Anxiety and the menstrual cycle in panic disorder. J Affect Disord 19:221–226, 1990

Dalton K: The Premenstrual Syndrome. Springfield, IL, Charles C. Thomas, 1964

Deutsch H: The Psychology of Women: A Psychoanalytic Interpretation. New York, Grune and Stratton, 1944

Digre K, Damasio H: Menstrual migraine: differential diagnosis, evaluation, and treatment. Clin Obstet Gynecol 30:417–430, 1987

Ellsworth A, Dugdale D, Witt D, et al: Medical Drug Reference. St. Louis, MO, Mosby-Year Book, 1997

Frank R: The hormonal causes of premenstrual tension. Arch Neurol Psychiatry 26:1053–1057, 1931

Gallant S: The role of psychological factors in the experience of premenstrual symptoms. Presented at the Society for Menstrual Cycle Research Biannual Meeting, Seattle, WA, March 1991

Gehlert S, Hartlage S: A design for studying the DSM-IV research criteria of premenstrual dysphoric disorder. J Psychosom Obstet Gynaecol 18:36–44, 1997

Gladis M, Walsh B: Premenstrual exacerbation of binge eating in bulimia. Am J Psychiatry 144:1592–1595, 1987

Graze K, Nee J, Endicott J: Premenstrual depression predicts future major depressive disorder. Acta Psychiatr Scand 81:201–205, 1990

Haen E (ed): Chronopharmacology of Reversible Airways Obstruction. Frankfurt, Germany, University of Munich, 1988

Halbreich U: Premenstrual dysphoric disorders: a diversified cluster of vulnerability traits to depression. Acta Psychiatr Scand 95:169–176, 1997

Halbreich U, Endicott J, Nee J: Premenstrual depressive changes: value of differentiation. Arch Gen Psychiatry 40:535–542, 1983

Halbreich U, Holtz I, Paul L: Premenstrual changes: impaired hormonal homeostasis. Neurol Clin 6:173–194, 1988

Hamilton J: Clinical pharmacology panel report, in Forging a Women's Health Research Agenda: Conference Proceedings. Edited by Blumenthal SJP, Parry B, Hamilton J, et al. Washington, DC, National Women's Health Resource Center, 1991, pp 1–27

Hamilton JA, Gallant SJ: Debate on late luteal phase dysphoric disorder. Am J Psychiatry 147:1106, 1990

Hamilton J, Gallant S, Lloyd C: Evidence for a menstrual-linked artifact in determining rates of depression. J Nerv Ment Dis 1779:359–365, 1989

Hammarback S, Backstrom T: Induced anovulation as treatment of premenstrual tension syndrome. Acta Obstet Gynecol Scand 67:159–166, 1988

Hanley S: Asthma variation with menstruation. Br J Dis Chest 75:306–308, 1981

Harris R, Laws A, Reddy V, et al: Are women using postmenopausal estrogens? A community survey. Am J Public Health 80:1266–1268, 1990

Hatcher R, Trussel J, Stewart F, et al: Contraceptive Technology. New York, Irvington, 1994

Hatotani N, Kitayama I, Inoue K, et al: Psychoneuroendocrine studies of recurrent psychoses, in Neurobiology of Periodic Psychoses. Edited by Hatotani N, Nomura J. Tokyo, Japan, Igaku-Shoin, 1983, pp 77–92

Hurt S, Schnurr P, Severino S, et al: Late luteal phase dysphoric disorder in 670 women. Am J Psychiatry 149:525–530, 1992

Jensvold M, Muller K, Putnam F, et al: Abuse and PTSD in PMS patients and controls. Presented at the International Society of Psychosomatic Obstetrics and Gynaecology Biannual Meeting, Amsterdam, Netherlands, May 1989

Jensvold MF, Reed K, Jarrett DB, et al: Menstrual cycle–related depressive symptoms treated with variable antidepressant dosage: a case report and case series. Journal of Women's Health 1:109–115, 1992

Johnson T: Premenstrual syndrome as a western culture-specific disorder. Culture, Medicine, and Psychiatry 11:337–356, 1987

Kawakami M, Arita J, Yoshida E: Loss of estrogen-induced daily surges of prolactin and gonadotropins by suprachiasmatic nucleus lesions in ovariectomized rats. Endocrinology 106:1087–1092, 1980

King C: Parallels between neurasthenia and premenstrual syndrome. Women Health 15:1–23, 1989

Kinney E, Trautmann J, Gold J, et al: Underrepresentation of women in new drug trials. Ann Intern Med 95:495–499, 1981

Kukopulos A, Minnai G, Muller-Oerlinghausen B: The influence of mania and depression on the pharmacokinetics of lithium: a longitudinal single-case study. J Affect Disord 8:159–166, 1985

Lokken C, Holm J, Myers T: The menstrual cycle and migraine: a time-series analysis of 20 women migraineurs. Headache 37:235–239, 1997

Magos A, Brincat M, Studd J: Treatment of the premenstrual syndrome by subcutaneous estradiol implants and cyclical oral norethisterone: placebo controlled study. BMJ 292:1629–1633, 1986

Martin E: The Woman in the Body. Boston, MA, Beacon Press, 1987

McClintock M: Estrous synchrony: modulation of ovarian cycle length by female pheromones. Physiol Behav 32:701–705, 1984

McDaniel W: Premenstrual exacerbation of bulimia (letter). Am J Psychiatry 146:807–808, 1989

McEwen B: Basic research perspective: ovarian hormone influence on brain neurochemical functions, in The Premenstrual Syndromes. Edited by Gise LH. New York, Churchill Livingstone, 1988, pp 21–33

McMillan M, Pihl R: Premenstrual depression: a distinct entity. J Abnorm Psychol 96:149–154, 1987

Morgan M, Rapkin A, Delia L, et al: Cognitive functioning in premenstrual syndrome. Obstet Gynecol 88:961–966, 1996

Morokoff P: Premenstrual Syndrome: Representation of a Cultural Conflict. Washington, DC, Society for Behavioral Medicine, 1991

Morse G: Effect of positive reframing and social support on perception of perimenstrual changes among women with premenstrual syndrome. Health Care Women Int 18:157–193, 1997

Mortola J: Premenstrual syndrome: pathophysiologic considerations. N Engl J Med 338:256–257, 1998

Oppenheim G: A case of rapid mood cycling with estrogen: implications for therapy. J Clin Psychiatry 45:34, 1984

Parry B: Psychobiology of premenstrual dysphoric disorder. Semin Reprod Endocrinol 15:55–68, 1997

Parry B, Wehr T: Therapeutic effect of sleep deprivation in patients with premenstrual syndrome. Am J Psychiatry 144:808–810, 1987

Parry B, Berga S, Mostofi N, et al: Plasma melatonin circadian rhythms during the menstrual cycle and after light therapy in premenstrual dysphoric disorder and normal control subjects. J Biol Rhythms 12:47–64, 1997

Pearlstein T, Frank E, Rivera-Tovar A, et al: Prevalence of Axis I and Axis II disorders in women with late luteal phase dysphoric disorder. J Affect Disord 20:129–134, 1990

Price W, Torem M, DiMarzio L: Premenstrual exacerbation of bulimia. Psychosomatics 28:378–380, 1987

Rivera-Tovar A, Frank E: Late luteal phase dysphoric disorder in young women. Am J Psychiatry 147:1634–1636, 1990

Rosenstein D, Kalogeras K, Kalafut M, et al: Peripheral measures of arginine vasopressin, atrial natriuretic peptide and adrenocorticotropic hormone in premenstrual syndrome. Psychoneuroendocrinology 21:347–359, 1996

Roy-Byrne P, Rubinow D, Hoban C, et al: TSH and prolactin responses to TRH in patients with premenstrual syndrome. Am J Psychiatry 144:480–484, 1987

Rubinow D, Hoban C, Grover G, et al: Changes in plasma hormones across the menstrual cycle in patients with menstrually related mood disorder and in control subjects. Am J Obstet Gynecol 158:5–11, 1988

Schmidt P, Nieman L, Grover G, et al: Lack of effect of induced menses on symptoms in women with premenstrual syndrome. N Engl J Med 324:1174–1179, 1991

Schmidt P, Nieman L, Danaceau M, et al: Differential behavioral effects of gonadal steroids in women with and in those without premenstrual syndrome. N Engl J Med 338:209–216, 1998

Severino S: Premenstrual dysphoric disorder: controversies surrounding the diagnosis. Harv Rev Psychiatry 3:293–295, 1996

Severino S, Moline M: Premenstrual Syndrome: A Clinician's Guide. New York, Guilford, 1989

Speroff L, Glass R, Kase N: Clinical Gynecologic Endocrinology and Infertility. Baltimore, MD, Williams and Wilkins, 1982

Spitzer RL, Severino SK, Williams JBW, et al: Late luteal phase dysphoric disorder and DSM-III-R. Am J Psychiatry 146:892–897, 1989

Stein M, Schmidt P, Rubinow D, et al: Panic disorder and the menstrual cycle: panic disorder patients, healthy control subjects, and patients with premenstrual syndrome. Am J Psychiatry 146:1299–1303, 1989

Steiner M: Premenstrual Syndromes. Annu Rev Med 48:447–455, 1997

Stewart D: Positive changes in the premenstrual period. Acta Psychiatr Scand 79:400–405, 1989

Stone A, Pearlstein T, Brown W: Fluoxetine in the treatment of late luteal phase dysphoric disorder. J Clin Psychiatry 52:290–293, 1991

Stout A, Steege J, Blazer D, et al: Comparison of lifetime psychiatric diagnosis in PMS clinic and community samples. J Nerv Ment Dis 174:517–522, 1986

Sullivan G, Lukoff D: Sexual side effects of antipsychotic medication: evaluation and interventions. Hospital and Community Psychiatry 41:1238–1241, 1990

Sundstrom I, Ashbrook D, Backstrom T: Reduced benzodiazepine sensitivity in patients with premenstrual syndrome: a pilot study. Psychoneuroendocrinology 22:25–38, 1997

Teichmann A: Influence of oral contraceptives on drug therapy. Am J Obstet Gynecol 163:2208–2213, 1990

Verri A, Nappi R, Vallero E, et al: Premenstrual dysphoric disorder and eating disorders. Cephalalgia 17(suppl 20):25–28, 1997

Wehr T, Sack D, Rosenthal N, et al: Rapid cycling affective disorder: contributing factors and treatment responses in 51 patients. Am J Psychiatry 145:179–184, 1988

Yonkers K: Anxiety symptoms and anxiety disorders: how are they related to premenstrual disorder. J Clin Psychiatry 58(suppl):62–69, 1997a

Yonkers K: The association between premenstrual dysphoric disorder and other mood disorders. J Clin Psychiatry 58(suppl):19–25, 1997b

Yonkers K, Halbreich U, Freeman E, et al: Symptomatic improvement of premenstrual dysphoric disorder with sertraline treatment: a randomized controlled trial. Sertraline Premenstrual Dysphoric Collaborative Study Group. JAMA 278:983–988, 1997

# Infertility and the New Reproductive Technologies

JENNIFER I. DOWNEY, M.D.

Infertility, defined as 1 year or more of unprotected coitus without pregnancy, is a common health problem. Medical authorities such as Speroff et al. (1994) estimated that 10%–15% of couples in the reproductive age group are affected by infertility. The only population-based survey of infertility in women, the National Survey of Family Growth, found in 1988 that the proportion of those who were infertile was 18% among childless couples in which the wife was 15–44 years of age (Mosher and Pratt 1990). The demand for infertility treatment is growing because of postponed childbearing, increases in the proportion of infertile couples seeking care, the shrinking supply of adoptable infants, new techniques for treating infertile couples, and heightened public awareness of these treatments. In the past, most infertility problems were attributed to women; in reality, 40%–50% of cases are wholly or in part due to a male factor (Jaffe and Jewelewicz 1991).

## Psychologic Effects of and Adjustment to Infertility

Menning (1980) proposed that infertility investigation and treatment bring on a life crisis because infertility poses a threat that is not solvable in the immediate future and that may tax the couple's existing problem-solving resources, threaten their achievement of important life goals, and awaken unresolved key difficulties from the past. She has described a series of feelings experienced by many couples, from surprise to denial, anger, isolation, guilt, and grief, followed by resolution if the feelings are worked through and overcome. Some couples may fail to resolve the problem and continue to seek new treatments, even after every potentially beneficial method has been tried. This model of infertility as a life crisis for many couples is helpful because it enables the clinician to think about the problem without pathologizing it and to organize data by phase in the process of resolving the problem.

The impact of infertility on marriage appears to vary greatly. It is unknown at present which couples are at risk for marital difficulties when facing involuntary childlessness. Cook et al. (1989) found that 71% of women participants reported that infertility had affected their marriage, but among those affected, the proportion of women who felt this impact to be positive was similar to the proportion who felt it it be negative. In some cases, the shared stress of infertility may strengthen a couple's bond. Medical diagnosis and phase of treatment may also affect the likelihood of harmful marital effects. For example, Connolly et al. (1987) found that marital difficulties were more likely if the cause of infertility was a male factor and that longer duration of treatment was associated with decreased emotional well-being of the couple.

When infertility affects a marriage, a key area that often deteriorates is sexual functioning and enjoyment. Negative effects on the sex life of couples have been widely reported, including impotence, anorgasmia, and lessened sexual desire (Berger 1980; Keye 1984; Lalos et al. 1985). Up to 10% of cases of infertility may be partially or completely explained by sexual dysfunctions of the man, such as premature ejaculation and impotence (Seibel and Taymor 1982). Among both women and men, planned intercourse for medical tests, such as the postcoital examination of cervical mucus, has been found to have an adverse impact on sexual functioning (DeVries et al. 1984; Drake and Grunert 1979).

Most investigators have found that women tend to be more distressed by infertility than are their male partners. Keye et al. (1981) reported that 57% of women but only 12% of men thought that infertility was the worst thing they had ever had to face in life. McEwan et al. (1987) found that 40% of women but only 13% of men evinced psychologic symptoms of clinical severity and that the women who were most disturbed were younger patients without a clear diagnosis of the infertility problem.

This difference in the level of reported distress between men and women is found throughout the phases of infertility evaluation and treatment. Wright et al. (1991) found that at the time of a couple's visit to an infertility clinic, women had significantly more overall psychiatric symptoms, depression, anxiety, and hostility and reported more stress and less self-esteem than did men. Assessing men and women after the failure of a first episode of in vitro fertilization (IVF) treatment—the other end of the spectrum usually reached after years of unsuccessful treatment—Newton et al. (1990) reported that 25% of women experienced mild or more serious depressions, as defined by scores on the Beck Depression Inventory (Beck 1978) of 10–18 for mild depression and scores of greater than 18 for serious depression. Only 10% of male participants were depressed, and most of these were only mildly so.

Effects on the infertile couple's family and social relationships can be profound. The couple's parents are often eager for grandchildren and apply spoken or unspoken pressure on their grown offspring to reproduce. Cultural and religious affiliations that place a high value on bearing children may increase the infertile couple's sense of failure and public embarrassment. Siblings and friends who have already conceived and borne children may be avoided because exposure to them exacerbates the infertile couple's sadness or because they are objects of envy. Because fertility is inevitably linked to sexual function, affected couples may feel embarrassed to reveal their problem or to have others allude to it. A frequent result is social isolation as the couple begins to avoid family gatherings at which their childless state may be mentioned and other social events at which pregnant women and small children may be present.

The financial burden of infertility can be considerable. Because of the ambiguous status of infertility as a medical problem, government-sponsored medical insurance programs such as Medicaid usually do not cover infertility treatment. Private insurance may reimburse only part of it; for example, treatments with IVF—which currently cost between $8,000 and $12,000 per cycle in the United States—are usually not covered. Adoption is also expensive: legal and other fees often average above $20,000 and may be considerably more if the adoption is privately arranged. As a result, infertility treatment is usually available only to couples of at least middle-class financial status, and couples undergoing treatment may make significant financial sacrifices such as foregoing vacations and using the money they had saved for a down payment on a house.

Months and sometimes years of infertility treatments affect patients' views of reality in sometimes subtle ways. Commonly, couples may become so focused on pregnancy as the concrete solution to their dilemma that they develop the attitude that all their life problems will be resolved if pregnancy occurs. Such patients can be particularly resistant to psychiatric interventions when needed because they believe that pregnancy is the only treatment necessary for whatever is bothering them.

Studies on the psychologic sequelae of successful fertility treatment are limited, but clearly the consequences can be deleterious. Pregnancy may be unexpectedly uncomfortable and fraught with excessive anxiety (Shapiro 1986). Parenthood may not have been anticipated in a realistic way. Use of the new reproductive technologies is associated with an increased incidence of multiple births, which carry their own risks of physical and psychologic morbidity (Attia and Downey 1992). These pregnancies are often complicated, with treatment requiring months of bed rest. Once the babies are born, the parents find that having more than one infant to care for can be physically, emotionally, and financially overwhelming. Garel et al. (1997), in a follow-up study of mothers with triplets, found that at 4 years after delivery all of the mothers were distressed and fatigued and that a significant minority regretted having triplets, were depressed, and were taking antidepressants.

Furthermore, it is unclear whether offspring conceived via infertility treatment grow up unharmed. The secrecy surrounding techniques such as artificial insemination by donor and the uncertainty about parentage that affects all involved parties when gametes are anonymously donated constitute risks to a happy childhood and family life (Sokoloff 1987). A small Australian study (Kovacs et al. 1993) of children aged 6–8 years who were conceived by donor insemination showed no abnormal findings on the Child Behavior Checklist (Achenbach 1978; Achenbach and Edelbrock 1983), but little other research has been done. More detailed and extensive studies on the psychologic well-being of children conceived using the new reproductive technologies are desperately needed.

## Specific Infertility Interventions and Their Psychologic Effects

Infertility evaluation usually begins with a history taken from the couple, a physical examination of the female partner, and a few basic studies. These include a basal body temperature chart kept by the woman for 1–2 months: the temperature is taken each morning before the woman rises and is charted on a graph; days on which intercourse occurs are also noted. The rationale for this study is that a rise in temperature signals the time of the surge of luteinizing hormone and ovulation, thus indicating the beginning of the woman's fertile period. Other early studies almost invariably include a postcoital examination or a sperm count. For the postcoital examination, a sample of cervical mucus, usually collected within 8 hours of the last intercourse, is assessed for its receptivity and for the number of sperm per high-power field that are present and moving. Semen specimens may also be examined to assess the number of motile sperm and the percentage of those sperm that has normal morphology.

These early studies may be repeated numerous times in the course of infertility evaluation and treatment, and although simple both in concept and execution, they are associated with psychologic morbidity. The need to take and chart one's temperature daily is a constantly repeated reminder of the couple's failure to conceive and leads in many cases to a loss of spontaneity and enjoyment in sexual intercourse, the timing of which is determined by "fertile days" on the chart. The postcoital examination also requires scheduled sexual activity and has the additional drawback of symbolically inviting a third person (the physician and/or laboratory technician) as an observer to the sexual act. Under these conditions, the incidence of both female anorgasmia and male impotence increases. Semen specimens usually must be studied within hours after collection, and production of semen by masturbation in a bathroom at the medical facility near the laboratory is often suggested. Under these conditions of intense performance anxiety, a significant number of men have difficulty obtaining the specimen, and the infertility evaluation becomes acutely embarrassing.

The female partner's failure to ovulate regularly is a relatively common cause of infertility, occurring in 40% of the cases in which the infertility is attributable to the woman. Treatment consists of one of several hormonal regimens. If the woman does not have ovarian failure (i.e., if she has not already undergone menopause, in which case no hormonal therapy will work), clomiphene, a nonsteroidal drug that blocks estrogen receptors, is usually the first drug used. The psychiatric side effects of this drug include nervousness, insomnia, and depression. Human menopausal gonadotropin preparations by daily injection are often used if clomiphene is ineffective. This treatment is expensive, however, costing several thousand dollars per cycle for the drug alone, and is associated with multiple ovulation: 30% or more of pregnancies achieved with the drug are multiple, and three or more fetuses are present in 5% of these cases. Ovarian hyperstimulation syndrome is a potentially life-threatening complication of treatment with human menopausal gonadotropins, and close monitoring by a knowledgeable physician is essential. As with clomiphene, ovulation and conception may not occur during the first cycle, in which case repeated cycles become necessary. In some cases, bromocriptine or gonadotropin-releasing hormone administered intravenously with a pump may be used to induce ovulation. (See the latest edition of Speroff et al.'s [1994]

*Clinical Gynecologic Endocrinology and Infertility* for additional information.)

To date, virtually no published reports exist that describe the psychiatric side effects of ovulation-inducing agents. The astute clinician will recognize, however, that hormonal treatments affecting the pituitary axis have the potential for effects on mood and thinking. Furthermore, the associated stresses are significant; these regimens of medication must be taken month after month despite multiple physical side effects, require close medical monitoring, are very expensive, require scheduled intercourse, have health risks, and may produce a multiple pregnancy if conception occurs. Thus, in the usual clinical situation, the couple will show signs of psychiatric distress, but the potential contributing factors to blame will not be immediately evident.

If the female partner has normal cervical mucus and appears to ovulate, and the male partner has normal sperm count and morphology, a hysterosalpingogram (radiographic examination of the female reproductive tract using radiopaque dye) and/or laparoscopy (direct visualization of the female reproductive organs performed under anesthesia during which a laparoscope is inserted through a small incision) may be performed to establish whether any anatomic abnormalities exist that might hinder the successful movement of an ovum through the fallopian tubes to the uterus. Such abnormalities include adhesions from previous pelvic surgery or infections, endometriosis from implants of the uterine lining that have seeded elsewhere in the reproductive tract, and congenital anomalies such as a bicornuate uterus. Obstruction of the fallopian tubes is a common factor in female infertility (30%–50% of cases). Thin adhesions and implants from endometriosis may be removed using the laparoscope. In other cases, hormonal therapy to shrink endometrial implants or surgery to restore the patency of the tubes (tuboplasty) may be attempted. Hormones used to suppress endometriosis include estrogen-progestin combinations (birth control pills) given continuously, medroxyprogesterone acetate, and danazol, an androgenic compound derived from the steroid 17α–ethinyltestosterone. All of these compounds may cause symptoms of depression or emotional lability. The success of tuboplasty, which may require microsurgical techniques, is variable depending largely on the preoperative condition of the tubes, and it cannot be relied on to produce a successful pregnancy.

About 5% of cases of infertility are attributed to "cervical factors" after a series of poor postcoital tests. This type of infertility is sometimes caused by excessively thick cervical mucus, which can be modified by treatment with low-dose estrogen or circumvented by the intrauterine insemination of sperm. In other cases, "sperm allergy," on the part of either the male or the female partner, may be suspected. Interventions have included corticosteroid therapy, use of condoms for periods of time to reduce exposure to semen, and intrauterine inseminations of washed sperm. All have been of equivocal benefit so far. A major contributing factor when postcoital tests are poor is often poor coital technique. A careful sexual history may reveal an impotence problem and that vaginal intercourse may not occur or that the couple is using vaginal lubricants, which may have a spermicidal effect.

Among the assisted reproductive technologies (ART) are IVF and gamete intrafallopian transfer (GIFT), interventions that are generally used after years of unsuccessful infertility treatment. With IVF, the woman is usually treated with ovulation-enhancing drugs and undergoes laparoscopy for the retrieval of eggs. The retrieved eggs are cultured, fertilized in vitro with the man's sperm, and implanted in the uterus. GIFT is a similar technique, except that fertilization takes place in the fallopian tube, into which follicles and sperm have been placed. In zygote intrafallopian transfer (ZIFT) the fertilized egg is returned to the tube. Such treatment is intense and expensive and success is uncertain. For years, pregnancy rates from a single cycle of IVF have hovered around 15%; a single cycle of GIFT yielded a viable pregnancy about 25% of the time (Society for Assisted Reproductive Technology and the American Fertility Society 1991). Technical advances are beginning to improve these odds, however.

Couples who conceive are at high risk of having a multifetal gestation, with its attendant increases in medical risks, rate of pregnancy loss, expense, and difficulties of simultaneously raising more than one child. Couples who fail to conceive after spending years and large amounts of money in a "go-for-broke" situation are at risk for significant psychologic sequelae. For instance, Newton et al. (1990) reported that both men and women experienced increased depressive and anxiety symptoms and depressive disorders after unsuccessful IVF treatment and that childless women were at particular risk.

The new reproductive technologies acquire an increased degree of psychologic risk when the gametes (sperm or eggs) are donated or a surrogate is involved to carry the pregnancy. Donor insemination (called artificial insemination by donor) is actually not new and is medically very simple to perform. It is also highly successful in producing pregnancy when the female partner's fertility is intact but the male partner has a low sperm count (oligospermia) or no viable sperm (azoospermia). Egg donation is a much newer and more elaborate procedure and involves locating an anonymous donor or a cooperative friend or relative. The donor and the infertile woman are then treated with medications to synchronize their cycles. At the appropriate time, the eggs are removed from the donor using a laparascope, and an IVF or GIFT procedure is used to fertilize the egg with the male partner's sperm. The infertile woman then carries the pregnancy. In cases where the infertile woman has sufficient eggs but for some reason cannot carry a pregnancy, a reverse of this procedure may be employed and a gestational surrogate may be found to "lend" her uterus for the duration of the pregnancy. In another variation, donor insemination is used to impregnate the surrogate, who then both contributes the egg and carries the pregnancy to delivery.

Oocyte donation was originally used in women of childbearing age who had experienced premature ovarian failure. More recently, it has been employed to impregnate women over 50 years of age who are postmenopausal (Sauer et al. 1995). This is an example of how infertility technology may outstrip an understanding of its consequences. We know that pregnancy for women past menopause has more physical hazards such as hypertension and gestational diabetes (Flamigni and Borini 1995), but the psychologic and social risks to the offspring conceived and to the couple (especially if both members are old) are not well understood (Ethics Committee of the American Society for Reproductive Medicine 1997).

After many years, during which treatments for male infertility remained scant, a new technique has recently become available. This procedure, intracytoplasmic sperm injection (ICSI), employs an IVF procedure in which eggs removed from the female partner under laparoscopic visualization are injected with carefully selected sperm. The sperm is delivered inside the cell membrane, thus enhancing chances of successful fertilization. An early report comparing couples who chose ICSI with those who chose donor insemination showed that couples employing ICSI did so because the technique allowed them to conceive a child who is biologically theirs, whereas couples choosing donor insemination did so because they could not afford IVF (Schover et al. 1996). This is another example of how economic factors play a major role in determining what kind of infertility treatment couples receive.

Berger (1980) has reported on the severe stress couples experience when the male partner is diagnosed as azoospermic or severely oligospermic. Of the men studied, 60% developed transient impotence, and their wives reported a high frequency of rageful dreams and fantasies of leaving the infertile partner. Donor insemination is so medically simple to perform that couples may proceed with it before fully exploring their feelings about incorporating a (usually) unknown man's genetic heritage into their relationship. In addition to the couple's shame at their deficiency, legal and religious ambiguity about the status of the procedure may induce the couple to try to keep it secret. Total secrecy is a burden to maintain, however, and in the heat of some family crisis, the fact of the insemination is likely to be blurted out in a harmful way (Sokoloff 1987), especially when couples who plan to keep donor insemination secret from the offspring confide in family and friends, as a significant percentage do. For instance, Amuzu et al. (1990) reported that 50% of couples conceiving through donor insemination had told at least one person in their social circle. Knowledge of one's genetic parentage is increasingly being seen in the United States as the birthright of every adult individual, a situation that complicates the task of maintaining secrecy.

On the other hand, when the donor of the gametes is known (which is much more likely if the donor is female), other complicating factors arise: the infertile couple's ongoing relationship with the donor, the donor's feeling of emotional proprietorship, and the possibility that the offspring may have "multiple parents" to deal with. Additionally, when the woman who carries the pregnancy will not keep the baby, she may encounter unforeseen difficulties in relinquishing it to the parents. This is understandable, because women who volunteer to be surrogates are often motivated not only by financial need, the desire to be pregnant, and the wish to give a baby to an infertile couple but also by the desire to master unresolved feelings about a previous pregnancy loss (Parker 1983; Schover et al. 1991).

## Psychologic Treatment Issues for Infertility Patients

Numerous studies have suggested that one response to infertility treatment, especially if unsuccessful, is depressive symptoms. An episode of depression by DSM-IV criteria (American Psychiatric Association 1994) must of course be distinguished from feelings of distress and discouragement that commonly occur and do not constitute an episode of depressive disorder (Downey et al. 1989). Mood swings may occur (with or without the presence of exogenous hormones and with or without a history of premenstrual mood symptoms) over the course of the month as women grow hopeful or anxious during the days before and after ovulation only to become frustrated and disappointed with the onset of menstruation. Women may appear to have moderately severe agitated depressions around the time of menses but become asymptomatic 2 weeks later and repeat this cycle every month.

Any complaint of depression needs careful evaluation, especially with regard to severity, because in a small number of infertility patients (both male and female) psychiatric illness may develop or be exacerbated by the stress of the infertility workup. Some episodes will be manageable with the physician's support and variations in the pace of infertility treatment. Others will require psychotherapy and, in a few, the addition of psychotropic medications. At this point, great tact on the part of the mental health practitioner is necessary (as well as the support of the gynecologist or urologist), because infertility treatment is often deferred when patients are receiving other medications and patients bent on achieving fertility may refuse any medication that would delay their efforts to conceive.

Although few women or men undergoing infertility treatment will develop a psychiatric disorder, many are so focused on achieving their goal of pregnancy that they will lose the ability to keep the problem in perspective with the rest of their lives. An infertile couple may feel that time is so pressing that even a respite of a few weeks during which they do not pursue treatment is unacceptable. The psychiatrist may be able to help such exhausted or symptomatic couples take a holiday from treatment. This is often the first intervention when distress seems to be building toward dysfunction, and in some cases it may be the only intervention needed.

It is important that the treating clinician not have preconceptions about how the infertility problem will affect the couple's relationship. Some women are more anxious about being childless than are their partners and feel isolated as a result. Other women find that facing this life crisis with their partners has strengthened their relationship. The emotional benefits of approaching infertility as a shared problem suggest that when one member of an infertile couple seeks psychologic help it is valuable for the clinician to see both partners, at least as part of the initial assessment, so that the less-symptomatic partner can be brought into the treatment as needed.

Couples undergoing infertility treatment may be under such pressure to perform sexually in order to comply with the many requirements of the evaluation and treatment that they begin to develop sexual dysfunctions such as impotence, anorgasmia, or lack of sexual desire. Frequently, the sexual symptoms will lessen with relatively simple interventions, such as limiting the taking of basal body temperature or taking 1–2 months' break from treatment. Persistent, severe sexual dysfunction needs more extensive exploration.

One of the most common problems infertility patients face has to do with the "relaxed attitude" often advised by their friends and family as an aid to enhancing fertility. It is innately stressful and not at all relaxing to be struggling to reach a difficult goal such as conception. Although it may be beneficial to learn relaxation techniques to enhance coping strategies, no good evidence has yet shown that relaxation enhances fertility. Adoption, although it may relieve the pressure to conceive, has also not been shown to enhance fertility beyond allowing additional time during which unprotected intercourse may lead to conception (Collins et al. 1983; Lamb and Leurgans 1979).

Couples seeking conception are prone to accept responsibility for the infertility problem when it does not have to do with their behavior, for instance, by assuming that conflicts about pregnancy may be causing their infertility. Clinicians can be most beneficial to such patients by clarifying that stress and conflicts do not ordinarily affect fertility, and that difficulties conceiving are not the patients' fault.

A perceived loss of control is perhaps the most common stress of infertility. For women accustomed to planning their careers and other aspects of their lives, infertility may be experienced as their first major disappointment and as an unjust shock. Envy of friends and family members who conceive easily is common: "Why them and not us?" couples ask. Anger toward the treating physician is also common, and one of the tasks of the mental health professional is helping the infertility patient determine when his or her expectations of the physician are unrealistic.

A central task in the clinical management of infertility patients is helping them to achieve a sense of mastery in managing their treatment. As more and more new reproductive technologies become available, it becomes increasingly difficult for patients to decide when "enough is enough" (Taylor 1990). The internal pressure to persist, no matter what the emotional and financial cost, is intense. As Becker and Nachtigall (1994) point out, it is common in our society for individuals to take risks by engaging in medical treatment to *avoid regret.*

As they seek a clear statement from the physician on the chances of achieving pregnancy, couples may need help from a mental health professional so that they can make an informed decision. Once they have this information, couples may need assistance in weighing the benefits and costs for themselves in relation to the other alternatives open to them, such as adoption or living without children.

The appropriate mode of psychiatric treatment, if indicated, will depend on the couples' or patients' presenting symptoms, their psychiatric history, and their characterologic strengths and deficits. Conjoint marital or sexual therapy may be indicated, as may individual psychotherapy or briefer periods of counseling. Support group–oriented therapies available in an infertility clinic setting (Stewart et al. 1992) or given under the aegis of RESOLVE (the national self-help organization for infertile couples) are appropriate when couples are willing to seek help in a group setting and are not too anxious and suggestible.

Speroff et al. (1994) have stated the goals of infertility treatment in their text for gynecologists: to seek out and correct the causes of infertility, to provide accurate information, to give emotional support for the couple, and to counsel them about the proper time to discontinue investigation and treatment.

Inherent in this advice is the idea that for all of us who treat patients with infertility problems, the goal is not to achieve pregnancy at any cost but rather to assist couples in resolving their infertility crisis and becoming able to move on in life. This may mean having a birth child, adopting or fostering a child or children, or living child-free in a manner in which their creativity and urge to contribute to the benefit of the next generation can find expression.

# References

Achenbach TM: The child behavior profile, 1: boys aged six–eleven. J Consult Clin Psychol 46:478–488, 1978

Achenbach TM, Edelbrock CS: Manual for the child behavior checklist and revised behavior profile. Burlington, VT, University of Vermont, 1983

American Psychiatric Association: Diagnostic and Statistical Manual of Mental Disorders, 4th Edition. Washington, DC, American Psychiatric Association, 1994

Amuzu B, Laxova R, Shapiro SS: Pregnancy outcome, health of children, and family adjustment after donor insemination. Obstet Gynecol 75:899–905, 1990

Attia E, Downey J: Psychological consequences of successful treatment: a case report of a pregnancy assisted by in vitro fertilization–embryo transfer. Psychosomatics 33:218–221, 1992

Beck AT: Depression Inventory. Philadelphia, PA, Center for Cognitive Therapy, 1978

Becker G, Nachtigall RD: "Born to be a mother": the cultural construction of risk in infertility treatment in the U.S. Soc Sci Med 39:507–518, 1994

Berger DM: Couples' reactions to male infertility and donor insemination. Am J Psychiatry 137:1047–1049, 1980

Collins JA, Wrixon W, Janes LB, et al: Treatment-independent pregnancy among infertile couples. N Engl J Med 309:1201–1206, 1983

Connolly KJ, Edelmann RJ, Cooke ID: Distress and marital problems associated with infertility. J Reprod Infant Psychol 5:49–57, 1987

Cook R, Parsons J, Mason B, et al: Emotional, marital and sexual functioning in patients embarking upon IVF and AID treatment for infertility. J Reprod Infant Psychol 7:87–93, 1989

DeVries K, Degani S, Eibschitz I, et al: The influence of the postcoital test on the sexual function of infertile women. J Psychosom Obstet Gynaecol 3:101–106, 1984

Downey J, Yingling S, McKinney M, et al: Mood disorder, psychiatric symptoms, and distress in women presenting for infertility evaluation. Fertil Steril 52:425–432, 1989

Drake TS, Grunert GM: A cyclic pattern of sexual dysfunction in the infertility investigation. Fertil Steril 32:542–547, 1979

Ethics Committee of the American Society for Reproductive Medicine: Ethical considerations of assisted reproductive technologies. Fertil Steril 67(suppl):i–iii, 1S–9S, 1997

Flamigni C, Borini A: Counseling post-menopausal women for donor in-vitro fertilization and hormone replacement therapy. Hum Reprod 10:1237–1241, 1995

Garel M, Salobir C, Blondel B: Psychological consequences of having triplets: a 4-year follow-up study. Fertil Steril 67:1162–1165, 1997

Jaffe SB, Jewelewicz R: The basic infertility investigation. Fertil Steril 56:599–613, 1991

Keye WR: Psychosexual responses to infertility. Clin Obstet Gynecol 27:760–766, 1984

Keye WR, Deneris A, Wilson T, et al: Psychosexual responses to infertility: differences between infertile men and women (abstract). Fertil Steril 36:426, 1981

Kovacs GT, Mushin D, Kane H, et al: A controlled study of the psychosocial development of children conceived following insemination with donor semen. Hum Reprod 8:788–790, 1993

Lalos A, Lalos O, Jacobsson L, et al: Psychological reactions to the medical investigation and surgical treatment of infertility. Gynecol Obstet Invest 20:209–217, 1985

Lamb EJ, Leurgans S: Does adoption affect subsequent fertility? Am J Obstet Gynecol 134:138–144, 1979

McEwan KL, Costello CG, Taylor PG: Adjustment to infertility. J Abnorm Psychol 96:108–116, 1987

Menning BE: The emotional needs of infertile couples. Fertil Steril 34:313–319, 1980

Mosher WD, Pratt WF: Fecundity and infertility in the United States, 1965–1988. Advance Data 192:1–6, 1990

Newton CR, Hearn MT, Yuzpe AA: Psychological assessment and follow-up after in vitro fertilization: assessing the impact of failure. Fertil Steril 54:879–886, 1990

Parker PJ: Motivations of surrogate mothers: initial findings. Am J Psychiatry 140:117–118, 1983

Sauer MV, Paulson RJ, Lobo RA: Pregnancy in women 50 or more years of age: outcomes of 22 consecutively established pregnancies for oocyte donation. Fertil Steril 64:111–115, 1995

Schover LR, Collins RE, Quigley MM, et al: Psychological follow-up of women evaluated as oocyte donors. Hum Reprod 6:1487–1491, 1991

Schover LR, Thomas AJ, Miller KF, et al: Preferences for intracytoplasmic sperm injection versus donor insemination in severe male factor infertility: a preliminary report. Hum Reprod 11:2461–2464, 1996

Seibel MM, Taymor ML: Emotional aspects of infertility. Fertil Steril 37:137–145, 1982

Shapiro CH: Is pregnancy after infertility a dubious joy? Social Casework 67:306–313, 1986

Society for Assisted Reproductive Technology and the American Fertility Society: In-vitro fertilization–embryo transfer (IVF–ET) in the United States during 1989. Fertil Steril 55:14, 1991

Sokoloff BZ: Alternative methods of reproduction: effects on the child. Clin Pediatr 26:11–17, 1987

Speroff L, Glass RH, Kase NG: Clinical Gynecologic Endocrinology and Infertility. Baltimore, MD, Williams & Wilkins, 1994

Stewart DE, Boydell KM, McCarthy K, et al: A prospective study of the effectiveness of brief, professionally led support groups for infertility patients. Int J Psychiatry Med 22:173–182, 1992

Taylor PJ: When is enough enough? Fertil Steril 54:772–774, 1990

Wright J, Duchesne C, Sabourin S, et al: Psychosocial distress and infertility: men and women respond differently. Fertil Steril 55:100–108, 1991

# Induced Abortion in the United States

NADA L. STOTLAND, M.D., M.P.H.

## Introduction and Definitions

The termination of a pregnancy is a powerful act, with significant psychologic meanings and implications arising from personal psychodynamics and experience, religion, interpersonal relationships, and biology. Induced abortion is an act enmeshed in its social surroundings in every respect: etiology, performance, and sequelae. Although, as elaborated in this chapter, pregnancies have been terminated at every time in history and on every continent of the world, the psychologic aspects of abortion are so closely culture bound that it is not possible either to discuss it generically or to do justice to more than one culture and its legal system. Therefore, this chapter focuses on induced abortion in the United States, which in itself contains a wide range of attitudes and practices.

Abortion is a medical intervention that evokes a great amount of feeling in the United States. Elections for public office are won and lost on the basis of candidates' positions toward abortion funding, access, availability, acceptable grounds, and the right of potentially concerned parties other than the pregnant woman herself to be informed of or to consent to the procedure (Tribe 1990). Both the intensity of feeling about abortion and the avoidance of the subject are reflected in confusing terminology. The term *abortion* is used by gynecologists to describe both induced abortion and spontaneous abortion, or miscarriage. *Induced* is a more accurate descriptor than *elective*; abortion is also induced in cases of fetal defects incompatible with life and of medical complications threatening the life of the mother. The term *abortion* as used in this chapter refers to induced abortion.

## Role of Psychiatry

The psychologic causes and experience of abortion are parallel to those of the other reproductive events discussed in this book, but with more publicity, passion, and misperception. Psychiatrists have been involved in access to the procedure, and organized psychiatry, as represented by the American Psychiatric Association (APA), has taken an official position on induced abortion. This position, adopted in 1978 and reconfirmed in 1992 and 1995, is as follows:

> The emotional consequences of unwanted pregnancy on parents and their offspring may lead to long-standing life distress and disability, and the children of unwanted pregnancies are at high risk for abuse, neglect, mental illness, and deprivation of the quality of life. Pregnancy that results from undue coercion, rape, or incest creates even greater potential distress or disability in the child and the parents. The adolescent most vulnerable to early pregnancy is the product of adverse sociocultural conditions involving poverty, discrimination, and family disorganization, and statistics indicate that the resulting pregnancy is laden with medical complications which threaten the well-being of mother and fetus. The delivery that ensues from teenage pregnancy is prone to prematurity and major threats to the health of mother and child, and the resulting newborns have a higher percentage of birth defects, developmental difficulties, and a poorer life and health expectancy than the average for our society. Such children are often not released for adoption and thus get caught in the web of foster care and welfare systems, possibly entering lifetimes of dependency and costly social interventions. The tendency of this pattern to pass from generation to generation is very marked and thus serves to perpetuate a cycle of social and educational failure, mental and physical illness, and serious delinquency.
>
> Because of these considerations, and in the interest of public welfare, the American Psychiatric Association 1) opposes all constitutional amendments, legislation, and regulations curtailing family planning and abortion services to any segment of the population; 2) reaffirms its position that abortion is a medical procedure in which physicians should respect the patient's right to freedom of choice—psychiatrists may be called on as consultants to the patient or physician in those cases in which the patient or physician requests such consultation to expand mutual appreciation of motivation and consequences; and 3) affirms that the freedom to act to interrupt pregnancy must be considered a mental health imperative with major social and mental health implications. (American Psychiatric Association 1978)

Several other medical specialty and practice organizations, including the American College of Obstetricians and Gynecologists, have taken a similar stance. The American Medical Association, after considerable debate, decided to leave attitudes about induced abortion to the individual physician. Although the official APA position probably represents the stance of a sizable majority of psychiatrists, there are those whose cherished values and beliefs are violated by it. They question the appropriateness of such a stance within a profession dedicated to the preservation of life, the relevance of abortion policy to psychiatry in particular, and the effectiveness of access to abortion in eliminating or reducing the problems to which the APA's statement addresses itself: child abuse, neglect, and deprivation. On the other hand, some psychiatrists regard abortion as such a fundamental human right that they threatened to boycott a psychiatric convention scheduled in a state in which the legislature had passed statutes limiting abortion access. Of particular importance to the practice of psychiatry are the psychosocial factors in unplanned pregnancies, the decision-making process, the effect of pregnancy and abortion on women's mental well-being, physician–patient confidentiality, the right and obligation of physicians to see that patients have access to and knowledge about all therapeutic options without barriers, and the autonomy of the pregnant woman, regardless of her age, to make decisions about her care in consultation with the health professionals who provide that care.

## Conceptual and Methodologic Issues

The issue of abortion is so contentious that fundamental realities are often overlooked. Consideration of these realities is essential not only for policymaking but also for clinical practice and scientific study. First of all, abortion is performed only on women who are pregnant. If an abortion is not performed (and barring complications such as spontaneous abortion), these women will go on to deliver. Study of the outcome of abortion without comparison with the sequelae of labor, delivery, and motherhood has very limited scientific validity and practical utility. The only truly appropriate control group for such studies is women who found their pregnancies similarly problematic, who sought abortion, and who were unable to obtain it. Findings from the few such studies that have been performed are summarized here. Women considering abortion are not only pregnant, but pregnant under circumstances they experience as untenable. The circumstances also make a substantive contribution to outcome; the abortion procedure does not have an impact in isolation. Last, the effects of social and medical context on the experience and outcome of abortion are often overlooked. These considerations are discussed further in the section on psychiatric issues.

## Gynecologic and Public Health Issues

Data in this section are taken from *Public Health Policy Implications of Abortion* (American College of Obstetricians and Gynecologists 1990), a handbook for health professionals that was developed collaboratively by a group of medical organizations, including the American College of Obstetricians and Gynecologists, the American Medical Association, and the APA, and published in January 1990. It can be obtained through those organizations. Statistics were derived from the Centers for Disease Control and Prevention (Koonin et al. 1998) and the National Center for Health Statistics.

Procedures to terminate a pregnancy vary somewhat by trimester. Until recently, second-trimester abortions were generally induced by the intrauterine instillation of chemical agents, such as urea or saline, that precipitated the onset of uterine contractions and the expulsion of the fetus. Currently, second-trimester pregnancies are also terminated by methods similar to those used in the first trimester: cervical dilation and uterine evacuation. Since 1981, 90% of all abortions have been performed using suction curettage. Under local anesthesia, the cervix is dilated and the uterine contents removed by suction. The procedure takes 10–12 minutes. This procedure cannot be performed late in pregnancy.

At least half of all induced abortions in the United States are performed within the first 8 weeks, and 90% within the first trimester, of pregnancy. During this time, the risk of medical complications is less than 0.5%. Abortions performed after 20 weeks of gestation constitute fewer than 1% of all such procedures; most of these occur at 21–23 weeks. Most abortions are performed in freestanding (nonhospital) clinics, where the cost is about one-third (average, $213) of that in a hospital, the safety is equivalent (for early and uncomplicated abortions), and the access and psychologic experience easier (unless complicated by the presence of protesters). Maternal mortality from abortion performed under safe conditions is 0.5 per 100,000 procedures; the rate from childbirth is 25 times greater. During the 1960s, before abortion was legalized in the United States, illegal abortion led to approximately 20% of pregnancy-related admissions to hospitals in major population centers and 20% of all deaths from pregnancy and childbirth. These kinds of statistics are still obtained in areas of the world where safe abortions are not available.

Access to abortion is geographically uneven; the vast majority of abortion providers are in urban areas. Of all counties in the United States, 82% lack a facility performing abortions; the 30% of women who live in a county without a provider obtain, on average, substantially fewer abortions than women in areas with a provider. Most general hospitals perform no abortions at all, and those that do perform very few. Other barriers to service include the federal ruling that Medicaid funds cannot be used for abortion services except to save the mother's life and requirements for notification or consent of the patient's parents. As growing numbers of women enter military service, the prohibition on abortion services at military hospitals, even when privately financed, affects greater numbers of women. Evidence indicates that such barriers deter timely and safe care and lead to adverse public health consequences (Berger 1978).

The antiprogestin mifepristone (RU 486) is 95% effective in inducing abortion when taken orally and followed by a dose of prostaglandin. It is associated with minimal side effects and with no known complications or long-term health implications. It is available and in use in China and in France; clinical trials are under way in other countries all over the world. The U.S. Food and Drug Administration has approved the use of mifepristone (Rosenblatt et al. 1995) and a private, nonprofit consortium has been founded to undertake the research and distribution of RU 486 within the United States. Antiabortion groups have reportedly threatened to initiate major actions, including boycotts, against any pharmaceutical company that seeks to market the drug in this country. Some women prefer surgical procedures because they are definitive and immediate, but most prefer medical abortion because it feels more private and less intrusive. There is a federal ban on the study of other abortifacients.

## Epidemiology

The World Health Organization estimates that as many as 53 million induced abortions are performed globally every year (World Health Organization 1997). Rates of induced abortion in the United States have been compiled according to race, age, and marital and reproductive status. The figures quoted here were published by the American College of Obstetricians and Gynecologists in 1990 and updated with the latest available figures from the Centers for Disease Control and Prevention (Koonin et al. 1998). Of women who undergo abortions, approximately 58% are white; 45% are nulliparous; 89% have two or fewer children; and 54% have not undergone an induced abortion previously. Seventy-nine percent of all women and 96% of teenage women obtaining abortions are unmarried. Marriage precipitated by pregnancy places teenagers at higher risk for abuse, school failure, and dependence on public support than their unmarried agemates (Zuravin 1991). Over 60% of women undergoing abortion are younger than 25 years; 42% of pregnancies in teenagers are terminated by induced abortion. Although women over 40 become pregnant more rarely and account for relatively few induced abortions, 51% of their pregnancies are terminated by induced abortion. The numbers and rates of induced abortion remained fairly constant throughout the 1980s and approximate those before abortion was legalized. In 1986, approximately 33 million legal and 27 million illegal abortions were performed throughout the world (Tietze and Henshaw 1986).

## History and Anthropology

Induced abortions have been performed throughout recorded history in every part of the world and in virtually every sort of culture. An exhaustive cross-cultural study performed by Devereux (1976) revealed a wide range of methods by which pregnancy termination is attempted or achieved and an equally wide range of social regulations, from those that proscribed abortion to those that mandated it under certain circumstances. Discussion of abortion practices and beliefs in selected cultures serves to put the practice into some perspective (Newman 1991). Induced abortion is mentioned—and proscribed—in the Hippocratic oath. Therefore, it must have been practiced and discussed in ancient Greece (Edelstein 1989). Moving to the twentieth century, in the former Soviet Union, an officially atheist state that sought to increase its population, abortions were provided by the state health system (although supplementary, sub rosa fees were required for anesthesia), and women underwent an average of nine abortions each (Page 1989). In China, it is reported that the number of induced abortions is at least equal to the number of live births. Population control is a national priority in China, and considerable pressure may be exerted on women or couples when conception has occurred without prior approval by their respective work group (Engelhardt 1989). Abortions are also widely performed in Roman Catholic countries, where they are illegal, only illicitly available, and lead to thousands of maternal deaths (Bromham and Oloto 1997).

In contrast, induced abortions are legal, common, safe, and accepted in Japan. This accepting social context is not associated with a lack of feeling and meaning, however (Klass and Heath 1997). Japanese religious and cultural beliefs hold that the soul of the embryo may cause health and other problems for the mother if not laid to rest in a religious observance. There is a goddess who takes a special interest in embryos and young children, and shrines dedicated to her are hung with offerings of baby toys and bibs (Ohnuki-Tierney 1984).

In the United States, abortion was first the province of the lay midwife who was responsible for most of women's reproductive health care. Around the middle of the nineteenth century, as medicine was increasingly professionalized and organized, obstetrics and gynecology became recognized as a medical specialty and physicians moved to establish hegemony over women's reproductive functions. Textbooks described menstruation and childbirth as debilitating events that made women vulnerable to medical disorders and unsuited to stresses such as those associated with higher education, lest their reproductive functions be impaired. Women of the lower classes, who performed heavy labor inside and outside the home even when pregnant and postpartum, were thought to have more primitive physiologies. With a focus on the middle and upper classes and the assumptions that childbearing within marriage was women's God-given duty and that conception outside marriage was sinful, abortion began to be decried by organized medicine. Eventually, it was outlawed.

Nevertheless, the practice of abortion continued. Women's magazines of the nineteenth and early twentieth centuries regularly carried thinly disguised advertisements for purported abortifacients. Abortion went underground, sometimes performed secretly by licensed physicians and more often by shadowy practitioners to whom women were referred by their physicians, friends, and relatives. In areas where legal scrutiny was tight, elaborate arrangements were made that involved meetings in out-of-the-way locations, blindfolded transport to unknown locations, and exchanges of cash. Anesthesia was rarely used because it lengthened the time for the clandestine procedure and made it difficult for the woman to flee in the case of a police raid. Serious complications and deaths were common; until the early 1970s most large hospitals had entire wards full of patients being treated for septic abortions. Care was complicated by the fact that the women were both unwilling and unable to give accurate histories when they presented hemorrhaging and/or infected for emergency care to often judgmental hospital staff. In cities such as Chicago, elaborate networks served to direct and bring women to quality physicians who would risk losing their medical licenses by performing abortions to prevent these dire complications.

Because many of the state laws prohibiting abortion allowed for exceptions when continued pregnancy was thought to threaten the life or, less commonly, the health of the woman, psychiatrists played a significant role in providing more affluent and/or sophisticated women access to medically safe abortion. As medical knowledge improved, medical illnesses once incompatible with successful pregnancy outcomes, such as diabetes, became manageable in the context of pregnancy. It was difficult to establish medical grounds for termination without blatant falsification of laboratory results and other verifiable findings. Psychiatric conditions, on the other hand, were not so verifiable. The earliest versions of DSM had just appeared, with highly subjective criteria for various diagnoses. If a psychiatrist asserted that a woman would commit suicide or suffer other psychiatric sequelae if her pregnancy were not terminated, there was little way to prove otherwise.

In many hospitals, committees were formed for the sole purpose of making decisions in these cases. Nearly always, a pregnant woman had to make her case to a panel of male physicians. Some of these women have written poignantly about the humiliation of presenting their painful stories to the gatekeepers who controlled access to the procedure they so desperately wanted. One of these women had three preschool children when she became pregnant for the fourth time. Her husband, who was the sole support of the young family, insisted that he would abandon the family if another child was born. This woman, Kate Michelman, went on to head the National Abortion and Reproductive Rights Action League.

## Legal Issues

Up to 1.5 million induced abortions are performed in the United States each year; this number was estimated to be much the same before the *Roe v. Wade* decision by the Supreme Court legalized abortion in 1973. The absolute numbers have fallen 15% since 1990, and the percentage of pregnancies terminated by induced abortion has continued to decline since 1987 (Koonin et al. 1998). The *Roe v. Wade* decision declared a right to privacy between a woman and her physician concerning the decision of whether to have an abortion and an unencumbered right to abortion during the first 12 weeks of pregnancy. During the second trimester, the state was permitted to regulate abortion only to protect maternal well-being.

The passage of *Roe v. Wade* has had some paradoxical consequences over the years. The collective memory of the consequences of outlawing abortion faded. People who favor rights to abortion became complacent. People who opposed abortion mobilized and made abortion an acknowledged and unacknowledged symbol of other social agendas. In response, the United States Congress has enacted legislation enjoining the use of federal funds to support abortion services. The Supreme Court, as its composition changes, has upheld various state laws limiting access to abortion. Laws requiring that the husband or father of the fetus be informed or give consent have been overturned. Other laws requiring that the parents of a pregnant girl under the age of majority be informed and/or give consent have been upheld—with the provision, called a *judicial bypass*, that the young woman can gain access to abortion by presenting herself to a judge with evidence that she is mature enough to make the decision and is independent of or abused or neglected by her parents.

Laws that require waiting periods between the time that abortion is sought and the time that it is performed are allowed, as are those requiring that government-generated statements be provided about the stages of gestation and the availability of support for mothers and children in the state. Under the guise of public health statistic-keeping, some states record the names of physicians who perform and patients who undergo abortions, data that is not kept for other procedures and that can be, and is, used to harass the physicians and patients and their families. The latest attempt to curtail access is the debate over late-term abortion (Epner et al. 1998). The successes of the antiabortion movement in obtaining restrictions on abortion have led some women to feel that the *Roe v. Wade* decision is more a facade than a guarantee of access; an impression that is to some degree accurate. However, the activities of antiabortion groups at women's clinics have also been constrained by legislation, generally precipitated by violence at those clinics, thus mitigating somewhat the additional stress imposed by clinic harassment.

# Ethical Perspectives

As mentioned, access to abortion services has become the subject of heated controversy. Irreconcilable factions argue that abortion is murder or that legal access is an imperative not only for justice for women but also for their very survival. Induced abortion has come to signify major social concerns and fears: the continuity of the nuclear family structure and traditional gender roles, the erosion of sexual morality, the liberation of women from oppression and abuse, and the opportunity for children to enter the world as wanted members of loving families with the resources to provide for them.

Cultural icons have crystallized around these positions: the fetus for groups self-identified as "pro-life," the bloody coat hanger of the back-alley abortionist for those who are "pro-choice." These symbols are also reflections of levels of discourse about the ethics of induced abortion. Because the opposing points are irreconcilable, no attempt to reconcile them is made here. It is important, however, that the issues be delineated. The levels of discourse reflect the medical, psychologic, and social complexities of the procedure (B. Brody 1982; Warren 1982). At the most basic level are the biologic, medical, and legal realities. Abortion is the termination of a pregnancy. Society has an interest in the successful propagation of the species; a particular pregnancy may advance or deter that goal. Pregnancy almost always occurs as the result of sexual intercourse between a man and a woman. This intercourse may be more or less consensual or coercive, and the sexual partners may have congruent, divergent, or contradictory investments in procreation and intentions with regard to the parenting of a potential child.

Fertilization may also take place deliberately, without intercourse, by recourse to more (in vitro fertilization) or less (artificial insemination by turkey baster) sophisticated technologic means. It always involves the genetic material of a male and a female human individual, although the genetic, gestational, and social parents may all be different persons. Because procreative maturity precedes legal maturity (the age of majority), pregnancy can and does occur in minor women whose capacity to weigh alternatives and whose moral rights to make decisions about their own care and futures is another ethical and legal question.

Another level of discourse concerns the ethical responsibilities of the medical profession. Induced abortion may be performed by a lay attendant, attempted by the pregnant woman herself, or carried out by a physician or other medically trained and licensed professional health care provider. This array of possibilities raises analogous ethical problems for the gynecologist and psychiatrist alike. Abortion may be viewed as a service that doctors are obligated to provide on request, a procedure for which physicians are the appropriate gatekeepers (many court decisions and official organization positions stipulate that the decision is to be made "by a woman and her doctor"), or a prima facie violation of medical ethics. The substantial dangers of abortion performed outside the medical system, an eventuality that seems unavoidable given the available anthropologic and demographic evidence, are sometimes weighed in ethical decisions as well (Jacobson 1988).

Another question concerns the woman's responsibility for conception and the embryo thus engendered. A more or less explicit image persists of the sexually wanton female who seeks to rid herself of the predictable outcome of her lifestyle at the expense of her child's life. In point of fact, however, many realities constrain women's control over sexual activity and contraception. These include not only rape and incest but also lack of access to information about reproduction and contraception, lack of access to contraceptive devices and medical services, and sexual activity in which financial, social, and psychologic coercion falls short of narrowly defined sexual assault (DaVanzo et al. 1991). Contraceptives also fail.

An alternative image exists, that of the virtuous woman who accepts responsibility, maintains the pregnancy once conceived, and makes the personal sacrifice involved in the experience of pregnancy, labor, delivery, and either child care or child relinquishment to adoption in the interest of her child (Vaux 1989). This stance imbues the woman in the earliest stages of pregnancy with the role and moral obligations of the parent of a child already born. It also raises the issue that pregnancy, delivery, parenthood, and the potential child become the instruments by which the woman is punished for sexual intercourse; the argument that most sentimentalizes attachment to the potential child sometimes conceptualizes that child as a retribution rather than a blessing.

The question of when human life begins overlaps with the question of the definition of "human life." A fertilized ovum is living matter with the genetic composition of a human being and the potential to develop into a human being. To date, however, that development can happen only within a woman's body. Embryologic research indicates that the differentiation of cells resulting in the formation of a normal organism can occur only in a given sequence and in the matrix and structure of embryonic development as a whole. The cells that are to differentiate into, for example, liver cells can do so only if the rest of development is proceeding normally around them at each of the requisite stages. Put another way—one relevant to the ethics of abortion—the cells and tissues of the preembryo and embryo are not inevitably destined to become a human being.

Even given the circumstances of normal development, no clear or consensual definition of human life exists. It may be defined by genetic composition, human form, the appearance of brain waves, the ability to experience sensation, or the awareness of the self and other people as human. What distinguishes human life from other forms of life, and what privileges, if any, does our humanity confer on us? Both humans and animals experience pleasure and pain, and both exert strenuous effort to stay alive. Although cells biopsied from human tissue are alive, capable of reproduction, and endowed with a full complement of human chromosomes, it would be difficult to argue that such a collection of cells constitutes human life or a human being. The assertion that any particular stage of human development constitutes the beginning of "human life" is fraught with problematic implications.

Fetal viability has been raised as an issue both by ethicists and lawmakers. Publicity about the survival of some infants born extremely prematurely has led the public to believe that the medical community is steadily moving back the point in pregnancy at which the fetus can live outside the mother. Scientific evidence does not support this belief, however, and some perinatologists think it likely that we have already approached the limits of our abilities to support extrauterine life in prematurely born infants.

All of these problems complicate attempts to apply the usual standards of beneficence, autonomy, and justice to the consideration of the ethics of abortion. The APA's position statement seems to imply that *not* allowing a potential child to come into being can be beneficent for that child. Abortion ends a potential or an actual life as well as the hopes and interests of those who wanted to see it realized, although it may further the good both of the woman whose pregnancy and potential motherhood are experienced as intolerable and of others for whom she is responsible or to whose lives she can make a contribution. The availability of abortion may hurt society because it undermines respect for potential life and for support during pregnancy and childrearing. It may benefit society because it diminishes the social burden of unwanted and poorly cared for children and the loss or injury of women who resort to unsafe attempts to terminate their pregnancies.

## Psychiatric Sequelae

Psychiatrists help patients make decisions about problem pregnancies and deal with their short- and long-term reactions to induced abortion. In 1988 C. Everett Koop, Surgeon General of the United States, was charged by President Bush to determine the medical and psychologic effects of abortion on American women and to publish a review of the findings. Dr. Koop, who was personally opposed to abortion, solicited opinions and scientific information from a wide variety of medical and interest groups, including the APA, and concluded that there was insufficient information to assert that abortion had negative sequelae (Koop 1991).

The public is nevertheless very concerned about the psychiatric sequelae of abortion. The popular press and antiabortion groups have published allegations that abortion causes serious, disabling, permanent psychologic damage: an "abortion trauma syndrome" (DeVeber et al. 1991). This term, which is absent from the peer-reviewed literature, seems to have been coined to resemble posttraumatic stress disorder. Allegations that the medical community is deliberately withholding or overlooking data supporting this position have also been made (Pro-Life Action Ministries, undated). Patients and the general public may turn to psychiatrists for accurate scientific findings concerning the psychologic sequelae of induced abortion (Stotland 1996).

Confusion often arises because of the failure to differentiate between passing negative feelings and psychiatric syndromes and because of the misattribution of the distress some women feel about an abortion. The first problem is compounded by semantic ambiguity; in the English language, *depression* is used both as a description of a mood and as a technical term to denote the diagnosis of a major psychiatric illness. With regard to the second problem, abortion is performed only on women who are pregnant–and pregnant in problematic circumstances. Women's reactions to induced abortion arise not only, and perhaps not mainly, from the procedure itself but also from psychologic, social (Major et al. 1997), and political circumstances and the communicated attitudes and behaviors of the personnel who perform the procedure.

The psychosocial impact of finding oneself to have conceived an unanticipated and undesired pregnancy is considerable. The process of arriving at the conclusion that the pregnancy cannot or should not be maintained is an additional stress, often involving confrontation with realities such as poverty; the implications of interrupting one's work or education; the end or threatened end of the relationship with one's partner, who may be the father of one's other children; genetic defects; or overwhelming burdens of caring for other young children. A woman's religion or significant others may disapprove of abortion, even to the point of excluding a woman who has undergone an abortion from membership in the religious community or from the protection and regard of the family. Abortion may be accessible only illicitly or only through a complex process such as obtaining parental approval, judicial bypass, or medical justification. Of particular importance for psychiatric study is the fact that women may choose abortions because they have psychiatric illnesses that make pregnancy and motherhood problematic. Given these realities, it is difficult or even impossible to assess the impact of the abortion in isolation.

Published studies of psychologic reactions to induced abortion have to some degree paralleled prevailing social attitudes and expectations. For example, a large (479 women) Swedish study revealed that 75% of the subjects had experienced no regrets or self-reproach and all of the 1% with psychiatric problems had had prior psychiatric illness (Ekblad 1955). Despite such findings, authors tended to assume negative effects until the early 1960s. Since that time, a succession of studies have been published, and methodology has been consistently improved. All studies agree that negative emotional effects are nearly always transient (Butler 1996), that most women who choose abortion tend to feel increasingly relieved and comfortable with their decisions, and that in many cases their overall life satisfaction and success are improved (Addelson 1973; H. Brody et al. 1971; Ford et al. 1971; Lask 1975; Marder 1970; Niswander and Patterson 1967; Osofsky and Osofsky 1972; Peck and Marcus 1966; Schusterman 1976; Simon et al. 1967; Whitmore 1995). Women who were denied abortion tended to have poorer outcomes, especially if the burdens of motherhood were compounded by great multiparity or lack of social support (Pare and Raven 1970).

The incidence of major psychiatric illness following induced abortion has been studied and compared with the occurrence of major psychiatric illness after delivery and in patients denied abortion. A large study in Great Britain reported that the incidence of psychosis was 0.3/1,000 after abortion and 1.7/1,000 postpartum (Brewer 1977). All other such studies report similar findings. A 1989 study performed by a researcher at Johns Hopkins University followed-up adolescents who presented to a school health clinic seeking pregnancy tests (Zabin et al. 1989). Some were not pregnant; of those who were, some chose to abort and some to carry to term. Those who terminated their pregnancies experienced the most favorable outcomes in terms of psychologic adjustment and completion of education—better outcomes than women who had not even been pregnant. The authors, surprised by this finding, theorized that vulnerability to unfounded fears of pregnancy might be correlated with other psychologic vulnerabilities.

No specific illness or pattern of pathologic response to induced abortion has been described, other than anecdotally, in the scientific literature. Risk factors for psychiatric illness following induced abortion include prior psychiatric illness, pressure or coercion to undergo the abortion, marked ambivalence about the decision, and a lack of social supports (Blumenthal 1991; Major et al. 1997). Negative attitudes of those who provide care during and after the procedure also increase patients' risk of psychiatric sequelae. Psychiatrists treating patients who are considering abortion can best help them by providing information and collaborating with them and with significant others of their choosing to arrive at autonomous but socially supported decisions that reflect their own circumstances, religious beliefs, and values.

The reactions of men to their partners' induced abortions have not been well studied. Male partners are often overlooked and their psychologic needs not attended to. In one study of men accompanying women to an urban hospital abortion service, the men reported that the circumstances surrounding the abortion had constituted a developmental challenge. Some men retreated to dependence on their parents, leaving their wives or girlfriends to obtain the necessary information and make the decision largely without their support. Most mastered the challenge, however, and emerged from the experience with an enhanced feeling of fatherliness and responsibility (Rothstein 1991). Like women who undergo abortion, they had decided that parenthood should be the result of a considered decision that one could provide for a child and should not be undertaken by chance.

## Psychiatric Implications of Legal Constraints

Restrictions on abortion services threaten all women with unintended motherhood or illegal abortion, outcomes likely to be psychologically stressful. Because restrictions limit access for some women but not others, they raise ethical and public health questions for all physicians. For example, the so-called Hyde Amendment passed by the United States Congress proscribes the use of federal funds for abortion services. Therefore, Medicaid funds other obstetric and gynecologic services but not abortion. Because few medical facilities operate without federal funds, this legislation affects a large proportion of the population, relegating them to second-class medical care. Women with social support, means, and sophistication have always been able to obtain safe abortions.

Why is abortion a psychiatric issue? There are several reasons. The procedure is medical, and psychiatrists are physicians. In times and places where abortion services are not freely available to women, abortion may be allowed only when deemed medically necessary in the interest of a woman's health. Where abortion is permitted only to save the mother's life, suicidal patients may qualify. Before abortion was generally legalized, sophisticated patients sometimes used psychiatrists to gain the consent of hospital review boards. As a result, psychiatric grounds were perceived by some authorities to be underjustified and overused, and some states and the military specifically disallowed psychiatric grounds for abortion. Other laws have been more liberal, allowing psychiatric factors to be considered on a par with other medical factors that have a significant likelihood of impairing the mother's health if the pregnancy continues (Shepler 1991).

Each of these circumstances is problematic for psychiatry. Excluding suicide or mental health indications isolates psychiatric illness from the rest of medicine and reinforces both the misconception that mental illnesses are not real and the stigma surrounding psychiatric patients and practitioners. Allowing psychiatric indications for abortions places psychiatrists in an untenable position. Suicidality and other adverse psychiatric outcomes, like all medical outcomes, are not entirely predictable, especially when the patient who is providing the data for the decision is in the midst of a crisis and has a vested interest in obtaining a particular procedure. Several decades ago it was possible for a psychiatrist to write a letter indicating that a patient was suicidal without entering this information in her permanent medical record. Today, a psychiatrist's observation that a patient is mentally ill and/or suicidal will follow her through life and may threaten her career opportunities and her ability to obtain life and health insurance. Given the current scrutiny of psychiatric care and the widespread role of religious groups opposed to abortion in supporting medical services, the psychiatrist who declares a pregnant patient suicidal may be constrained to hospitalize her for a time or even until she delivers. The psychiatrist may be in a bind because the clinical evidence in a case may not warrant the conclusion that the patient is suicidal although the patient or the psychiatrist (or both) may feel strongly that an abortion would be in the patient's best interest. The psychiatrist must then either lie about the findings or see the patient denied abortion. Studies indicate that patients who are denied abortions requested on psychiatric or psychosocial grounds, as well as their children, suffer adverse outcomes as compared with control families but that these patients seldom complete the act of suicide during the pregnancy (Dagg 1991).

Psychiatrists have a particular interest and expertise in the circumstances associated with the unplanned pregnancies. These circumstances range from ignorance, poverty, and lack of contraceptives to abuse, immaturity and impulsivity, various degrees of interference with reality testing, and more individual and interpersonal psychodynamics. Psychiatrists treat patients with histories of severe psychiatric complications of pregnancy and delivery. We treat patients who appear or have been shown to be unable to master the responsibilities of motherhood, including patients who have suffered terrible emotional pain and exacerbations of psychiatric illness after losing custody of children in the past. We treat patients for whom we have prescribed psychotropic medications in the early days and weeks before pregnancy could be diagnosed, with unknown effects on the embryo and fetus (see Chapter 5), and patients who require psychotropic drugs to forestall repeated decompensations.

Limitations on access to abortion may put the psychiatrist in another sort of legal bind as well. The 1989 United States Supreme Court decision affirming the Missouri law in the case of *Webster v. Reproductive Health Services* let stand language stating that public funds may not be used to advise or counsel a woman to have an abortion. This language, which has been repeated in the laws of other states, could be interpreted to mean that a psychiatrist caring for a woman with a history of severe postpartum psychiatric illness, loss of custody, severe psychiatric vulnerability, or treatment with psychotropic drugs in early pregnancy may not inform the patient of the full range of therapeutic options. When a patient's care is publicly funded, or takes place in a publicly funded facility (few medical facilities, including private offices, have no public funding), such a law may proscribe the discussion of abortion. Antiabortion activists have threatened to visit doctors' offices with simulated psychiatric histories in order to expose physicians who violate the law.

As noted earlier, U. S. Supreme Court decisions since *Roe v. Wade* in 1973 have precipitated the passage of state laws restricting abortion access. Some legislative and judicial restrictions on abortion are couched in terms of notification and consent of third parties. The Pennsylvania legislature passed a bill requiring the signature of a woman's husband that was vetoed by the governor. Several states have enacted laws requiring the notification and/or consent of the parents of a minor woman seeking abortion that have been found to be constitutional so long as they include a provision for judicial bypass (Shepler 1991). These laws have a clear emotional appeal to the public's sentiments about parental protection of minor children and the sanctity of the family. However, they ignore realities about adolescent development, troubled families, and the judicial process. All of the major medical organizations endorse the physician's role in advising and helping pregnant young women to inform and enlist the support of their families when that is in their best interest. Most young women do so. Unfortunately, adolescents from abusive and neglectful families are at increased risk of unintended pregnancy; forcing them to tell their parents further exposes them to the risk of abuse, expulsion from the home, and self-destructive behavior, including suicide. Mandating parental involvement is also a contratherapeutic intrusion in the physician–patient relationship, whether the physician in question is an obstetrician, pediatrician, family practitioner, or psychiatrist.

Judicial bypass requires than an adolescent without adequate family support, and in the middle of the crisis precipitated by an unwanted pregnancy, be aware of the judicial bypass procedure. She must locate the court, make excuses for her absence from home and/or school, and present herself at the court. In rural areas, she may have to travel a considerable distance. Once at the court, she must make her intentions known to staff so that she can be directed to the appropriate room. The law requires that this process be confidential, but in rural areas both the courts staff and the judge may well know her and her family personally. In Minnesota, such a law was found to produce no positive outcome. Judges who heard these cases almost invariably allowed the abortion to take place. In other states, judges have granted virtually no requests for abortion. For these reasons, major medical societies, including the American Academy of Pediatrics, have taken official positions against parental notification laws.

Although it recognizes the deeply felt religious and moral aversions of some psychiatrists to induced abortion and the profound decision most feel abortion to be, the APA, in concert with other medical and public interest organizations, has taken a strong stance opposing legislation that places dangerous and inequitable restrictions on women's access to safe abortion services as well as limitations on all physicians' ability to discuss, recommend, and provide services for their patients. It is truly tragic that psychosocial ignorance and inadequacies lead to so many problem pregnancies in a world that has the scientific knowledge to prevent them.

# References

Addelson F: Induced abortion: source of guilt or growth? Am J Orthopsychiatry 43:815–823, 1973

American College of Obstetricians and Gynecologists: Public Health Policy Implications of Abortion: A Government Relations Handbook for Health Professionals. Washington DC, American College of Obstetricians and Gynecologists, 1990

American Psychiatric Association: Position Statement on Abortion. Washington DC, American Psychiatric Association, 1978

American Psychiatric Association: APA actions on reproductive rights. Am J Psychiatry 149:723, 1992

American Psychiatric Association: Board of Trustees Meeting, March, 1995

Berger LR: Abortions in America: the effects of restrictive funding. N Engl J Med 398:1474–1477, 1978

Blumenthal SJ: Psychiatric consequences of abortion: overview of research findings, in Psychiatric Aspects of Abortion, Edited by Stotland NL. Washington DC, American Psychiatric Press, 1991, pp 17–37

Brewer C: Incidence of post-abortion psychosis: a prospective study. BMJ 1:476–477, 1977

Brody B: The morality of abortion, in Contemporary Issues in Bioethics, 2nd Edition. Edited by Beauchamp TL, Walters L. Belmont CA, Wadsworth Publishing, 1982, pp 201–211

Brody H, Meikle S, Gerritse R: Therapeutic abortion: a prospective study. Am J Obstet Gynecol 109:347–352, 1971

Bromham D, Oloto E: Trying to prevent abortion. Eur J Contracept Reprod Health Care 2:81–87, 1997

Butler C: Late psychological sequellae of abortion: questions from a primary care perspective. J Fam Pract 43:396–401, 1996

Dagg P: The psychological sequelae of therapeutic abortion: denied and completed. Am J Psychiatry 148:578–585, 1991

DaVanzo J, Parnell AM, Foege WH: Health consequences of contraceptive use and reproductive patterns: summary of a report from the U.S. National Research Council. JAMA 265:2692–2696, 1991

DeVeber LL, Ajzenstat J, Chisholm D: Post abortion grief: psychological sequelae of induced abortion. Humane Medicine 7:203–208, 1991

Devereux G: A Study of Abortion in Primitive Societies, Revised Edition. New York, International Universities Press, 1976

Edelstein L: The Hippocratic oath: text, translation, and interpretation, in Cross-Cultural Perspectives in Medical Ethics: Readings. Edited by Veatch R. Boston, MA, Jones & Bartlett, 1989, pp 6–24

Ekblad M: Induced abortion in psychiatric grounds: a follow-up study of 479 women. Acta Psychiatr Scand Suppl 99:1–238, 1955

Engelhardt HT: Bioethics in the People's Republic of China, in Cross-Cultural Perspectives in Medical Ethics: Readings. Edited by Veatch R. Boston, MA, Jones & Bartlett, 1989, pp 112–119

Epner J, Jonas H, Seckinger D: Late-term abortion. JAMA 280:724–729, 1998

Ford CV, Castelnuovo-Tedesco P, Long KD: Abortion: is it a therapeutic procedure in psychiatry? JAMA 218:1173–1178, 1971

Jacobson JL: Choice at any cost. World Watch Mar/Apr:30–38, 1988

Klass D, Heath A: Grief and abortion: Mizuko Kuyp, the Japanese ritual resolution. Journal of Death and Dying 34:1–14, 1997

Koonin LM, Smith JC, Ramick M, et al: Abortion surveillance: United States. MMWR Surveill Summ 47:31–40, 1998

Koop CE: Former Surgeon General Koop speaks out on health care reform and policy. Hospitals 65:57–58, 1991

Lask B: Short-term psychiatric sequelae to therapeutic termination of pregnancy. Br J Psychiatry 126:173–177, 1975

Major B, Zubek J, Cooper M, et al: Mixed messages: implications of social conflict and social support within close relationships for adjustment to a stressful life event. J Pers Soc Psychol 72:1349–1363, 1997

Marder L: Psychiatric experience with a liberalized therapeutic abortion law. Am J Psychiatry 126:1230–1236, 1970

Newman LF: Historical and cross-cultural perspectives on abortion, in Psychiatric Aspects of Abortion. Edited by Stotland NL. Washington, DC, American Psychiatric Press, 1991, pp 39–49

Niswander K, Patterson R: Psychologic reaction to therapeutic abortion. Obstet Gynecol 29:702–706, 1967

Ohnuki-Tierney E: Illness and Culture in Contemporary Japan: An Anthropological View. Cambridge England, Cambridge University Press, 1984

Osofsky JD, Osofsky HJ: The psychological reaction of patients to legalized abortion. Am J Orthopsychiatry 42:48–60, 1972

Page B: Eastern Europe in the twentieth century, in Cross-Cultural Perspectives in Medical Ethics: Readings. Edited by Veatch R. Boston, MA, Jones & Bartlett, 1989, pp 98–105

Pare C, Raven H: Follow-up of patients referred for termination of pregnancy. Lancet 1:635–658, 1970

Peck A, Marcus H: Psychiatric sequelae of therapeutic interruption of pregnancy. J Nerv Ment Dis 143:417–425, 1966

Pro-Life Action Ministries: What They Won't Tell You at the Abortion Clinic. St. Paul, MN, Pro-Life Action Ministries, undated

Rosenblatt R, Mattis R, Hat G: Abortions in rural Idaho: physicians' attitudes and practices. Am J Public Health 85:1423–1425, 1995

Rothstein A: Male experience of elective abortion: psychoanalytic perspectives, in Psychiatric Aspects of Abortion. Edited by Stotland NL. Washington, DC, American Psychiatric Press, 1991, pp 145–158

Schusterman LR: The psychosocial factors of the abortion experience: a critical review. Psychology Women's Quarterly 1:79–106, 1976

Shepler LT: The law of abortion and contraception: past and present, in Psychiatric Aspects of Abortion. Edited by Stotland NL. Washington, DC, American Psychiatric Press, 1991, pp 51–73

Simon N, Senturia A, Rothman D: Psychiatric illness following therapeutic abortion. Am J Psychiatry 124:59–65, 1967

Stotland N: Conceptions and misconceptions: decisions about pregnancy. Gen Hosp Psychiatry 18:238–243, 1996

Tietze C, Henshaw SK: Induced Abortion: A World Review, 6th Edition. New York, Alan Guttmacher Institute, 1986

Tribe LH: Abortion: The Clash of Absolutes. New York, Noston, 1990

Vaux K: Birth Ethics: Religious and Cultural Values in the Genesis of Life. New York, Crossroad, 1989

Warren DG: The law of human reproduction: an overview. J Leg Med 3:1–57, 1982

Whitmore E: Abortion, in Psychological Aspects of Women's Reproductive Health. Edited by O'Hara M, Reiter R, Johnson S, et al. New York, Springer, 1995, pp 207–223

World Health Organization: Medical methods for termination of pregnancy: report of a WHO Scientific Group. World Health Organ Tech Rep Ser 871:i–vii, 1–110, 1997

Zabin LS, Hirsch MB, Emerson MR: When urban adolescents choose abortion: effects on education, psychological status, and subsequent pregnancy. Fam Plann Perspect 21:248–255, 1989

Zuravin SJ: Unplanned childbearing and family size: their relationship to child neglect and abuse. Fam Plann Perspect 23:155–161, 1991

# Menopause

## Myths and Realities

BARBARA B. SHERWIN, PH.D.

$M$enopause is both a natural and a universal event in the human female life cycle. A set of defining characteristics for this biologic event was formulated at the first International Congress on Menopause (Utian and Serr 1976). According to this formulation, the climacteric marks the transition from the reproductive to the nonreproductive stage of life in women that spans several years. Menopause occurs during the climacteric, at a mean age of 51 years, and is defined by the last menstrual period. In addition, decreased ovarian activity and sociocultural and psychologic factors could act individually or in concert to produce climacteric symptoms.

Because menopause is a universal phenomenon, it is curious that it was not until 1976 that an international definition of this event was first formulated and published. One explanation may be related to changes in statistics regarding female life expectancy. In 1900 the average life span of a woman living in the United States was approximately 50 years; in 1995, 40% of white American women reached 85 years of age. It is projected that this percentage will continue to rise with time (U.S. Bureau of the Census 1990). Therefore, many women now live one-third of their lives beyond cessation of their reproductive capacity, and the quality of life during the latter one-third of the life span has, understandably, become a major issue of concern to both health professionals and women themselves.

Surgical menopause occurs when both ovaries are removed before natural menopause has occurred. Before the 1970s, bilateral oophorectomy was performed fairly commonly in association with hysterectomy undertaken for benign gynecologic conditions. The rationale underlying this was the prevention of ovarian cancer and the belief that ovarian function was expendable if pregnancy was no longer possible. Epidemiologic evidence suggesting that, in the absence of a family history, women have a low risk of ovarian cancer served to curtail this practice of indiscriminately removing normal-appearing ovaries. An even more compelling reason for retaining the ovaries in premenopausal women emerged when it became clear that acceleration of cardiovascular disease (Parrish et al. 1967) and osteoporosis (Lindsay et al. 1980) were associated with early oophorectomy. For these reasons, conservation of normal ovaries at hysterectomy has become the more common practice in North America.

Consistent with the 1976 definition of the climacteric syndrome (Utian and Serr 1976), the etiology and frequency of symptoms that may occur at this time are discussed in this chapter from neurohormonal, sociocultural, and psychologic perspectives and an attempt is made to synthesize this material.

# Neurohormonal Processes

## Change in Sex Hormone Secretion in Menopausal Women

In premenopausal women, the ovary secretes 95% of the estradiol that enters the circulation (Lipsett 1986). After menopause, the ovary virtually stops producing estradiol. Estrone, a much weaker estrogen, becomes the predominant estrogen arising from peripheral conversion of androstenedione (Longcope 1981). Although it was once thought that the drastic decrease in ovarian estradiol secretion at menopause was due solely to follicle depletion and ovarian senescence, it is now clear that age-related alterations in hypothalamic function also occur (Wise et al. 1989). Thus, the transition to menopause is a multifactorial process involving both neural and ovarian factors.

In women, both the adrenal glands and the ovaries contain the biosynthetic pathways necessary for androgen synthesis and secretion. The ovary produces approximately 25% of plasma testosterone, 60% of androstenedione, and 20% of dehydroepiandrosterone (DHEA), whereas the adrenal produces 25% of circulating testosterone, 40% of androstenedione, 50% of DHEA, and 90% of DHEA sulfate. The remainder of circulating androgens in the female are thought to arise through peripheral conversion, which probably accounts for the production rate of 50% of testosterone and 25% of DHEA (Longcope 1986). Although ovarian production of estrogens decreases drastically, about 50% of women produce even greater amounts of androgens after menopause because of ovarian stromal hyperphasia that occurs under the influence of high levels of luteinizing hormone (Judd et al. 1974). When it occurs, however, this increase in ovarian testosterone production is time limited, so that eventually testosterone levels decrease in all women.

## Neurobiologic Effects of Estrogen and Androgen

Estrogen has both inductive and direct effects on neurons. It induces RNA and protein synthesis through genomic mechanisms that, in turn, cause changes in levels of specific gene products, such as neurotransmitter synthesizing enzymes (Luine et al. 1975). Other prolonged neuronal regulatory effects include the expression of gonadal hormone receptors in specific brain areas. The direct effects of estrogen on the brain appear to take place more rapidly. For example, estrogens can alter the electrical activity of neurons in the hypothalamus (Kelly et al. 1977).

Autoradiographic studies have demonstrated that neurons containing specific cytosolic receptors for estrogen are found in specific areas of the brain, predominantly in the pituitary, hypothalamus, limbic forebrain (including the amygdala and lateral septum), and the cerebral cortex (McEwen 1980). Estrogen has widespread effects throughout the brain, including the brainstem and midbrain catecholaminergic neurons, midbrain serotonergic pathways, and the basal forebrain cholinergic system (McEwen 1999).

Autoradiographic studies have also demonstrated that specific cytosolic receptors for testosterone predominantly are found in the preoptic area of the hypothalamus, with smaller concentrations in the limbic system (amygdala and hippocampus) and cerebral cortex (Chamness et al. 1979). Moreover, the brain contains aromatizing enzymes necessary to convert androgens to estrogens. The anterior hypothalamus is the most active aromatizing central tissue, although limbic system structures also convert androgens to estrogens (Naftolin and Ryan 1975). It is important to note that the limbic system, especially the amygdala, plays a critical role in emotion; the fact that sex steroid receptors are found in these brain structures supports the idea that these hormones may influence emotion and affect.

## Peripheral Effects of Estrogen

Because the tissue integrity of the female reproductive tract is dependent on estrogen, degenerative changes in these structures ensue when levels of estrogen decrease after menopause. The vaginal mucosa of postmenopausal women who do not receive estrogen therapy becomes attenuated and pale because of decreased vascularity. Marked atrophic changes may result in atrophic vaginitis, in which the vaginal epithelium is very thin and may become inflamed or even ulcerated (Bergman and Brenner 1987). These changes, in turn, may lead to a severe diminution in vaginal lubrication and/or dyspareunia. The urethral epithelium is also estrogen dependent (Ostergard 1980), and urge incontinence is a frequent complaint in untreated postmenopausal women (Brenner 1988).

## Consequences of Hormonal Changes at Menopause

### Physical Symptoms

Because estrogen affects a multitude of organ systems, the drastic changes in the hormonal milieu that occur around the time of menopause may have consequences for both physical and psychologic functions. Hot flushes, the cardinal menopausal symptom, occur in 60%–90% of menopausal women, albeit with a high degree of variability in their frequency and intensity. For 65% of postmenopausal women, the vasomotor phenomena of hot flashes and cold sweats persist for at least 1 year, and for 20% these symptoms continue for more than 5 years (Brenner 1988). Because hot flashes occur more frequently at night, sleep is often disrupted. Hot flashes are reliably relieved by estrogen replacement therapy (Coope et al. 1975), and although some researchers have noted a simultaneous beneficial effect of exogenous estrogen on hot flashes and sleep quality (Schiff et al. 1980), others have found these two things to be dissociable (Sherwin and Gelfand 1984). If sleep disturbance is associated with frequent awakenings during the night because of hot flashes, it seems clear that estrogen administration will probably eliminate both symptoms. The efficacy of exogenous estrogen is less well established, however, for sleep disturbance not associated with nocturnal flushes.

### Psychologic Symptoms

Historically, myriad psychologic symptoms have been associated with menopause, the most prominent of which are depression, irritability, and mood lability. It is now thought that affective disorders occurring during menopause do not constitute a distinct subtype of depression. Winokur (1973) found that women were not at greater risk for a first episode of depression at menopause than they were other times during the life span. In that study, however, more stringent severity criteria for the diagnosis of depression during menopause were used because of the high frequency of depression and nervousness symptoms that occurred in this sample of menopausal patients. The circularity of this reasoning makes the results difficult to interpret. In a sample of female outpatient admissions diagnosed with major nonbipolar depression, it was concluded that there was insufficient evidence to consider onset of depression at menopause as a distinct entity (Weissman 1979), despite the fact that 47% of the depressed menopausal women and 65% of the depressed postmenopausal women had no history of depression.

Although some epidemiologic studies have failed to find an increased incidence of depression and minor psychologic symptoms in peri- and postmenopausal women (Kaufert and Syrotuik 1981; Ballinger 1990; Thompson et al. 1973), others have documented an increase in the prevalence of depressive symptoms at this time (Bungay et al. 1980; Greene and Cooke 1980; Hunter and Whitehead 1989). Increases in the prevalence of depression are more pronounced in the perimenopausal compared with menopausal years (Charney and Stewart 1997). Of women who seek medical consultation for menopausal symptoms, 79% have physical symptoms and 65% have varying degrees of depression (Anderson et al. 1987). In surveys of general populations, the occurrence of a depressive episode was positively associated with a surgical but not with a natural menopause (McKinlay et al. 1987). Moreover, a history of depressive episodes prior to menopause was a strong predictor of an episode at menopause (Avis et al. 1994).

Measuring changes in mood in premenopausal women before and after a trial of hormone replacement therapy (HRT) is the experimental technique most commonly used to investigate the effects of sex steroids on affect. Many earlier studies were uncontrolled with respect to blindness (George et al. 1973), the presence of malignant disease (Chakravarti et al. 1977), and concurrent psychiatric illness (Dennerstein et al. 1979), thus rendering their findings difficult to interpret. In more-controlled studies, reported discrepancies may be related to both the psychiatric status of the populations investigated and the doses of estrogen administered.

Several studies of nonpsychiatric populations of postmenopausal women have reported changes in affect to be a function of circulating levels of sex hormones. In two prospective studies of women who had undergone oophorectomy, depression scores covaried inversely with circulating levels of both estradiol and testosterone (Sherwin 1988; Sherwin and Gelfand 1985). Moreover, depression scores increased when a placebo was substituted for estrogen in these surgically menopausal women. These results therefore confirmed the positive association between mood and plasma sex hormone levels in healthy nondepressed women. It is important to note that, in both studies, women never became clinically depressed, and the doses of hormones administered induced circulating levels that were within the physiologic range for women of reproductive age.

In another study, affective responses to exogenous estrogen were investigated in postmenopausal women who differed at pretreatment with regard to the intensity of their depression (Schneider et al. 1977). Of 10 women whose pretreatment depression scores were in the mildly, or subclinically, depressed range, nine improved after treatment with 1.25 mg of conjugated equine estrogen daily, whereas 6 of the 10 women who were more severely, or clinically, depressed before treatment actually became more depressed with the same dose of exogenous estrogen. When women with severe, refractory depression were given very large pharmacologic doses of conjugated equine estrogen (15–25 mg/day), depression scores decreased in most of the women after 3 months (Klaiber et al. 1979). On the basis of these findings and those of our own studies of nondepressed women (Sherwin 1988; Sherwin and Gelfand 1985), it now seems reasonable to suggest that the administration of estrogen in doses conventionally used to treat menopausal symptoms enhances mood in nondepressed women but is therapeutically ineffective with respect to mood disturbances of a clinical magnitude. Recent work suggests that treatment-resistant depression during menopause may be alleviated in some women by antidepressant augmentation with physiologic doses of estradiol (Stahl 1998).

Several mechanisms of estrogenic action on indolamine metabolism could account for its mood-enhancing effect. First, it has been demonstrated that exogenous estrogen decreases monoamine oxidase activity in the amygdala and hypothalamus of rats (Luine et al. 1975). Because monoamine oxidase is the enzyme that catabolizes serotonin, the net effect of estrogen administration would be to maintain higher serotonin levels in the brain. Indeed, it has been found that regularly cycling depressed women have higher levels of plasma monoamine oxidase activity than do nondepressed women (Klaiber et al. 1972).

A second mechanism of action is related to estrogen's impact on tryptophan in plasma. Tryptophan, the precursor of serotonin, is displaced from its binding sites to plasma albumin by estrogens both in vitro and in vivo (Aylward 1973), thereby allowing more free tryptophan to be available to the brain, where it is metabolized to serotonin. A significant negative correlation between depression scores and free plasma tryptophan was reported in women who had undergone oophorectomy and whose mood and free tryptophan levels were enhanced after treatment with exogenous estrogen (Aylward 1976). The results of this clinical study provide some, albeit indirect, support for an estrogenic effect on neurotransmitter concentrations.

Finally, a prospective study of surgically menopausal women found an increase in the density of tritiated imipramine binding sites on platelets coincident with higher estradiol levels and lower depression scores (Sherwin and Suranyi-Cadotte 1990). To the extent that estrogen increases serotonin concentrations or the amount of time this neurotransmitter remains in the synapse, it will, in accordance with the biogenic amine hypothesis of depression (Schildkraut 1965), enhance mood.

# Gynecologic Aspects

## Gynecologic Assessment

The premenopausal period is characterized by changes in the regularity of the menstrual cycle and in the duration and volume of menstrual bleeding. Menopause is said to have occurred when 12 successive menstrual cycles have been missed. Gonadotropin levels increase because of the lack of positive feedback resulting from the vastly diminished ovarian production of estradiol. Follicle-stimulating hormone levels of greater than 50 IU/mL and luteinizing hormone levels of greater than 35 IU/mL are considered, in the absence of organic disease, to be diagnostic of menopause (Jaffe 1989). The vaginal epithelium becomes atrophic, and decreased lubrication may be apparent. When the endometrium is biopsied with a curette after menopause, atrophy of this tissue in noted (Benirschke 1986). In time, a decrease in the size of the uterus and breasts occurs. Hair on the upper lip and the chin may increase in some women, probably because of testosterone production by the postmenopausal ovary that is unopposed by the premenopausal levels of estrogen (Jaffe 1989). Because menopausal women are in a high-risk age group for breast cancer, most gynecologists recommend breast self-examination and yearly mammography for menopausal and postmenopausal women.

## Hormone Replacement Therapy

The ideologic dispute as to whether menopause is a normal reproductive event, an endocrine deficiency disease, or an endocrinopathy requiring medical intervention continues to rage. Does menopause need to be "managed," or is it a reproductive event, like menarche, to be simply experienced? Indeed, it is unlikely that this dispute will ever be resolved, because it is a conceptual and not an empirical issue. The differing conceptualizations of menopause have a major impact on whether medical intervention ought to play a role. Perhaps a more dispassionate and more useful approach is one that weighs the short- and long-term consequences of estrogen depletion for each individual woman.

The variability among women with respect to the intensity and frequency of the early symptoms of hot flashes and cold sweats means that some are greatly disturbed by these vasomotor phenomena, whereas others experience them so mildly that they do not have any negative influence on daily functioning. Highly symptomatic women may be treated with HRT for a limited period until its gradual withdrawal does not provoke a resurgence of vasomotor disturbances. Another consideration is that, regardless of the severity of these vasomotor symptoms, all untreated women will in time develop atrophy of the estrogen-dependent urogenital tissues, which may give rise to symptoms such as atrophic vaginitis and urge incontinence. Whether a woman wishes to begin HRT to effectively alleviate these symptoms usually depends on her own assessment of the degree of discomfort she is experiencing. On the other hand, evidence now indicates that HRT can protect against degenerative diseases that seriously compromise the quality of life beyond the sixth decade. The two most compelling reasons for using long-term HRT are 1) that estrogen helps to maintain bone density, thereby protecting against osteoporosis (Lindsay et al. 1980) and 2) that estrogen administration reduces mortality from cardiovascular disease by two-thirds (Bush et al. 1987) and ultimately reduces mortality from all causes by 10%–60% (Henderson et al. 1991). Evidence from epidemiologic studies suggests (but does not prove) that HRT may also reduce the risk of Alzheimer's disease in women by 30%–50% (Paganini-Hill and Henderson 1996). The accumulated research findings therefore strongly suggest that postmenopausal women who receive HRT experience both increased longevity and an enhanced quality of life during the latter decades of their life span.

## Risks of Hormone Replacement Therapy

It became clear in 1975 that the use of unopposed estrogen was associated with a marked increase in the incidence of endometrial cancer (Weiss et al. 1976). Adding a progestin to the therapy for 10–12 days each month effectively protects the endometrium from the stimulatory effects of estrogen (Gelfand and Ferenczy 1989), and estrogen-progestin regimens given either continuously or in cyclic sequence are now recommended as HRT for women with an intact uterus.

Orally administered estrogen induces changes in hepatic metabolism that could have adverse influences. Among these potential changes are increased production of renin substrate and decreased production of antithrombin III (DeLignieres et al. 1986). No increased incidence of hypertension or thrombosis has been noted, however, in postmenopausal women receiving oral estrogen replacement (Ettinger 1988).

Considerable controversy has existed regarding the association between HRT and the incidence of breast cancer in postmenopausal women. A qualitative review of studies on estrogen and breast cancer published between 1970 and 1995 concluded that short-term use of estrogen (5 years or less) does not increase breast cancer risk, whereas longer durations of use may be associated with a small but significant increase in risk (Ewertz 1996).

Despite the knowledge gained during the past 10 years with respect to the beneficial effects of HRT for postmenopausal women, its use is not mandated for all such women. For example, not every women is at risk for the development of osteoporosis. Indeed, it has been established that tall, slim, small-boned Caucasian women who smoke are at greatest risk. The decision as to whether an individual woman is a suitable candidate for HRT should, therefore, be predicated on assessing her risks and providing her with information so that she can be a full partner in the decision-making process.

# Psychosocial Issues for Women in Midlife

## Psychologic Theories

Historically, psychologic theorizing with respect to the etiology of menopausal symptoms first occurred within the psychoanalytic framework. The psychologic loss theory of menopause is based on the contention that the ability to bear children is central to the meaning of a woman's life. Logically, then, to lose this ability is to lose life's meaning (Deutsch 1945). Other Freudians have expressed the view that menopause is "symbolic castration" (Benedek 1950) and deprives the woman of any means of compensating for the anger, hopelessness, and frustration she has always felt at not being born a male (Prados 1967). With regard to treatment of symptoms that arise at this time, psychoanalytic theory is geared toward helping women accept the "mortification of menopause" (Deutsch 1944).

## Sociocultural Theories

The sociocultural model posits that the major determinants of psychologic disturbance at the time of menopause are role changes and cultural attitudes toward aging. The culture of a given society may be regarded as that which attributes meaning to reality and thereby transforms a natural or biologic event into a cultural event. It follows that the psychologic impact of menopause will be strongly influenced by the importance a particular culture attaches to procreation, fertility, aging, and female roles (van Keep and Prill 1975). Cross-cultural studies have shown that menopause is indeed experienced differently in different cultures. In cultures in which women receive rights at menopause that were denied them during their fertile period (e.g., some castes in India), menopausal symptoms are minimal (Flint 1975; Maoz et al. 1977). Because North American society is youth oriented and stereotypes of aging women are largely negative, our culture does not provide a supportive environment for menopausal women.

Level of education and socioeconomic factors also seem to influence the experience of menopause. Several authors from different countries have reported that menopausal women with less education and from lower socioeconomic classes have a higher degree of symptoms at menopause than do more advantaged women (Jaszmann et al. 1969; Maoz et al. 1977; van Keep and Kellerhals 1974).

## Postparental Phase and Other Transitional Phenomena

Menopause, of course, occurs during midlife, a time that is commonly regarded as a period of psychosocial transition and readjustment. Women who heretofore had heavily invested their emotion and energy in childbearing are forced to redefine their role at menopause because the children are growing up and leaving the home and reproductive capacity ceases. From the perspective of role theory, it would be important at this time to develop new, alternate roles in order to maintain self-esteem when old roles lose importance (Havighurst 1966). The departure of grown children from the parental home, which tends to occur coincident with menopause, has come to be known as the postparental stage of life. Some authors hold that this change inevitably constitutes a psychologic loss because the mother loses one of her major roles and thus the rewards that accompanied it (Blood and Wolfe 1960). This formulation, therefore, points to the conclusion that depression occurring during menopause may be caused by empty-nest syndrome.

In fact, a careful reading of the literature suggests that this conclusion is a function of the population studied. For example, menopausal women who are hospitalized with a major depressive disorder after their last child has left home have been characterized as having had overprotective or overinvolved relationships with their offspring (Bart 1971; Bart and Grossman 1978). Results of general population surveys tell another story. In nonclinical populations, middle-aged women whose children had left home reported somewhat greater happiness, enjoyment of life in general, and greater marital harmony than did women of similar age with at least one child still living at home (Glenn 1975). The findings of this cross-sectional study are consistent with those of retrospective (Deutscher 1964) and longitudinal (Clausen 1972) investigations of the postparental stage in nonclinical populations. This evidence indicates that, for previously well-functioning middle-aged women, the so-called "crisis of the empty nest" is mythical.

Certain life stresses may be temporally linked with menopause. Some of the negative events that may occur in a woman's life at this time include onset of a major illness or disability in her spouse, death of her spouse, employment uncertainty for either partner, the need to care for one's own elderly parent(s), and loss of support from important friends or family through illness, death, or geographic relocation. It is clear that stressful life events, particularly losses or bereavements, may lead to somatic or psychologic symptoms for women during the climacteric (Greene and Cook 1980) just as they do during other life phases.

Studies of the impact of marital status on the experience of menopause are equivocal, probably because it is the quality and not the fact of the relationship that determines whether it serves as a buffer against other life stresses (Gove et al. 1983). Studies in the United States (McKinlay et al. 1987) and England (Hunter 1990) have found that single women were least likely to be depressed, followed by married women and those who were widowed, divorced, or separated. Moreover, less well-educated women who were widowed, divorced, or separated were the most likely to be depressed (Hunter 1990).

## Sexuality

Survey data generally show a considerable incidence of problems in various aspects of sexual functioning in postmenopausal women. Various studies have reported a 10%–85% decrease in sexual interest (Cutler et al. 1987; Mc-Coy and Davidson 1985) and a 16%–47% decrease in the frequency of orgasm (Hallström 1977; Kinsey et al. 1953) in menopausal women. Although numerous studies have found that exogenous estrogen alleviates atrophic vaginitis and associated dyspareunia and increases vaginal lubrication (Morrell et al. 1984; Myers and Morokoff 1986), exogenous estrogen failed to increase sexual desire or libido. Several prospective studies of surgically menopausal women, however, have demonstrated that the addition of test-osterone, which is normally produced by the ovaries, to an estrogen replacement regimen increased sexual desire, sexual arousal, and the frequency of sexual fantasies compared with women treated with estrogen alone (Sherwin et al. 1985; Sherwin and Gelfand 1987). The consistency between these findings and those of investigators in England (Cardozo et al. 1984) and Australia (Burger et al. 1984) who used subcutaneously implanted pellets containing both estradiol and testosterone strongly suggests that in women, as in men, testosterone is the sex steroid that is critical for the maintenance of sexual desire.

Numerous nonhormonal factors may also influence sexual functioning in postmenopausal women. Clearly, one such factor is the desire and capacity of the partner for sexual activity (Davidson et al. 1983). A positive relationship also exists between previous sexual interest or importance of sex and the frequency of sexual activity in later middle life (Pfeiffer and Davis 1972). Finally, cultural and societal notions of sexual attractiveness and attitudes concerning the expression of sexuality beyond the reproductive years also have a significant influence on the maintenance of sexual activity in middle-age and elderly women.

## "Life Begins at Fifty"

With so much emphasis on the negative impact of the changing hormonal milieu and the losses and life stresses that often occur coincident with menopause, the fact that this reproductive event is welcomed as a positive event by many women is frequently ignored. For example, the departure of children from the home also means that women are able to redirect their time and energy to tasks and activities that bring other important sources of gratification. Reentering the work force or devoting more time to an already established career, travel, and other leisure activities are all potential benefits of the postparental years. Solid marital relationships may become closer and more intimate at a time when a couple has more opportunity to spend time alone together. Moreover, the absence of menstrual cycles and the accompanying freedom from the need to be concerned about birth control methods may serve to enhance the sexual relationship. Although the climacteric can be characterized as potentially offering the opportunity for freedom to explore new roles, it should be noted that this freedom presumes both the time and the personal and economic resources for such explorations, which a middle-class bias often ignores.

## Menopause and the Mental Health Professional

The most common reason for referring a menopausal woman to a mental health professional is for the diagnosis and treatment of a depressive disorder associated with the endocrine changes occurring during this reproductive event. Recent studies have failed to confirm the existence of involutional melancholia as a distinct subtype of depressive illness, leading to its removal from current psychiatric nomenclature. A great deal of evidence has shown, however, that depressive symptoms—if not a distinctive syndrome—are experienced by many women at the time of menopause. Clinical observations suggest that women who experienced premenstrual syndrome during their reproductive years and those with a history of depressive illness may be at a greater risk for the development of a depressive episode at the time of menopause than are women without such a history.

The initial approach to the management of mood and behavioral information on disturbances in menopausal women requires information on the woman's symptoms and the hormonal context in which they occur, a personal history of depression, a family history of affective disorder, feelings about aging and mortality, and concurrent life stresses. If a woman is experiencing distressing signs of estrogen deficiency, such as hot flashes and vaginal dryness, has no contraindications to HRT (such as a history of breast cancer), and does not fulfill diagnostic criteria for a major depressive disorder, then a trial of HRT may be indicated as a first approach. Women who have undergone surgical menopause usually experience more severe symptoms of estrogen deficiency, owing to the abruptness of the change in their hormonal milieu. In the absence of contraindications, HRT would be particularly important for these women. In these cases, it is also critical to explore the psychologic impact of the hysterectomy and bilateral oophorectomy and the reasons that necessitated the surgery.

Because of the demonstrated ability of estrogen to alter the concentrations or availability of neurotransmitters in the synapse, it is possible that menopausal women with affective symptoms in the presence of mild or minimal hypoestrogenic somatic symptoms may also respond to a trial of HRT. It is important to note, however, that presently no evidence suggests that a major depressive illness will be significantly alleviated by the doses of estrogen conventionally used to treat postmenopausal women. The decision to institute adjunctive psychopharmacotherapy will depend on the severity and duration of the depressive symptoms and on the premorbid and family history of affective illness.

## Acknowledgment

The preparation of this manuscript was supported by a grant from The Medical Research Council of Canada (No. MA-11623) awarded to B.B. Sherwin.

## References

Anderson E, Hamburger S, Liu JH, et al: Characteristics of menopausal women seeking assistance. Am J Obstet Gynecol 156:428–433, 1987

Avis N, Brambilla D, McKinlay SM, et al: A longitudinal analysis of association between menopause and depression: results from the Massachusetts women's health study. AEP 4:15–21, 1994

Aylward M: Plasma tryptophan levels and mental depression in postmenopausal subjects: effects of oral piperazine-oestrone sulphate. IRCS Journal of Medical Science 1:30–34, 1973

Aylward M: Estrogens: plasma tryptophan levels in perimenopausal patients, in The Management of the Menopause and Post-Menopausal Years. Edited by Campbell S. Baltimore, MD, University Park Press, 1976, pp 135–147

Ballinger CB: Psychiatric aspects of the menopause. Br J Psychiatry 156:773–787, 1990

Bart PB: Depression in middle-aged women, in Women in Sexist Society. Edited by Gornick V, Morgan BK. New York, Basic Books, 1971, pp 163–186

Bart PB, Grossman M: Menopause, in The Woman as Patient. Edited by Notman M, Nadelson C. New York, Plenum, 1978

Benedek T: Climacterium: a developmental phase. Psychoanal Q 11:19–26, 1950

Benirschke K: The endometrium, in Reproductive Endocrinology, 2nd Edition. Edited by Yen SSC, Jaffe RB. Philadelphia, PA, WB Saunders, 1986, pp 385–405

Bergman A, Brenner PF: Alterations in the urogenital system, in Menopause: Physiology and Pharmacology. Edited by Mishell DR. Chicago, IL, Year Book Medical, 1987, pp 67–75

Blood RO, Wolfe DM: Husbands and Wives: The Dynamics of Married Living. New York, Free Press, 1960

Brenner PF: The menopause syndrome. Obstet Gynecol 72(suppl):6–11, 1988

Bungay GT, Vessey MP, McPherson CK: Study of symptoms in middle-life with special reference to the menopause. BMJ 2:181–183, 1980

Burger HG, Hailes J, Menelaus M, et al: The management of persistent menopausal symptoms with oestradiol-testosterone implants: clinical, lipid and hormonal results. Maturitas 6:351–358, 1984

Bush TL, Barrett-Connor E, Cowan LD, et al: Cardiovascular mortality and noncontraceptive use of estrogen in women: results from the Lipid Research Clinics Program Follow-Up Study. Circulation 6:1102–1109, 1987

Cardozo L, Gibb DMF, Tuck SM, et al: The effects of subcutaneous hormone implants during the climacteric. Maturitas 5:177–184, 1984

Chakravarti S, Collins WP, Newton JR: Endocrine changes and symptomatology after oophorerectomy in premenopausal women. Br J Obstet Gynecol 84:769–776, 1977

Chamness GC, King TW, Sheridan PJ: Androgen receptors in the rat brain: assays and properties. Brain Res 161:267–273, 1979

Charney DA, Stewart DE: Psychiatric aspects, in A Clinician's Guide to Menopause. Edited by Stewart DE, Robinson G. Washington, DC, American Psychiatric Press, 1997, pp 129–144

Clausen JA: The life course of individuals, in Aging and Society, Vol 3. Edited by Riley MW, Johnson M, Foner A. New York, Russel Sage Foundation, 1972

Coope J, Thompson J, Poller L: Estrogen administration and hot flushes in menopausal women. BMJ 4:139–143, 1975

Cutler WB, Garca CR, McCoy NL: Perimenopausal sexuality. Arch Sex Behav 16:225–234, 1987

Davidson JM, Chen JJ, Crapo L, et al: Hormonal changes and sexual function in aging men. J Clin Endocrinol Metab 51:19–28, 1983

DeLignieres B, Basdevant A, Thomas G, et al: Biological effects of estradiol-17 beta in postmenopausal women: oral versus percutaneous administration. J Clin Endocrinol Metab 62:536–541, 1986

Dennerstein L, Burrows GD, Hyman GJ: Hormone therapy and affect. Maturitas 1:247–259, 1979

Deutsch H: The Psychology of Women. New York, Grune & Stratton, 1944

Deutsch H: The Psychology of Women, Vol 2. New York, Grune & Stratton, 1945

Deutscher J: The quality of postparental life. Journal of Marriage and the Family 26:52–59, 1964

Ettinger B: Optimal use of postmenopausal hormone replacement therapy. Obstet Gynecol 82(suppl):31–36, 1988

Ewertz M: Hormone therapy in the menopause and breast cancer risk: a review. Maturitas 23:241–246, 1996

Flint M: The menopause: reward or punishment? Psychosomatics 16:161–173, 1975

Gelfand MM, Ferenczy A: A prospective one-year study of estrogen and progestin in postmenopausal women: effects on the endometrium. Obstet Gynecol 74:398–402, 1989

George GCW, Beaumont PJV, Beardwood CJ: Effects of exogenous estrogens on minor psychiatric symptoms in postmenopausal women. S Afr Med J 47:2387–2388, 1973

Glenn ND: Psychological well-being in the postparental stage: some evidence from national surveys. Journal of Marriage and Family 32:105–110, 1975

Gove WR, Hughes M, Style CB: Does marriage have positive effects on the psychological well-being of the individual? J Health Soc Behav 24:122–131, 1983

Greene JG, Cooke DJ: Life stress and symptoms at the climacterium. Br J Psychiatry 136:486–491, 1980

Hallström T: Sexuality in the climacteric. Clin Obstet Gynecol 4:227–239, 1977

Havighurst RJ: Changing roles of women in the middle years, in Potentialities of Women in the Middle Years. Edited by Gross J. Lansing, MI, Michigan State University Press, 1966

Henderson BE, Paganini-Hill A, Ross RK: Decreased mortality in users of estrogen replacement therapy. Arch Intern Med 151:75–78, 1991

Hunter MS: Psychological and somatic experience of the menopause: a prospective study. Psychosom Med 52:357–367, 1990

Hunter MS, Whitehead MJ: Psychological experience of the climacteric and postmenopause, in Menopause: Evaluation, Treatment, and Health Concerns. Edited by Hammond CB, Haseltine FP. New York, Alan R. Liss, 1989, pp 211–224

Jaffe RB: The menopause and postmenopausal period, in Menopause: Evaluation, Treatment, and Health Concerns. Edited by Hammond CB, Haseltine FP. New York, Alan R. Liss, 1989, pp 406–423

Jaszmann L, Van Lith WD, Zoat JL: The perimenopausal syndrome: the statistical analysis of a survey. Medical Gynecology 4:268–272, 1969

Judd HL, Judd GE, Lucas WE, et al: Endocrine function of the postmenopausal ovary: concentrations of androgens and estrogens in ovarian and peripheral vein blood. J Clin Endocrinol Metab 139:1020–1026, 1974

Kaufert P, Syrotuik J: Symptom reporting at the menopause. Soc Sci Med 15:173–184, 1981

Kelly MJ, Mass RL, Dudley CA: The effect of microelectrophoretically applied estrogen, cortisol, and acetylcholine on medial preoptic-septal unit activity through the estrous cycle of the female rat. Exp Brain Res 30:53–64, 1977

Kinsey AC, Pomeroy WB, Martin CE, et al: Sexual Behavior in the Human Female. Philadelphia, PA, WB Saunders, 1953

Klaiber EL, Broverman DM, Vogel W, et al: Effects of estrogen therapy on plasma MAO activity and EEG driving responses of depressed women. Am J Psychiatry 128:1492–1498, 1972

Klaiber EL, Broverman DM, Vogel W, et al: Estrogen therapy for severe persistent depression in women. Arch Gen Psychiatry 36:550–554, 1979

Lindsay R, Hart DM, Forrest C, et al: Prevention of spinal osteoporosis in oophorectomized women. Lancet 2:1151–1154, 1980

Lipsett MB: Steroid hormones, in Reproductive Endocrinology, Physiology, Pathophysiology and Clinical Management. Edited by Yen SSC, Jaffe RB. Philadelphia, PA, WB Saunders, 1986

Longcope C: Metabolic clearance and blood production rates in postmenopausal women. Am J Obstet Gynecol 111:779–785, 1981

Longcope C: Adrenal and gonadal steroid secretion in normal females. J Clin Endocrinol Metab 15:213–220, 1986

Luine VN, Khylchevskaya RJ, McEwen B: Effect of gonadal steroids on activities of monoamine oxidase and choline acetylase in rat brain. Brain Res 86:293–306, 1975

Maoz B, Antonovsky A, Apter A, et al: The perception of menopause in five ethnic groups in Israel. Acta Obstet Gynaecol Scand 65:69–76, 1977

McCoy NL, Davidson JM: A longitudinal study of the effects of menopause on sexuality. Maturitas 7:203–209, 1985

McEwen BS: The brain as a target organ of endocrine hormones, in Neuroendocrinology. Edited by Kreiger DT, Hughes JS. Sunderland, MA, Sinauer Associates, 1980, pp 33–42

McEwen BS: The molecular and neuroanatomical basis for estrogen effects in the central nervous system. J Clin Endocrinol Metab 84:1790–1797, 1999

McKinlay JB, McKinlay SM, Brambilla D: The relative contribution of endocrine changes and social circumstances to depression in mid-aged women. J Health Soc Behav 28:345–363, 1987

Morrell MJ, Dixon JM, Carter S, et al: The influence of age and cycling status on sexual arousability in women. Am J Obstet Gynecol 148:166–174, 1984

Myers LS, Morokoff PJ: Physiological and subjective sexual arousal in pre- and postmenopausal women taking replacement therapy. Psychophysiology 23:283–290, 1986

Naftolin F, Ryan KJ: The metabolism of androgens in central neuroendocrine tissues. J Steroid Biochem 6:993–997, 1975

Ostergard DR: Embryology and anatomy of the female bladder and urethra, in Gynecologic Urology: Therapy and Practice. Edited by Ostergard DR. Baltimore, MD, Williams & Wilkins, 1980, pp 3–10

Paganini-Hill A, Henderson VW: Estrogen replacement therapy and risk of Alzheimer's disease. Arch Intern Med 156:2213–2217, 1996

Parrish HM, Carr CA, Hall DG, et al: Time interval from castration in premenopausal women to development of excessive coronary atherosclerosis. Am J Obstet Gynecol 99:155–162, 1967

Pfeiffer E, Davis GC: Determinants of sexual behavior in middle and old age. J Am Geriatr Soc 4:151–160, 1972

Prados M: Emotional factors in the climacterium of women. Psychother Psychosom 15:231–244, 1967

Schiff I, Regenstein Q, Schinfeld J, et al: Interactions of oestrogens and the hours of sleep on cortisol, FSH, LH, and prolactin in hypogonadal women. Maturitas 2:179–183, 1980

Schildkraut JJ: The catecholamine hypothesis of affective disorders: a review of supporting evidence. Am J Psychiatry 122:509–522, 1965

Schneider MA, Brotherton PL, Hailes J: The effect of exogenous oestrogens on depression in menopausal women. Med J Aust 2:162–163, 1977

Sherwin BB: Affective changes with estrogen and androgen replacement therapy in surgically menopausal women. J Affect Disord 14:177–187, 1988

Sherwin BB, Gelfand MM: Effects of parenteral administration of estrogen and androgen on plasma hormone levels and hot flushes in the surgical menopause. Am J Obstet Gynecol 148:552–557, 1984

Sherwin BB, Gelfand MM: Sex steroids and affect in the surgical menopause: a double-blind cross-over study. Psychoneuroendocrinology 10:325–335, 1985

Sherwin BB, Gelfand MM: The role of androgen in the maintenance of sexual functioning in oophorectomized women. Psychosom Med 49:397–409, 1987

Sherwin BB, Suranyi-Cadotte BE: Upregulatory effect of estrogen on platelet 3H-imipramine binding sites in surgically menopausal women. Biol Psychiatry 28:339–348, 1990

Sherwin BB, Gelfand MM, Brender W: Androgen enhances sexual motivation in females: a prospective, cross-over study of sex steroid administration in the surgical menopause. Psychosom Med 47:339–351, 1985

Stahl SM: Basic psychopharmacology of antidepressants, part 2: estrogen as an adjunct to antidepressant treatment. J Clin Psychiatry 59(suppl 4):15–24, 1998

Thompson B, Hart SA, Durno D: Menopausal age and symptomatology in a general practice. J Biosoc Sci 5:71–82, 1973

U.S. Bureau of the Census: Projections of the population of the United States: 1977 to 2050. Curr Pop Rep Series P-25, No 704, 1990

Utian W, Serr D: The climacteric syndrome, in Consensus on Menopause Research. Edited by van Keep PA, Greenblatt R, Fernet A. Lancaster, UK, MTP Press, 1976, pp 1–4 van Keep PA, Kellerhals JM: The impact of sociocultural factors on symptom formation. Psychother Psychosom 23:251–263, 1974

van Keep, Prill HJ: Psychosociology of menopause and postmenopause, in Estrogen in the Postmenopause. Edited by Lauritzen C, van Keep PA. Basel, Switzerland, Karger, 1975

Weiss NS, Szekely R, Austin DF: Increasing evidence of endometrial cancer in the United States. N Engl J Med 294:1259–1262, 1976

Weissman MM: The myth of involutional melancholia. JAMA 242:742–744, 1979

Winokur G: Depression in the menopause. Am J Psychiatry 130:92–93, 1973

Wise PM, Weiland NG, Scarbrough K, et al: Changing hypothalamopituitary function: its role in aging of the female reproductive system. Horm Res 31:39–44, 1989

# Chronic Gynecologic Pain

JOHN F. STEEGE, M.D.
ANNA L. STOUT, PH.D.

This chapter reviews vulvovaginitis and chronic pelvic pain, two of the most vexing problems in clinical gynecology. Both problems are marked by their often chronic and intractable natures as well as by the frequent contribution of psychologic factors to their severity. They represent opportunities for effective collaboration between the gynecologic and mental health specialties.

## Types of Chronic Gynecologic Pain

### Vulvovaginitis

Vaginal yeast infections, trichomoniasis, and the mixed infection of bacterial vaginosis are extremely common. Monilial (yeast) vaginitis typically is marked by a white, cheesy discharge; trichomoniasis (*Trichomonas vaginalis* infection) by a frothy, mildly malodorous discharge; and bacterial vaginosis by a chronic, intermittent, irritating, and malodorous discharge. Women with such clearly identifiable acute symptoms and signs will seldom require mental health consultation. Many women with these disorders, however, may later develop chronic continuing vaginal and vulvar symptoms, even though the bacteriologic precipitants may have been brought under control. The possible role of psychologic factors in perpetuating symptoms may lead to referral for psychologic evaluation.

More troubling than these entities is the patient who undergoes careful, frequent examinations with no pathogenic organisms visualized. Gynecologists often recognize that such individuals may be unduly focused on any perceived irregularities of vaginal sensation or secretion. Intense symptoms of vaginal discomfort may be a "calling card" or presenting symptom for affective disorders, anxiety disorders, marital discord, somatization tendencies, or sexual dysfunction. For example, continued dyspareunia may be caused by vaginismus triggered by repeated uncomfortable vaginal events associated with vaginitis. When pain persists, the patient may return to her physician, claiming that her "vaginitis is back," assuming that any pain in this area must be caused by recurrent infection. This situation may benefit from collaboration between the gynecologist and the mental health clinician.

In the postmenopausal patient, specific vaginal infections are far less common, except for atrophic vaginitis in women who are not receiving estrogen replacement therapy. Postmenopausal women, however, are prone to the development of vulvar dystrophies, which can present with intense vulvar burning and itching in the absence of any significant vaginal infection. These distressing symptoms can become such an impediment to normal functioning that they may precipitate depressive episodes. Conversely, vulvar symptoms may represent a depressive equivalent.

## Chronic Pelvic Pain

Pelvic pain is usually defined as chronic when it has lasted for 6 months or more on a continuous or a cyclic basis. It may be useful to distinguish between patients who have pain that is chronic and those who have a true chronic pain syndrome. In chronic pain syndrome, the pain is accompanied by impaired function in recreational activities and household responsibilities, possible vegetative signs of depression (especially sleep disturbance), and significant alterations in the patient's roles within her family (Steege et al. 1991). Psychologic evaluation and treatment are often helpful in such patients.

## Dyspareunia

Dyspareunia, or painful intercourse, is usually described as being either introital (in the area around the opening of the vagina) or deep (Steege 1984). Patients often describe introital dyspareunia as pain "at the opening" or as "trouble getting in" during intercourse. The pain is usually continuous but can be exacerbated perimenstrually in the presence of contributing factors, such as recurrent nonilial vaginitis or inflammation of the vestibule. Deeper pelvic pain is often described as "pain inside" or by noting that the partner's penis feels as though it "hits something." Traditionally, deep dyspareunia has been felt by gynecologists to be more likely causd by organic factors, whereas introital dyspareunia is more often psychologically based. Although these generalizations are still partly valid, enough exceptions occur to impel careful inquiry into all aspects of the problem. A careful history should delineate the location of the pain, the relationship of the pain to the sexual response cycle, and any alterations of the sexual response cycle. Tactful inquiry should be made regarding any variation of symptoms with different sexual partners.

## General Pelvic Pain

Pain that is present over the entire lower pelvic area, sometimes greater in intensity on one side than on the other, may occur on either a cyclic or a continuous basis. Cyclic discomforts are more typically associated with en-dometriosis, although pain associated with pelvic adhesive disease can also be somewhat cyclic, being worse before and during menstruation. Similarly, pain that is possibly attributable to pelvic congestion (overdistention of the pelvic venous system) will often be worse premenstrually (Beard et al. 1989). Worsening endometriosis often starts out as cyclic dysmenorrhea, with the pain gradually subsuming more and more of the menstrual month as time goes on. Continuous pain is more often caused by adhesive disease that is ei-ther postinfectious or postsurgical in nature. Dyspareunia may be present, along with chronic daily pain. It is more common when the pelvic pathology is central in location rather than in the adnexal areas.

The role of organic pathology in the pathophysiology of chronic pelvic pain is poorly understood despite research efforts (Steege et al. 1991). Most series in the literature report that no abnormal laparoscopic findings are present in approximately 10%–60% of women undergoing this procedure for evaluation of chronic pelvic pain. These numbers, however, may be an over-estimation of the percentage of negative pelvic findings, because most of the studies were published before it was recognized that endometriosis can present in atypical or unpigmented forms. A woman with negative findings on laparoscopy may nevertheless have some physical contributions to her pain, such as trigonitis, urethritis, functional pelvic musculoskeletal problems, postural changes, or irritable bowel syndrome. Some of the studies describing psychologic profiles in women with negative laparoscopies fail to describe evaluations for such problems.

Sizable fractions of women with organic pathology also demonstrate sub-stantial psychologic changes on psychometric testing and clinical or struc-tured interview (Castelnuovo-Tedesco and Krout 1970). This confusing picture makes it clinically difficult to decide in an individual case whether the primary difficulty is physiologic or psychologic. For example, several studies document that women with organic pathology, most often endometriosis or adhesions, will more often have pelvic pain than those without any organic pathology. Although the location of the pain often correlates with the location of the pathology, the intensity of the pain demonstrates no quantitative relationship to the amount of tissue change present (Fedele et al. 1990; Stout et al. 1991). It therefore remains a matter of difficult clinical judgment to decide on the appropriate medical or surgical treatments of the organic pathology.

## Diagnosis and Treatment

### Vulvovaginal Symptoms

#### *Vulvovaginitis*

A complete evaluation of vulvovaginitis includes a careful history of sexually transmitted diseases, use of intrauterine devices, the medical risk factors described previously in this chapter, and a sexual history. Physical examination should include a complete routine pelvic examination as well as a microscopic examination of the vaginal secretions for the detection of *Trichomonas*, a search for the clue cells indicative of bacterial vaginosis, and a rough quantitation of yeast forms. Specific cultures for yeast are seldom of benefit, because they are often positive in asymptomatic women and do not provide a quantitative measure. *T. vaginalis* cultures may be useful in the rare instance when symptoms appear to be typical of that disease, but the microscopic test is not diagnostic. Cultures for bacterial vaginosis are useful only on a research basis.

In the postmenopausal woman with intense vulvar symptoms, careful visual inspection of the vulva is essential. A biopsy should be performed to evaluate any suspected abnormalities. Vulvar carcinoma is notoriously difficult to recognize visually, and the vulvar dystrophies are so varied in appearance that biopsy is often necessary for proper diagnosis.

In many situations these diagnostic tests are indeterminate, yet the symptoms persist. Often, the gynecologist in this situation may prescribe topical steroids and other vaginal medications as therapeutic trials. When the mental health professional sees such a patient, it is often useful to initiate a candid dialogue with the gynecologist to better understand the degree to which bacteriologic or fungal diagnoses are truly well established.

## Vulvodynia

Vulvar pain without any evidence of visual or intraepithelial change is a perplexing problem for both the gynecologist and the mental health professional. Investigation by routine histologic and culture techniques is often unrevealing. Present studies are focused on the potential role of human papillomavirus in this disorder, but results are far from conclusive. Although allowing the possibility of as-yet undiscovered organic etiologies, health professionals must be prepared to deal with the often simultaneous problems of significant depression and despair for such patients in the face of continuing symptoms. These symptoms may also be somatic symptoms of a primary psychiatric condition.

## Chronic Pelvic Pain

Adequate assessment of chronic pelvic pain includes a careful chronologic history of pain development as it affects the woman's daily life. Disability often develops gradually, and particular inflection points in the curve of disability may be punctuated by external life events or events within the family. A careful history should also include the chronology of the development of any particular sexual dysfunctions. Although such dysfunctions may be initially triggered by organic events, they may become chronic. Sexual dysfunctions may be more apt to occur in women with previous difficulties in sexual adjustment.

In a careful physical examination for chronic pelvic pain, the examiner should systematically look for vulvar epithelial changes and sensitivity, vaginal introital muscle tone and control, levator plate tension, cervical motion tenderness, and general pelvic tenderness during the bimanual and rectovaginal examinations. The two conditions most often associated with chronic pelvic pain—endometriosis and adhesions—are often difficult to detect by physical examination and imaging techniques. Laparoscopy should be freely used for diagnosis and probably for treatment of these conditions. In one encouraging report of laparoscopic adhesiolysis, long-term relief was noted in 75% of women without a chronic pain syndrome as defined previously in this chapter and in 40% of those with chronic pain syndrome (Steege and Stout 1991). Other reports have noted improvement rates of 50%–85% following such procedures (Daniell 1989; Sutton and MacDonald 1990), depending to some extent on the degree of adhesive disease treated.

Psychologic Aspects of Chronic Gynecologic Pain

Early reports in the medical literature implied that women who reported chronic pelvic pain had a high degree of feminine identity problems arising from conflicts regarding adult sexuality (Gidro-Frank et al. 1960), psychiatric disturbance characterized by mixed character disorders with predominant schizoid features (Castelnuovo-Tedesco and Krout 1970), and high neuroticism and unsatisfactory relationships (Beard et al. 1977). Studies by Duncan and Taylor (1952) and Benson et al. (1959) reported an association between the onset of symptoms of pelvic pain and emotional stress.

Although these initial studies identified the importance of psychologic factors in patients with chronic pelvic pain, some of their generalizations about psychopathology have been questioned from several perspectives. Because some physical abnormalities that cannot be identified on pelvic examination can often be observed on laparoscopic surgery, women who were considered to have normal pelvic examinations in early studies may be diagnosed with some type of organic pathology if evaluated by currently accepted diagnostic procedures. In a study of 1,200 women undergoing diagnostic laparoscopy for pelvic pain, Cunanan et al. (1983) found that 63% of the women with normal pelvic examinations before diagnostic laparoscopy had abnormal findings on diagnostic laparoscopy. On the other hand, questions have been raised about the assumption of a cause-and-effect relationship between physical findings and pain symptoms. Kresch et al. (1984) identified some possible pathologic conditions in 29% of asymptomatic women who underwent laparoscopic surgery for tubal ligation. Recent work with diagnostic laparoscopy under conscious sedation technique, with the purpose of "mapping" the association of pain with pelvic organs and their pathology, may provide clinically useful information about both the patient's general level of visceral and somatic sensitivity and the role of pelvic pathology in causing pain (Palter et al. 1996; Steege 1997).

Conclusions of previous studies suggesting the high prevalence of psychopathology are called into question by other methodologic issues, including 1) a selection bias in the sample of patients studied psychologically, because of the high refusal rates for psychologic assessment reported in some studies, 2) a potential bias of psychologic evaluators not blinded to the presence or absence of organic disease, and 3) a lack of appropriate control groups to establish population base rate data for psychosocial factors, such as marital and sexual adjustment difficulties. In all of the studies of which we are aware, limited information is available on the psychologic status of pelvic pain samples before onset of pain.

Some of the confusion about the relative contribution of psychologic factors in chronic gynecologic conditions has probably arisen because of the varying definitions of chronic pelvic pain and other gynecologic conditions. At least three different operational definitions of chronic pelvic pain appear in the literature with some frequency. These definitions focus on different aspects of the chronic condition: 1) duration (chronic pelvic or gynecologic pain that has lasted 6 months or longer, a time marker used in other chronic pain conditions); 2) anatomic-chronic (pelvic or gynecologic pain lacking an apparent physical cause sufficient to explain it); and 3) affective-behavioral (pain accompanied by significant disturbance of mood and altered physical activities such as work, recreational, or sexual activity).

Studies in which psychologic inquiry has focused on patients for whom no apparent physical findings can be identified may reflect more psychologic contributions to the pain. Obviously, chronic pelvic pain samples selected on the basis of accompanying affective disturbance may be expected to reflect a strong association with depressive symptoms. Other studies that have selected patients with chronic pelvic pain on the basis of pain duration may include women with documented organic pathology, most commonly endometriosis and pelvic adhesive disease; however, these women may report varying levels of pain severity and impairment. Stout et al. (1991) reported that the extent of physical disease evaluated by diagnostic laparoscopy did not correlate significantly with ratings of pain levels or several other indices of impairment. These findings confirmed the need for exploration of other factors such as psychologic variables, which have been shown to account for a significant portion of individual differences in functional impairment in other pain conditions.

In the literature on chronic pain, investigators have examined several personality variables, including anxiety, depression, and certain patterns on personality inventories that have been described as neurotic, particularly those characterized by hypochondriasis and somatization tendencies (Sternbach 1974). In several studies (Chaturvedi 1988; Papciak et al. 1987; Postone 1986), alexithymia (lack of words for feelings) has been investigated as a personality characteristic that may promote and maintain pain symptoms. Bradley et al. (1981) pointed out that an important shortcoming of many personality studies is that most such studies of patients with chronic pain present composite responses, therefore fostering an inaccurate picture of homogeneity in these patients. Keefe et al. (1986) found that depression was a significant predictor of pain behavior in patients with low-back pain independent of demographic or medical status variables. However, psychologic variables (depression, anxiety, helplessness) were not found to be independent predictors of pain behaviors in patients with rheumatoid arthritis (Anderson et al. 1988), pointing out the danger of generalizing from one chronic population to another.

In reviewing studies of chronic pelvic pain (specifically focusing on those in which diagnostic laparoscopy was used to investigate the organic component) and other chronic gynecologic conditions, an association has been noted between these conditions and certain psychologic variables. Rosenthal et al. (1984) administered the Minnesota Multiphasic Personality Inventory (MMPI) (Hathaway and McKinley 1970) to 163 consecutive patients referred for chronic pelvic pain, 60 of whom underwent diagnostic laparoscopy. The most frequent finding was a "somatizing" pattern (elevations on scales 1 and 3). Abnormal physical findings were present in 75% of the women who underwent diagnostic laparoscopy; however, 75% of those patients thought to have an organic cause for their pain also had evidence of psychopathology on the MMPI. The MMPI was therefore a poor predictor of organic pathology.

Magni et al. (1986) examined the psychologic characteristics of 30 women who underwent diagnostic laparoscopies for chronic pelvic pain and 30 matched controls using the Middlesex Hospital Questionnaire (Crown and Crisp 1966) and the Zung Self-Rating Depression Scale (Zung 1965). No differences in somatization scores were observed in patients with chronic pelvic pain with or without organic pathology, although both groups had higher scores than did control subjects. Patients with pelvic pain and without observed physical pathology were, however, more depressed than were patients with organic pelvic pain and controls.

Harrop-Griffiths et al. (1988) used a structured psychiatric interview (the National Institute of Mental Health Diagnostic Interview Schedule; Robbins et al. 1981) in a study of 25 women with chronic pelvic pain and 30 women with other gynecologic concerns. They found that patients with chronic pelvic pain had a significantly higher prevalence of lifetime major depression, current major depression, lifetime substance abuse, adult sexual dysfunction, and somatization. Stout and Steege (1991) found that 50% of 294 women seeking evaluation at a pelvic pain clinic scored in the depressed range ($<16$) on the Center for Epidemiologic Studies Depression Scale (Radloff 1977) at the time of their initial visit. Slocumb et al. (1989) found that patients with abdominal pelvic pain syndrome scored higher as a group on the Hopkins Symptom Checklist (Derogatis et al. 1974) scales of anxiety, depression, anger-hostility, and somatization; they also pointed out, however, that 56% of the patients with pain rated themselves within the normal range on all scales. Stewart et al. (1990) found that women with clinically unconfirmed vulvovaginitis were significantly more emotionally distressed than were the women with confirmed vulvovaginitis and healthy control subjects.

Sexual history has been explored in several inquiries, indicating that women seeking treatment have a high incidence of sexual trauma, including molestation, incest, and rape (Beard et al. 1977; Duncan and Taylor 1952; Gross et al. 1980; Haber and Roos 1985; Raskin 1984; Reiter and Gambone 1990; Schei 1991; Walker et al. 1988). In the study by Harrop-Griffiths et al. (1988), the two groups undergoing diagnostic laparoscopies were also administered a structured interview on sexual abuse. Patients with chronic pelvic pain with or without positive laparoscopy findings were more likely than control subjects to have experienced childhood and adult sexual abuse. In the study by Reiter and Gambone (1990), 48% of 106 women with chronic pelvic pain had a history of major psychosexual trauma (molestation, incest, and rape), as compared with 6.5% in a control group of 92 pain-free control subjects presenting for annual routine gynecologic examinations ($P < 0.001$). Rapkin et al. (1990) did not find a higher prevalence of childhood or adult sexual abuse in a group of women with chronic pelvic pain than in women with chronic pain in other locations or in control subjects, although women with chronic pelvic pain reported a higher prevalence of childhood physical abuse. The authors concluded that their findings did not support the hypothesis that pelvic pain is specifically and psychodynamically related to sexual abuse and suggested that abusive experiences, whether physical or sexual, may promote the chronicity of many different painful conditions.

As might be expected, many of these same studies also report a high incidence of marital distress. Stout and Steege (1991) found that 56% of 220 married women presenting for evaluation of chronic pelvic pain scored in the maritally distressed range ($< 100$) on the Locke-Wallace Marital Adjustment Scale (Locke and Wallace 1959).

Women presenting with chronic gynecologic conditions often present with concomitant sexual dysfunction, particularly dyspareunia. Although establishing accurate baseline functioning is difficult, some women report satisfactory sexual functioning before the onset of pain symptoms, whereas others appear to have long-standing sexual difficulties. In any case, sexual dysfunction is likely associated with chronic gynecologic pain, either as an antecedent or as a consequence. Decreased sexual desire and conditioned vaginismus are correlates of this problem that often need specific intervention in addition to any indicated medical treatment.

Because studies to date have been cross-sectional in design, it is not possible to determine whether the negative psychologic states reported are a predisposing factor or a reaction to the pain condition. It is important to note that no significant differences in personality or psychosocial variables have been found in most studies of women with chronic pelvic pain with or without identified organic pathology, perhaps suggesting that chronic pelvic pain in some women may be more closely associated with psychosocial factors than with organic factors. In reviewing the literature regarding the relationship between chronic pain and depression, Romano and Turner (1985) concluded that at least two distinct groups of chronic pain patients may exist: one subgroup in which pain and depression are a final common presentation reached by a number of pathways and a second group in which depression develops in reaction to pain, as occurs in some other acute and chronic medical diseases. Patients with chronic gynecologic conditions also appear to be a heterogeneous group; however, the high prevalence of sexual trauma, marital and sexual dysfunction, and emotional distress in previously studied samples of these patients warrants specific attention to these areas in any clinical evaluation. Further research is needed to explore whether these psychosocial factors have a specific relationship to the development and persistence of chronic gynecologic conditions.

## Management of Chronic Gynecologic Pain

In current gynecologic practice, the woman usually referred for psychiatric care has had negative laparoscopy results—that is, the referring physician believes that gynecologic causes have been "ruled out." Unfortunately, it is far more common for the patient to have some organic pathology and to have been repeatedly subjected to medical and surgical measures in pursuit of pain relief. Many of these women have developed a chronic pain condition, characterized by significant changes in mood and activities, that needs behavioral and psychologic approaches as well as psychopharmacologic treatment in some cases. This group of patients with chronic pain presents an opportunity for fruitful collaboration between the gynecologic and mental health specialties. In most of these cases it is clinically difficult to diagnose any particular underlying psychopathology as the precise cause for the pain. More often, clinical judgment will determine that attention to both physical and psychologic factors may be important, that both should proceed simultaneously, and that the hope of assigning a particular degree of responsibility to either element must be surrendered. In some cases, the treatment of intrapelvic pathology by laparoscopic approaches, such as lysis of adhesions or vaporization of endometriosis, may be useful. When the parameters of chronic pain syndrome described here are also present, however, behavioral and psychologic assistance is also required.

Reports of controlled trials of psychologic interventions specifically for chronic pelvic pain are very limited; however, increasing evidence substantiates the belief that combined medical and psychologic approaches are likely to result in greater improvement than are gynecologic treatments alone in many women with chronic pelvic pain. Pearce et al. (1987) reported the results of a prospective, randomized, controlled trial of two different psychologic interventions in the treatment of chronic pelvic pain. Seventy-eight women with chronic pelvic pain of at least 6 months' duration and with no obvious pathology observed on laparoscopy were allocated to a pain analysis, a stress analysis, or a minimal-intervention control group. All groups received an explanation of the pain as being caused by abnormalities in pelvic blood flow. In addition, the stress analysis group received training in identifying and implementing alternative cognitive and behavioral responses to concerns other than pain and in applying Jacobsonian relaxation strategies in stressful situations. The pain analysis group focused on monitoring and modifying events antecedent and consequent to pain, graded exercise, and reinforcement of "well behaviors." Both the stress analysis and the pain analysis group reported significantly lower pain intensity ratings at 6-month follow-up visits than did the control group.

In studies by Kames et al. (1990) and Peters et al. (1991), significant improvement in pain ratings and functioning was reported after multidisciplinary pain management approaches. Peters et al. (1991) randomly assigned 106 patients with chronic pelvic pain to either a standard-approach group or an integrated-approach group. The standard approach consisted of excluding organic pathology by diagnostic laparoscopy and then referring the patient for psychologic treatment if no somatic cause was found. The integrated approach included attention to somatic, psychologic, dietary, environmental, and physiotherapeutic factors from the beginning of the evaluation. After a 1-year interval, women in the integrated-approach group showed significantly greater improvement in their general pain experience, in the disturbance of their daily activities, and in the associated pain symptoms. Because the particular types of treatments applied to any individual patient were not standardized in either of these studies, it is unfortunately not possible to identify the effective therapeutic components in these combined approaches.

In general, the psychologic treatment component of chronic gynecologic conditions appears to be most effective when psychosocial factors are evaluated simultaneously with organic factors. Although patients with chronic pelvic pain are often unwilling to view their pain symptoms as other than organically based, many individuals are aware of some factors that worsen their pain, such as worry, muscle tension, or depression. A crucial aspect of successful psychotherapeutic intervention is making a connection with the patient at her own level of conceptualization of the pain problem.

Therapeutic interventions for the patient with chronic pelvic pain usually focus initially on exploring behavioral and cognitive patterns that exacerbate the pain symptoms and developing coping strategies to interrupt these patterns. New information is often obtained by having the patient record pain ratings across the day. Depending on the relative influence of particular factors on pain ratings, psychologic treatment interventions have often included relaxation training directed at reducing muscle tension components, stress analysis to identify difficult life areas, assertiveness training to teach skills for dealing more directly with people or circumstances that may be controlled or avoided by the patients' complaints of pain, and cognitive interventions directed at specific emotional responses to pain that may feed back to increase anxiety, depression, and perceived pain.

Psychologic approaches may also involve spouses or families to assist in defining a valued role in the family despite some possible limitations in previous activities. Changes in sexual activity often accompany pelvic pain, and specific education and counseling may be required to allow the patient to return to a level of comfort. Sexual counseling suggestions often include information about adequate physiologic arousal, changes in sexual positions, and instruction in vaginal relaxation exercises to treat a conditioned vaginismus response. As a trusting therapeutic relationship is established and coping skills are developed, some women may be receptive to pursuing psychotherapeutic approaches that are inclusive of broader issues related to unresolved emotional issues from past experiences.

Medical management of chronic pelvic pain may include the use of antidepressants, although therapeutic trials of these agents in treating this condition are lacking. Tricyclic antidepressants and the newer serotonergic agents are used by many clinics providing care for patients with chronic pelvic pain. Although analgesic prescriptions should be limited to nonnarcotic agents, chronic pain is better treated by the continuous use of such medications, thereby eliminating the tendency for medication to act as a reinforcer of pain behaviors or complaints. Other medications aimed at the symptomatic relief of bladder and bowel dysfunction are often additive. We have found that it is often better to treat various contributing factors simultaneously. When narcotics are found to be necessary, it is useful to prescribe them on a "contract" basis—that is, from one physician, one pharmacy, and at a strictly prescribed rate with no early refills.

Nonpharmacologic methods are also useful in selected individuals. Alterations of gait or stance that might be traced to a musculoskeletal problem can be best evaluated by a physical therapist. Chronic spasm of the levator, psoas, and piriformis muscles can frequently contribute to chronic pelvic pain. Appropriate muscle strengthening, stretching, and relaxation exercises can also help. Transcutaneous nerve stimulators have been used sparingly in patients with pelvic pain but are sometimes useful.

When pain and related disabilities are severe, many clinicians feel that intensive inpatient treatment is warranted (Fogel and Stoudemire 1986; Maruta et al. 1989; Stoudemire and Fogel 1986). In such a case, a multispecialty team, particularly on a combined medical-psychiatric unit, is the most productive approach because it may best maintain a balanced approach to the often complicated and integrated psychologic and physical components to chronic pelvic pain.

## Conclusions

Chronic pelvic pain is a common complaint. Although a minority of women will present with this problem in the absence of any organic pathology, chronic pain in most women will have developed in the presence of disease processes, such as adhesions and endometriosis. It is often clinically impossible to assign specific degrees of responsibility to physical and psychologic contributions to pain. Clinical care is therefore facilitated when needs in both areas are addressed as clinically appropriate and efforts to assign degrees of responsibility are suspended. This approach requires close collaboration between the gynecologist and the mental health professional.

The patient experiencing chronic pain in the total absence of organic pathology presents a more difficult problem and often represents more long-standing and complicated psychopathologic processes. Again, collaborative management will be useful to evaluate and minimize unnecessary treatment while continuing to offer psychologic assistance aimed at helping the patient and her family cope with her difficulties.

References

Anderson KO, Keefe FJ, Bradley LA, et al: Prediction of pain behavior and functional status of rheumatoid arthritis patients using medical status and psychological variables. Pain 33:25–32, 1988

Beard RW, Belsey EM, Lieberman BA, et al: Pelvic pain in women. Am J Obstet Gynecol 128:566–570, 1977

Beard W, Reginald PW, Wadsworth J: Clinical features of women with chronic lower abdominal pain and pelvic congestion. Br J Obstet Gynecol 95:153–161, 1989

Benson RC, Hanson KH, Matarazzo JD: Atypical pelvic pain in women: gynecologic and psychiatric considerations. Am J Obstet Gynecol 77:806–825, 1959

Bradley LA, Prokop CK, Gentry WD, et al: Assessment of chronic pain, in Medical Psychology: Contributions to Behavioral Medicine. Edited by Prokup CK, Bradley LA. New York, Academic Press, 1981, pp 35–52

Castelnuovo-Tedesco P, Krout BM: Psychosomatic aspects of chronic pelvic pain. Int J Psychiatry Med 1:109–126, 1970

Chaturvedi SK: Chronic pain patients with and without alexithymia. Can J Psychiatry 33:830–833, 1988

Crown S, Crisp AH: A short clinical diagnostic self-rating scale for psychoneurotic patients: the Middlesex Hospital Questionnaire. Br J Psychiatry 112:917–923, 1966

Cunanan RG, Courey NG, Lipes J: Laparoscopic findings in patients with pelvic pain. Am J Obstet Gynecol 146:589–591, 1983

Daniell JF: Laparoscopic enterolysis for chronic abdominal pain. J Gynecol Surg 5:61–66, 1989

Derogatis LR, Lipman RS, Rickels K, et al: The Hopkins Symptom Checklist (HSCL): a self-report symptom inventory. Behav Sci 19:1–15, 1974

Duncan CH, Taylor HC: A psychosomatic study of pelvic congestion. Am J Obstet Gynecol 64:1–12, 1952

Fedele L, Parazzini F, Bianchi S, et al: Stage and localization of pelvic endometriosis and pain. Fertil Steril 53:155–158, 1990

Fogel BS, Stoudemire A: Organization and development of combined medical-psychiatric units, II. Psychosomatics 27:417–428, 1986

Gidro-Frank L, Gordon T, Taylor HC Jr: Pelvic pain and female identity: a survey of emotional factors in 40 patients. Am J Obstet Gynecol 79:1184–1202, 1960

Gross R, Doerr J, Caldirola D, et al: Borderline syndrome and incest in chronic pelvic pain patients. Int J Psychiatry Med 10:79–96, 1980

Haber J, Roos C: Effects of spouse abuse and/or sexual abuse in the development and maintenance of chronic pain in women, in Advances in Pain Research and Therapy, Vol 9. Edited by Fields HL, Dubner R, Cervero F. New York, Raven, 1985, pp 889–895

Harrop-Griffiths J, Katon W, Walker E, et al: The association between chronic pelvic pain, psychiatric diagnoses, and childhood sexual abuse. Obstet Gynecol 71:589–594, 1988

Hathaway SR, McKinley JC: Minnesota Multiphasic Personality Inventory, Revised. Minneapolis, University of Minnesota, 1970

Kames LD, Rapkin AJ, Naliboff BD, et al: Effectiveness of an interdisciplinary pain management program for the treatment of chronic pelvic pain. Pain 41:41–46, 1990

Keefe FJ, Wilkins RH, Cook WA, et al: Depression, pain and pain behavior. J Consult Clin Psychol 54:665–669, 1986

Kresch AJ, Seifer DB, Sachs LB, et al: Laparoscopy in 100 women with chronic pelvic pain. Obstet Gynecol 64:672–674, 1984

Locke MJ, Wallace KM: Short marital adjustment and predictions tests: their reliability and validity. Marriage and Family Living 21:251–255, 1959

Magni G, Anderoli C, de Leo D, et al: Psychological profile of women with chronic pelvic pain. Arch Gynecol Obstet 237:165–168, 1986

Maruta T, Vatterott MK, McHardy MJ: Pain management as an antidepressant: long-term resolution of pain-associated depression. Pain 36:335–337, 1989

Palter SF, Olive DL: Office microlaparoscopy under local anesthesia for chronic pelvic pain. J Am Assoc Gynecol Laparosc 3:359–364, 1996

Papciak AS, Feuerstein M, Belar CD, et al: Alexithymia and pain in an outpatient behavioral medicine clinic. Int J Psychiatry Med 16:347–357, 1987

Pearce S, Matthews AM, Beard RW: A controlled trial of psychological approaches to the management of pelvic pain in women. Paper presented at the 8th annual scientific sessions of the Society of Behavioral Medicine, Washington, DC, March, 1987

Peters AAW, van Horst E, Jellis B, et al: A randomized clinical trial to compare two different approaches in women with chronic pelvic pain. Obstet Gynecol 77:740–744, 1991

Postone N: Alexithymia in chronic pain patients. Gen Hosp Psychiatry 8:163–167, 1986

Radloff LS: The CES-D Scale: a self-report depression scale for research in the general population. Applied Psychological Management 1:385–410, 1977

Rapkin AJ, Kames LD, Darke LL, et al: History of physical and sexual abuse in women with chronic pain. Obstet Gynecol 76:92–96,1990

Raskin DE: Diagnosis in patients with chronic pelvic pain (letter). Am J Psychiatry 141:824, 1984

Reiter RC, Gambone JC: Demographic and historic variables in women with idiopathic chronic pelvic pain. Obstet Gynecol 75:428–432, 1990

Robbins LN, Helzer JD, Croughan J, et al: National Institute of Mental Health Diagnostic Interview Schedule: its history, characteristics and validity. Arch Gen Psychiatry 38:381, 1981

Romano JM, Turner JA: Chronic pain and depression: does the evidence support a relationship? Psychol Bull 97:18–34, 1985

Rosenthal RH, Ling FW, Rosenthal TL, et al: Chronic pelvic pain and laparoscopic findings. Psychosomatics 25:833–841, 1984

Schei B: Sexual factors in pelvic pain. J Psychosom Obstet Gynaecol 12(suppl):99–108, 1991

Slocumb JC, Kellner R, Rosenfeld RC, et al: Anxiety and depression inpatients with the abdominal pelvic pain syndrome. Gen Hosp Psychiatry 11:48–53, 1989

Steege JF: Dyspareunia and vaginismus. Clin Obstet Gynecol 23:750–759, 1984

Steege JF: Microlaparoscopy, in Chronic Pelvic Pain: An Integrated Approach. Edited by Steege JF, Metzger DA, Levy BS. Philadelphia, PA, WB Saunders, 1998, pp 337–346

Steege JF, Stout AL: Resolution of chronic pelvic pain following laparoscopic adhesiolysis. Am J Obstet Gynecol 165:278–283, 1991

Steege JF, Stout AL, Somkuti SG: Chronic pelvic pain in women: toward an integrative model. J Psychosom Obstet Gynaecol 12(suppl):3–30, 1991

Sternbach RA: Pain Patients: Traits and Treatment. New York, Academic Press, 1974

Stewart DE, Whelan CL, Fong IW, et al: Psychosocial aspects of chronic, clinically unconfirmed vulvovaginitis. Obstet Gynecol 76:852–856, 1990

Stoudemire A, Fogel BS: Organization and development of combined medical-psychiatric units, I. Psychosomatics 27:341–345, 1986

Stout AL, Steege JF: Psychosocial and behavioral self-reports of chronic pelvic pain patients. Paper presented at the meeting of the American Society of Psychosomatic Obstetrics and Gynecology, Houston, TX, March, 1991

Stout AL, Steege JF, Dodson WC, et al: Relationship of laparoscopic findings to self-report of pelvic pain. Am J Obstet Gynecol 164:73–79, 1991

Sutton C, MacDonald R: Laser laparoscopic adhesiolysis. J Gynecol Surg 6:155–159, 1990

Walker EW, Katon W, Harrop-Griffiths J, et al: Relationship of chronic pelvic pain to psychiatric diagnoses and childhood sexual abuse. Am J Psychiatry 145:75–80, 1988

Zung WWK: A self-rating depression scale. Arch Gen Psychiatry 12:63–70, 1965

# Gynecologic Disorders and Surgery

PAULA J. ADAMS HILLARD, M.D.

Gynecologic disorders and gynecologic surgery have the potential to evoke significant emotional responses. A sexually transmitted disease (STD) contracted from a partner with whom a woman had been intimate suggests betrayal and violation of trust and self. That some STDs are incurable and have the potential for carcinogenesis or death as a consequence is understandably terrifying. From the time of menarche, women learn to identify monthly cycles and rhythms of menstrual function, and disturbances of normal functioning may be distressing. Surgeries on the genital organs threaten childbearing potential, sense of feminine identity, and sexual functioning. This chapter provides background information on several of these common gynecologic concerns and a discussion of the impact that they may have. Although the potential for adverse psychologic consequences for the individual is significant and the number of individuals with these common gynecologic problems is large and increasing, little attention has been directed toward the psychologic consequences of many of these problems.

## Sexually Transmitted Diseases

The current complement of STDs is an alphabet soup of acronyms, including infections caused by the following organisms: *Neisseria gonorrhea* (GC for gonococcus), herpes simplex virus (HSV), human papillomavirus (HPV), HIV, *Chlamydia trachomatis* (as yet without a common acronym), and *Treponema pallidum*. An increasing number of individuals have experienced disease related to one of these organisms, with some types of infections reaching epidemic proportions, primarily among young adults and adolescents. Although some bacterial infections are easily treated and cured with antibiotics, viral infections are usually incurable and may have potential sequelae for future health and fertility, as with chlamydia-associated pelvic inflammatory disease. The potential for HPV-associated cervical, vulvar, and vaginal intraepithelial neoplasia may be significant, and the potential lethality of HIV infection is well known. Individuals who initiate sexual activity at an early age and those who have had multiple sexual partners are at greater risk for contracting an STD. Sexually active adolescents and young adults are a particularly high-risk group (Bell and Hein 1984; Institute of Medicine 1997).

Public health reporting of STDs is required in all states for *N. gonorrhea*, syphilis, and AIDS (not HIV seropositivity). The incidences of HSV, HPV, and chlamydia are estimates only, although an increasing number of states are mandating report of these infections (Webster et al. 1993). Nationally, the rates for gonorrhea and primary and secondary syphilis have declined since 1990, reaching low points in 1993 that were below or approaching year-2000 objectives (225 cases or fewer of gonorrhea and 10 cases or fewer of primary and secondary syphilis per 100,000 persons). However, rates for both diseases remained higher than the year-2000 objectives for certain population subgroups: adolescents and young adults, minorities (especially blacks), and persons living in the southern United States (Centers for Disease Control and Prevention 1994b). The greatest number of cases of gonorrhea occurred in the ages 20–24 group (Centers for Disease Control and Prevention 1996b). *Chlamydia trachomatis* causes an estimated 3–5 million infections annually in the United States (Centers for Disease Control and Prevention 1994a; Judson 1985). Sexually active adolescents and young adults are at particular risk for chlamydia infections (Bell 1990). From 1986 to 1990, an epidemic of syphilis occurred in the United States, primarily among drug users who traded drugs for sex (Webster and Rolfs 1993), and a concomitant increase occurred in the incidence of congenital syphilis (Dunn et al. 1993). Subsequently, rates of syphilis have declined (Centers for Disease Control and Prevention 1994b).

## Herpes Simplex Virus

It has been estimated that more than 2 million cases of genital herpes occur annually in the United States (Droegemueller et al. 1987). From 1988 to 1994, the seroprevalence of genital herpes (herpes simplex virus type II, or HSV-II) in the United States was 22%, corresponding to 45 million infected people. The seroprevalence was higher among women (25.6%) than among men (17.8%) and higher among blacks (45.9%) than among whites (17.6%). Less than 10% of those who were seropositive reported a history of genital herpes infection (Fleming et al. 1997), which means that many individuals have been infected with the virus and are potentially infectious to sexual partners but have no history of a typical lesion.

## Human Papillomavirus

The rate of consultations with private physicians for HSV and for genital warts (HPV infections) has increased markedly (Becker et al. 1987); nearly 1.2 million office visits for genital warts were reported in 1988. Cervical HPV infection is associated with cervical dysplasia and abnormal Pap smears, the reported rates of which appear to be increasing, especially among adolescents (P. J. Hillard et al. 1989b), and the degree of abnormality reported on the Pap smear may range from mild squamous atypia to frankly invasive carcinoma. This spectrum of abnormalities is often not appreciated by the lay public, who may view the Pap (or "cancer") smear as having only one of two possible results—normal or indicative of cancer. Thus the potential exists for the generation of significant anxiety. Providing patients with accurate information about this spectrum of abnormalities, the procedures necessary to evaluate abnormal results (colposcopy and biopsy), and any planned treatment and expected outcome can help to alleviate this concern (P. J. Hillard et al. 1989a).

In selected patients with mild cervical abnormalities on biopsy results, observation without specific therapy may be recommended because spontaneous regression may occur in up to 60%–80% of patients (American College of Obstetricians and Gynecologists 1994). Compliance with recommendations for subsequent Pap smears is essential, because progression may also occur. Fear about possible progression may sometimes paradoxically result in failure to keep subsequent appointments or in other maladaptive behaviors (Biro et al. 1991). It has been argued that because mild cervical dysplasia can be effectively eradicated with a single treatment in a high percentage of patients, this treatment should be considered for all such patients to spare them the psychologic and emotional trauma of repeated abnormal cervical cytology on follow-up (Tay and Yong 1995). Most clinicians feel that the potential for morbidity from treatment modalities outweighs any psychologic risk for most women; however, treatments should be individualized.

Higher-grade abnormalities (cervical intraepithelial neoplasia [CIN] 2, moderate dysplasia and CIN 3, severe dysplasia, or carcinoma in situ) generally require ablative therapy, which may range from office laser vaporization to cervical cryotherapy, hysterectomy, or excision using an electrical current. Cervical cryotherapy and laser vaporization have been shown to have essentially similar rates of lesion cure or eradication (in the range of 85%–90%)

(Townsend and Richart 1983), and thus have largely replaced hysterectomy as therapy for cervical dysplasia (in the absence of other gynecologic problems that would warrant a hysterectomy). Reassurances of this fact should be given at the onset of a diagnostic work-up because the patient's fear of hysterectomy, with its real and perceived losses, may be an unstated concern. Loop electrical excision is a newer technique; its efficacy appears to be comparable with that of cryotherapy or laser vaporization (T. C. Wright et al. 1992). The type of treatment recommended depends primarily on the preferences of the treating physician and the modalities available.

In patients who do not fulfill the criteria for outpatient ablative therapy, cervical conization is necessary. This procedure preserves childbearing potential with little or no detrimental effect on future fertility or childbearing. Criteria for conization include inability to visualize the lesion completely with disease of the endocervical canal or significant discrepancy between Pap smear and biopsy results. Cervical conization involves the removal of a cone-shaped biopsy specimen using a laser or conventional scalpel. This procedure is usually performed in an operating room with the patient under general or regional anesthetic. In the absence of complications, the patient can be admitted and discharged on the same day. The potential for resolution of cervical dysplasia is good with therapy, but follow-up is critical because recurrences are possible.

As with other STDs, it is important for women to be aware that their risk of HPV acquisition is determined not only by their own sexual history and number of partners but also by those of their partners. Evidence suggesting that HPV-associated genital lesions are not eradicated by treatment is psychologically distressing for the patient, and the prospect of an incurable disease is often associated with anxiety. How HPV-related disease is transmitted, how infectious it is, and the degree of risk of progressive disease remain in great part unknown (although generally considered to be sexually transmissible, the possibility of nonsexual transmission has been raised). It is distressing that these questions, with very practical implications, remain unanswered by scientific evidence, and medical professionals who acknowledge the uncertainties related to HPV are sometimes viewed as incompetent or insensitive to the patient's concerns.

## HIV Infection

HIV infection is a major cause of morbidity and mortality among women and children in the United States. In 1995, women accounted for 19% of the reported cases of AIDS. HIV infection is the third leading cause of death among all women aged 25–44 years in the United States and the leading cause of death among black women in this age group. An estimated 7,000 infants are born to HIV-infected women in the United States each year; without treatment, approximately 15%–30% of these infants would be infected (Centers for Disease Control and Prevention 1996a). HIV counseling and testing services are important for women to reduce their risk of infection or, if already infected, to initiate early treatment and prevent HIV transmission to others, including their infants. Attention has been given to the psychologic factors motivating STD risk reduction and HIV prevention (Darrow 1997; Gillespie 1997). In addition, the body of literature focusing on the risks of HIV infection among the seriously and chronically mentally ill is increasing because the risks of HIV and other STDs are higher in this population (Carey et al. 1997; Weinhardt et al. 1997). As HIV infection becomes a chronic disease, the psychosocial factors related to coping behaviors become important to understand (Nannis et al. 1997). A complete discussion of the psychiatric conditions associated with HIV infection and AIDS is beyond the scope of this chapter, but mood disorders, substance use, and organic mental disorders are common (Judd et al. 1997).

## Psychologic Effects

The psychologic effects of STDs have been systematically addressed in only a limited manner. STDs have been characterized as "among the most stigmatizing diseases that most Americans . . . acquire" (Darrow and Pauli 1984). The effects have been most extensively studied for genital herpes infections, but to some extent, psychologic reactions described with herpes may also occur with any of the other STDs. Psychologic distress related to herpes was first characterized in a report of herpes self-help groups (Luby and Gillespie 1981).

With herpes, as with other serious disease, the initial diagnosis of the infection may be shocking for the patient; the impact of an STD diagnosis may be differentiated from that of other infectious diseases by the stigma associated with STDs in general (Darrow and Pauli 1984). Once the diagnosis is made, the patient often searches for a cure; he or she subsequently may be overcome with a sense of isolation and loneliness when, as with HSV or HPV, the incurable nature of the disease is realized (Luby and Gillespie 1981). A diagnosis of a curable STD, such as gonorrhea or chlamydia, may not result in such feelings, but HIV infection, with its ultimately fatal outcome, has great potential for psychologic distress. As concerns increase, anger becomes important. Initially, the patient's anger is directed toward the infecting partner, but it may also be directed toward the physician who is unable to cure the viral disease. Anxiety and fears about the infectious nature of the disease, its impact on future childbearing and fertility, and the potential risks of cancer may generalize to other areas of the individual's life. Fears about the impact of the disease on sexual activity, sexuality, and sexual performance begin to surface. Some individuals go on to feel that they are contagious or dangerous—a "leper" effect. Patients may become self-involved, decide to become celibate, or engage in "anti-sexual" or moralistic behavior. Depression, feelings of helplessness, or guilt may increase over time in some patients and they may ask "why me?" (Luby and Gillespie 1981), a reaction similar to that of patients diagnosed with life-threatening illnesses, such as cancer.

One study (Orr et al. 1989) has reported an association between STDs and low self-esteem among adolescents, although it is not clear whether problems with self-esteem are a cause or effect of STD acquisition. Elevated levels of psychologic disturbance among patients in STD clinics have been noted (Ikkos et al. 1987), and in some individuals the sequelae of an STD such as herpes may include a reactivation of underlying psychopathology. The extent to which these reactions occur and their severity and duration vary among individuals; however, an awareness of possible psychologic reactions will aid the physician in helping patients develop the skills to cope with their disease.

Several studies of herpes have reported elevated levels of psychologic distress with adverse effects on sexuality, self-image, and love relationships lasting many months after the diagnosis or initial episode of the disease (J. R. Hillard et al. 1989). Concern that herpes affects young people "at a critical phase of psychosocial development as they are attempting to develop lasting attachments" has been expressed (Luby and Klinge 1985, p. 494). Attempts to define individuals or populations at greater risk of significant and long-lasting psychiatric distress have not been particularly successful, and thus all individuals who contract herpes (and by extension, other STDs) should be considered to be at risk for persistent psychologic symptoms (J. R. Hillard et al. 1989).

## Effects of Diethylstilbestrol

The association between in utero exposure to diethylstilbestrol (DES), a synthetic estrogen, and vaginal clear cell adenocarcinoma was first described in

1971, and it has not generally been prescribed during pregnancy since that date. Thought to decrease the risk of pregnancy loss and miscarriage, DES was ultimately shown to be ineffective for this indication. Many thousands of women were exposed to DES before birth, but vaginal adenocarcinoma fortunately remains rare, with an estimated risk in exposed women of 1/1,000 or less (Berek and Hacker 1989). Vaginal, uterine, and cervical structural abnormalities have also been associated with DES, and infertility and pregnancy loss, including preterm delivery, have been correlated with DES exposure (Herbst et al. 1981). The prognosis for a good pregnancy outcome in women exposed to DES is generally good, with reports suggesting that about 80% will have a live-born child (Herbst and Holt 1990).

Mothers who received DES during pregnancy must deal with feelings of anxiety, guilt, and anger, particularly if their daughters also have reproductive problems. Their daughters may themselves be anxious about their own future fertility and may feel anger toward their mothers and toward the medical profession that prescribed the treatment. In one study, however, 80% of DES-exposed daughters felt trust and alliance with their mothers and doctors and only a minority reacted with hostility or fear, a finding that ran contrary to the investigators' expectations (Burke et al. 1980). An appropriate physician–patient relationship may be particularly important in minimizing the adverse emotional sequelae for mothers and daughters exposed to DES.

# Psychologic Preparation for Gynecologic Procedures

## Preoperative Preparation for Gynecologic Surgery

Psychologic preparation is an important part of preoperative preparation for any type of surgery, but particularly so for gynecologic procedures (Youngs and Wise 1980). A woman's first reaction to gynecologic problems depends on the severity of the diagnosis, its potential or imagined sequelae (life or fertility threatening), the extent of the required treatment (office biopsy, ambulatory surgery, major surgery), and the woman's own psychologic make-up and reactions to stress in general. The practicing psychiatrist or other mental health professional can address gynecologic concerns most effectively if he or she has a basic understanding of the most frequently encountered gynecologic problems, their management, and the potential issues that commonly surface.

In any situation involving gynecologic pathology and the recommendation for operative intervention, informed consent and medical decision making are critical (American College of Obstetricians and Gynecologists 1993; Rockwell and Peitone-Rockwell 1979). The term *informed refusal* has been proposed as another dimension of this concept (American College of Obstetricians and Gynecologists Committee on Professional Liability 1996). The acronym BRAIDED has been proposed as a mnemonic for remembering the basic components of informed consent (Hatcher et al. 1990). Patients should have a clear understanding of expected **B**enefits, potential **R**isks, and **A**lternatives (both medical and surgical); of their right and responsibility to make **I**nquiries about the physician's recommendations; and of their right to make the **D**ecision to withdraw from procedure, to have an **E**xplanation of the type of surgery planned and its indications, and to have **D**ocumentation of all informed-consent components. Although some physicians consider the informed consent process to be a mere formality, it is essential to patient understanding and acceptance of surgery and minimizes the potential for subsequent misunderstanding or, even worse, a lawsuit. Although this medicolegal aspect of informed consent may be foremost in consideration, the benefits to subsequent physician–patient communication, understanding, and trust should not be underestimated. Computer-aided CD-ROM programs are now available that provide preoperative patient educational material, print responses to questions about the surgical procedure, and serve as an informed consent document (American College of Obstetricians and Gynecologists 1995); however, these programs do not replace face-to-face physician–patient discussions about the potential risks and benefits of the surgery.

Psychologic preparation prior to surgery has been addressed relative to cognitive coping techniques (Ridgeway and Mathews 1982). The logistics of surgery–how long hospitalization is expected to last and the average period of recovery or time off from work–are important to convey to every patient. Specifics about pre- and postoperative procedures may be helpful for some patients (Johnson et al. 1985; Ridgeway and Mathews 1982). The ability to predict which women benefit most from which type of preoperative preparation would be useful, but most of the studies that address coping styles have been unable to identify predictive factors.

Involving the family or partner in discussions of surgery may be helpful if the woman chooses to do so. The patient's resources and previous coping skills should be assessed. It should be emphasized that surgery is stressful for the patient and will require the mobilization of personal resources, including family and friends (Youngs and Wise 1980). Following a surgical procedure, psychologic characteristics and coping styles may affect the perception of pain, the use of pain medication, and other characteristics of postoperative recovery (Ridgeway and Mathews 1982; Thomas et al. 1995; Wilson 1981). The gynecologist may recognize women at higher risk for adverse psychologic sequelae and refer them for evaluation, counseling, or therapy prior to surgery (Stellman 1990). If the patient's degree of anxiety is judged by the gynecologist to exceed that usually noted, surgery should be deferred (if possible) pending a referral for psychiatric evaluation (Schwab 1971).

Preoperative preparation includes a discussion of the specific pathology and indications for the surgery. The type of surgery to be performed should be described in terms that are understandable but not condescending. For procedures such as oophorectomy, this discussion should include the expected benefits, risks, and alternatives as well as the effect on physiology in terms of the production of ovarian steroid hormones. The need for hormone replacement therapy should be addressed. With a hysterectomy, it is important that the woman understand the basics—that she will no longer experience menses and will not be able to have children.

## Dilation and Curettage

Disturbances in menstrual regularity, sometimes accompanied by excessively heavy flow, are common at the extremes of reproductive life, particularly in the perimenopausal years prior to the cessation of menses. Because the risks of uterine fibroids and endometrial pathology (including hyperplasia, polyps, and malignancy) increase with age, histologic sampling of the endometrium is warranted for abnormal bleeding in women who are over age 40 or who have other risk factors such as obesity, chronic anovulation, or polycystic ovarian disease.

In the past, endometrial sampling typically required a dilation and curettage (D&C), an outpatient procedure typically performed in an operating room setting under general anesthesia. However, new endometrial sampling techniques have allowed endometrial biopsies to be performed in the physician's office, and thus fewer patients require a D&C (Grimes 1982); women also tend to cope better with the less-invasive endometrial biopsy than with a D&C. Hysteroscopy, in which the endometrial cavity is visualized directly using fiber optics, is an additional diagnostic tool that may be performed in lieu of or in addition to a D&C. Evidence for the efficacy of D&C as a therapeutic technique is not well established despite its widespread use (Grimes 1982).

## Sterilization

Female sterilization is now the most frequently chosen contraceptive option among married and formerly married women (Abma et al. 1997; Mosher and Pratt 1990). Female sterilization may be performed in the immediate postpartum period or as an interval outpatient procedure. Techniques of tubal occlusion include use of suture, cautery, plastic rings, or clips. Women considering sterilization should be counseled about alternative methods of contraception, including male sterilization, which has a significantly lower risk of morbidity and mortality. Women often feel that because they have assumed the health risks and discomforts of pregnancy and childbirth, their partner should assume his share of responsibility by obtaining a vasectomy. However, some women remain protective of the concerns their partners express regarding a vasectomy as a threat to his potency, virility, and manhood. Some women are pragmatic in their desire to end childbearing and assume the responsibility for permanent sterilization just as they have for reversible methods of contraception. A woman in a physically abusive relationship with an obsessively jealous and controlling man may experience an increase in abuse when making a decision for sterilization if the abusive partner attempts to preserve his control over her by forbidding such a procedure.

Sterilization should be considered to be permanent, although recent studies have suggested that the procedure's risk of failure is higher than previously recognized (Peterson et al. 1996). Less permanent but still long-lasting methods of contraception such as an implantable subdermal device (Norplant) or an intrauterine device may be appropriate alternatives for women who are not ready for sterilization. Regret after sterilization procedures is infrequent, ranging from less than 1% to 3% (Huggins and Sondheimer 1984), but certain groups appear to be at higher risk for subsequent regret. Women who are younger at the time of the procedure and who later changed partners, those who made the decision for socioeconomic reasons, and those who had the procedure at the time of an abortion or immediately postpartum may be somewhat more likely to regret sterilization (Huggins and Sondheimer 1984). Some childless women express a strong desire for sterilization and should not arbitrarily be denied the procedure. The woman's motivation and expectations regarding sterilization should be explored to ascertain that the decision is not based on misinformation (e.g., the idea that the "tubes will come untied" after a period of time), unrealistic expectations of benefits (e.g., the expectation that a faltering marriage will be saved), or a hastily made decision.

## Laparoscopy

Laparoscopy is a surgical procedure usually performed on an outpatient basis. It involves the use of fiber optics to visualize the pelvic and abdominal organs in order to explore possible causes of pelvic pain, such as adhesions or endometriosis, or for other surgical indications. Laparoscopy may also be considered to be therapeutic when techniques such as laser ablation of endometriosis or lysis of adhesions are performed under laparascopic visualization. Laparoscopy, or pelviscopic surgery, is increasingly replacing traditional open laparotomy procedures, which has resulted in decreased hospital stays, decreased pain, and possibly decreased costs for the patient. In addition, the psychologic sequelae of these less-extensive surgeries may be reduced, although this issue has not been addressed systematically. Laparoscopy is now frequently used to diagnose and remove ectopic pregnancies, and other pelviscopic techniques such as ovarian cystectomies, oophorectomies, or myomectomies are being performed laparoscopically by a growing number of gynecologists. Laparoscopically assisted vaginal hysterectomy is a newer technique that may be used to avoid an abdominal hysterectomy.

## Surgical Procedures to Correct Anatomic Stress Urinary Incontinence or Pelvic and Vaginal Relaxation

In many women, damage to uterine and vaginal supporting structures during childbirth and changes related to aging often result in some degree of pelvic and vaginal relaxation, including cystocele, urethrocele, rectocele, enterocele, or uterine prolapse. *Cystocele* refers to the loss of bladder support; *urethrocele* involves loss of urethral support; *rectocele* includes weakening of the supporting fascia in the rectovaginal septum; *enterocele* is a herniation of the pouch of Douglas cul de sac into the rectovaginal septum; and *uterine prolapse* is a weakening of uterine support and uterine descent into the vagina to the vaginal introitus or beyond. A significant degree of pelvic and vaginal relaxation is not typically seen in nulliparous women. These conditions may be asymptomatic or may have symptoms, such as stress urinary incontinence, that are extremely limiting and distressing. Surgery to correct symptomatic pelvic relaxation is almost always a purely elective procedure; that is, the decision for surgery should be dictated by the woman herself, based on the degree to which her activities are disrupted by her symptoms or the extent of her social disability as a result of urinary incontinence. Women should be made aware that incontinence is not an inevitable consequence of aging, and that an evaluation of the specific cause frequently leads to therapies, including surgery, that are helpful or curative.

The types of surgery used for vaginal/pelvic relaxation vary depending on the anatomic alterations involved. An anterior and posterior colporrhaphy are frequently performed to correct a cystocele and rectocele, respectively, and are usually performed in conjunction with a vaginal hysterectomy to correct the accompanying uterine prolapse. The diagnosis of anatomic stress incontinence is confirmed by cystometric and dynamic testing, which is used to rule out other possible causes such as neurologic problems or hyperactive bladder contractions. If anatomic stress urinary incontinence is a factor, a retropubic bladder neck suspension may be performed. Sexual dysfunction may occur after vaginal vault procedures because of vaginal shortening or alteration of the vaginal axis (Amias 1975; Bachmann 1990b; Masters and Johnson 1966; Sloan 1978).

Expectations for the results of surgery should be discussed prior to the procedure, because no surgery for stress urinary incontinence is 100% successful. In addition, it is important for the woman to understand that although unlikely, it is possible that her voiding problems will be worse after surgery or that the problem will recur, making it necessary that a second surgical procedure be performed.

Nonsurgical therapies for pelvic relaxation include the use of pessaries, which provide mechanical support for the pelvic organs. Nonsurgical therapies for stress urinary incontinence include electrical stimulation, urethral plugs, or vaginal weights and exercises to strengthen the muscles of the pelvic floor (Newman and Burns 1997; Rackley and Appell 1997). Other behavioral methods including timed voiding and fluid restriction are frequently helpful for mild stress urinary incontinence. Most major cities have centers at which specialists address incontinence problems with sensitivity and expertise.

## Hysterectomy

Hysterectomy is the one surgical procedure that has most defined the field of gynecologic surgery. Hysterectomy rates have declined since 1970 (Easterday et al. 1983), although a number of factors including physician gender, training, acceptance of alternatives to hysterectomy, and community practice patterns effect marked variations in the rate (Bachmann 1990a).

Hysterectomy involves the removal of the uterus, including the uterine cervix, and may be performed transvaginally or transabdominally. Vaginal hysterectomy is generally accompanied by less postoperative pain and a more rapid return to normal function. Factors that influence the route of surgical approach include anatomy, specific pathologic conditions, previous surgery, physician skill and experience, and the need for associated procedures (such as a retropubic bladder suspension).

Before the risks of cervical malignancy and premalignancy were recognized, supracervical or subtotal hysterectomy with removal of the uterine corpus, leaving the cervix in situ, was much more commonly performed. In recent years, supracervical hysterectomy has been performed solely in situations of excessive hemorrhage or severe pelvic pathology in which further attempts to remove the cervix have been judged to involve life-threatening risk. However, some resurgence of interest in the supracervical procedure has occurred; proponents argue that retaining the cervix offers fewer adverse effects on sexual function and less potential for subsequent pelvic relaxation (Cutler 1988; Kilkku et al. 1983; Munro 1997; Scott et al. 1997). Opponents argue that these potential benefits have not been proven and that leaving the cervix in situ entails the risk of subsequent cervical intraepithelial neoplasia or invasive cancer.

Women may be confused about which type of hysterectomy their gynecologist has proposed. This confusion arises because the medical term *total hysterectomy,* meaning removal of the uterus and the cervix, is often interpreted by women to mean removal of the uterus and ovaries, the medical term for which is *total hysterectomy with bilateral salpingo-oophorectomy.* The literature on adverse reactions to hysterectomy is obfuscated by reports that do not take this distinction into account. In a premenopausal woman, removing the ovaries results in a surgical menopause that is usually rapid in onset and has severe symptoms.

Gynecologists are divided as to the benefits versus the risks of ovary removal at hysterectomy (Garcia and Cutler 1984). Proponents of ovarian conservation argue that many normal ovaries would need to be removed to significantly reduce the death rate from ovarian cancer and that normal ovaries continue to produce valuable hormones prior to or even beyond menopause (Underwood 1976). Ovarian steroid hormones significantly impact many body functions, influence the health of the female genital organs (i.e., the vagina and urethra), play a critical role in the preservation of bony mass and the prevention of osteoporosis, and reduce the risks of cardiovascular disease (Barrett-Connor and Bush 1991). Thus, the removal of these hormones without adequate replacement has important adverse health consequences. Meijer and van Lindert (1992) provided a quantitative model for assessing risks and benefits of prophylactic oophorectomy, taking into account the risks of various types of ovarian and breast malignancy, osteoporosis, and cardio-vascular disease as well as the risks of noncompliance with hormone therapy.

Hormone replacement therapy can often be accomplished with oral or parenteral (transdermal patch) estrogen and progestin. However, such treatment does have potential side effects in addition to its problems of ongoing compliance and cost (Speroff et al. 1991).

It has been assumed that the postmenopausal ovary is not hormonally active. However, data have shown continued secretion of ovarian androgens that may support the well-being and general health (including libido) of post-menopausal women (Garcia and Cutler 1984). Studies have suggested that oophorectomy (with or without hormone replacement therapy) is associated with adverse effects on libido, vaginal lubrication, and pleasure with coitus, although one study found no correlation between psychosexual variables and biochemical androgen markers (Nathorst-Boos and von Schoultz 1992). It has been suggested that androgen replacement as well as estrogen replacement after hysterectomy and oophorectomy may result in fewer physical and psychologic symptoms, although this issue remains controversial (Sherwin and Gelfand 1985).

The argument favoring an oophorectomy is that ovarian conservation entails the risk of subsequent ovarian cancer (Travis 1985). Of all gynecologic cancers, ovarian cancer is the most insidious in onset and frequently eludes detection in its early stages; 60%–75% of ovarian cancers present in advanced stages (Knapp and Berkowitz 1986). It is frequently argued that the 2%–5% risk of developing ovarian cancer or requiring a second surgery for residual ovarian disease warrants an oophorectomy at the time of hysterectomy, particularly if the woman is approaching menopause (Terz et al. 1967). The average age of menopause is 51–a fact that is relatively unknown among the lay public, who frequently assume menopause arrives in the mid-40s. Age 45 or even 40 is commonly cited as the age beyond which many physicians would recommend a prophylactic oophorectomy.

### Alternatives to Hysterectomy

In most developed countries increased skepticism has arisen about not only the necessity for oophorectomy but also that for hysterectomy itself. Nonsurgical hormonal therapy should be considered as the initial treatment for many gynecologic conditions, including abnormal bleeding or menorrhagia (Chuong and Brenner 1996). Alternatives to hysterectomy, such as myomectomy or endometrial ablation by laser, electrical means, or thermal energy, have been proposed and are gaining acceptance in the medical community.

Women are becoming aware that alternatives to hysterectomy exist and are asking their clinicians about these options. Although some of these procedures may ultimately prove to be appropriate surgical management, the final word based on definitive, long-term follow-up studies is not yet in.

Myomectomy, or removal of uterine leiomyomata, is gaining in popularity as an alternative to hysterectomy for women with uterine fibroids, even among women who have completed childbearing and who would not have traditionally been considered for such a procedure. Some women note that the sensation of uterine contractions accompanying orgasm is pleasurable, and for these women, myomectomy may be appropriate. Other women feel that the monthly reassurances of menses are important to them. Myomectomy can be accompanied by risks similar to those of hysterectomy, including the potential for excessive blood loss; it is incorrect for women to believe that this is a "minor" surgical procedure. In addition, studies suggest that about one-third of women who have a myomectomy have recurrent fibroids and that the need for a hysterectomy subsequent to myomectomy is 20%–25% (Te Linde 1977).

Endometrial ablation, as an alternative to hysterectomy, involves the destruction of the endometrium through the cervix using an electric current, a laser, or a balloon that transmits heat to the endometrium. The main indication for endometrial ablation is heavy menstrual blood loss in the absence of organic disease (Garry 1995). Most of these techniques have involved preoperative hormonal treatment to thin the endometrium, use of a general anesthetic, hysteroscopically directed laser, or electrical removal or destruction of the endometrium followed by a short postoperative hospital stay. The advantages of these procedures include a significant reduction in hospital stay and a potential to minimize the morbidity associated with hysterectomy (Bachmann 1990a; Easterday et al. 1983). The goal of endometrial ablation is to completely destroy the endometrium, thus eliminating or significantly decreasing menses. Currently, endometrial ablation is performed much less frequently than hysterectomy. Future studies will document the actual magnitude of risks and complications associated with the procedure, and it may prove to be a useful technique (American College of Obstetricians and Gynecologists Committee on Quality Assessment 1996). In December 1997, the U.S. Food and Drug Administration granted pre-market approval for the use of a uterine balloon therapy system for endometrial ablation. This and similar devices offer the potential for a simple office procedure as an alternative to hysterectomy. Long-term studies are lacking, and caution is indicated prior to widespread adoption of this technique.

Patients who request alternative surgical procedures deserve accurate information about hysterectomy as well as the alternative procedures (Bachmann 1990a) because their reasons for avoiding a hysterectomy may be based on misconceptions about the procedure. Although it has been suggested that alternative procedures are less likely to have psychologic consequences than hysterectomy, this assertion has not been studied carefully (Goldfarb 1990; J. B. Wright et al. 1996). One prospective, randomized, controlled trial found that hysteroscopic surgery and hysterectomy had a similar effect on psychiatric and psychosocial outcomes and found no evidence that hysterectomy led to postoperative psychiatric illness (Alexander et al. 1996). Other studies have reported greater satisfaction among women who had a hysterectomy than among those those who had endometrial ablation (Crosignani et al. 1997; O'Connor et al. 1997).

However, hysterectomy remains an important alternative when conservative treatment fails (Carlson et al. 1994b). Quality of life measures suggest that women having a hysterectomy for leiomyomas, abnormal bleeding, and chronic pelvic pain report improvement over time when compared with those who receive nonsurgical management (Carlson et al. 1994a, 1994b). Other studies attempting to assess the consequences of hysterectomy in women's lives have found reports of improvement in general and sexual outcomes in the short term (3 months postoperatively), but less positive reports in the longer term (2 years) (Bernhard 1992). Quality of life and overall satisfaction are difficult to measure; one study with 2–10 year follow-up found generally high levels of self-reported satisfaction after the procedure (Schofield et al. 1991).

## Psychologic Reactions to Hysterectomy

For many women, removal of the uterus has unique medical, emotional, and sexual significance and meaning (Bachmann 1990b; Polivy 1978). Its relationship to childbearing or childbearing potential is a factor for many women as is its association with femininity and completeness (Polivy 1974). Loss of menses may be perceived as a specific benefit of the surgery, particularly if the indications include abnormal or excessive bleeding or pain (Schofield et al. 1991); however, some women feel that menses represent a familiar and comforting rhythm or monthly cycle or that menstruation cleanses the body (Bachmann 1990a). Misconceptions about anatomy and sexual functioning are common, with women expressing the concern that a hysterectomy actually involves removal of the vagina, rendering sexual activity impossible postoperatively. Concerns about a decrease in sexual attractiveness as a woman or to one's partner may be culturally related (Bachmann 1990b).

Sexual responsiveness after hysterectomy has been addressed in several studies (Dennerstein et al. 1977; Zussman et al. 1981). The physical effects of hormone deficiency from oophorectomy contribute to symptoms of vaginal dryness, dyspareunia, or decreased genital sensation. However, in the absence of oophorectomy or estrogen deficiency, several studies have suggested no adverse effect of hysterectomy on sexual function (Bachmann 1990b; Helstrom et al. 1993). One study found that the presence of preoperative psychiatric problems had little influence on postoperative sexuality (Helstrom et al. 1994).

The psychologic, social, and sexual consequences of hysterectomy on women's partners has been largely ignored. One recent study showed a positive effect not only on the sexual life but also on the overall quality of life of most men (Lalos and Lalos 1996).

There is a current move championing supracervical or subtotal hysterectomy, with the view that the cervix itself triggers orgasm or affects the capacity to experience orgasm (Cutler 1988), although relatively little data exist (Kilkku et al. 1983; Munro 1997; Scott et al. 1997). It is also argued that retaining the cervix reduces the likelihood of painful coitus (Sloan 1978). These arguments are not well accepted among those gynecologists who believe careful surgical attention to minimizing loss of vaginal length will prevent subsequent dyspareunia.

Despite the suggestion that hysterectomy adversely effects sexual functioning, several studies have shown either no change or a beneficial effect (Clarke et al. 1995; Dennerstein et al. 1977; King et al. 1993; Lalinec-Michaud and Engelsmann 1985, 1989). Historically, the belief that removing the uterus could precipitate mental illness has been advanced; in 1890, Kraft-Ebing described his observation that psychoses were more frequently caused by hysterectomy than by any other type of surgery. Although posthysterectomy depression is widely believed to occur (Ananth 1978), several review articles have questioned the frequency of its occurrence (Bachmann 1990a; Cohen et al. 1989; Newton and Baron 1976; Patterson 1963; Polivy 1974). Psychologic distress has recently been reported to be *less* frequent after hysterectomy, with decreased symptoms (Ryan et al. 1989). Several recent studies have found no evidence that hysterectomy leads to postoperative psychiatric illness (Alexander et al. 1996). It is likely that recent changes in gynecologic practice resulting in more stringent indications for hysterectomy as well as the move toward recognizing, acknowledging, and respecting the patient as a partner in decision making, have contributed to a lower frequency of adverse sequelae than had been reported previously (Gath et al. 1995).

Some studies have compared the risk of postoperative psychiatric depression or referral for psychiatric services and hospitalization after hysterectomy with the risks after other surgical procedures such as cholecystectomy or cardiac surgery (Ananth 1978; Bachmann 1990a; Gould and Wilson-Barnett 1985; Polivy 1974; Roos 1984). Some of the older studies suffer from significant flaws, including studying small samples, containing little statistical data, or being based on anecdotal information. Other studies are retrospective, with problems of recall and bias. Many were published in the 1960s, when the indications and frequency of the procedure were different. Some studies have varying and often short (as little as 6 weeks) follow-up periods, whereas others have long (3–5 years) follow-up periods but have problems with conclusions of causality. Many studies lack control groups for age, parity, or menopausal status; the meaning of a hysterectomy for a 20-year-old nulligravid woman is likely to be different than it is for a 60-year-old woman. Education and social class may also affect a woman's reactions to any type of surgery. Many studies have failed to control for whether the hysterectomy procedure included an oophorectomy. In addition, some studies do not separate subjects by the indications for hysterectomy; a hysterectomy for malignant disease evokes more anxiety and legitimate concerns of mortality than does a hysterectomy for benign indications (Drellich 1956; Walton 1979). Adjunctive therapies for malignancy, such as chemotherapy or radiotherapy, may have an impact on the risk of sexual dysfunction (Corney et al. 1993; Flay and Matthews 1995; Schover et al. 1989).

Studies may not control for the route of the procedure (e.g., vaginal versus abdominal); surgical morbidity varies by the type and route of the procedure (Easterday et al. 1983). Psychiatric morbidity may also vary. The definition of adverse psychologic sequelae is frequently not clear; some studies use vague terms such as *emotional problems*, and *depression* is a term used loosely in some studies. Other problems include cultural and social assumptions about women's primary role and the functions of childbearing.

From the literature, it appears that some women may be at high risk for adverse psychologic reactions or psychiatric sequelae from hysterectomy (Ananth 1978); this most notably and consistently includes women who have had previous psychiatric problems or psychiatric care (Iles and Gath 1989; Martin et al. 1980; Moore and Tolley 1976; Polivy 1974; Salter 1985). This group appears to have a several-fold increased risk over women without such a history. An association between abnormal menses and anxiety or depression has also been reported, which may be important in predicting a reaction to hysterectomy (Salter 1985; Thornton et al. 1997). A history of sexual abuse may also be predictive of an adverse reaction (Wukasch 1996).

An optimal level of preoperative anxiety may also occur (Drellich 1956); an attitude of casual unconcern may suggest a significant level of denial that will ultimately result in symptoms (Ridgeway and Mathews 1982).

Women who have a hysterectomy at a young age are at an increased risk for adverse reactions (Kaltreider et al. 1979). In psychologic terms, it has been stated that this may be caused by a disruption of sexual/gender self-concepts that were not yet well established. An associated risk factor is that of an emergency procedure, as there may be little time to psychologically prepare for the hysterectomy (Tang 1985).

Poor social support may also be a predictor of adverse psychologic sequelae (Webb and Wilson-Barnett 1983a, 1983b; Wolf 1970). It appears that hysterectomy functions as does any stress, with a need for support from family, friends, and partner (Kraaimaat and Veeninga 1984). Preoperative marital problems may be a predictor of postoperative problems (Polivy 1974). Low socioeconomic status and less-well-educated women also seem to have higher risks of adverse reactions, perhaps related to misconceptions and fears (Wolf 1970).

Women with a history of multiple surgeries or chronic pelvic pain constitute another high-risk group (Bachmann 1990a). It has been said that "Some women have psychic conflicts sailing under a gynecologic flag" (Rogers 1950) and some suggest that if no pathologic diagnosis is found from the surgical specimen, the risk of adverse psychologic sequelae is higher (Barker 1968). It has also been said, however, that "women are not as concerned about unnecessary hysterectomies as defined by others as they are about unwanted hysterectomies as defined by themselves" (Burchell 1977).

Preoperative preparation for hysterectomy, with a focus on the groups of women at higher risk, may prove helpful in minimizing the likelihood of adverse psychologic reactions (Coppen et al. 1981; Stellman 1990). The patient's own anticipation of the effects of surgery should be explored; negative expectations about hysterectomy in particular have been correlated with deterioration in sexual functioning (Dennerstein et al. 1977). Many women want and appreciate a preoperative discussion of the potential effects of hysterectomy on sexual function (Krueger et al. 1979).

Hysterectomies have been categorized as being emergent, mandatory, urgent, advisable, or elective (Easterday et al. 1983). Particularly for advisable surgery, which constitutes the majority of hysterectomies, patient participation in the decision-making process will facilitate an appropriate or adaptive response to the surgery. Hysterectomies performed to prevent problems or for premalignant disease should be clearly indicated. With a hysterectomy, women must take into account several quality-of-life considerations (Easterday et al. 1983; Roeske 1979) that are influenced by her own psychologic and emotional health and by her own past experiences. She is often in the best position to consider these factors, but she may need guidance from her gynecologist or a therapist.

It is important to state the risks versus the benefits of the procedure. Preoperative preparation for surgery, with education and counseling by both gynecologists and other clinicians, is particularly important for hysterectomy (Williamson 1992). The most effective manner in which to accomplish this preparation—whether in written form, verbally, or using new computer technology—is not yet well established (American College of Obstetricians and Gynecologists 1995; Young and Humphrey 1985).

It is also important to state very clearly which symptoms will be alleviated by the surgery and to foster realistic expectations (Williamson 1992). Premenopausal women in whom a hysterectomy without oophorectomy is planned should be advised to expect some persistence of cyclic symptoms (e.g., premenstrual syndrome or premenstrual dysphoric disorder) related to ovarian hormone production if these symptoms were present prior to hysterectomy. However, several studies report amelioration of symptoms after hysterectomy (with ovarian conservation) in women with premenstrual tension, implicating psychologic factors associated with the menstrual cycle in the etiology of symptoms (Metcalf et al. 1992; Osborn and Gath 1990; Silber et al. 1989). Hysterectomy with oophorectomy and subsequent hormone replacement therapy has been suggested in rare situations for the relief of severe premenstrual symptoms (Casper and Hearn 1990).

## Liaison Between Psychiatrist and Obstetrician/Gynecologist

Direct communication between the therapist and the obstetrician/gynecologist is important; miscommunications sometimes arise if the physicians rely solely on the patient for information about the gynecologic diagnosis or recommendations for treatment. When hospitalization is planned, psychiatric follow-up during the inpatient stay may be appropriate or indicated. Psychiatric care may be even more critical than gynecologic care in the weeks to months after surgery. Gynecologists may feel that their care has been completed by the time of the standard 4–6 week postoperative office visit. However, this may not be sufficient follow-up for individuals at risk for depression or other severe psychiatric sequelae.

A psychiatrist or psychologist who has an ongoing relationship with a patient may need to ensure that preoperative preparation for any planned gynecologic procedure is adequate. The therapist will want first to understand the patient's understanding and expectations and then to explore the underlying meaning to the individual woman. The patient may have misconceptions about the procedure. Ideally, the gynecologist will have given the patient accurate information about the nature of the diagnosis and the recommended treatment; the psychiatrist may, however, need to address basic issues of anatomy, physiology, pathology, and therapy or to speak with the gynecologist if it appears that the patient has significant misunderstandings. Although assumptions about the patient's underlying concerns may prove to be false, common concerns such as those related to loss of sexual function, reproductive capability, or femininity may be suggested and explored as an initial effort to understand the issues for the individual.

A planned surgery may sometimes prompt the gynecologist to refer a patient for preoperative preparation, although it may be more common for the psychiatrist to be consulted when problems arise postoperatively. Prevention and attempts to alleviate psychiatric risks are always preferable to consultation after a problem becomes severe (Schwab 1971).

Psychiatric problems after a hysterectomy or other gynecologic procedure should be evaluated in the same way as problems presenting after other life events (Dennerstein and van Hall 1986). Depression should be evaluated, and treatment should be initiated with antidepressants or other appropriate medications (including hormone replacement therapy) if indicated. Suicide potential should be assessed. Psychotherapy is often most useful in conjunction with the use of antidepressants. The issue of hysterectomy or other surgery as a precipitating factor for psychiatric symptoms and the significance that the patient ascribes to her uterus can be explored during the course of therapy (Dennerstein and van Hall 1986).

# References

Abma J, Chandra A, Mosher WD, et al: Fertility, family planning, and women's health: new data from the 1995 National Survey of Family Growth. Vital Health Stat 23:1–114, 1997

Alexander DA, Naji AA, Pinion SB, et al: Randomised trial comparing hysterectomy with endometrial ablation for dysfunctional uterine bleeding: psychiatric and psychosocial aspects. BMJ 312:280–284, 1996

American College of Obstetricians and Gynecologists: Ethical dimensions of informed consent. Womens Health Issues 3:1–10, 1993

American College of Obstetricians and Gynecologists: Genital human papillomavirus infections. American College of Obstetricians and Gynecologists Technical Bulletin, Vol 193, 1994

American College of Obstetricians and Gynecologists: New CD-ROM informed-consent program set for launch at ACM. American College of Obstetricians and Gynecologists Newsletter, Vol 39, 1995

American College of Obstetricians and Gynecologists Committee on Professional Liability: ACOG Committee Opinion: informed refusal. Int J Gynaecol Obstet 53:84–85, 1996

American College of Obstetricians and Gynecologists Committee on Quality Assessment. Endometrial ablation. Int J Gynaecol Obstet 52:99–100, 1996

Amias AG: Sexual life after gynaecological operations, II. BMJ 2:680–681, 1975

Ananth J: Hysterectomy and depression. Obstet Gynecol 52:724–730, 1978

Bachmann GA: Hysterectomy: a critical review. J Reprod Med 35:839–862, 1990a

Bachmann GA: Psychosexual aspects of hysterectomy. Womens Health Issues 1:41–49, 1990b

Barker MG: Psychiatric illness after hysterectomy. BMJ 2:91–95, 1968

Barrett-Connor E, Bush TL: Estrogen and coronary heart disease in women. JAMA 265:1861–1867, 1991

Becker TM, Stone KM, Alexander ER: Genital human papillomavirus infection: a growing concern. Obstet Gynecol Clin North Am 14:389–396, 1987

Bell T: *Chlamydia trachomatis* infections in adolescents. Med Clin North Am 74:1225–1233, 1990

Bell T, Hein K: Adolescents and sexually transmitted diseases, in Sexually Transmitted Diseases. Edited by Holmes K, Mardh PA, Sparling P, et al. New York, McGraw-Hill, 1984

Berek JS, Hacker NF: Practical Gynecologic Oncology. Baltimore, MD, Williams & Wilkins, 1989

Bernhard LA: Consequences of hysterectomy in the lives of women. Health Care Women Int 13:281–291, 1992

Biro FM, Rosenthal SL, Wildey LS, et al: Self-reported health concerns and sexual behaviors in adolescents with cervical dysplasia: a pilot study. J Adolesc Health 12:391–394, 1991

Burchell RC: Decision regarding hysterectomy. Am J Obstet Gynecol 127:113–117, 1977

Burke L, Apfel RJ, Fisher S, et al: Observations on the psychological impact of diethylstilbestrol exposure and suggestions on management. J Reprod Med 24:99–102, 1980

Carey MP, Carey KB, Weinhardt LS, et al: Behavioral risk for HIV infection among adults with a severe and persistent mental illness: patterns and psychological antecedents. Community Ment Health J 33:133–142, 1997

Carlson KJ, Miller BA, Fowler FJ Jr, et al: The Maine Women's Health Study, I: outcomes of hysterectomy. Obstet Gynecol 83:556–565, 1994a

Carlson KJ, Miller BA, Fowler FJ Jr, et al: The Maine Women's Health Study, II: outcomes of nonsurgical management of leiomyomas, abnormal bleeding, and chronic pelvic pain. Obstet Gynecol 83:566–572, 1994b

Casper RF, Hearn MJ: The effect of hysterectomy and bilateral oophorectomy in women with severe premenstrual syndrome. Am J Obstet Gynecol 162:105–109, 1990

Centers for Disease Control and Prevention: Chlamydia prevalence and screening practices: San Diego County, California, 1993. MMWR 43:366–369, 1994a

Centers for Disease Control and Prevention: Summary of notifiable diseases, United States, 1993. MMWR 42:i–xvii, 1–73, 1994b

Centers for Disease Control and Prevention: HIV testing among women aged 18–44 years: United States, 1991 and 1993. MMWR 45:733–737, 1996a

Centers for Disease Control and Prevention: Ten leading nationally notifiable infectious diseases: United States, 1995. MMWR 45:883–884, 1996b

Chuong CJ, Brenner PF: Management of abnormal uterine bleeding. Am J Obstet Gynecol 175:787–792, 1996

Clarke A, Black N, Rowe P, et al: Indications for and outcome of total abdominal hysterectomy for benign disease: a prospective cohort study. Br J Obstet Gynaecol 102:611–620, 1995

Cohen SM, Hollingsworth AL, Rubin M: Another look at psychologic complications of hysterectomy. Image J Nurs Sch 21:51–53, 1989

Coppen A, Bishop M, Beard RJ, et al: Hysterectomy, hormones, and behavior: a prospective study. Lancet 1:126–128, 1981

Corney RH, Crowther ME, Everett H, et al: Psychosexual dysfunction in women with gynaecological cancer following radical pelvic surgery. Br J Obstet Gynaecol 100:73–78, 1993

Crosignani PG, Vercellini P, Apolone G, et al: Endometrial resection versus vaginal hysterectomy for menorrhagia: long-term clinical and quality-of-life outcomes. Am J Obstet Gynecol 177:95–101, 1997

Cutler WB: Hysterectomy: Before and After. New York, Harper and Row, 1988

Darrow WW: Health education and promotion for STD prevention: lessons for the next millennium. Genitourin Med 73:88–94, 1997

Darrow WW, Pauli ML: Health behavior in sexually transmitted diseases, in Sexually Transmitted Diseases. Edited by Holmes K, Mardh PA, Sparling P, et al. New York, McGraw-Hill, 1984

Dennerstein L, van Hall E: Psychosomatic Gynecology: A Total Approach to Women's Health Problems. Park Ridge, NJ, Parthenon Publishing, 1986

Dennerstein L, Wood C, Burrows GD: Sexual response following hysterectomy and oophorecomy. Obstet Gynecol 49:92–96, 1977

Drellich MG: The psychological impact of cancer and cancer surgery, VI: adaptation to hysterectomy. Cancer 9:1120–1126, 1956

Droegemueller W, Herbst AL, Mishell DR, et al: Comprehensive Gynecology. St. Louis, MO, CV Mosby, 1987

Dunn RA, Webster LA, Nakashima AK, et al: Surveillance for geographic and secular trends in congenital syphilis: United States, 1983–1991. MMWR CDC Surveill Summ 42:59–71, 1993

Easterday CL, Grimes DA, Riggs JA, et al: Hysterectomy in the United States. Obstet Gynecol 62:203–212, 1983

Flay LD, Matthews JH: The effects of radiotherapy and surgery on the sexual function of women treated for cervical cancer. Int J Radiat Oncol Biol Phys 31:399–404, 1995

Fleming DT, McQuillan GM, Johnson RE, et al: Herpes simplex virus type 2 in the United States, 1976 to 1994. N Engl J Med 337:1105–1111, 1997

Garcia CR, Cutler WB: Preservation of the ovary: a reevaluation. Fertil Steril 42:510–514, 1984

Garry R: Good practice with endometrial ablation. Obstet Gynecol 86:144–151, 1995

Gath D, Rose N, Bond A, et al: Hysterectomy and psychiatric disorder: are the levels of psychiatric morbidity falling? Psychol Med 25:277–283, 1995

Gillespie CC: Women's HIV risk reduction efforts and traditional models of health behavior: a review and critique. Womens Health 3:1–30, 1997

Goldfarb HA: A review of 35 endometrial ablations using the Nd:YAG laser for recurrent menometrorrhagia. Obstet Gynecol 76:833–835, 1990

Gould D, Wilson-Barnett J: A comparison of recovery following hysterectomy and major cardiac surgery. J Adv Nurs 10:315–323, 1985

Grimes DA: Diagnostic dilation and curettage: a reappraisal. Am J Obstet Gynecol 142:1–6, 1982

Hatcher RA, Guest F, Stewart F, et al: Contraceptive Technology: 1990-91. New York, Irvington, 1990

Helstrom L, Lundberg PO, Sorbom D, et al: Sexuality after hysterectomy: a factor analysis of women's sexual lives before and after subtotal hysterectomy. Obstet Gynecol 81:357–362, 1993

Helstrom L, Weiner E, Sorbom D, et al: Predictive value of psychiatric history, genital pain, and menstrual symptoms for sexuality after hysterectomy. Acta Obstet Gynecol Scand 73:575–580, 1994

Herbst AL, Holt LH: Clinical Aspects of in utero DES exposure, in Obstetrics and Gynecology. Edited by Sciarra JJ. Philadelphia, PA, JB Lippincott, 1990

Herbst AL, Hubby MM, Azizi F, et al: Reproductive and gynecologic surgical experience in diethylstilbestrol-exposed daughters. Am J Obstet Gynecol 141:1019–1028, 1981

Hillard JR, Hillard PA, Kitchell C, et al: Natural history of psychological reaction to genital herpes: a prospective study of woman university students. J Psychosom Obstet Gynaecol 10:147–156, 1989

Hillard PJ, Biro FM, Wildey LS, et al: Cervical dysplasia and human papillomavirus: evaluation in an adolescent dysplasia clinic. Adolescent and Pediatric Gynecology 2:32–36, 1989a

Hillard PJ, Biro FM, Wildey LS, et al: The value of an adolescent dysplasia clinic. Adolescent and Pediatric Gynecology 2:43–46, 1989b

Huggins GR, Sondheimer SJ: Complications of female sterilization: immediate and delayed. Fertil Steril 41:337–355, 1984

Ikkos G, Fitzpatrick R, Frost D, et al: Psychological disturbance and illness behaviour in a clinic for sexually transmitted diseases. Br J Med Psychol 60:121–126, 1987

Iles S, Gath D: Psychological problems and uterine bleeding. Baillieres Clin Obstet Gynaecol 3:375–389, 1989

Institute of Medicine: The Hidden Epidemic: Confronting Sexually Transmitted Diseases. Washington, DC, National Academy Press, 1997

Johnson JE, Christman NJ, Stitt C: Personal control interventions: short- and long-term effects on surgical patients. Res Nurs Health 8:131–145, 1985

Judd FK, Cockram A, Mijch A, et al: Liaison psychiatry in an HIV/AIDS unit. Aust N Z J Psychiatry 31:391–397, 1997

Judson FN: Assessing the number of genital chlamydial infections in the United States. J Reprod Med 30:269–272, 1985

Kaltreider NB, Wallace A, Horowitz MJ: A field study of the stress response syndrome: young women after hysterectomy. JAMA 242:1499–1503, 1979

Kilkku P, Gronroos M, Hirronen T, et al: Supravaginal uterine amputation vs hysterectomy: effects on libido and orgasm. Acta Obstet Gynecol Scand 62:147–152, 1983

King MC, Torres C, Campbell D, et al: Violence and abuse of women: a perinatal health care issue. AWHONNS Clin Issues Perinat Womens Health Nurs 4:163–172, 1993

Knapp RC, Berkowitz RS: Gynecologic Oncology. New York, MacMillan, 1986

Kraaimaat FW, Veeninga AT: Life stress and hysterectomy-oophorectomy. Maturitas 6:319–325, 1984

Krueger JC, Hassell J, Goggins DB, et al: Relationship between nurse counseling and sexual adjustment after hysterectomy. Nurs Res 28:145–150, 1979

Lalinec-Michaud M, Engelsmann F: Anxiety, fears, and depression related to hysterectomy. Can J Psychiatry 30:44–47, 1985

Lalinec-Michaud M, Engelsmann F: Cultural factors and reaction to hysterectomy. Soc Psychiatry Psychiatr Epidemiol 24:165–171, 1989

Lalos A, Lalos O: The partner's view about hysterectomy. J Psychosom Obstet Gynaecol 17:119–124, 1996

Luby E, Gillespie D: The Helper: A Quarterly Publication of the Herpes Resource Center 3:3–4, 1981

Luby E, Klinge V: Genital herpes: a pervasive psychosocial disorder. Arch Dermatol 121:494–497, 1985

Martin RL, Roberts WV, Clayton PJ: Psychiatric status after hysterectomy: a one-year prospective follow-up. JAMA 244:350–353, 1980

Masters WH, Johnson V: Human sexual response. Boston, MA, Little, Brown, 1966

Meijer WJ, van Lindert AC: Prophylactic oophorectomy. Eur J Obstet Gynecol Reprod Biol 47:59–65, 1992

Metcalf MG, Braiden V, Livesey JH, et al: The premenstrual syndrome: amelioration of symptoms after hysterectomy. J Psychosom Res 36:569–584, 1992

Moore JT, Tolley DH: Depression following hysterectomy. Psychosomatics 17:86–89, 1976

Mosher WD, Pratt WF: Use of contraception and family planning services in the United States, 1988. Am J Public Health 80:1132–1133, 1990

Munro MG: Supracervical hysterectomy: a time for reappraisal. Obstet Gynecol 89:133–139, 1997

Nannis ED, Patterson TL, Semple SJ, et al: Coping with HIV disease among seropositive women: psychosocial correlates. Women Health 25:1–22, 1997

Nathorst-Boos J, von Schoultz B: Psychological reactions and sexual life after hysterectomy with and without oophorectomy. Gynecol Obstet Invest 34:97–101, 1992

Newman DK, Burns PA: New approaches for managing stress incontinence in women. Lippincotts Prim Care Pract 1:382–387, 1997

Newton N, Baron E: Reactions to hysterectomy: fact or fiction? Prim Care 3:781–801, 1976

O'Connor H, Broadbent JA, Magos AL, et al: Medical Research Council randomised trial of endometrial resection versus hysterectomy in management of menorrhagia. Lancet 349:897–901, 1997

Orr DP, Wilbrandt ML, Brack CJ, et al: Reported sexual behaviors and self-esteem among young adolescents. Am J Dis Child 143:86–90, 1989

Osborn MF, Gath D: Psychological and physical determinants of premenstrual symptoms before and after hysterectomy. Psychol Med 20:565–572, 1990

Patterson RM: Misconceptions concerning the psychological effects of hysterectomy. Am J Obstet Gynecol 85:104–111, 1963

Peterson HB, Xia Z, Hughes JM, et al: The risk of pregnancy after tubal sterilization: findings from the U.S. Collaborative Review of Sterilization. Am J Obstet Gynecol 174:1161–1168, 1996

Polivy J: Psychological reactions to hysterectomy: a critical review. Am J Obstet Gynecol 118:417–426, 1974

Polivy J: Quality of life and factors affecting the response to hysterectomy. Fam Pract 3:483–488, 1978

Rackley RR, Appell RA: Evaluation and medical management of female urinary incontinence. Cleve Clin J Med 64:83–92, 1997

Ridgeway V, Mathews A: Psychological preparation for surgery: a comparison of methods. Br J Clin Psychol 21:271–280, 1982

Rockwell DA, Peitone-Rockwell F: The emotional impact of surgery and the value of informed consent. Med Clin North Am 63:1341–1351, 1979

Roeske NC: Hysterectomy and the quality of a woman's life. Arch Intern Med 139:146–147, 1979

Rogers FS: Emotional factors in gynecology. Am J Obstet Gynecol 59:321–327, 1950

Roos NP: Hysterectomies in one Canadian province: a new look at risks and benefits. Am J Public Health 74:39–46, 1984

Ryan MM, Dennerstein L, Pepperell R, et al: Psychological aspects of hysterectomy: a prospective study. Br J Psychiatry 154:516–522, 1989

Salter JR: Gynaecological symptoms and psychological distress in potential hysterectomy patients. J Psychosom Res 29:155–159, 1985

Schofield MJ, Bennett A, Redman S, et al: Self-reported long-term outcomes of hysterectomy. Br J Obstet Gynaecol 98:1129–1136, 1991

Schover LR, Fife M, Gershenson DM: Sexual dysfunction and treatment for early stage cervical cancer. Cancer 63:204–212, 1989

Schwab JJ: The psychiatric consultation: problems with referral. Dis Nerv Syst 32:447–452, 1971

Scott JR, Sharp HT, Dodson MK, et al: Subtotal hysterectomy in modern gynecology: a decision analysis. Am J Obstet Gynecol 176:1186–1191, 1997

Sherwin BB, Gelfand MM: Differential symptom response to parenteral estrogen and/or androgen administration in the surgical menopause. Am J Obstet Gynecol 151:153–160, 1985

Silber M, Carlstrom K, Larsson B: Premenstrual syndrome in a group of hysterectomized women of reproductive age with intact ovaries. Adv Contracept 5:163–171, 1989

Sloan D: The emotional and psychosexual aspects of hysterectomy. Am J Obstet Gynecol 131:598–605, 1978

Speroff T, Dawson NV, Speroff L, et al: A risk–benefit analysis of elective bilateral oophorectomy: effect of changes in compliance with estrogen therapy on outcome. Am J Obstet Gynecol 164:165–174, 1991

Stellman RD: Psychological aspects of gynecologic surgery, in Gynecology and Obstetrics. Edited by Sciarra JJ. Philadelphia, PA, LB Lippincott, 1990

Tang GW: Reactions to emergency hysterectomy. Obstet Gynecol 65:206–210, 1985

Tay SK, Yong TT: High long-term cure rate justifies routine treatment of cervical intraepithelial neoplasia grade I. Aust N Z J Obstet Gynaecol 35:192–195, 1995

Te Linde RW (ed): Te Linde's Operative Gynecology. Philadelphia, PA, JB Lippincott, 1977

Terz JJ, Barber HR, Brunschwig A: Incidence of carcinoma in the retained ovary. Am J Surg 113:511–515, 1967

Thomas V, Heath M, Rose D, et al: Psychological characteristics and the effectiveness of patient-controlled analgesia. Br J Anaesth 74:271–276, 1995

Thornton EW, McQueen C, Rosser R, et al: A prospective study of changes in negative mood states of women undergoing surgical hysterectomy: the relationship to cognitive predisposition and familial support. J Psychosom Obstet Gynaecol 18:22–30, 1997

Townsend DE, Richart RM: Cryotherapy and carbon dioxide laser management of cervical intraepithelial neoplasia: a controlled comparison. Obstet Gynecol 61:75–78, 1983

Travis CB: Medical decision making and elective surgery: the case of hysterectomy. Risk Anal 5:241–251, 1985

Underwood PB Jr: Ovarian conservatism. South Med J 69:405–408, 1976

Walton LA: The stress of radical pelvic surgery: a review. Biochemical, psychological, gastrointestinal, hepatic, and cardiac effects. Gynecol Oncol 7:25–35, 1979

Webb C, Wilson-Barnett J: Hysterectomy: a study in coping with recovery. J Adv Nurs 8:311–319, 1983a

Webb C, Wilson-Barnett J: Self-concept, social support, and hysterectomy. Int J Nurs Stud 20:97–107, 1983b

Webster LA, Rolfs RT: Surveillance for primary and secondary syphilis: United States, 1991. MMWR CDC Surveill Summ 42:13–19, 1993

Webster LA, Greenspan JR, Nakashima AK, et al: An evaluation of surveillance for Chlamydia trachomatis infections in the United States, 1987–1991. MMWR CDC Surveill Summ 42:21–27, 1993

Weinhardt LS, Carey MP, Carey KB: HIV risk reduction for the seriously mentally ill: pilot investigation and call for research. J Behav Ther Exp Psychiatry 28:87–95, 1997

Williamson ML: Sexual adjustment after hysterectomy. J Obstet Gynecol Neonatal Nurs 21:42–47, 1992

Wilson JF: Behavioral preparation for surgery: benefit or harm? J Behav Med 4:79–102, 1981

Wolf SR: Emotional reaction to hysterectomy. Postgrad Med 47:165–169, 1970

Wright JB, Gannon MJ, Greenberg M: Psychological aspects of heavy periods: does endometrial ablation provide the answer? Br J Hosp Med 55:289–294, 1996

Wright TC Jr, Gagnon S, Richart RM, et al: Treatment of cervical intraepithelial neoplasia using the loop electrosurgical excision procedure. Obstet Gynecol 79:173–178, 1992

Wukasch RN: The impact of a history of rape and incest on the posthysterectomy experience. Health Care Women Int 17:47–55, 1996

Young L, Humphrey M: Cognitive methods of preparing women for hysterectomy: does a booklet help? Br J Clin Psychol 24:303–304, 1985

Youngs DD, Wise TN: Psychological sequelae of elective gynecologic surgery, in Psychosomatic Obstetrics and Gynecology. Edited by Youngs DD, Ehrhardt AA. New York, Appleton-Century-Crofts, 1980

Zussman L, Zussman S, Sunley R, et al: Sexual response after hysterectomy-oophorectomy: Recent studies and reconsideration of psychogenesis. Am J Obstet Gynecol 140:725–729, 1981

# Gynecologic Oncology

LINDA HAMMER BURNS, PH.D.

Sweet weight,
in celebration of the woman I am
and of the soul of the woman I am
and of the central creature and its delight
I sing for you.

Anne Sexton, *In Celebration of My Uterus*

Each year in the United States, 81,000 women are newly diagnosed and approximately 26,500 die from gynecologic cancer, and 180,200 women are newly diagnosed and 43,900 die from breast cancer (Parker et al. 1997). In short, although many more women contract breast cancer, proportionately, more women *die* of gynecologic cancer. Gynecologic cancer is defined as carcinoma of the female reproductive organs (e.g., uterine, ovarian, cervical, vaginal, vulvar) and is usually treated by a specialist in gynecologic oncology.

Increasingly, screening of healthy, asymptomatic women for some gynecologic cancers through Papanicolaou (Pap) smears (and increasingly sonography) is becoming fundamental to the routine care of women. Within the array of gynecologic cancers exists variation in diagnosis, treatment, and options. For example, more than two-thirds of cervical cancers in the United States are detected in situ, largely as a result of the Pap smear, and are highly curable. By contrast, ovarian cancer is the most deadly gynecologic cancer, and yet no effective screening method exists. Ovarian cancer typically affects older women who present with vague symptoms in advanced stages of the disease, when it is most difficult to treat. Cervical cancer is now largely considered a sexually transmittable disease, with sexual history and socioeconomic status as major factors in its development, whereas ovarian cancer is more likely to be related to genetic factors, reproductive history, obesity, and age. Treatment of gynecologic cancers may include surgery, radiation therapy, and/or chemotherapy; for example, early cervical cancers may involve a single minor surgery (colposcopy) using laser or cryotherapy with little long-term impact on functioning or well-being, whereas some more-advanced cancers involve total pelvic exenteration that dramatically affects the woman's long-term health, psychologic adjustment, sexuality, and reproductive life.

## Psychosocial Aspects of Gynecologic Cancer

Throughout history, the uterus has had special meaning to women and men. The importance of the uterus as a psychosexual organ varies from woman to woman, culture to culture, and encompasses a broad range of meanings: a childbearing organ, an excretory organ, a regulator and controller of body processes, a sexual organ, a source of female competency, a reservoir of strength and vitality, and maintainer of youth and attractiveness (Bachman 1990). Even for women who have children, premature loss of childbearing ability may create worries about accelerated aging, inadequacy, incompleteness, altered sexual experiences, and loss of femininity (Bachman 1990). Despite ambivalent feelings about the discomfort or inconvenience of menstruation, many women value it as a means of setting the rhythm of life, as an important cleansing process, and/or as a reassurance of health and well-being. As such, it is understandable how the loss of these organs can have complex and significant meanings for women that affect not only their response but also their psychologic adjustment to the disease.

It is not uncommon for a woman to feel that gynecologic cancer is punishment for past sexual "misdeeds" (e.g., promiscuity, contraction of a sexually transmitted disease) or reproductive "failures" (e.g., elective abortion, miscarriage, or infertility). These issues become particularly complex if a woman's gynecologic cancer *is* related to her sexual behavior or that of her partner (e.g., cervical). It is noteworthy that the woman's sexual experiences are the only sexual risk factor often considered, even though she assumes the risk of her partner and his previous/current sexual partners. A monogamous woman who develops cervical cancer is often assumed to have been promiscuous while her partner's sexual risk behavior is disregarded! When issues of infidelity do arise, the result can be relationship and psychologic distress, social stigma, or misconceptions that the cancer was self-inflicted or preventable and as such does not warrant support. Feelings of guilt and self-recrimination may follow the diagnosis, although these feelings may not be openly shared. Equally difficult is the cancer diagnosis that may have a genetic etiology (e.g., ovarian), prompting family discussion and/or risk identification of first-degree relatives. As with many genetic conditions, women often feel guilty and responsible for "passing on bad genes" and putting their loved ones in jeopardy. In addition, many women still fear that cancer is contagious or an automatic death sentence and, as a result, fear telling family and friends because they are afraid of rejection, abandonment, or reproach. Finally, some women, especially those who have lived healthy, low-risk lifestyles, simply cannot believe the cancer diagnosis and respond with denial, avoidance, or minimization, which may affect compliance and other health behaviors.

Newsom et al. (1996) found that cancer patients who believe that they could have prevented their illness may be at greater risk for depression. In a study of 120 adults with recurrent cancer, five domains of control were identified: 1) self-blame, 2) control over cancer onset, 3) control over symptoms, 4) control over the course of the illness, and 5) overall control over life events. Although self-blame was not found to be related to symptoms of depression, perceived control over cancer onset predicted subsequent depression. The authors concluded that helping cancer patients resolve feelings of regret and remorse is an important intervention.

Today, a diagnosis of cancer is less likely to mean a precipitously shortened life and is more likely to mean a chronic illness. Because many patients are cured by initial therapy, psychologic response is less likely to involve preparation for death and dying and more likely to entail adjustment to what may be extensive, invasive, and prolonged medical treatment. The losses of gynecologic cancer are, therefore, more likely to be loss of health, lifestyle, reproductive ability, or sexual satisfaction.

## Cross-Cultural Issues

Cross-cultural issues have increasingly gained attention in the care of cancer patients as an important aspect of medical and psychosocial care, because cultural beliefs and values necessarily influence the patient's reaction to illness, treatment choices, illness behavior, and psychologic response. In a review of the major cultural considerations in the optimal care of patients with chronic medical illness, Trill and Holland (1993) found the following factors to be influential in health-related behaviors: family function, gender roles, language, disclosure of disease-related information, pain, attitudes toward illness and health practices, immigration, religion, autonomy versus dependency, and death and bereavement. Finally, many patients straddle two cultures and it is often difficult to assess which cultural practices and beliefs they (or their family members) have retained from their original culture and which they have adopted from the new culture.

Culturally defined gender roles may affect a woman's coping mechanisms, the response of others, and the caregivers' response. Gender role expectations can be highly significant for women with gynecologic cancer in a culture that highly values women for their reproductive ability. A (or *the*) major loss for many young women with cancer is the loss of reproductive ability. Although alternative forms of childbearing or family building may be considered, the loss remains significant for most women—although it is not often addressed in the early stages of cancer treatment. In some cultures, women are expected to suffer silently and stoically (e.g., Scandinavian, American Indian), whereas in other cultures women are expected to relinquish their autonomy and become completely dependent on male family members and caregivers (e.g., some Hispanic cultures). Family beliefs about illness, including family involvement in patient care and acceptable levels of patient dependence on family members, are also influenced by cultural values and are important factors in treatment planning and implementation.

The need for autonomy or dependency appears to be strongly influenced by cultural values, with significant implications for caregivers and medical decision making. Religion is another area that can determine patient acceptance of illness, the suffering it entails, and acceptable behaviors regarding death and dying. Finally, acceptable practices regarding dying and bereavement vary significantly across cultures, with behaviors and customs often having significantly different meanings.

## Developmental Life Stages

Although women of all ages may have some feelings about the loss of reproductive organs, the stage of a woman's life may influence the degree of her feelings. Typically, an older woman who has completed her childbearing will respond differently to the loss of her reproductive organs than will a younger, childless woman. Erikson's (1963) developmental life stage model outlines normal developmental milestones and describes how failure to achieve developmental stage goals threatens a women's normal and healthy maturation. Psychologic issues of cancer across the developmental lifespan involve altered relationships, dependence versus independence, achievement disruptions, integrity of body image, and existential issues (Rowland 1989).

## Young Adulthood (Age 19–30)

According to Erikson (1963), the developmental tasks of young adulthood are *separation and individuation* and *intimacy versus isolation*; during this period, the young person establishes an autonomous and stable sense of self. Cancer interrupts these tasks—at a time when a young woman should have increased autonomy and independence, she must rely instead on her parents for physical as well as psychologic care. Life goals must be readjusted or redirected, limitations integrated, and relationships realigned, all within the context of complex medical treatment and side effects (e.g., alopecia, nausea, vomiting, surgical scars, weight loss/gain, fatigue, ostomies, vaginal stenosis, fistulas, anxiety, or depression).

### Sexual Functioning

Gynecologic cancer interrupts a young woman's establishment of healthy, intimate, and romantic relationships by challenging the integrity of her body image (e.g., impaired feelings about oneself as a sexual person, dampening of sexual feelings) and by altering established relationships (e.g., unsteady romances unable to weather the demands of cancer). Cancer may strike before the young woman has become sexually active, established a stable sexual identity, explored romantic relationships, or explored reproductive goals. Postoperative psychosexual problems in women who have had a hysterectomy appear to be more prevalent in women with the following profiles: 1) preoperative history of depression, sexual dysfunction, or other psychologic disturbances; 2) age less than 35–40 years; 3) limited education; 4) conflict about future childbearing; 5) poor understanding of the surgery and its consequences; 6) belief that the uterus has unique psychologic and sexual importance; and 7) absence of pelvic pathology (Bachman 1990). In evaluating sexual problems in the young woman, it is important to determine her sense of her sexual self; her previous sexual functioning; the extent of her physical impairment because of the disease; the etiology of the sexual problem; and the status of her romantic relationship(s).

## Family Relationships and Reproduction

Although young women with gynecologic cancer have more reproductive choices than ever before, the issue of reproductive loss remains primary and fundamental. Today, assisted reproductive technologies offer many women (depending on the type of cancer) the opportunity to extend or preserve their reproductive ability. Patients increasingly expect caregivers to protect their reproductive options and/or consider their reproductive futures as part of treatment. Gynecologic cancer can be less traumatizing when caregivers offer information on family-building alternatives such as in vitro fertilization, donor oocytes, surrogacy, and/or gestational carrier.

## Work

Achievement disruptions during this era typically involve postponement or relinquishment of education or career goals and redefinition of life plans and long-held hopes and dreams. The completion of education and/or the establishment of a career are important tasks of this stage; failure to proceed on course puts many young women out of synch with their peers, thus increasing social and economic pressure and precipitating reassessment of original goals and life plans.

## Existential Issues

Existential issues focus on the question "how and why me?"; on feelings about death or dying; and on incorporation of the illness and its consequences into one's sense of self. The specter of potential death does not fit into young people's schema of life and/or that of their peers. Combined with the typical self-absorption and egocentricity of this stage, it is understandable that many young women feel isolated and detached, even from caring friends and family. Issues of survivorship may enhance feelings of inability to relate to peers or difficult romantic attachments. Having lost important friendships and relationships, these women may gain an altered perspective, a new internal schema and inner strength, and a better sense of their internal resources, all of which affect their relationships with others as well as with themselves.

## Mature Adulthood (Ages 31–45)

Often considered the most stable era of life, mature adulthood is characterized by personal maturity, consolidation of career, and development of stable relationships, including nurturance of the younger generation through either parenthood or mentorship. Erikson (1963) defined this stage as *generativity versus stagnation*, contending that failure to achieve a productive and creative sense of self leads to personal impoverishment, pseudointimacy, excessive dependence, or premature disengagement from society. Emphasis on generativity during this era highlights the childbearing losses of women who had postponed childbearing or had experienced infertility or childbearing losses (e.g., miscarriage). Although unusual, gynecologic cancer during pregnancy is considered a reproductive crisis, especially if the pregnancy lost is the woman's only or final pregnancy.

## Sexual Functioning

The impact of cancer on sexuality is largely determined by the type of cancer and its treatment, (e.g., cervical dysplasia treated by cone biopsy versus invasive vulvar cancer requiring total exenteration). Both estrogen and/or testosterone deficiency caused by absent ovarian function due to surgical or radiation-induced menopause (resulting in vaginal shrinking and reduced lubrication) may contribute to sexual problems and feelings of being "old before my time." Side effects of cancer treatment such as scarring, depression and anxiety, hot flashes, ostomies, or the use of vaginal dilators are often interpreted as insults to one's sense of self and body integrity. The most common sexual problems encountered by women with gynecologic cancer are painful intercourse, lack of arousal, less satisfaction with sex, and less enjoyment of intercourse (Anderson and deProsse 1989a, 1989b; Krumm and Lamberti 1993). Women who do not follow advice regarding the use of vaginal dilators and/or do not resume their preillness level of sexual functioning are more likely to develop physical and sexual changes that ultimately affect sexual satisfaction. Interestingly, most women believe that cancer could be transmitted through sexual intercourse—a factor often overlooked in caregiver discussions of sexual functioning with women and their partners (Krumm and Lamberti 1993). Suggestions for enhancing sexual functioning include arousal-enhancing rather than anxiety-reducing techniques; lubricants (e.g., Astroglide); variation of sexual positions; controlled depth of penetration to manage pain; and the use of vaginal dilators (Schover 1997).

## Family Relationships and Reproduction

For women who are mothers, their role as mother is often significantly affected by cancer. Women are typically distressed and anxious about their inability to care for their children, find trustworthy caregivers, and deal with their children's response to their illness as well as the possibility that they may not live to raise their children. Many women feel guilty for being irritable with normal childish behaviors (e.g., bickering, pushing limits) or disappointed by their children's inability to provide *them* with comfort and support. In a study of children's responses to their mother's cancer (Hilton and Elfert 1996), the developmental level of the child was the definitive factor. With preschoolers, the dependency needs of the child made childcare a primary concern, whereas with teenagers, increased home and caregiving demands interrupted the adolescent's moves toward independence, creating role confusion and increasing family tension. Furthermore, parents were unaware of increased distress or psychologic symptoms in their children.

## Work

For many women, diminished productivity at work represents myriad losses: personal fulfillment, financial remuneration, a social sphere, personal direction, and life structure, meaning, or purpose. Anderson and deProsse (1989b) found that although women with cancer were not able to work as many hours as their healthy counterparts, their career paths remained intact. Nevertheless, cancer treatment often results in missed raises or promotions, lost opportunities to change positions, pressure to make up for time away, and fatigue that prevents work performance at previous standards (Petzel et al. [in press]). Furthermore, both illness-related job disruptions and the high cost of medical care may threaten long-term personal and familial financial commitments (e.g., children's educations, mortgages) (Rowland 1989).

## Existential Issues

Cancer is a traumatic event in which many women experience a "shattering of assumptions" about themselves and the world in which they live: 1) the world is benevolent; 2) the world is meaningful; and 3) the self is worthy (Janoff-Bulman 1992). The existential struggle involves giving meaning to the cancer experience and regaining a belief in a predictable and benevolent world.

# Midlife or Older Adulthood (Age 46–65)

According to Erikson (1963), the developmental task of midlife is *integrity versus despair*, characterized by achieving a balance between the triumph of one's accomplishments and the despair of one's failures. Inadequate resolution during this era results in despair about one's achievements and disappointments. Although midlife is often a stage of reflection and self-examination during which individuals redirect energies and replot life goals, cancer can trigger identity crises and distress in women who fear aging or for whom womanhood and/or feminine identity is linked to reproductive ability, sexual organs, and/or sexuality. Cancer treatments may accelerate aging at a time when many women are already adjusting to typical midlife changes such as increased weight, diminished skin elasticity, or musculoskeletal problems. In fact, some women simply cannot tolerate the physical limitations or alterations in appearance imposed by cancer and/or aging, thus precipitating serious psychologic distress.

## Sexual Functioning

Anderson and deProsse (1989a), in a longitudinal study, found that although sexual functioning was significantly disrupted for women with gynecologic cancer, their marital and other social relationships remained satisfactory. In a study of cancer patients' spouses (Sabo et al. 1986), men assumed the supportive role preferred by their wives, but the women interpreted this role reversal as rejecting and insensitive, thus leading to relationship distress. However, in a study of experiences of the male partners of women with gynecologic cancer, Lalos et al. (1995) found that both partners experienced sexual intercourse as much more negative after treatment had been completed, and most men reported impaired sexual desire. Men found it difficult to know how to behave and communicate with their wives, with most reporting that they had nobody to whom they could speak openly about their wife's cancer. Furthermore, most men had not obtained basic information about their partner's disease, leading many researchers to conclude that increased involvement of spouses in cancer treatment and decision making leads to better adjustment in both the patient and the spouse (Anderson and deProsse 1989a; Schover 1997).

## Family Relationships and Reproduction

It is not uncommon for women to operate as the emotional "kingpin" in families, providing emotional connection, stability, and direction in the family system. Not surprisingly, when these women are unable to perform their various roles as mother, daughter, sister, and/or wife, they experience discomfort and the family system is destabilized, often with distressing results. Cancer has the potential for affecting a woman's "unfinished business" with family members or triggering the reemergence of old issues or conflicts. Relationship distress may affect multiple relationships or be confined to a single relationship (e.g., marriage, parent/child) and may include recognition of a chronically unhappy marriage (spouses who are unavailable, unreliable, or uninterested as the demands of cancer treatment and emotional dependence intensify). Cancer often precipitates long-postponed personal reflection or relationship examination that results in the realignment of personal priorities, revamping of relationships, or resetting of personal goals in an attempt to make one's remaining years as meaningful, productive, and pleasant as possible.

Women in this stage are typically less involved in beginning parenthood and more likely to be launching children. However, whether their children are very young, adolescents, or independent adults, women's roles as mothers and caretakers often remain significant and they may grieve the loss of these roles. Alternatively, during this era many women have responsibility for the care of parents or older family members. Within this context, cancer may trigger family adjustments such as the placing of older family members in residential care, which often triggers feelings of guilt, regret, or worry. Relinquishing these important nurturing roles can be very difficult for many women, especially if it also means relinquishing their own independence and autonomy (e.g., having to live with their own children).

## Work

Anger, frustration, and disappointment may arise when cancer requires curtailment of career goals, precipitates early retirement, or creates financial insecurity. Women may feel frustrated by their inability to pursue career goals or enjoy a pleasant and worry-free retirement. Feelings of discouragement and depression are understandable when women must spend their golden years being ill and watching their hard-earned retirement savings go to medical bills. Some patients choose less-expensive medical treatments or even contemplate suicide as a means of protecting their spouse and family from financial ruin (Rowland 1989).

## Existential Issues

Characteristic of the midlife era is heightened introspection and reflection, which may lead to potential despair about failures, unattained goals, or the meaning of one's life (Rowland 1989). Depression may be associated with less denial and greater recognition of death as a possible outcome of the disease. Overemphasis on death, despair about one's lack of accomplishments, or introspection may put a woman at risk of self-imposed isolation or of premature surrender to the illness (Rowland 1989). Struggles with existential issues often involve such questions as "is this what I lived and worked for?"; "why me?"; and "what now?"

## Aging Adulthood (Age 66 and older)

Late adult transition involves reworking the past, finding a balance between social and self-involvement, making peace with inner and external enemies, and coping with death (Levinson 1986). It also involves adapting to changes associated with normal aging, such as physical and mental deterioration or limitations imposed by other health problems.

### Family Relationships

Aging and illness often involve relinquishing status and authority within the family and within society. For many women, cancer precipitates the abdication of leadership roles: they are no longer the primary family caretakers, but rather the responsibility of the younger generation. Issues of autonomy and independence often surface as women grapple with feelings of "being a burden" to spouses, children, or grandchildren. An important task is finding new purposes in life and adapting to losses of health, work, friends, and family, which for many women involves creating a legacy for their families or getting their affairs in order.

### Sexual Functioning

Thranov and Klee (1994) investigated the extent of sexual problems and the prevalence of sexual activity in women aged 52–63 with gynecologic cancer. Little or no desire for sexual relations was the most common sexual problem found (74% of women and 42% of their partners), although 54% of the women were sexually active. Only 22% of the women with a partner expressed dissatisfaction with their sexual life or lack thereof. Sexual activities were not related to diagnosis or stage of disease. Despite decreased sexual desire and dyspareunia, a large percentage of women continued to be sexually active, leading the study authors to conclude that patients and their partners should be given information on sexual changes caused by their disease, reassured about regaining sexual capacity, and informed about the feasibility of sexual satisfaction.

## Work

Retirement, a normal transition at this stage, typically involves yielding of authority and status and the review of one's life successes and failures. These normal transitions can be complicated by abrupt changes or interruption of an enjoyable retirement by illness, medical treatment, or adapting to physical disabilities, decreased income, or limited mobility.

## Existential Issues

In one recent study (Cicirelli 1997) of 388 adults over age 60, most expressed a wish to continue living if they faced a terminal illness or nonterminal illness that resulted in sustained lower quality of life (immobility, extreme dependency, pain, or loss of mental faculties). A minority (10%) favored ending their life under such circumstances; these adults tended to be of higher socioeconomic status, less religious, more lonely, placed a higher value on the quality of life, and expressed greater fear of the dying process. Brown et al. (1994) asked women with gynecologic cancer about their reactions to a poor prognosis and their preferences for withdrawing or withholding life-sustaining technologies. Only 5% anticipated giving up, whereas 78% expressed resolve to continue the fight against their disease. Most preferred receiving in-home care and would refuse artificial life-sustaining measures such as ventilator support (90%), surgery for another life-threatening condition (34%), artificial nutrition (37%), and antibiotics (22%). These women anticipated managing their disease with a fighting spirit; although many would reject life-sustaining measures, far fewer would take active measures to shorten their lives.

## Disturbed Psychologic Response

Although several studies suggest that the initial, short-term response to cancer may include psychologic distress and impaired social functioning, most cancer patients adjust successfully and, over time, do not differ on most psychologic outcome measures from individuals with benign disease. The vast majority of psychologic problems in women with cancer involve the efforts of psychologically stable individuals to adjust to cancer and its treatment. Women at risk for disturbed response are more likely to have a history of maladaptive coping strategies, previous severe psychiatric disorder, low levels of social support, and/or a history of previous suicide attempts. The most common types of psychologic disturbances in cancer patients are depression and anxiety. Most cancer patients experience heightened anxiety and depression at diagnosis and at crisis points in the disease or treatment. However, up to 50% of women develop a psychiatric disorder, most of which are adjustment disorders and mood problems (Derogatis et al. 1983) that can result in poor reporting of medical symptoms, poor adherence or refusal of treatment, deterioration of relationships, and delayed return to preillness functioning because of loss of motivation and pessimistic outlook. Preexisting psychiatric problems can worsen during treatment-complicating care (e.g., patients with a history of chemical dependency or abuse requiring special attention). Psychologic symptoms in cancer patients also warrant a search for organic causes (see Table 15–1). Social problems in families relating to alcoholism, criminal activity, cultural pressures, poverty, physical or sexual abuse, and other forms of maltreatment should be considered—especially in elderly or vulnerable patients.

## Depression

When sadness becomes depression, women must not only manage the burden of cancer but the consequences of depression, which often increase the level of disability, decrease compliance, increase suicidality, and lead to poorer outcome (Roth and Holland 1994). Major depression occurs in approximately 25% of cancer patients, with the highest prevalence in those with the greatest disability and most distressing symptoms (McCoy 1996; Valente et al. 1994). Women at increased risk of depression have a history of affective disorder or alcoholism, poorly controlled pain, concurrent illness, advanced illness, poor prognosis, and severely disfiguring treatments and are being treated with medications that produce depressive symptoms (Bukberg et al. 1984; Massie 1989b; Massie and Holland 1989).

Psychiatric consultation should be considered when depressive symptoms last longer than 2 weeks, worsen rather than improve, or interfere with the patient's ability to function or cooperate with treatment (see Tables 15–2 and 15–3). Prolonged and severe depressive symptoms usually require combined psychotherapy and somatic treatment. Typically, the decision to prescribe a psychotropic medication depends on the level of distress and how significantly the patient's symptoms impair her daily functioning. It should be remembered that inadequate attention and detection are the biggest barriers to effective treatment.

The most commonly used antidepressants for cancer patients in the past were the tricyclic antidepressants (e.g., amitriptyline, nortriptyline, imip-

**TABLE 15–1.** Medications that may induce depression

**Analgesics/anti-inflammatory**
Ibuprofen
Indomethacin*
Baclofen
Cocaine
Opiates* (morphine, codeine)
Pentazocine
Penacetin
Phenylbutazone

**Anticonvulsants**
Carbamazepine
Ethosuximide
Phenobarbital*
Phenytoin*
Primidone*

**Antihistamines**

**Antihypertensive agents***
Clonidine
Guanethidine
Hydralazine
Hydrochlorothiazide
Methyldopa*
Propranolol
Reserpine*
Spironolactone

**Antimicrobials**
Ampicillin
Cycloserine
Dyapsone

Griseofulvin
Isoniazid
Metronidazole
Nalidixic acid
Nitrofurantoin
Procaine penicillin
Streptomycin
Sulfonamide
Tetracycline

**Antineoplastics**
Arathioprine
6-Azouridine
L-Asparaginase
Bleomycin
Cisplatin
Cyclophosphamide
Doxorubicin
Mithramycin
Vinblastine
Vincristine

**Antiparkinsonian agents**
Amantidine
Bromocriptine
Levodopa*

**Hormones**
ACTH*
Corticosteroids*
Estrogens/oral contraceptives

**Immunosuppressive agents**

**Miscellaneous**
Amphetamine withdrawal*
Caffeine
Cimetidine
Digitalis
Disulfuram
Halothane
Inderal*
Metoclopramide (where?)
Methysergide
Methrizamide
Phenylephrine

**Neuroleptics**
Fluphenazine*
Haloperidol
Prochlorperazine

**Sedatives/tranquilizers**
Barbiturates*
Chloral hydrate
Diazepam*
Ethanol
Flurazepam*
Major tranquilizers
Minor tranquilizers*
Triazolam*
Alprazolam

**Stimulants**
Amphetamine* (abuse)
Diethylproprion
Fenfluramine (abuse)
Methylphenidate

*Drugs that have a high incidence of depressive side effects.
*Source.* Valente SM, Saunders JM, Cohen MZ: Evaluating depression among patients with cancers. *Cancer Practice* 2:65–71, 1994. Reprinted with permission.

ramine) (Massie 1989b) (see Table 15–4), which were started in low doses (25–50 mg) given at bedtime and increased slowly over days to weeks until symptoms improved (usually the peak dose is lower than that tolerated by physically healthy patients). Heterocyclic antidepressants, including the second-generation antidepressants (e.g., trazadone), have been found useful as sedating medications in agitated patients and those with insomnia. The

**TABLE 15–2.** Discriminators of depression from medical illness

Guilt and self-reproach

Psychomotor retardation

Recurrent suicidal thoughts

Difficulty concentrating, confusion, forgetfulness

Social withdrawal, isolation

Increased irritability, problematic anger

Increased relationship disruption, disturbances

Anhedonia

Preoccupation with (or obsessive) negative thoughts

Anxiety, panic attacks, newly emergent phobias

**TABLE 15–3.** Assessment guide for major depression in cancer patients

| Risk factors | Precipitants | Symptoms |
|---|---|---|
| *History (past/present)* | *Stress from* | |
| Affective disorder | Meaning of cancer | Sad facial expression/mood |
| Chemical dependency | Unmet needs | Decreased interest in self |
| Physical abuse/self-injury | Pain/symptom distress | Anhedonia |
| Poor control of pain/ symptoms | Anxiety/fears | Social withdrawal |
| Advanced stages of cancer | Financial concerns | Somatic symptoms: anorexia, insomnia, fatigue |
| Medications with depressive side effects | Automatic negative thinking | |
| Inadequate social supports | Drugs causing depression | Slow thought, concentration |
| Impaired body image | | Thoughts of suicide |
| Changed work/family roles | | |

*Source.* Valente SM, Saunders JM, Cohen MZ: Evaluating depression among patients with cancers. *Cancer Practice* 2:65–71, 1994. Reprinted with permission.

most commonly used antidepressants for cancer patients at present are selective serotonin reuptake inhibitors (e.g., fluoxetine, sertraline, paroxetine, fluvoxamine), which have fewer side effects (lower cardiac risks, hypertension, and anticholinergic effects) than do the tricyclic antidepressants. Newer anti-

**TABLE 15–4.** Medications commonly used to treat depression

| Medications | Dosages start dose/ daily dose, *mg* | Primary side effects and comments |
|---|---|---|
| **Tricyclic antidepressants (TCAs)** All TCAs may cause cardiac arrhythmias; blood levels are available for all but doxepin. Get baseline EKG. | | |
| Amitriptyline (Elavil) | 10–25/50–100 | Sedation; anticholinergic; orthostasis |
| Imipramine (Tofranil) | 10–25/50–150 | Intermediate sedation; anticholinergic; orthostasis |
| Desipramine (Norpramin) | 25/75–150 | Little sedation or orthostasis; moderate anticholinergic |
| Nortriptyline (Pamelor) | 10–25/75–150 | Little anticholinergic or orthostasis intermediate sedation; therapeutic window |
| Doxepin (Sinequan) | 25/75–150 | Very sedating; orthostatic; intermediate anticholinergic; potent antihistamine |
| **Heterocyclics** | | |
| Amoxapine (Asendin) | 25/100–150 | Sedation; risk of tardive dyskinesia; extrapyramidal side effects |
| Maprotiline (Ludiomil) | 25/50–75 | Moderate sedation; risk of seizures |
| **Second-generation antidepressants** | | |
| Buproprion (Wellbutrin) | 15/200–450 | May cause seizures in those with low threshold; initially activating |
| Trazodone (Desyrel) | 50/150–200 | Sedating; not anticholinergic |
| **Selective serotonin reuptake inhibitors** Serotonin reuptake inhibitors have no anticholinergic or cardiovascular side effects | | |
| Fluoxetine (Prozac) | 20/20–60 | Headache, nausea, anxiety, insomnia, very long half-life, may be even longer in debilitated patients |
| Sertraline (Zoloft) | 50/50–150 | Nausea, insomnia, diarrhea |
| Paroxetine (Paxil) | 20/20–60 | Nausea, somnolence, asthenia, muscle spasm |

**TABLE 15–4.** Medications commonly used to treat depression *(continued)*

| Medications | Dosages start dose/ daily dose, *mg* | Primary side effects and comments |
|---|---|---|
| **Psychostimulants** Should be given in two divided doses at 8 AM and noon; can be used as antidepressant, analgesic adjuvant, and to counter sedation of opiates | | May cause nightmares, insomnia, psychosis, anorexia, agitation, restlessness |
| d-Amphetamine (Dexedrin) | 2.5/5–30 | |
| Methylphenidate (Ritalin) | 2.5/5–30 | |
| Pemoline (Cylert) | 18.75/37.5–150 | Follow liver tests |
| **Monoamine oxidase inhibitors (MAOIs)** MAOIs are orthostatic; risk of hypertensive crisis; strict dietary and medication restrictions; should *never* be used with meperidine | | |
| Isocarboxazid (Marplan) | 10/20–40 | Hypertensive/hypotensive |
| Phenelzine (Nardil) | 15/30–60 | Drug/diet interactions |
| Tranycypromine (Parnate) | 10/20–40 | |

*Source.* Roth AJ, Holland JC: Treatment of depression in cancer patients. *Primary Care and Cancer* 14:23–29, 1994. Reprinted with permission of *Primary Care and Cancer*, Melville, NY.

depressants such as nefazodone (Sersone) and bupropion (Wellbutrin) promise relief for depression without sexual side effects. Psychostimulants (e.g., methylphenidate) are being used increasingly to treat depression in cancer patients, especially those suffering from depressed mood, apathy, low energy, poor concentration, and weakness. In small doses they are helpful in countering the effects of morphine, and response is more rapid than that for tricyclic antidepressants. Finally, psychopharmacology with cancer patients requires alertness for interaction with other medications, chemotherapy, and medical conditions (see Table 15–4).

## Anxiety and Panic Disorders

Anxiety is ubiquitous in cancer patients, typically occurring at turning points of illness such as diagnosis, recurrence, treatment failure, and even at termination of successful curative treatment when patients fear the loss of close monitoring or the supportive relationships of medical staff. Anxiety can also be situational secondary to pain, underlying medical conditions, hormone-secreting tumors, medications, treatment (e.g., hospitalization, needles), or as a side effect of medications (Massie 1989a). The most common preexisting chronic anxieties (predating cancer diagnosis) are phobias (e.g., claustrophobia) and panic disorders, although anxiety disorders such as generalized anxiety disorder and posttraumatic stress disorder are often activated by cancer or its treatment.

Anxiety is often complicated by pain, nausea, and depression. Evaluation of the cause of anxiety may lead to immediate control of symptoms, with the long-term outcome dependent on etiology. Psychotherapy, medication, and behavioral interventions are usually effective in the short term, but are least effective in the management of long-standing anxiety disorders. Anxiolytic or antidepressant medications are often effective. Self-regulatory therapies (e.g., hypnosis, meditation, biofeedback, progressive relaxation, guided imagery, and cognitive behavioral techniques) have also been effective with anxiety disorders.

## Nausea, Vomiting, and Pain

Symptoms such as nausea, vomiting, and anticipatory nausea may develop either before or during chemotherapy. Patients differ in how prone they are to nausea and vomiting depending on their neurologic makeup and their anxiety level. Some chemotherapeutic medications are more likely to cause nausea than others. Approximately 45% of cancer patients experience nausea, vomiting, or both within the 24 hours before chemotherapy. These symptoms appear to be caused by the interplay of associative learning and the stress associated with chemotherapy.

Cancer pain regrettably continues to be undertreated, and severe pain is experienced in 60%–90% of patients with advanced cancer. Poorly controlled pain results in heightened levels of anxiety and depression. Despite patient beliefs or myths, cancer patients rarely abuse pain medications or become addicted to them. Psychologic techniques such as hypnosis, relaxation training, biofeedback, distraction, guided imagery, acupuncture, acupressure, massage therapy, biofeedback, and sensation redefinition may assist in pain control. Antidepressant medications are often used successfully as an additional pain management technique (Mastrovito 1989).

# Psychologic Treatment

The first psychiatric group in the United States devoted to the study of the psychosocial consequences of cancer and surgical treatment was established by Sutherland in 1950 (Holland 1989). The emerging field of psychooncology has two dimensions: 1) the impact of cancer on the psychologic function of the patient, the patient's family, and staff; and 2) the role that psychologic and behavioral variables may have in cancer risk and survival (Holland 1989). Care of cancer patients increasingly involves a team of professionals specializing in oncology, including psychooncologists—psychiatrists, psychologists, social workers, and psychiatric nurses with special interest and/or training in the psychologic aspects of cancer and its treatment. Psychooncologists are familiar with cancer diagnosis, prognosis, and treatment; the psychosocial issues of cancer for the patient and her family; and their own personal responses to patients who have a life-threatening illness.

Consultation-liaison psychiatry developed in the early 1970s when psychiatrists, acting as hospital consultants for inpatients, expanded their responsibilities to include a liaison role. They conducted multidisciplinary teaching rounds and groups that focused on psychologic and behavioral problems, ethical dilemmas, and conflicts between patients and staff and among staff members (Artiss and Levine 1973). Psychiatrists, as psychooncologists, provide consultation-liaison services as well as outpatient psychopharmacologic care and psychotherapy. Multidisciplinary teams including social workers, psychologists, specially trained nurses, and clergy may offer support groups for patients and their families as well as individual patient care.

Components of effective interventions include an emotionally supportive context in which to address fears about the disease, information about the disease and its treatment, behavioral and cognitive coping strategies, relaxation training to lower arousal and enhance sense of control, focused interventions for disease-specific problems, and social support (Anderson 1997). Five patterns of coping with cancer were identified by Dunkel-Schetter et al. (1992): 1) seeking or using social support, 2) focusing on the positive, 3) distancing, 4) cognitive escape-avoidance, and 5) behavioral escape-avoidance. They found that women with cancer use a large repertoire of behaviors to cope flexibly rather than rigidly adhering to a particular coping style, with distancing being the most commonly used pattern.

The goals of psychotherapy are to help the patient regain a sense of self-worth, to correct misconceptions, to integrate the present illness into a continuum of life experiences, and to provide practical help in managing treatment side effects (Roth and Holland 1994). Psychotherapy emphasizes past strengths, supports previously successful ways of coping, and mobilizes inner resources. The length of therapy must be tailored to the patient to reduce symptoms to a tolerable level. In addition, family members may be helpful as part of the therapy, or group attendance may be beneficial. Adjuvant psychologic therapy emphasizes fostering a positive attitude, helping the patient adhere and cope with treatment, and reducing emotional distress (Moorey and Greer 1989). It is a cognitive-behavioral therapy based on the cognitive model of adjustment to cancer in which appraisals, interpretations, and evaluations that the individual makes about cancer determine her behavioral reactions. Therapy involves mobilizing coping behaviors (fighting spirit, denial, fatalism, helplessness/hopelessness, anxious preoccupation) and finding problem-oriented solutions; the problems encountered may be emotional (e.g., depression), interpersonal (e.g., problems communicating with spouse), or related to the cancer type (e.g., body image problems of vulvar cancer patients).

Self-help and mutual support programs date from the 1940s, when the American Cancer Society began its volunteer visitor programs offering practical help for patients at home (Mastrovito et al. 1989). These patient–visitor programs offer a dimension of help beyond the scope of professional practitioners. Support volunteers (e.g., Gilda's Club) typically have personal experience with cancer, good communication skills, emotional stability, the ability to model good coping skills, sensitivity, empathy, and good listening skills.

Alternative or complementary cancer therapies are increasingly being used, although safety and efficacy standards have not been developed in these products or approaches. Cassileth et al. (1984) reported the six most widely used alternative therapies today to be metabolic therapy, diet treatments, megavitamins, mental imagery approaches, spiritual or faith healing, and immunotherapy. Patients also report the use of homeopathic therapies, massage, tai chi, acupuncture, acupressure, nutrition, and herbal therapies. These treatments may have direct effects, placebo effects, side effects, and/or potential drug interactions. When taking a patient's history and developing a treatment plan, it is important to consider any alternative treatments the patient may be using (e.g., St. John's wort).

## Conclusion

For women of all ages, gynecologic cancers are responsible for a significant amount of mortality and morbidity, including physical suffering and psychosocial distress. Adding to the distress for women are the high degree of uncertainty of the illness, its prognosis, and its treatment as well as the lack of social awareness or community support. Breast cancer often steals the limelight of women's cancer; gynecologic cancers often linger in the shadows, receiving much less attention, funding, support, or consumer education. Yet the toll of gynecologic cancers on the reproductive, sexual, and psychologic lives of women (both young and old) is profound. Therefore, it is important that caregivers be cognizant of the complex lives women live, the unique and powerful meanings of their reproductive organs, the potentially devastating impact of gynecologic cancer and its treatment on their physical and psychologic health and well-being, and the social costs in their lives. The grief expressed by women with gynecologic cancer is not simply for the loss of good health, it is also for the loss of the parts of themselves that some feel make them uniquely women.

# References

Anderson BL, de Prosse C: Controlled prospective longitudinal study of women with cancer, I: sexual functioning outcomes. J Consult Clin Psychol 57:683–691, 1989a

Anderson BL, de Prosse C: Controlled prospective longitudinal study of women with cancer, II: psychological outcomes. J Consult Clin Psychol 57:692–697, 1989b

Anderson BL: Psychological interventions for individuals with cancer. Clinician's Research Digest Supplemental Bulletin, Vol 16, 1997

Artiss LK, Levine AS: Doctor–patient relation in severe illness: a seminar for oncology fellows. N Engl J Med 288:1210–1214, 1973

Bachman GA: Psychosexual aspects of hysterectomy. The Jacobs Institute of Women's Health. 1:41–49, 1990

Brown D, Roberts JA, Elkins TE, et al: Hard choices: the gynecologic cancer patient's end-of-life preference. Gynecol Oncol 55:355–362, 1994

Bukberg JD, Penman D, Holland JC: Depression in hospitalized cancer patients. Psychosom Med 46:199–212, 1984

Cassileth B, Lusk EJ, Strouse BA, et al: Contemporary unorthodox treatments in cancer medicine. Ann Intern Med 101:105–112, 1984

Cicirelli VG: Relationship of psychosocial and background variables to older adults' end-of-life decisions. Psychol Aging 12:72–83, 1997

Derogatis LR, Morrow GR, Fettig J, et al: The prevalence of psychiatric disorders among cancer patients. JAMA 249:751–757, 1983

Dunkel-Schetter C, Feinstein LG, Taylor SE, et al: Patterns of coping with cancer. Health Psychol 11:79–87, 1992

Erikson EH: Childhood and Society, 2nd Edition. New York, Norton, 1963

Hilton BA, Elfert H: Children's experiences with mothers' early breast cancer. Cancer Pract 4:96–104, 1996

Holland JC: Historical overview, in Handbook of Psychooncology. Edited by Holland JC, Rowland JH. New York, Oxford, 1989, pp 3–12

Janoff-Bulman R: Shattered Assumptions: Toward a New Psychology of Trauma. New York, Free Press, 1992

Krumm S, Lamberti J: Changes in sexual behavior following radiation therapy for cervical cancer. J Psychosom Obstet Gynaecol 14:51–63, 1993

Lalos A, Jacobsson L, Lalos O, et al: Experiences of the male partner in cervical and endometrial cancer: a prospective interview study. J Psychosom Obstet Gynaecol 16:153–166, 1995

Levinson DJ: A conception of adult development. American Psychologist 41:3–13, 1986

Massie MJ: Anxiety, panic, and phobias, in Handbook of Psychooncology. Edited by Holland JC, Rowland JH. New York, Oxford, 1989a, pp 300–309

Massie MJ: Depression, in Handbook of Psychooncology. Edited by Holland JC, Rowland JH. New York, Oxford, 1989b, pp 283–290

Massie MJ, Holland JC: Overview of normal reactions and prevalence of psychiatric disorders, in Handbook of Psychooncology. Edited by Holland JC, Rowland JH. New York, Oxford, 1989, pp 273–282

Mastrovito R: Behavioral techniques: progressive relaxation and self-regulatory therapies, in Handbook of Psychooncology. Edited by Holland JC, Rowland JH. New York, Oxford, 1989, pp 492–501

Mastrovito R, Moynihan R, Parsonnet L: Self-help and mutual support programs, in Handbook of Psychooncology. Edited by Holland JC, Rowland JH. New York, Oxford, 1989, p 502–507

McCoy DM: Treatment considerations for depression in patients with significant medical morbidity. J Fam Pract 43:S35–S44, 1996

Moorey S, Greer S: Psychological Therapy for Patients with Cancer: A New Approach. Washington, DC, American Psychiatric Institute, 1989

Newsom JT, Knapp JE, Schulz R: Longitudinal analysis of specific domains of internal control and depressive symptoms in patients with recurrent cancer. Health Psychol 15:323–331, 1996

Parker SL, Tony T, Bolder S, et al: Cancer statistics, 1997. CA Cancer J Clin 47:5–27, 1997

Petzel SV, Burns LH, Hampl A, et al: Self-management, psychological adjustment, and coping during treatment for ovarian cancer: a feasibility and adherence study. submitted for publication, 1997

Roth AJ, Holland JC: Treatment of depression in cancer patients. Primary Care and Cancer 14:23–29, 1994

Rowland JH: Developmental stage and adaptation: adult model, in Handbook of Psychooncology. Edited by Holland JC, Rowland JH. New York, Oxford, 1989, pp 25–43

Sabo D, Brown J, Smith C: The male role and mastectomy: support groups and men's adjustment. J Psychosoc Oncol 4:19–31, 1986

Schover LR: Sexuality and Fertility After Cancer. New York, John Wiley & Sons, 1997

Thranov I, Klee M: Sexuality among gynecologic cancer patients: a cross-sectional study. Gynecol Oncol 52:10–13, 1994

Trill MD, Holland JC: Cross-cultural differences in the care of patients with cancer: a review. Gen Hosp Psychiatry 15:21–30, 1993

Valente SM, Saunders JM, Cohen MZ: Evaluating depression among patients with cancer. Cancer Practice 2:65–71, 1994

# Women and HIV Infection

Jan Moore, Ph.D.

Dawn K. Smith, M.D., M.S., M.P.H.

## Epidemiology of HIV/AIDS in Women

### Global HIV/AIDS Epidemiology

The World Health Organization (1998) estimated that of the 5.2 million adults (age > 15 years) infected with HIV in 1998 worldwide, 40% were women. Of the 32.2 million adults living with HIV/AIDS, 43% were women. Women as a proportion of new HIV infections in 1998 ranged from 5% in Australia and New Zealand to 50% in sub-Saharan Africa, with other regions in the 15%–35% range.

More than 95% of HIV-infected people live in the developing world. Sub-Saharan Africa, which contains only 10% of the world's population, was home to 70% of those infected in 1998 and the site of 80% of HIV/AIDS deaths that year. In 1998, AIDS was responsible for an estimated 2 million deaths—5,500 funerals a day. An estimated 1/7 HIV infections in sub-Saharan Africa and 1/10 infections worldwide occurred in 1998 alone. Half of these African infections occurred in women. In India, HIV infection rates among antenatal women are greater than 1% in urban areas of at least five states and 13.6% among women in Pune with sexually transmitted diseases (STDs) who reported that their only risk factor was sex with their husbands.

In most regions of the world, it is estimated that more than 90% of HIV infections among women are acquired heterosexually, often from husbands or regular sex partners. An additional contributor in some regions (e.g., Africa, Asia) is unsafe blood transfusion, which is of particular concern for women in association with pregnancy and childbirth. In North America and Europe, intravenous drug use contributes significantly to the HIV epidemic in women.

Although less than 1% of new infections globally in 1998 occurred in the United States, most of our data about disease trends, manifestions, and progression in women come from the United States and, to a lesser extent, Europe.

## AIDS Case Surveillance in the United States

Reported AIDS cases are the most commonly used measure of the HIV/AIDS epidemic in the United States. Through December 1997, 98,468 cases of AIDS in women had been reported to the Centers for Disease Control and Prevention—15% of all persons ever reported with AIDS in the United States (Centers for Disease Control and Prevention 1997b). In 1997 alone, 13,105 cases of AIDS in women were reported, accounting for 22% of the AIDS cases reported that year.

In 1997, most of the women reported to have AIDS were black (60%) or Hispanic (20%) (Centers for Disease Control and Prevention 1997b). Compared with the 1997 AIDS incidence rate per 100,000 population for white women, the rate for black women was nearly 13 times higher and that for Hispanic women was 7 times higher (Table 16–1A).

## HIV Case Surveillance in the United States

Three factors have led to a decreased ability to rely on reported AIDS cases as a primary indicator of the size and trends in the epidemic of HIV infection. First, the time from HIV infection to the development of AIDS can extend for 10 years or longer, so that even accurate AIDS surveillance does not give a timely indication of trends in HIV infection. Second, because of the recent availability and increasing use of highly active antiretroviral therapy and prophylaxis for opportunistic infections, which delay the onset of AIDS in many HIV-infected people, reported AIDS cases are now declining while the numbers of HIV-infected people living without having developed AIDS are increasing (Centers for Disease Control and Prevention 1997d). Last, these same medical therapies are reducing mortality among people with AIDS, thus increasing the number of people living with AIDS. The combination of

TABLE 16–1A. Female adult/adolescent AIDS cases reported in the United States in 1997[a]

| | Black, n (%) | Hispanic, n (%) | White, n (%) | Asian/Pacific Islander, n (%) | American Indian/ Alaska Native, n (%) |
|---|---|---|---|---|---|
| Intravenous drug use | 2,511 (32) | 750 (29) | 907 (36) | 11 (17) | 14 (39) |
| Heterosexual | 2,790 (35) | 1,174 (46) | 991 (40) | 30 (47) | 13 (36) |
| Blood product | 122 (2) | 31 (1) | 41 (2) | 5 (8) | 2 (6) |
| No identified risk reported[b] | 2,457 (31) | 623 (24) | 546 (22) | 18 (28) | 7 (19) |
| Total number | 7,880 | 2,578 | 2,485 | 64 | 36 |
| Rate/100,000 | 38.8 | 21.3 | 3.0 | 1.5 | 4.7 |

[a]Table excludes 133 women with unknown race/ethnicity.
[b]At time of AIDS case report.

these factors means that reported AIDS cases no longer provide a representative picture of the HIV epidemic. For these reasons, the Centers for Disease Control and Prevention has recommended that all states develop routine, confidential HIV surveillance systems to more accurately measure the epidemic. Annual data for 1997 were reported for the 27 states that have surveillance for HIV among adults (Table 16–1B), but the reporting states do not include several states with high rates of infection among women (e.g, New York), so the data are not yet nationally representative.

In the 27 states that had integrated HIV and AIDS surveillance from January 1994 through June 1997, the number of people reported with HIV infection (not AIDS) was compared with the number first reported after they had already developed AIDS. Of people in whom HIV infection was the initial diagnosis, 28% were women (compared with 17% of AIDS diagnoses), 57% were black (compared with 45% of AIDS diagnoses), and 32% were aged 13–29 (compared with 14% of AIDS diagnoses). Of HIV diagnoses among people aged 13–24 years, 44% were women and 63% were black. These data strongly suggest that young women, especially black women, are continuing to be infected with HIV at high rates (Centers for Disease Control and Prevention 1998b).

## Modes of Exposure to HIV for Women in the United States

In 1997, 32% of women reported with AIDS had a history of intravenous drug use and were assumed to have become infected with HIV through this route (see Table 16–1A) (Centers for Disease Control and Prevention 1997b). Heterosexual contact accounted for 38% of AIDS cases in women, this proportion having steadily increased from approximately 15% in 1983. The number of women infected with HIV through heterosexual contact may be underestimated. Women who inject drugs frequently have male sex partners who also inject drugs or have other risk factors; therefore, these women may have become infected with HIV through sexual contact. Additionally, approximately 28% of women who have AIDS report that they have none of the established risk factors. At least a portion of these cases includes women who were heterosexually infected by partners whose HIV status or risk history was unknown to the woman, including sexual contact with a bisexual male.

Women who have multiple sex partners are at increased risk for HIV because their chance of encountering an HIV-infected partner is greater than

**TABLE 16–1B.** Female adult/adolescent HIV (not AIDS) cases reported in the United States in 1997[a]

| | Black, *n* (%) | Hispanic, *n* (%) | White, *n* (%) | Asian/Pacific Islander, *n* (%) | American Indian/ Alaskan Native, *n* (%) |
|---|---|---|---|---|---|
| Intravenous drug use | 386 (13) | 57 (19) | 204 (21) | 1 (7) | 9 (43) |
| Heterosexual | 992 (33) | 112 (37) | 375 (39) | 4 (29) | 5 (24) |
| Blood product | 23 (1) | 2 (1) | 13 (1) | 0 (0) | 0 (0) |
| No identified risk reported[b] | 1,615 (54) | 134 (44) | 362 (38) | 9 (64) | 7 (33) |
| Total number | 3,016 | 305 | 954 | 14 | 21 |

[a]From 27 states that reported HIV cases among adults in 1997. Table excludes 269 women with unknown race/ethnicity.
[b]At time of AIDS case report.

that for women with fewer partners. These women are also at increased risk for acquiring other STDs that may facilitate HIV transmission, thus contributing to a higher incidence of HIV infection (Holmberg et al. 1989; Royce et al. 1997). Finally, although recent data suggest some leveling, the National Survey of Family Growth has shown that first sexual experiences are occurring at younger ages (Centers for Disease Control 1991). The literature suggests that women who begin sexual intercourse at a young age are more likely to have multiple partners and thus to be at greater risk for HIV infection than are women who delay intercourse (Greenberg et al. 1992). These factors may contribute to a significant increase in the still small number of AIDS cases among adolescent and young adult women, the latter of whom may presumably have been infected as adolescents.

Transfusion recipients and recipients of other blood products now account for a small and declining percent of women with AIDS (4%). Virtually all new cases of transfusion-related AIDS are associated with the receipt of blood before 1985 (i.e., before HIV antibody screening of blood donations was implemented) (Ward et al. 1988).

Female-to-female sexual transmission of HIV has been of interest and concern to health care providers and HIV-infected women. Three cases of female-to-female transmission have been reported in the medical literature (Marmor et al. 1986; Monzon and Capellan 1987; Perry et al. 1989). However, a review of AIDS cases in 164 women who reported having sex only with other women revealed that in all cases another risk factor was present: 93% of the women had a history of intravenous drug use and 7% had a history of blood transfusion before March 1985 (Chu et al. 1992). None of these cases was attributable to female-to-female sexual transmission.

## HIV/AIDS Mortality in the United States

Mortality rates clearly demonstrate the severe impact of AIDS on women, particularly black women. As early as 1990, AIDS and HIV-related diseases were the sixth leading cause of death among women aged 25–44 years in the United States (Centers for Disease Control and Prevention 1993b) and the leading cause of death among black women of this age group. In 1996, HIV/AIDS was the fourth leading cause of death among all women aged 15–44 and continued to be the leading cause of death among black women (Figure 16–1).

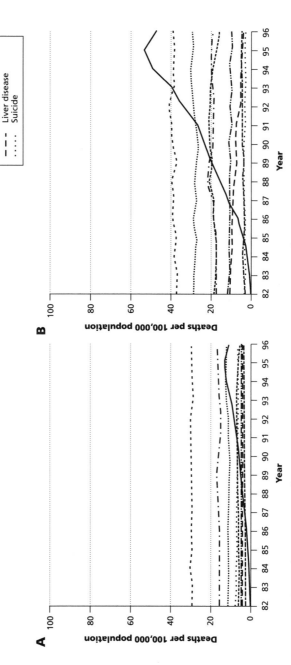

**FIGURE 16-1.** A, Death rates among *all* women ages 25-44 years (1982-1996). B, Death rates among African-American women ages 25-44 years (1982-1996).

# Manifestations of HIV Infection in Women

The first case of AIDS in a woman in the United States was reported in August 1981 (Centers for Disease Control 1981), and the first description of the clinical and epidemiologic characteristics of women with AIDS appeared in May 1982 (Masur et al. 1982). However, because of the early severe impact of the epidemic on homosexual/bisexual male communities, almost all early studies of the natural history of HIV infection were conducted in cohorts of white homosexual men living in AIDS epidemic centers such as New York and San Francisco. Studies of blood transfusion recipients and intravenous drug users have included women but not in sufficient numbers to definitively examine gender differences in HIV disease progression.

In recent years, several studies have followed-up with groups of women over varied periods of time and have attempted to describe aspects of the course and clinical manifestations of HIV infection in women, including two large prospective cohort studies of women with HIV infection and behaviorally matched, uninfected women (Barkan et al. 1998; Smith et al. 1997). Except for gynecologic findings and mental health, these studies have shown few gender-based differences in HIV disease manifestations and disease progression. Recent findings suggest that the clinical implications of viral load may differ by gender (Farzadegan et al. 1998; Sterling et al. 1998), but confirmatory studies are not yet completed.

## Non-AIDS-Defining Conditions

Following the occurrence of acute antiretroviral illness in some patients at the time of HIV infection (Flanigan et al. 1992; Kinloch-de Loës et al. 1993; Schacker et al. 1998; Tindall and Cooper 1991), a long period of asymptomatic HIV infection occurs during which HIV establishes a chronic infection, primarily involving lymph nodes. Over several years, untreated HIV infection leads to the gradual impairment of the immune system by several mechanisms, eventually leaving the infected person susceptible to the many opportunistic infections and malignancies that define AIDS.

The hallmark of HIV disease progression, a decline over time in $CD4^+$ T lymphocytes, has been prospectively studied in a few cohorts of women and heterosexual men; these studies have suggested no substantial difference between HIV-infected men and women in immunologic decline (Chaisson et al. 1992; Selwyn et al. 1992). Because women experience a mild form of immunosuppression during pregnancy, including a decline in $CD4^+$ T lymphocytes

(Biggar et al. 1989), the effect of pregnancy on disease progression in women was a matter of concern at first. However, larger prospective controlled studies have shown no increase in disease progression associated with pregnancy, suggesting that pregnancy has little or no independent effect on the progression of HIV disease (Brettle and Leen 1991; Deschamps et al. 1993).

Several studies report that the prevalence and persistence of human papillomavirus infection are higher in HIV-infected women than in uninfected women and are strongly associated with the development of cervical dysplasia, the precursor to invasive cervical cancer (Feingold et al. 1990; Wright and Sun 1996). Other studies of HIV-infected women have shown an association between immunosuppression and severe grades of dysplasia on Pap smear or cervical biopsy results (Maiman et al. 1991; Schafer et al. 1991). In addition, studies of treated cervical dysplasia suggest that HIV-infected immunosuppressed women have high rates of recurrence or persistence of dysplasia after receiving standard therapies (Fruchter et al. 1996; Maiman et al. 1990).

## AIDS-Defining Conditions

The occurrence of AIDS-defining conditions differs somewhat for men and women, but the available data suggest more similarities than differences. A recent analysis of gender differences among AIDS cases diagnosed from 1988 through mid-1991 indicated similar prevalence for most, but not all, AIDS-defining conditions when differences in race/ethnicity and the mode of transmission were controlled. In a comparison of 7,183 female and 21,776 male intravenous drug users, only esophageal candidiasis, herpes simplex virus (HSV), and cytomegalovirus were significantly more frequent among women than among men, whereas toxoplasmosis, cryptococcosis, histoplasmosis, Kaposi's sarcoma, and lymphomas were significantly less common in women (Fleming et al. 1993).

Few studies have been published about the causes of death among HIV-infected women, either alone or in comparison with those of HIV-infected men. Among women in the United States aged 15–44 years who died in 1987 and whose death certificates mention HIV/AIDS, the leading causes of death were drug abuse (26.5%), followed by *Pneumocystis carinii* pneumonia (19.7%), other pneumonia (14.1%), and septicemia (9.8%) (Chu et al. 1990).

## HIV/AIDS Manifestations in Developing Countries

Few studies have examined the manifestations and progression of HIV disease in representative cohorts of women in developing countries. The limited data available suggest no significant differences in survival rates of women compared with men (Morgan et al. 1997a) but suggest survival rates for adults of both genders may be half that of adults in developed countries (Mocroft et al. 1996; Todd et al. 1997). Similarly, time to AIDS appears shorter in developing countries (Anzala et al. 1995; Morgan et al. 1997b). Studies have not rigorously examined potential gender differences in the manifestations of HIV disease in these populations, but all gender-specific conditions described in North American and European women (e.g., HPV infection/cervical dysplasia, vaginal candidiasis, pelvic inflammatory disease) have also been found in women in developing countries.

# Health Care Issues for Women with HIV Infection

Critical to optimal medical, psychologic, and social service care for women are 1) the early diagnosis of HIV infection; 2) the provision of education both about HIV disease and the importance of early care; and 3) access to and adherence support for the use of highly active antiretroviral therapy and prophylaxis for opportunistic infections.

Accumulating evidence indicates that many opportunities for identifying women with HIV infection are missed (Boekeloo et al. 1993; Schoenbaum and Webber 1993). Standard recommendations for HIV testing rely largely on the patient's history of behaviors associated with a risk of HIV infection. However, standard risk history questions failed to identify most asymptomatic HIV-infected women in studies in which results from blinded testing are available. Providers are often reluctant to ask sensitive questions about sexual and drug use behaviors and women are frequently unwilling to disclose such behaviors to providers whom they do not know or trust (Boekeloo et al. 1993; Centers for Disease Control and Prevention 1994; Schoenbaum and Webber 1993). In addition, women may be unaware of behaviors of their sexual partners that place them at risk of heterosexual transmission (Doll et al. 1991).

## HIV Infections in Pregnancy

Recent medical advances in the ability to reduce HIV transmission from mother to infant have increased the emphasis on routine HIV counseling and testing of pregnant women. The Public Health Service issued recommendations in 1995 that all pregnant women be counseled and offered voluntary

HIV testing in prenatal settings (Centers for Disease Control and Prevention 1995). Early data suggest that most women in prenatal care in the United States are being offered HIV testing (Royce et al. 1998) and that approximately 80% accept (Fernandez et al. 1998; Royce et al. 1998). Surveillance data on HIV-infected pregnant women indicate that about 80% know their HIV status by the time of delivery (Wortley et al. 1998). Interventions to overcome barriers to prenatal HIV testing (e.g., lack of prenatal care, misperceptions of no risk for HIV by women and their health care providers, and logistical problems related to getting a test) are being planned and are expected to result in even higher rates of testing. Widespread HIV testing of pregnant women is hoped to not only decrease rates of perinatal transmission but also to ensure that HIV in women is diagnosed and treated earlier in the course of the disease.

## Treatment of HIV Infection in Women

After HIV infection is diagnosed, several conditions must exist for women to receive appropriate treatment for the infection and its related conditions: 1) providers of high-quality health care services must be available; 2) women must have financial access to these services; and 3) these women must use accessible services and adhere to recommended follow-up and therapy.

Health care professionals experienced both in women's health care and HIV-related treatment are not easily found. For example, providers may be very knowledgeable about the treatment of HIV, but because of their inexperience with socioeconomically disadvantaged women, they alter treatment decisions based on expectations derived from the sociodemographic rather than the clinical characteristics of their patients (Centers for Disease Control and Prevention 1994; Stein et al. 1991). Providers experienced in women's health care frequently are not familiar with HIV-related treatment issues and so may not prescribe the most effective antiretroviral or prophylaxis therapies (Boekeloo et al. 1993); this situation is especially worrisome because mortality rates of patients with AIDS appear to be related to the level of experience of medical personnel in the treatment of AIDS (Stone et al. 1992).

Treatment of HIV infection in women is not gender specific, and published guidelines for the content and periodicity of physical and laboratory examinations, vaccinations, and the selection of appropriate drug therapies should be followed (Centers for Disease Control and Prevention 1997a, 1997e, 1998e, 1998f). Recommendations for screening and treatment of gynecologic and obstetric conditions in HIV-infected women are also available

(Centers for Disease Control and Prevention 1997a, 1998c, 1998f).

Recent advances in the use of potent antiretroviral combination therapies have provided unprecedented delays in the progression of HIV disease (Collier et al. 1996; Deeks et al. 1997; Palella et al. 1998). To achieve this benefit, however, patients must adhere to complex drug regimens. Nonadherence to antiretroviral therapy may result not only in treatment ineffectiveness but also in the development of drug-resistant HIV strains. Particular concern has been raised about nonadherence by HIV-infected persons living in disadvantaged situations. Data collected on poor, inner-city, HIV-infected women indicate that they are less likely to be taking antiretroviral medication than are infected men (Solomon et al. 1998). It is unclear, however, how much of this gender difference can be attributed to the unwillingness of health providers to prescribe state-of-the-art drugs to disadvantaged persons, some of whom use illicit drugs, and how much can be attributed to women's failure to fill prescriptions and adhere to prescribed treatments.

All patients, regardless of gender, race/ethnicity, or income have reported difficulty in following the current recommended regimens for HIV treatment (Cramer and Mattson 1991; Epstein and Cluss 1982; Glasgow 1991). HIV-infected women who have many competing life stresses are likely to have great difficulty maintaining drug regimens. They may need assistance in working out a realistic schedule for taking medications and in developing support networks to assist them in maintaining highly complex treatment regimens. Without these supportive services women may be unable to fully benefit from available medical advances in treatment.

## Principles of Care in Developing Countries

Widespread availability of affordable HIV testing is not found in most developing countries; thus, identifying HIV infection in women prior to serious illness is uncommon. With increasing availability of inexpensive rapid testing technologies and the dissemination of HIV test counseling protocols appropriate to these settings, it is anticipated that greater numbers of women (and their male partners) will learn their HIV status in a timely fashion. Because long-term use of antiretroviral medications is not logistically or financially feasible in most developing countries, treatment issues are focused on prevention, early identification, and treatment of opportunistic or comorbid infections, especially tuberculosis, bacteremia, and diarrheal disease (DeCock et al. 1993; Grant et al. 1997; Lucas et al. 1993). In addition, recent documentation of the effectiveness of short, relatively inexpensive courses of antiretroviral treatment in late pregnancy for reducing perinatal transmission (Centers for Disease Control and Prevention 1998a) is anticipated to increase access to HIV testing for women and thus their use of the prevention and treatment therapies available to them.

## Psychosocial Issues and HIV Infection Among Women in the United States

Although all serious, debilitating illnesses have been shown to affect psychologic and social functioning (Anderson et al. 1989; Manne and Zautra 1990; Revenson and Felton 1989), HIV infection may have a greater impact than most medical conditions. The stigma associated with the disease and the activities related to its acquisition (e.g., illicit drug use, sexual behavior), the potential for discrimination against oneself and one's family, and the greater likelihood that members of one's family or social circle are also infected present unique psychologic and social challenges for HIV-infected people. Most research on the psychosocial effects of HIV has been conducted with gay men, the population initially most affected by the AIDS epidemic. Gay men affected by HIV in the early phase of the epidemic, however, tended to be white, well-educated, and to have substantial financial and social resources. Because the epidemic has moved to intravenous drug users and women, the socioeconomic face of the epidemic has changed dramatically (Centers for Disease Control and Prevention 1993a, 1995); those most affected by the second wave of the epidemic have been poor and from racial/ethnic minority groups. Poor, urban, minority women (a group already experiencing myriad stressful life events, elevated psychologic distress, and few social and economic resources) have been hit particularly hard by HIV and AIDS. Because of the vulnerability of this group, particular concerns have been raised about many women's ability to cope with the added stress of living with HIV infection or the prospect of becoming infected.

In this section of the chapter, we review the limited literature available on the psychologic and social issues for women related to getting an HIV test, receiving test results, adjusting to a positive diagnosis, and living with HIV infection. Issues that present particular challenges to HIV-infected women compared with infected men are addressed, including 1) confronting one's risk for HIV; 2) disclosing HIV status to sex partners, other adults, and children; 3) changing sexual behavior; 4) making reproductive decisions; and 5) making plans for the future.

# HIV Antibody Testing

Nonpregnant women typically are not offered HIV testing unless they present to the medical system with HIV-related symptoms. Studies have shown that approximately one-half of HIV-infected women are not diagnosed until they enter the health care system with HIV-related symptoms or an AIDS-defining illness (Beevor and Catalan 1993). Women, nonwhites, and people at heterosexual risk are likely to be detected later in their course of disease than are men, whites, drug users, and gay men (Sorvillo et al. 1998). A primary reason women are not tested earlier is that their risk for HIV is frequently overlooked or not assessed by health care providers (Schoenbaum and Webber 1993). Additionally, women may overlook or misperceive their own risk for HIV and thus fail to seek testing. Recent studies have shown that failure to acknowledge risk for HIV is the primary reason that people, including women, delay or do not obtain HIV testing (Lehman et al. 1998).

Confronting HIV risk may be particularly difficult for women. Not only must they assess their own behavioral risk but they must also examine the potential risk behaviors of male partners (i.e., intravenous drug use or sex with other partners). Although some women are unaware of the risk behaviors of their sex partners (Doll et al. 1991), others deny or overlook evidence of their partners' HIV risk. In a study including high-risk, uninfected women, approximately 63% reported inconsistent condom use in the 6 months prior to the study (Moore et al. 1998b). When asked the reasons for nonuse of condoms at last incident of unprotected intercourse, approximately 85% said that their partner was not at risk, although only a small proportion actually knew the HIV status of their partner and many had earlier acknowledged their partners' involvement in risk behaviors.

Confronting partners with their risk behavior can cause considerable turmoil in a relationship. Anticipation that the relationship will be disrupted or the partner will be made upset may prevent women from initiating any discussion with their partner about HIV (Harrison et al. 1995). In a study of women who knew or suspected that their partner had other sex partners, the most frequently reported reasons for not broaching the issues of partner's risk behavior or of his getting an HIV test were concerns that the partner would feel accused of infidelity or of having a disease and that he would be displeased with the woman for bringing up the subject (Moore et al. 1995). Many health care professionals and researchers have written about women's fear of violence from their partner as a primary obstacle to initiating discussions about HIV. Data available on the subject suggest that although fear of abuse may be the reason for lack of confrontation for some women, many more women do not bring up issues related to HIV for fear of displeasing or upsetting the partner (Harrison et al. 1995; Moore et al. 1998b). Additionally, recent data suggest that only a small proportion of women decline HIV testing for fear of abusive repercussions from male partners (Maher et al. 1998). The threat of violence, however, is a real concern for at least a portion of women at risk for HIV (Gielen et al. 1997; Moore et al. 1995), and health care professionals must be mindful of this possibility as they help women face their own and their partners' HIV risk.

Women may need support not only in deciding to obtain an HIV test but also in taking the steps to get the test. They may have informational needs such as where to go for a test, what to expect from the testing situation, and the implications of different test results. Once women have been tested and are waiting for test results, support needs are likely to be even greater. Research suggests that waiting for HIV test results is highly stressful for both men and women, particularly for persons perceiving themselves to be at high risk for HIV (Ickovics et al. 1994; Jacobsen et al. 1990). People with few social supports and a history of prior psychiatric difficulties are typically more distressed during this time (Kelly et al. 1993; Perry et al. 1990b). Women without sufficient internal or external resources to deal with the waiting period are likely to need help generating internal coping strategies and external sources of social support to get through this time. Pretest counseling often includes helping women identify persons to whom they can disclose that they are awaiting HIV test results and who could offer support during the waiting period. They also may need help anticipating and planning how they would cope with a positive test result.

## Receiving HIV Test Results

### Negative Results

Depression, anxiety, and suicidal thoughts tend to decrease in most people after notification of negative results; emotional stabilization is a well-established positive outcome of learning one's status (Ostrow et al. 1989; Perry et al. 1990a, 1990c). Reduced depression and anxiety, however, are sometimes accompanied by a return to old patterns of risk behavior. Research has shown that both men and women reduce high-risk sexual activity after testing and while awaiting results, but gradually resume risk behaviors after receiving a negative diagnosis (Ickovics et al. 1994; G. Marks, "Length of Time Since Testing HIV Seropositive and Prevalence of Sexual Activity," unpublished data, 1993). Ickovics et al. (1994) interviewed women about sexual risk behavior prior to HIV testing, when they returned for results 2 weeks later, and again 3 months after receiving negative results. The authors found that sexual risk-taking decreased during the waiting period but returned to pretest rates at the 3-month assessment. In some cases, receiving a negative test result may actually confer a feeling of invulnerability or immunity, resulting in an increase in risk behaviors above those seen prior to testing.

Women receiving negative test results need support in maintaining the reductions in risk behavior they achieved while waiting for test results. They may need reminders that a negative test result does not mean they cannot nor will not become infected with HIV in the future, nor does it mean that their sex partner is uninfected. Women who receive negative HIV test results should encourage sex partners to be tested. Until the partner receives a negative test result and the couple decides to practice monogamy, protection should be used during each sexual episode.

## Positive Results

Women's advocates, health care providers, and public health professionals have been concerned that a positive HIV diagnosis may cause severe psychologic reactions (i.e., anxiety, depression, suicide) and social ramifications (i.e., loss of partners, children, friends, family, job, and health care benefits) for women who have relatively few internal and external resources to help them cope (Chung and Magraw 1992; Ickovics and Rodin 1992). Particular concerns have been raised about the consequences of a positive HIV diagnosis for pregnant women, a group already vulnerable to adverse psychologic and social events (Lester et al. 1995).

Only limited data have been published on the psychologic consequences of an HIV diagnosis for women. Studies from mixed gender samples and other populations (e.g., gay men, intravenous drug users) have shown that many people experience depressive symptoms and anxiety when they learn of their HIV infection (Cleary et al. 1993; Jacobsen et al. 1990; Ostrow et al. 1989); however, most persons do not experience severe psychiatric disorders such as clinical depression or suicidal thoughts and attempts. When these disorders do occur, they do so more often in people with a prior history of psychiatric disorder (Perry et al. 1993). Additionally, after a period of adaptation to the diagnosis, most newly diagnosed people return to levels of depressive symptoms and anxiety typical of similar uninfected populations (Dew et al. 1990; Perry et al. 1990a). For example, Perry et al. (1990) found that 2 months after HIV testing, people diagnosed with HIV did not differ on suicidal thoughts, wishes, and intent from those receiving a negative diagnosis. For both HIV-infected and uninfected people, lower scores on psychopathology ratings were found at the 10-week follow-up compared with scores prior to learning their serostatus. Studies comparing men and women are rare, but the available data suggest that women experience more distress and depression after diagnosis than do infected men (Cleary et al. 1993; Fleishman and Fogel 1994; Perry et al. 1993), although gender differences tend to be less striking when socioeconomic status and drug use are similar between the two groups. Brown and Rundell (1993) reported few occurrences of depression, suicidal ideation, or other psychiatric disorders among a group of HIV-infected women in the military; 41% of these women qualified as having a psychiatric diagnosis, but hyposexuality or sexual dysfunction constituted the majority of these cases.

Few studies have reported on the adverse social events and losses experienced by women after receiving a positive HIV diagnosis. Early studies of gay men reported some loss of health care benefits, confidentiality, economic resources (i.e., housing, income, and insurance), and social support and relationships (Bayer et al. 1986; Lo et al. 1989). Advocates and public health practitioners have been particularly concerned about the social and economic repercussions of HIV testing of pregnant women, a group already at social and economic risk. Lester et al. (1995) followed-up 22 HIV-infected pregnant women and a comparison group of 20 uninfected pregnant women. They found no evidence of increased economic loss among infected women and greater satisfaction with social supports among infected than among uninfected women. HIV-infected women, however, reported higher levels of health care discrimination, personal isolation, and anxiety than did uninfected women. Additional data on this issue among pregnant and nonpregnant women are sorely needed to assess potential negative, unintended consequences of HIV testing and to ensure that newly diagnosed HIV-infected women receive the social support services they need.

Disclosure of test results is of primary concern to newly diagnosed men and women (Hays et al. 1993; Marks et al. 1991; Semple et al. 1993). In a study of the psychobiologic stressors of HIV-infected women, Semple et al. (1993) reported that most women viewed disclosure as one of their most pressing concerns following HIV diagnosis. Data indicate that most HIV-infected women disclose their status to at least one person (Gielen et al. 1997; Lester et al. 1995; Simoni et al. 1995). Generally, disclosure is made most frequently to partners/spouses/lovers, with rates reported between 85% and 100% in various studies (Gielen et al. 1997; Lester et al. 1995; Simoni et al.

1995); disclosure is then made to close friends and immediate family members, followed by extended family, coworkers, and acquaintances.

Most women cite fear of abandonment or rejection as their primary reason for failing to disclose HIV status to other adults (Gielen et al. 1997; Simoni et al. 1995). Available data suggest, however, that women frequently receive supportive reactions from others when they disclose (Simoni et al. 1995), and in one study, HIV-infected women reported more satisfaction with social support from friends and family than did uninfected women (Lester et al. 1995). Several studies have reported disrupted relationships, primarily with sex partners, following women's disclosure of HIV results. Simoni et al. (1995) found that 6 of 30 male partners reacted to the woman's disclosure of her serostatus by leaving the relationship. Gielen et al. (1997) reported that 8% of newly diagnosed women anticipated violent reactions from their partner on disclosure of their HIV infection. Of those expecting violence, 4% actually experienced some violent reaction when the partner was told and another 4% who had not anticipated such a reaction reported violence at follow-up. Violent reactions from partners were not direct physical attacks to the woman but instead involved activities such as throwing objects against the wall or kicking the television.

Women frequently need assistance in deciding when and how to tell sex partners about their HIV status and in anticipating partner reactions. In some states, infected persons must tell their sex partners of their serostatus or authorities will locate partners and inform them of their exposure to HIV. Women's advocates have suggested that partner notification laws may place women at risk for violence from male sex partners who learn of their exposure to HIV (North and Rothenberg 1993). Although data suggest that partner violence is not a frequent reaction to disclosure (Gielen et al. 1997), women should be assisted in anticipating partner response and in planning when, where, and how to tell partners, particularly those with a history of domestic violence. Additionally, women may need information about where to go for help if their partner becomes violent.

Women also must decide if and when to talk to their children about their HIV infection. Few data are available on the extent to which infected women disclose their HIV status to their children, but much has been written about mothers' concerns with regard to informing children (Armistead and Forehand 1995; Semple et al. 1993). Armistead and Forehand (1995) interviewed HIV-infected women about decisions and challenges they faced, and found that women perceived disclosure to children as the most emotionally difficult issue they faced. The authors discussed several reasons mothers may choose not to disclose their HIV status to their children, including 1) desire to protect children; 2) fear that children will feel stigmatized by their illness; 3) concern about children's feelings toward them and the way they contracted HIV; and 4) concern about children's ability to keep a secret and not tell others about their disease. Women must take into account several factors when making the decision to disclose to a child, including the child's age, coping ability, the status of mother's illness and functioning, and the likelihood that the child will hear about the mother's illness from others. Women are likely to need assistance in thinking through repercussions to children and in deciding what the child should be told. Few data are available to guide women in their decisions. Draimen (1993), writing about the professional's role in helping mothers decide about disclosure to children, states that "Although professionals can help the parent explore the consequences related to disclosure and nondisclosure, whether or not to disclose is a highly personal and demanding choice about which the parent is the best judge" (p. 21).

## Living with HIV

### Coping and Adjustment

Few data have been reported on adjustment and coping by women living with HIV infection. Available data suggest that asymptomatic HIV-infected women and uninfected women from similar socioeconomic backgrounds differ little in their social and psychologic functioning (Lipsitz et al. 1994; Moore et al. 1999; Pergami et al. 1993). For example, Moore et al. (1999), in a study that included HIV-infected and uninfected women, reported high levels of depressive symptoms and adverse social events in both groups, with no difference in the number of depressive symptoms between the groups and more adverse social events in the uninfected group (e.g., insufficient money for necessities, physical assaults, and removal of children from the home). Intravenous drug and crack use were more important predictors of psychosocial dysfunction than was HIV status; however, the women in this study were at a relatively early stage of infection. Studies of men have shown that distress increases with the onset of HIV-related symptoms or with a diagnosis of AIDS (Belkin et al. 1992; Rabkin et al. 1991). Most studies of HIV infection in women have not followed participants to the later stages of disease and the development of AIDS. HIV-infected women are likely to show higher levels of psychosocial dysfunction as they become more sick, and differences between infected and uninfected women may become more striking.

Considerable attention has been given by AIDS researchers to the effects of psychosocial stress on HIV disease progression. Psychologic stressors have been shown to affect the onset of illness by negatively impacting the immune system (Herbert and Cohen 1993; Persky et al. 1987), and thus researchers have speculated about the possible effect of stress on people with HIV infection (Glaser and Kiecolt-Glaser 1987). Data collected from men's cohort studies throughout the United States present an inconsistent picture of the importance of social and psychologic factors on rates of immunologic decline (Burack et al. 1993; Lyketsos et al. 1993), although it appears that if an effect exists, it is likely to be small (Perry and Fishman 1993). This topic has been of great interest to researchers and clinicians of HIV-infected women because of the high levels of psychosocial stress found in this population. Data addressing this issue in women have not been published, although they should soon become available from the ongoing longitudinal studies of HIV-infected women.

## Sexual Behavior

Many HIV-infected women modify their sexual behavior after learning their diagnosis (Hankins et al. 1998; Moore et al. 1998c). Although most remain sexually active (i.e., approximately 70% in the early stages of disease), more HIV-infected women than uninfected women (matched on sociodemographics and risk behaviors) report being abstinent (Hankins et al. 1997; Zierler et al. 1999). Additionally, more infected (54%) than uninfected women (26%) report always using condoms with male partners (Moore et al. 1998a). Among infected women not consistently using condoms, Moore et al. (1998b) found that approximately one-half reported having an HIV-infected partner. Of those women with an uninfected partner, approximately half used condoms for all episodes of vaginal sex. Among the inconsistent users or nonusers of condoms, approximately 60% indicated that their uninfected partner knew of the woman's HIV status but elected not to use condoms. Currently, the only methods of HIV protection known to be effective are abstinence and use of the male condom. Because men wear condoms, they can elect not to use them and thus not to protect themselves. These data point to the importance of involving uninfected partners of HIV-infected women in safe-sex counseling to ensure that they understand the risks they are taking and work to change unsafe sexual behaviors. Without the male partner's cooperation, HIV-infected women will be unable to ensure that their sex partners are protected.

## Reproductive Decision Making

HIV-infected women are faced with difficult decisions about continuing a current pregnancy or becoming pregnant in the future. In the early phase of the HIV epidemic, the possibility of transmission from mother to child was expected to greatly change the childbearing plans of infected women and result in pregancy termination among those already pregnant. Early studies, however, reported that HIV serostatus was not associated with pregnancy termination (Johnstone et al. 1990; Selwyn et al. 1989) nor with becoming pregnant in the future (Barbacci et al. 1989; Sunderland et al. 1992). More recent studies suggest that HIV-infected women have less desire and intention to become pregnant than do matched, uninfected women (Lester et al. 1995) and that infected women may change childbearing plans after learning their serostatus (Hankins et al. 1998). It is unclear how these desires and intentions affect contraceptive behavior and pregnancy rates.

With the publication of the AIDS Clinical Trials Group 076 (1998) results, which showed a two-thirds reduced risk of perinatal HIV transmission with a zidovudine regimen, more infected women may see pregnancy as a realistic option. Data collected after the publication of 076 results are not yet available on women's decisions to terminate pregnancy or avoid future pregnancies. The decision to bear a child is likely to be difficult for HIV-infected women despite medical advancements that have greatly reduced chances of having an infected child (Centers for Disease Control and Prevention 1997c). Women still must deal with issues related to their own mortality and the effect that this disease will have on the child's quality of life. With the advent of new medications to improve length and quality of life of infected persons, women may feel they have a better chance of raising their children, and thus more infected women may decide to reproduce.

## Planning for the Future

Despite promising new therapies, many HIV-infected women will face declining health and the prospect of early death. The needs of people preparing for disability or death have been written about extensively (Kastenbaum and Aisenberg 1972; Kübler-Ross 1969, 1975). Because HIV-infected women are relatively young compared with many other women with declining health, they have the additional need to plan for the future of dependent children. In many families with children, the HIV-infected mother has been the only parent providing care (Schable et al. 1995), and so an alternative placement must be sought for children when the mother becomes debilitated.

Contemplating the alternative care of one's children can be an overwhelming task for mothers. Armistead and Forehand (1995) discuss reasons HIV-infected women may delay or avoid planning for the future of their children, including 1) having to face their own impending death; 2) a lack of alternative caregivers whom the mother trusts to raise her children; 3) negative experiences with welfare agencies; and 4) lack of access to legal services necessary for making formal custody arrangements. In some large metropolitan areas, agencies have been organized for the specific purpose of helping women make decisions about the future of their children and ensuring that these plans are legally documented and carried out when the woman can no longer care for her children. New York City's Early Permanency Planning Program, for example, assists HIV-infected mothers in planning for future placement of children and assists children in making the transition to the new family (Levine 1995). These programs are relatively new, concentrated in only a few metropolitan areas, and may reach relatively few HIV-infected women. One study has shown that most HIV-infected women with children are unaware of or have not contacted available child care agencies (Schable et al. 1995). Other studies report that most infected women do not make formal plans for transferring guardianship of children, and thus the fate of children is left primarily to surviving relatives (Lester et al. 1995; Levine 1995). HIV-infected women repeatedly indicate that the well-being of their children is their most pressing concern (Armistead and Forehand 1995; Semple et al. 1993). Legal, social service, and psychologic assistance are needed to help them confront, plan for, and transition their children into acceptable alternative placements.

# Summary

As the number of HIV-infected women in need of health care services swells in the coming years, these biomedical and psychosocial issues will become increasingly salient to medical providers caring for women's health. It is imperative that care providers, administrators, funders, and advocates build the expertise and services necessary to improve HIV counseling and testing services for women, the risk-reduction interventions to lower the rates of new infections, and the medical, psychologic, and social service care for women who are already infected.

# References

AIDS Clinical Trial Group 076: Public Health Service Task Force recommendations for the use of antiretroviral drugs in pregnant women infected with HIV-1 for maternal health and for reducing perinatal HIV-1 transmission in the United States. CDC MMWR 47(RR-2):1–30, 1998

Anderson B, Anderson B, deProsse C: Controlled prospective longitudinal study of women with cancer, II: psychological outcomes. J Consult Clin Psychol 57:692–697, 1989

Anzala OA, Nagelkerke NJD, Bwayo JJ, et al: Rapid progression to disease in African sex workers with human immunodeficiency virus type 1 infection. J Infect Dis 171:686–689, 1995

Armistead L, Forehand R: For whom the bell tolls: parenting decisions and challenges faced by mothers who are HIV seropositive. Clinical Psychology: Science and Practice 2:239–250, 1995

Barbacci M, Chaisson R, Anderson J, et al: Knowledge of HIV serostatus and pregnancy decisions (abstract no. MBP10), in Abstracts of the International Conference on AIDS, Vancouver, Canada, June 4–9, 1989

Barkan SE, Melnick SL, Preston-Martin S, et al: The Women's Interagency HIV Study: WIHS Collaborative Study Group. Epidemiology 9:117–125, 1998

Bayer R, Levine C, Wolf SM: HIV antibody screening: an ethical framework for evaluating proposed programs. JAMA 256:1768–1774, 1986

Beevor AS, Catalan J: Women's experience of HIV testing: the views of HIV positive and HIV negative women. AIDS Care 5:177–186, 1993

Belkin GS, Fleishman JA, Stein MD, et al: Physical symptoms and depressive symptoms among individuals with HIV infection. Psychosomatics 33:416–427, 1992

Biggar RJ, Pahwa S, Minkoff H, et al: Immunosuppression in pregnant women infected with human immunodeficiency virus. Am J Obstet Gynecol 161:1239–1244, 1989

Boekeloo BO, Rabin DL, Coughlin SS, et al: Knowledge, attitudes, and practices of obstetrician-gynecologists regarding the prevention of human immunodeficiency virus infection. Obstet Gynecol 81:131–136, 1993

Brettle RP, Leen CLS: The natural history of HIV and AIDS in women. AIDS 5:1283–1292, 1991

Brown GR, Rundell JR: A prospective study of psychiatric aspects of early HIV disease in women. Gen Hosp Psychiatry 15:139–147, 1993

Burack JH, Barrett DC, Stall RD, et al: Depressive symptoms and CD4 lymphocyte decline among HIV-infected men. JAMA 270:2568–2573, 1993

Centers for Disease Control: Follow-up on Kaposi's sarcoma and *Pneumocystis* pneumonia. MMWR 30:409–410, 1981

Centers for Disease Control: Premarital sexual experience among adolescent women: United States, 1970–1988. MMWR 39:929–931, 1991

Centers for Disease Control and Prevention: Update: acquired immunodeficiency syndrome: United States, 1992. MMWR 42:547–557, 1993a

Centers for Disease Control and Prevention: Update: mortality attributable to HIV infection/AIDS among persons aged 25–44 years: United States, 1981–1991. MMWR 42:481–486, 1993b

Centers for Disease Control and Prevention: HIV prevention practices of primary-care physicians: United States, 1992. MMWR 42:988–992, 1994

Centers for Disease Control and Prevention: HIV/AIDS Surveillance Report, Vol 7. Centers for Disease Control and Prevention, Atlanta, Georgia, 1995. Available online at http://www.cdc.gov/hiv/stats/hasrlink.htm

Centers for Disease Control and Prevention: Anergy skin testing and preventive therapy for HIV-infected persons: revised recommendations. MMWR 46:1–12, 1997a

Centers for Disease Control and Prevention: HIV/AIDS Surveillance Report, Vol 7. Centers for Disease Control and Prevention, Atlanta, Georgia, 1997b. Available online at http://www.cdc.gov/hiv/stats/hasrlink.htm

Centers for Disease Control and Prevention: Update: Perinatally acquired HIV/AIDS: United States, 1997. MMWR 46:2–8, 1997c

Centers for Disease Control and Prevention: Update: trends in AIDS incidence: United States, 1996. MMWR 46:861–867, 1997d

Centers for Disease Control and Prevention: USPHS/IDSA guidelines for the prevention of opportunistic infections in persons infected with human immunodeficiency virus. MMWR 46:1–46, 1997e

Centers for Disease Control and Prevention: Administration of zidovudine during late pregnancy and delivery to prevent perinatal HIV transmission: Thailand, 1996–1998. MMWR 47:151–154, 1998a

Centers for Disease Control and Prevention: Diagnosis and reporting of HIV and AIDS in states with integrated HIV and AIDS surveillance: United States, January 1994–June 1997. MMWR 47:309–314, 1998b

Centers for Disease Control and Prevention: 1998 guidelines for treatment of sexually transmitted diseases. MMWR 47:1–115, 1998c

Centers for Disease Control and Prevention: Public Health Service Task Force recommendations for the use of antiretroviral drugs in pregnant women infected with HIV-1 for maternal health and for reducing perinatal HIV-1 transmission in the United States. MMWR 47:1–30, 1998e

Centers for Disease Control and Prevention: Report of the NIH panel to define principles of therapy of HIV infection and guidelines for the use of antiretroviral agents in HIV infected adults and adolescents. MMWR 47:1–82, 1998f

Chaisson RE, Taylor E, Margolick JB, et al: Immune serum markers and CD4 cell counts in HIV-infected intravenous drug users. J AIDS 5:456–460, 1992

Chu SY, Buehler JW, Berkelman RL: Impact of the human immunodeficiency virus epidemic on mortality in women of reproductive age, United States. JAMA 264:225–229, 1990

Chu SY, Hammett TA, Buehler JW: Update: epidemiology of reported cases of AIDS in women who report sex only with other women: United States, 1980–1991. AIDS 6:518–519, 1992

Chung JY, Magraw MM: A group approach to psychosocial issues faced by HIV-positive women. Hospital and Community Psychiatry 43:891–894, 1992

Cleary PD, Devanter NV, Rogers TF, et al: Depressive symptoms in blood donors notified of HIV infection. Am J Public Health 83:534–539, 1993

Collier AC, Coombs RW, Schoenfeld DA, et al: Treatment of human immunodeficiency virus infection with saquinavir, zidovudine, and zalcitabine. N Engl J Med 334:1011–1017, 1996

Cramer J, Mattson R: Monitoring compliance with antiepileptic drug therapy, in Patient Compliance in Medical Practice and Clinical Trials. Edited by Cramer J, Spilker B. New York, Raven, 1991, pp 123–137

DeCock KM, Luca SB, Lucas S, et al: Clinical research, prophylaxis, therapy, and care for HIV disease in Africa. Am J Public Health 83:1385–1389, 1993

Deeks SG, Smith M, Holodnly M: HIV-1 protease inhibitors: a review for clinicians. JAMA 277:145–153, 1997

Deschamps MM, Pape JW, Desvarieux M, et al: A prospective study of HIV seropositive asymptomatic women of childbearing age in a developing country. J AIDS 6:446–451, 1993

Dew A, Ragni M, Nimorwicz P: Infection with human immunodeficiency virus and vulnerability to psychiatric distress. Arch Gen Psychiatry 47:737–744, 1990

Doll LS, Petersen LR, White CR, et al: Human immunodeficiency virus type 1–infected blood donors: behavioral characteristics and reasons for donation. Transfusion 31:704–709, 1991

Draimen B: Adolescents in families with AIDS: growing up with loss, in A Death in the Family: Orphans of the HIV Epidemic. Edited by Levine C. New York, United Hospital Fund, 1993, pp 13–23

Epstein LH, Cluss PA: A behavioral medicine perspective on adherence to long-term medical regimens. J Consult Clin Psychol 50:950–971, 1982

Farzadegan H, Hoover DR, Astemborski J, et al: Gender differences in the relationship between HIV-1 load and progression to AIDS (abstract no. 133784), in Abstracts of the 12th World AIDS Conference, Geneva, Switzerland, June 28–July 3, 1998

Feingold AR, Vermund SH, Burk RD, et al: Cervical cytologic abnormalities and papillomavirus in women infected with human immunodeficiency virus. J AIDS 3:896–903, 1990

Fernandez MI, Wilson T, Moore J, et al: Acceptance of HIV testing among women in prenatal care in Miami, New York city, and Connecticut (abstract no. 43142), in Abstracts of the 12th World AIDS Conference, Geneva, Switzerland, June 28–July 3, 1998

Flanigan TP, Imam N, Lange N, et al: Decline of CD4 lymphocyte counts from the time of seroconversion in HIV-positive women. J Womens Health 1:231–234, 1992

Fleishman JA, Fogel B: Coping and depressive symptoms among people with AIDS. Health Psychol 13:156–169, 1994

Fleming PL, Ciesielski CA, Byers RH, et al: Gender differences in reported AIDS-indicative diagnoses. J Infect Dis 168:61–67, 1993

Fruchter RG, Maiman M, Sedlis A, et al: Multiple recurrences of cervical intraepithelial neoplasia in women with the human immunodeficiency virus. Obstet Gynecol 87:338–344, 1996

Gielen AC, O'Campo P, Faden RR, et al: Women's disclosure of HIV status: experiences of mistreatment and violence in an urban setting. Women Health 25:19–31, 1997

Glaser R, Kiecolt-Glaser J: Stress-associated depression of cellular immunity: implications for acquired immune deficiency syndrome (AIDS). Brain Behav Immun 1:107–112, 1987

Glasgow RE: Compliance to diabetes regimens: conceptualization, complexity, and determinants, in Patient Compliance in Medical Practice and Clinical Trials. Edited by Cramer J, Spilker B. New York, Raven, 1991, pp 209–224

Grant AD, Djoman G, Smets P, et al: Profound immunosuppression across the spectrum of opportunistic disease among hospitalized HIV-infected adults in Abidjan, Côte d'Ivoire. AIDS 1:1357–1364, 1997

Greenberg J, Magder L, Aral S: Age at first coitus: a marker for risky sexual behavior in women. Sex Transm Dis 19:331–334, 1992

Hankins C, Gendron S, Tran T, et al: Sexuality in Montreal women living with HIV. AIDS Care 9:261–271, 1997

Hankins C, Tran T, Lapointe N, et al: Sexual behavior and pregnancy outcome in HIV-infected women. J Acquir Immune Defic Syndr Hum Retrovirol 18:479–487, 1998

Harrison JS, Moore JS, Deren S: HIV-related communication and condom use among Hispanic women and their male partners. Presented at the HIV Infection in Women Conference, Washington, DC, February 1995

Hays RB, McKusick L, Pallack L, et al: Disclosing HIV seropositivity to significant others. AIDS 7:425–431, 1993

Herbert TB, Cohen S: Depression and immunity: a meta-analytic review. Psychol Bull 113:472–486, 1993

Holmberg SD, Horsburgh CR Jr, Ward JW, et al: Biologic factors in the sexual transmission of human immunodeficiency virus. J Infect Dis 160:116–125, 1989

Ickovics JR, Rodin J: Women and AIDS in the United States: epidemiology, natural history, and mediating mechanisms. Health Psychol 11:1–16, 1992

Ickovics JR, Morrill AC, Beren SE, et al: Limited effects of HIV counseling and testing for women: a prospective study of behavioral and psychological consequences. JAMA 272:443–448, 1994

Jacobsen PB, Perry SW, Hirsch DA: Behavioral and psychological responses to HIV antibody testing. J Consult Clin Psychol 58:31–37, 1990

Johnstone FD, Brettle RP, MacCallum LR, et al: Women's knowledge of their HIV antibody state: its effect on their decision whether to continue the pregnancy. BMJ 300:23–24, 1990

Kastenbaum R, Aisenberg RB: The Psychology of Death. New York, Springer, 1972

Kelly JA, Murphy DA, Bahr GR, et al: Factors associated with severity of depression and high-risk sexual behavior among persons diagnosed with human immuno-deficiency virus (HIV) infection. Health Psychol 12:215–219, 1993

Kinloch-de Loës S, de Saussure P, Saurat J-H, et al: Symptomatic primary infection due to human immunodeficiency virus type 1: review of 31 cases. Clin Infect Dis 17:59–65, 1993

Kübler-Ross E: On Death and Dying. New York, Macmillan, 1969

Kübler-Ross E: Death: The Final Stage of Growth. Englewood Cliffs, NJ, Prentice-Hall, 1975

Lehman JS, Hecht FM, Fleming PL, et al: HIV testing behavior among at-risk popu-lations: why do persons seek, defer, or avoid getting tested in the United States? (abstract no. 43103), in Abstracts of the 12th World AIDS Conference, Geneva, Switzerland, June 28–July 3, 1998

Lester P, Partridge JC, Chesney M, et al: The consequences of a positive prenatal HIV antibody test for women. J AIDS Hum Retrovirol 10:341–349, 1995

Levine C: Orphans of the epidemic: unmet needs in six U.S. cities. AIDS Care 7:S57–S62, 1995

Lipsitz JD, Williams JBW, Rabkin JG, et al: Psychopathology in male and female intravenous drug users with and without HIV infection. Am J Psychiatry 151:1662–1668, 1994

Lo B, Steinbrook R, Cooke M, et al: Voluntary screening for human immunodeficiency virus (HIV) infection: weighing the benefits and harms. Ann Intern Med 110:727–733, 1989

Lucas SB, Hounnou A, Peacock C, et al: The mortality and pathology of HIV infection in a West African city. AIDS 7:1569–1579, 1993

Lyketsos CG, Hoover DR, Guccione M, et al: Depressive symptoms as predictors of medical outcomes in HIV infection. JAMA 270:2563–2567, 1993

Maher, J, Seeman, GM, Peterson, J, et al: Partner violence and women's decision to have an HIV test (abstract no. 43110), in Abstracts of the 12th World AIDS Conference, Geneva, Switzerland, June 28–July 3, 1998

Maiman M, Fruchter RG, Serur E, et al: Human immunodeficiency virus infection and cervical neoplasia. Gynecol Oncol 38:377–382, 1990

Maiman M, Tarricone N, Vieira J, et al: Colposcopic evaluation of human immuno-deficiency virus seropositive women. Obstet Gynecol 78:84–88, 1991

Manne SL, Zautra AJ: Couples coping with chronic illness: women with rheumatoid arthritis and their healthy husbands. J Behav Med 13:327–342, 1990

Marks G, Richardson JL, Maldonado N: Self-disclosures of HIV infection to sexual partners. Am J Public Health 81:1321–1322, 1991

Marmor M, Weiss LR, Lyden M, et al: Possible female-to-female transmission of human immunodeficiency virus (letter). Ann Intern Med 105:969, 1986

Masur H, Michelis MA, Wormser GP, et al: Opportunistic infection in previously healthy women: Initial manifestations of a community-acquired cellular immun-odeficiency. Ann Intern Med 97:533–539, 1982

Mocroft A, Johnson MA, Phillips AN. Factors affecting survival in patients with the acquired immunodeficiency syndrome. AIDS 10:1057–1065, 1996

Monzon OT, Capellan JMB: Female-to-female transmission of HIV (letter). Lancet 2:40–41, 1987

Moore J, Harrison JS, Kay KL, et al: Factors associated with Hispanic women's HIV-related communication and condom use with male partners. AIDS Care 7:415–427, 1995

Moore J, Schuman P, Schoenbaum E, et al: Severe adverse life events and depressive symptoms among women with, or at risk for, HIV infection in four cities in the United States of America. AIDS 13:2459–2468, 1999

Moore J, Saul J, vanDevanter N, et al: Factors influencing relationship quality of HIV-serodiscordant heterosexual couples, in HIV and Social Interaction. Edited by Derlega VJ, Barbee AP. Thousand Oaks, CA, Sage Publications, 1998a, pp 165–192

Moore J, Schoenbaum E, Warren D, et al: Barriers to condom use identified by HIV-infected and at-risk women (abstract no. 23420), in Abstracts of the 12th World AIDS Conference, Geneva, Switzerland, June 28–July 3, 1998b

Moore J, Schoenbaum E, Warren D, et al: Patterns of condom use reported by HIV-infected and at-risk women at three time periods (abstract no. 23404), in Abstracts of the 12th World AIDS Conference, Geneva, Switzerland, June 28–July 3, 1998c

Morgan D, Malamba SS, Maude GH, et al: An HIV-1 natural history cohort and survival times in rural Uganda. AIDS 11:633–640, 1997a

Morgan D, Maude GH, Malamba, et al: HIV-1 disease progression and AIDS-defining disorders in rural Uganda. Lancet 350:245–250, 1997b

North RL, Rothenberg KH: Partner notification and the threat of domestic violence against women with HIV infection. N Engl J Med 329:1194–1196, 1993

Ostrow DG, Monjan A, Joseph J, et al: HIV-related symptoms and psychological functioning in a cohort of homosexual men. Am J Psychiatry 146: 737–742, 1989

Palella FJ, Delaney KM, Moorman AC, et al: Declining morbidity and mortality among patients with advanced human immunodeficiency virus infection. N Engl J Med 338:853–860, 1998

Pergami A, Gala C, Burgess A, et al: The psychosocial impact of HIV infection in women. J Psychosom Res 37:687–696, 1993

Perry S, Fishman B: Depression and HIV: how does one affect the other? JAMA 270:2609–2610, 1993

Perry S, Jacobsberg L, Fogel K: Orogenital transmission of HIV. Ann Intern Med 111:951–952, 1989

Perry S, Jacobsberg L, Fishman B: Suicidal ideation and HIV testing. JAMA 263:679–682, 1990a

Perry S, Jacobsberg L, Fishman B, et al: Psychiatric diagnosis before serological testing for the human immunodeficiency virus. Am J Psychiatry 147:89–93, 1990b

Perry S, Jacobsberg L, Fishman B, et al: Psychological responses to serological testing for HIV. AIDS 4:145–152, 1990c

Perry S, Jacobsberg L, Card CAL, et al: Severity of psychiatric symptoms after HIV testing. Am J Psychiatry 150:775–779, 1993

Persky VW, Kempthorne-Rawson J, Shekelle RB: Personality and risk of cancer: 20-year follow-up of the Western Electric Study. Psychosom Med 49:435–444, 1987

Rabkin JG, Williams JBW, Remien RH, et al: Depression, distress, lymphocyte subsets, and human immunodeficiency virus symptoms on two occasions in HIV-positive homosexual men. Arch Gen Psychiatry 48:111–119, 1991

Revenson T, Felton BJ: Disability and coping as predictors of psychological adjustment to rheumatoid arthritis. J Clin Consult Psychol 57:344–348, 1989

Royce RA, Sena A, Cates W Jr, et al: Sexual transmission of HIV. N Engl J Med 337:1072–1078, 1997

Royce RA, Walter E, Fernandez I, et al: HIV counseling and testing among parturients sampled at four U.S. sites: preliminary findings (abstract no. 43117), in Abstracts of the 12th World AIDS Conference, Geneva, Switzerland, June 28–July 3, 1998

Schable B, Diaz, T, Chu SY, et al: Who are the primary caretakers of children born to HIV-infected mothers? Results from a multi-state surveillance project. Pediatrics 95:511–515, 1995

Schacker TW, Hughes JP, Shea T, et al: Biological and virologic characteristics of primary HIV infection. Ann Intern Med 128:613–620, 1998

Schafer A, Friedmann W, Mielke M, et al: The increased frequency of cervical dysplasia-neoplasia in women infected with the human immunodeficiency virus is related to the degree of immunosuppression. Am J Obstet Gynecol 164:593–599, 1991

Schoenbaum EE, Webber MP: The underrecognition of HIV infection in women in an inner-city emergency room. Am J Public Health 83:363–368, 1993

Selwyn PA, Carter RJ, Schoenbaum EE, et al: Knowledge of HIV antibody status and decisions to continue or terminate pregnancy among intravenous drug users. JAMA 261:3567–3571, 1989

Selwyn PA, Alcabes P, Hartel D, et al: Clinical manifestations and predictors of disease progression in drug users with human immunodeficiency virus infection. N Engl J Med 327:1697–1703, 1992

Semple SJ, Patterson TL, Temoshok LR, et al: Identification of psychobiological stressors among HIV-positive women. Women Health 20:15–36, 1993

Simoni JM, Mason HRC, Marks G, et al: Women's self-disclosure of HIV infection: rates, reasons, and reactions. J Consult Clin Psychol 63:474–478, 1995

Smith DK, Warren DL, Vlahov D, et al: Design and baseline participant characteristics of the Human Immunodeficiency Virus Epidemiology Research (HER) Study: a prospective cohort study of human immunodeficiency virus infection in U.S. women. Am J Epidemiol 146:459–469, 1997

Solomon L, Stein M, Flynn C, et al: Health services use by urban women with or at risk for HIV-1 infection: the HIV epidemiologic research study (HERS). J Acquir Immune Defic Syndr Hum Retrovirol 17:253–261, 1998

Sorvillo F, Kerndt P, Bunch G, et al: Early HIV detection: successes and failures (abstract no. 43104), in Abstracts of the 12th World AIDS Conference, Geneva, Switzerland, June 28–July 3, 1998

Stein MD, Piette J, Mor V, et al: Differences in access to zidovudine (AZT) among symptomatic HIV-infected persons. J Gen Intern Med 6:35–40, 1991

Sterling T, Lyles C, Quinn TC, et al: Gender-specific differences in HIV-1 RNA level in a longitudinal study of HIV-1 seroconverters (abstract no. 13379), in Abstracts of the 12th World AIDS Conference, Geneva, Switzerland, June 28–July 3, 1998

Stone VE, Seage GR, Hertz T, et al: The relation between hospital experience and mortality for patients with AIDS. JAMA 268:2655–2661, 1992

Sunderland A, Minkoff HL, Handte J, et al: The impact of human immunodeficiency virus serostatus on reproductive decisions of women. Obstet Gynecol 79:1027–1031, 1992

Tindall B, Cooper DA: Primary HIV infection: host responses and intervention strategies. AIDS 5:1–14, 1991

Todd J, Balira R, Grosskurth H, et al: HIV-associated adult mortality in a rural Tanzanian population. AIDS 11:801–807, 1997

Ward JW, Holmberg SD, Allen JR, et al: Transmission of human immunodeficiency virus (HIV) by blood transfusion screened as negative for HIV antibody. N Engl J Med 318:473–478, 1988

World Health Organization: AIDS epidemic update: December 1998. Available online at http://www.who.int/emc-hiv/december1998/wadr98e.pdf. Accessed August 22, 2000

Wortley PM, Fleming PL, Lindegren ML, et al: Prevention of perinatal transmission in the U.S.: a population-based evaluation of prevention efforts in 4 states (abstract no. 23282), in Abstracts of the 12th World AIDS Conference, Geneva, Switzerland, June 28–July 3, 1998

Wright TC Jr, Sun XW: Anogenital papillomavirus infection and neoplasia in immunodeficient women. Obstet Gynecol Clin North Am 23:861–893, 1996

Zierler S, Mayer K, Moore J, et al: Sexual practices in a cohort of U.S. women with and without human immunodeficiency virus. J Am Med Womens Assoc 54:79–83, 1999

# General Issues

# Reproductive Choices and Development

## Psychodynamic and Psychoanalytic Perspective

MALKAH TOLPIN NOTMAN, M.D.

CAROL C. NADELSON, M.D.

Reproductive choices profoundly affect an individual's life. Some are made almost automatically in the course of the life cycle, whereas others are made inadvertently, influenced by social expectations, life experiences, and unconscious factors. Even if choices are conscious and deliberate, however, they express deep-seated attitudes, beliefs, and expectations about oneself, one's gender role, and one's relationship to society.

In the past several decades social changes have influenced the size of families and the timing of pregnancies. Increased career opportunities and the rise in the number of women working outside the home have affected reproductive decisions. The desire to have children is very powerful for both men and women; however, women have traditionally defined themselves and been defined more by their family roles than by their work. Women also experience a pregnancy more intimately and their wishes for children have more closely expressed the primary fulfillment of female gender role and aspirations. A recent study (Ravin et al. 1997) reported that when asked to choose between a gestational or genetic tie with a child, women more often chose the gestational tie, whereas men chose the genetic tie. This supports the longstanding view that the experience of pregnancy has greater significance for women, and that men and women have different reproductive perspectives.

For a woman, a pregnancy also has a developmental significance. It evokes her identification with and relationship with her mother. The woman with a troubled or ambivalent relationship with her mother can experience a pregnancy, particularly a first pregnancy, as distressing. It marks her transition from a daughter to a mother, and she may feel anxious that she will repeat her mother's problematic mothering. It also may cause angry feelings toward her mother to surface (Bibring et al. 1961).

If a woman's relationship with her mother is positive, pregnancy provides a less conflicted shift between daughterhood and motherhood and is also a step toward a concept of adulthood. Intrapsychially, the baby represents a separate individual and calls for the development of care and responsibility for another person apart from oneself. This process is intensified once the baby is born and taking care of it is less automatic than during the pregnancy. In her identification with the baby, the mother can feel gratified in her new role as caretaker. The baby also represents its father as well as others in the family; if the mother is angry or ambivalent toward the father, this can be expressed as anger or ambivalence toward the baby. These feelings are sometimes expressed during pregnancy and delivery.

Wishes to conceive and carry a pregnancy and to deliver a baby, however, do not necessarily reflect a grasp of the real tasks of parenting, with its accompanying demands, responsibilities, and personal life changes. Instead, they can represent a fantasy of the fulfillment of an identity as a man or a woman or other fantasies such as passing on one's genes and in some way achieving immortality. Even for those who choose not to have children, knowing that one has the capacity to do so is an important part of the adult gender identity.

The societal importance of producing children varies to some extent with differing economic conditions and values. In all cultures, however, women's roles as mothers and nurturers of young children remain central, although there is an enormous range in the other roles and activities that each culture assigns to men and women (LeVine 1991). In most cultures, women are the primary caretakers of infants and children whether they stay at home or work in the fields, factories, or offices. This role is an extension of pregnancy and nursing. Pregnancy, childbirth, and nursing establish a bond between infant and mother that is not available in the same way to the father; they are unique experiences for women who will always be known as the child's mother even if the father is not known.

The "reproductive clock" and the knowledge that fertility is time limited also form a background context for many women's choices in a way that has no equivalent for men. Women are aware of their capacity to have babies from early childhood, and they also learn during the course of their development that they have a biologic clock, although they may not think consciously of it until well into adulthood. A woman's sexual behavior is always affected by the possibility of pregnancy, whether she is consciously thinking about it or not. This possibility creates both a promise and vulnerability.

Cessation of fertility at menopause also has a different impact on women in different cultures and in different life circumstances, but it is universal in marking an end to childbearing possibilities. Recent technology has extended the time frame for pregnancy beyond normal menopause through the use of egg donation and hormone treatment, but it is unlikely that geriatric-age childbearing will become widespread. Many women actually end their childbearing well before menopause occurs. Knowing that fertility is time limited, however, affects many decisions before the menopause. A feeling of loss dominates the menopausal years despite the fact that for many women cessation of childbearing comes with relief and the positive impetus for a new period of life and psychologic development.

The reality that reproductive capacity is finite also influences other life choices. Most women maintain an awareness of their biologic clock as it affects their career and marital choices and their wishes to experiment with work and lifestyles. Often this awareness is not conscious until it becomes a pressing issue, usually when a woman reaches her 30s (Nadelson 1989; Notman 1973, 1979).

As career opportunities for women have expanded, health status has improved, and technology has advanced, first pregnancies at a later age have become more common. Infertility, however, has also become more common and is a psychologically stressful experience for most couples. Women feel particularly vulnerable. It is not unusual to feel deeply responsible for infertility, and many women blame themselves consciously or unconsciously for delaying attempts at pregnancy, for past sexual behaviors, or even for fantasies and feelings that they feel guilty for having. Many women also have negative feelings toward their bodies that can come into play if they discover they are infertile. This can be true even if the man bears the responsibility for the infertility.

Development of new reproductive technologies has had complex effects, but these technologies are often sought, and most women have been grateful to be offered new possibilities when fertility seemed foreclosed. The most difficult aspects have been the cycles of hope and intense disappointment that many women experience. Despite the many possible causes of fertility problems, women have traditionally been seen as responsible and they have felt burdened and guilty for failing to conceive. This has begun to change in the face of newer data that indicate a high prevalence of male factors responsible for infertility (Rosenthal and Goldfarb 1997).

## Decisions About Marriage

Despite enormous social change over the past three decades, marriage is still perceived by many women as their central adult role. Women can be independent but have psychologic needs for intimacy and connection that are met in marriage and childbearing. Other activities, especially work, continue to be regarded by women as temporary or subordinate to family functions and identifications. This expectation has not been the same for men. Nevertheless, more than 50% of mothers of young children are working, and women are earning a substantial proportion of family income.

In the 1970s, Bernard (1991) and others (Gove and Tudor 1973) documented that marriage improves mental health and satisfaction for men but not for women. Data indicated that more married than unmarried women were depressed, whereas more unmarried than married men were depressed. This probably reflected the social constraints of marriage in the 1950s and 1960s, when women were dependent on men for financial support, had few activities outside the home, and were expected to put their husbands' wishes first. Opportunities for self-realization, independence, and development outside the family were limited.

Women have always experienced considerable social pressure to marry. In the past, their social and economic status depended on the status of the men who were responsible for them—that is, their fathers and husbands. The decision for a woman was usually not whether to marry, but whom and when to marry. Loss of self-esteem and damage to her pride and her family's reputation when a woman remained unmarried led to the familiar desperation of women who became "old maids." This was not so for an unmarried man, whose status as bachelor had a more positive ring and was seen as involving choice and self-determination. The expectation was that a man could choose to marry—and a woman was chosen (Bernard 1991; Nadelson and Notman 1981).

When Kuhn, in 1955, studied a group of men and women who had not married, their reasons for doing so were often expressed negatively—hostility toward marriage or toward members of the opposite sex; dependency on parents; poor health; feelings of physical unattractiveness; unwillingness or inability to assume responsibility; social inadequacy; perception of marriage as a threat to career goals; economic problems; and geographic, educational, or occupational isolation that limited the chances of meeting an eligible mate (Nadelson and Notman 1981). Two decades later, a shift was noted: being single was more often stated as a positive choice. Both men and women spoke of increased freedom and enjoyment of life, opportunities to meet people, economic independence, and a chance for personal development (Stein 1976). In addition, people more openly stated their wishes about not wanting children, about their homosexuality, and about their negative family experiences.

Unconscious and conflictual issues such as strong dependency needs, difficulty forming a stable and secure identity alone, or an intolerable fear of isolation or loneliness also influence the motivation to marry. The desire for children is a strong motivator for marriage, and many conscious and unconscious factors influence the decision to have or not have children. Some people have little interest in actually being with children or in parental roles. Others believe that they cannot be good parents. Some explicitly prefer the freedom of childlessness or want to invest their energy in careers, although this may also be a way of covering deeper anxieties about parenting. Sometimes women fear pregnancy despite a strong wish for children. Others struggle with their unresolved, difficult, and/or ambivalent relationships with their mothers, which affects their confidence in becoming mothers themselves (Nadelson and Notman 1981; Veevers 1979). They may fear that becoming a mother would draw them back to a regressive or devalued position, or they may identify with the negative aspects of their mother's experience. In this era of recombined families, many couples exist in which one partner has had children in a previous marriage and does not want more, leaving the other partner without children of his or her own. Sometimes the decision not to have children is not explicitly stated. Some couples postpone the decision until a future time that never arrives. Sometimes personal circumstances such as careers in dance, athletics, or other demanding professions communicate an ideology that negates childbearing or makes it difficult. Homosexuality had been a determinant of childlessness in the past, but recently the number of lesbian women becoming pregnant has increased. Veevers (1979) noted that "with the exception of race, childlessness tends to be influenced by the major socioeconomic determinants known to influence fertility in general: education, urbanity, socioeconomic status, religious beliefs" (p. 208). However, this does not address the psychologic determinants. Social changes have made childlessness more acceptable.

Women who remain childless may feel bereft and need to mourn what parenthood meant to them. Sometimes these feelings do not emerge until later, and the process of working through them involves a shift in orientation and a search for other experiences to fulfill needs. Infertile women also face the narcissistic injury that usually accompanies that realization, which can threaten their sense of femininity and even their perception of fully being an adult because adulthood is so often closely associated with parenthood (Mazor 1978).

## Gender Identity and Development

It is useful at this point to review ideas about gender development and its relationship to reproduction. *Gender identity*, or the awareness of one's gender, was thought at one time to be established when a young child becomes aware of his/her genitals and of the differences between males and females. In Freud's (1905/1961) early formulations, this process took place later in childhood than current data suggest (Tyson and Tyson 1990). The influences that shape gender identity begin before birth with the parents' expectations and beliefs about gender, particularly when the prenatal determination of the gender of the baby is made.

Classic Freudian theory held that girls had long-standing penis envy, and that this was an organizing and driving force in female development. From this perspective, girls think of their mothers—and of all women—as being defective because they lack a penis (Freud 1905/1961). Contemporary psychoanalytic thinking, informed by developmental observations and research, recognizes that although penis envy exists in some women, it is not the central organizer of development and that the greater power and value that society gives to men plays the major role in some women's sense of self.

Furthermore, according to early psychoanalytic theory, girls blamed their mothers for the missing penis and subsequently turned to their fathers as love objects. This was the initiation of the female Oedipus complex. Other factors also drew girls to their fathers, such as their expanded interests in the world and their desire for their fathers' approval and affection. Fathers were more active and more related to the world outside the family than were mothers. Girls were thought to develop erotic feelings toward and to fantasize about having a baby by their fathers, which led them to both identify and compete with their mothers (expressed in the wish to "marry daddy when I grow up"). These feelings placed girls at risk of alienating their mothers. Forming their own identities and negotiating these competitive and aggressive feelings while at the same time remaining close to their mothers, whom they need and identify with, was a developmental challenge for girls.

Contemporary theory about development suggests that a complex process occurs during the first years of life. Children begin developing their gender identity from birth, influenced by the external environment as well as by genetics and prenatal hormones. Both boys' and girls' early development occurs within the context of a close relationship with their mothers, who are usually their primary caretakers. For girls, the relationship with the parent of the same gender facilitates a different kind of mutual identification than for boys. A mother identifies with her daughter and sees herself in the girl baby, and a girl gradually identifies with the mother. This identification remains a powerful force throughout life, although it is not without conflict. Thus, a girl's gender identity develops from identification with her mother and also with her mother's feminine roles and activities in whatever way the particular culture presents these (and with many individual variations). Turning toward her father is also supported by her identification with her mother, who, after all, preceded her in this (Clower 1976; Freud 1933/1964; Notman et al. 1991; Person 1980).

Boys also have close relationships with their mothers, but because mothers are different from them, boys need a male identification figure. To develop a sense of masculinity, boys distance themselves from early attachments to and identification with their mothers and, to some extent, from their childhood activities; they relinquish and build emotional barriers to these early attachments, including what are perceived to be "feminine ways" (Chodorow 1978). At the same time, envy of the capacity to have babies is found in little boys, and in their development toward a masculine identity they must abandon this possibility (Fast 1984; McDougall 1989). Both mothers and fathers behave differently toward their female and male children from earliest infancy (Block 1976; Moss 1967). These behaviors transmit cultural patterns that promote and consolidate gender differences. Personality differences between men and women are also shaped by these processes as well as by biologic factors.

Although the development of gender identity continues throughout childhood and is consolidated in a more permanent way in adolescence, it does not depend primarily on the awareness of genital differences. One's body image does play an important role in one's sense of self; it incorporates the multiple identifications and learning that take place from early life, including the powerful effects of socialization. Yet gender identity also includes the cognitive awareness of the behavior and attitudes that go with being female or male and the way these roles are shaped in a given culture (Silverman 1981; Stoller 1976). Some cultures have preadolescent and adolescent rituals to mark the transition into the more adult roles. For boys, these can involve abrupt separation from their mothers and other women and initiation into the company and behaviors of men.

Gender identity development also includes ideas about reproductive capacity, which are more elaborated for girls. Girls' thoughts about their ability to have children are both concrete and the subject of fantasies. Their reproductive capacities are thought of as being fulfilled in the future, when they reach sexual maturity. Their breasts are not apparent until puberty. Boys have a somewhat different experience than girls in that although their genitals change in size and shape, their external genitalia are outwardly visible and present at birth. Many women have negative feelings toward their bodies. This has been studied in relation to feelings of defectiveness about not being male, to social pressures toward thinness and bodily perfection, to the devaluation of women, and to identification with a depressed mother.

Pregnancy and parenthood are sources of emotional maturation for both parents (Anthony and Benedek 1970; Cath et al. 1989). In parenthood, identification with parents is revived for both men and women. Although the father of the child does not participate as intimately in pregnancy, having a child is an important confirmation of potency and masculinity (Benedek 1979; Bibring et al. 1961; Notman and Lester 1988). For women who do not become pregnant or mothers, other pathways exist for reworking their identification with their mothers and consolidating their female gender identity. Some adopt children, others work with children, and still others identify with other aspects of maternal roles.

## Sexuality

Ideas that women were sexually unresponsive and that sexual passivity was normal and desirable for women have been replaced with a better understanding of sexual functioning. Contraception has also made it possible to separate sexuality from reproduction to some extent in most western cultures.

Resistance to contraception can be based on religious prohibitions or cultural values that promote a concept of masculinity dependent on producing children. Although seeking sexual gratification has become more acceptable for women, some differences appear to exist in men's and women's attitudes and experiences of sexuality. For women, sexual functioning is more often linked to intimacy in a relationship than to pure genital gratification (Person 1980). For men, sexual performance consolidates gender identity. It is not clear how much the physiologic differences in male and female sexual response cycles affect psychologic experiences.

## Homosexuality

Just as patterns of heterosexual behavior vary, so do patterns of homosexual behavior. A wide range of personalities and characteristics of relationships exists among homosexuals just as among heterosexuals. Psychoanalytic understanding of homosexuality has changed considerably, and the idea that homosexuality is inevitably pathologic has generally given way to an appreciation of the complexity of homosexual choices and styles and an awareness that this is a variation of orientation.

It is likely that most people have some potential to respond erotically under certain circumstances to individuals of the same gender. A spectrum of homosexuality to heterosexuality appears to exist: for some individuals only a homosexual or heterosexual orientation seems possible, whereas others appear to be bisexual. Individuals with homosexual orientations sometimes marry and have children and later act on these homosexual feelings and "come out," often breaking up their marriages. Some have ongoing homosexual relationships during a marriage but remain married and even continue to be heterosexually active. Sometimes the feelings of emotional and sexual attraction to individuals of the same gender are unconscious until some experience of life circumstance mobilizes them. Sometimes they are conscious but not acted on.

The issue of having children is complex for many homosexuals. Some lesbians choose to have children by adoption or donor insemination. Some have arranged for known donors, whereas others have chosen anonymous donors. Gay men may seek out a partner in order to have a child or may adopt. Different kinds of relationships have been emerging as these families develop.

## Contraception

The effectiveness of contraception depends on both the effectiveness of the individual method of contraception and how well the method fits the lifestyle and preferences of the person using it. Many effective contraceptive methods conflict with individual preferences and may not be used as intended; thus, they may not be as effective in practice as a less foolproof method to which there is less resistance. For example, a woman who hesitates to touch or explore her genitals may be inhibited in using a diaphragm. For a contraceptive decision to be made, it is important to take these factors into account as well as the nature of the sexual relationship between the two people.

The only available reliably reversible method of contraception for men is the condom, which has the additional benefit of protection from sexually transmitted diseases, including AIDS. Because it must be used during and interrupts each act of sexual intercourse, however, some couples find it awkward to use. It is perceived to interfere with spontaneity, romance, and sensation. For a man who has anxieties about sexual performance, these problems can forestall condom use.

Vasectomy has been used by some men worldwide. It is sometimes, but not reliably, reversible with microsurgical techniques. The decision for sterilization is often made because the couples and/or individuals feel that they have the number of children they want. They may later regret their decision when a subsequent marriage or the death of a child evokes new desires for parenthood. Women sometimes also choose more permanent methods, such as tubal ligation or even hysterectomy; a hysterectomy marginally indicated for medical reasons is sometimes welcomed by a woman who has religious prohibitions against contraceptives. Reasons for choosing sterilization can range from failure with other methods to feeling overwhelmed by one or more childbirths and wanting to avoid more pregnancies. For some people it is a "politically correct" choice for the man to have the contraceptive procedure.

Other important considerations in assessing which contraceptives to use are the individual's capacity for planning or impulsiveness, the actual availability of various methods, and unconscious resistances that may be present. A person's life circumstances can also contribute to the appropriateness of a particular method. For example, a young girl living with parents who do not know and would not approve of her sexual activity is likely to have trouble with a diaphragm because she must obtain a medical prescription and must keep it hidden, which may be difficult and make its use less reliable. A condom is much more readily available.

Oral contraceptives, although generally safe and effective, are often less acceptable to women who are not in stable relationships, who are sporadically sexually active, who have concerns about long-term effects or side effects, or who have other medical contraindications. Instances have also been reported in which instructions have been given to take the pill regularly, but women use it episodically or only with a sexual encounter. Barrier methods such as the diaphragm and spermicidal creams or jellies require planning as well as a willingness to interrupt sexual activity, which can be particularly difficult for adolescents. The expectation of intercourse implied by the use of these methods can be difficult for some women to acknowledge.

Some men may consciously state that they want to use contraceptives but have an unconscious resistance related to the link between masculinity, potency, and their ability to impregnate a woman. Interference with pregnancy may thus be experienced as a threat to masculinity. Some men also resent having to pay attention to contraception because he sees it as "a woman's job" and the resulting pregnancy as her concern. For women, unconscious wishes for pregnancy may interfere with contraceptive use; becoming pregnant may be an unconscious way of reacting to a loss or a disappointment (Notman and Lester 1988). Women who experience conflicts about a career choice may become pregnant in an unconscious attempt to avoid the conflict.

## Consultative Interaction

New data about contraception, pregnancy, induced abortion, sterilization, rape, menopause, and sexual functioning have challenged widely held myths and provided new insights and information that are often not well known to patients or those providing primary care (Nadelson et al. 1985). Formal consultation in these areas is not often sought because these problems are not usually defined as psychiatric or may involve the relationship between a physician and patient (e.g., because of noncompliance with medication or a regimen or because of differences between the priorities and wishes of patient and physician).

Reproduction and sexuality are emotionally charged subjects. Physicians providing obstetric or gynecologic care are vulnerable to their own emotional responses and may avoid investigating these concerns with patients. Emotionally related problems may be avoided by physicians and referred to others with less experience or knowledge in the specifics of these health care issues. Obstetrician/gynecologists function as primary care physicians for many women during their reproductive years; thus, attention to sexuality and the emotional aspects of gynecologic problems is especially important. Yet gynecologists are often not prepared for a sensitive discussion of sexual problems;

information about sex and reproduction is often not integrated into the education of health providers in a way that specifically addresses the kinds of problems faced by physicians in practice.

Gynecologists must also become accustomed to new realities, such as the possibility of sexually transmitted diseases in a wide cross-section of patients, requests for contraceptive services, infertility treatment and sexual counseling for unmarried couples, and gynecologic care of patients who are bisexual or lesbian. New reproductive technologies have raised clinical as well as ethical issues for which the gynecologist and psychiatrist may be unprepared. Physicians have neither the data nor the ethical position to be gatekeepers to services, but prejudices can nevertheless intrude. Infertile couples may request fertility techniques although they seem "unsuitable" to the gynecologist because of socioeconomic or psychiatric factors. Fertility procedures can be very stressful and hospital and clinic personnel may not always be responsive to the patients' sensitivities. The intense cycles of hope and disappointment that such procedures inspire can cause patients to make emotional and/or gynecological demand that gynecologists are not prepared to meet. Physicians may also have personal beliefs about the appropriateness of pregnancy for some individuals (e.g., lesbians) that affect the way they provide services.

Today, challenges are being made to the provision of thoughtful and adequate care. Constraints imposed by managed care and other medical care systems may make obtaining consultations or performing some procedures difficult and may limit the time a physician has to spend with a patient. Physicians may often be asked to perform a permanent procedure, such as sterilization, in which he/she acts merely as a technician. Thus, as the role and responsibility of the physician, patient, institutions, and society are questioned from ethical, political, medical, psychologic, and economic perspectives, being informed about the issues involved in reproduction becomes even more important.

## References

Anthony EJ, Benedek T: Summing up, in Parenthood: Its Psychology and Psychopathology. Edited by Anthony EJ, Benedek T . Boston, MA, Little, Brown, 1970, pp 599–603

Benedek T: The psychobiology of pregnancy, in Parenthood: Its Psychology and Psychopathology. Edited by Anthony EJ, Benedek T. Boston, MA, Little, Brown, 1979, pp 137–151

Bernard J: Ground rules for marriage: perspectives on the pattern of an era, in Women and Men: New Perspectives on Gender Differences. Edited by Notman MT, Nadelson CC. Washington, DC, American Psychiatric Press, 1991, pp 89–115

Bibring G, Dwyer T, Huntington D, et al: A study of the psychological processes in pregnancy and of the earliest mother–child relationship. Psychoanal Study Child 16:9–72, 1961

Block J: Assessing sex differences: issues, problems, and pitfalls. Merrill Palmer Quarterly 22:54–69, 1976

Cath S, Gurwitt A, Ginsberg L: Fathers and Their Families. Hillsdale, NJ, Analytic Press, 1989

Chodorow N: The Reproduction of Mothering: Psychoanalysis and the Sociology of Gender. Berkeley, CA, University of California Press, 1978

Clower V: Theoretical implications in current views of masturbation in latency girls. J Am Psychoanal Assoc 24:109–125, 1976

Fast I: Gender Identity: A Differentiation Model. Hillsdale, NJ, Analytic Press, 1984

Freud S: Three essays on the theory of sexuality (1905), in The Standard Edition of the Complete Psychological Works of Sigmund Freud, Vol 7. Translated and edited by Strachey J. London, England, Hogarth, 1961, pp 171–179

Freud S: Femininity (1933), in The Standard Edition of the Complete Psychological Works of Sigmund Freud, Vol 22. Translated and edited by Strachey J. London, England, Hogarth, 1964, pp 112–135

Gove WR, Tudor JF: Adult sex roles and mental illness. Am J Sociol 78:812–835, 1973

LeVine RA: Gender differences: interpreting anthropological data, in Women and Men: New Perspectives on Gender Differences. Edited by Notman MT, Nadelson, CC. Washington, DC, American Psychiatric Press, 1991, pp 1–8

Mazor M: The problem of infertility, in The Woman Patient, Vol 1: Medical and Psychological Interfaces. Edited by Notman MT, Nadelson CC. New York, Plenum, 1978, pp 137–160

McDougall J: The dead father. Int J Psychoanal 70:205–219, 1989

Moss H: Sex, age, and state as determinants of mother–infant interaction. Merrill Palmer Quarterly 13:19–36, 1967

Nadelson CC: Issues in the analyses of single women in their thirties and forties in the middle years, in New Psychoanalytic Perspectives. Edited by Oldham S, Liebert R. New Haven, CT, Yale University Press, 1989, pp 105–122

Nadelson CC, Notman MT: To marry or not to marry: a choice. Am J Psychiatry 138:1352–1356, 1981

Nadelson CC, Notman MT, Ellis EA: Psychosmatic aspects of obstetrics and gynecology, in Psychosomatic Illness Review. Edited by Dorfman W, Crisofar L. New York, Macmillan, 1985, pp 162–179

Notman MT: Pregnancy and abortion: implications for career development of professional women. Ann N Y Acad Sci 208:205–210, 1973

Notman MT: Midlife concerns of women: implications of the menopause. Am J Psychiatry 136:1270–1274, 1979

Notman MT, Lester E: Pregnancy: theoretical considerations. Psychoanalytic Inquiry 8:139–159, 1988

Notman MT, Klein R, Jordan JV, et al: Women's unique developmental issues across the life cycle, in American Psychiatric Press Review of Psychiatry, Vol 10. Edited by Tasman A, Goldfinger SM. Washington, DC, American Psychiatric Press, 1991, pp 556–577

Person E: Sexuality as a mainstay of identity: psychoanalytic perspectives, in Women: Sex and Sexuality. Edited by Stimpson C, Person E. Chicago IL, University of Chicago, 1980, pp 36–61

Ravin AJ, Mahowald MB, Stocking CB: Genes or gestation? Attitudes of women and men about biologic ties to children. J Women Health 6:639–648, 1997

Rosenthal M, Goldfarb J: Infertility and assisted reproduction technology: an update for mental health professionals. Harv Rev Psychiatry 5:169–172, 1997

Silverman M: Cognitive development and female psychology. J Am Psychoanal Assoc 29:581–605, 1981

Stein PL: Single in America. Englewood Cliffs, NJ, Prentice-Hall, 1976

Stoller RJ: Primary femininity. J Am Psychoanal Assoc 24:59–78, 1976

Tyson P, Tyson R: Psychoanalytic Theories of Development. New Haven, CT, Yale University, 1990

Veevers J: Voluntary childlessness: a review of issues and evidence. Man and Family Review 2:1–26, 1979

# Female Sexual Disorders

ROBERT TAYLOR SEGRAVES, M.D., PH.D.
KATHLEEN BLINDT SEGRAVES, PH.D.

$S$exual function is influenced by complicated and interactive biologic and psychologic factors. Thus, the diagnosis of sexual dysfunction is complicated because of the numerous diverse etiologies that must be considered. The differential diagnosis of sexual disorders is not widely understood by physicians. Because of the interaction between biologic and psychologic factors, evaluation of many disorders of female sexual function by necessity involves close collaboration between practitioners in obstetrics and gynecology and those in psychiatry. The psychiatric clinician will focus on a careful sexual and psychiatric history, attempting to ascertain the specific nature of the psychologic problem (e.g., affective disorder, marital discord, or transient stress) and whether it appears to be secondary to other psychiatric disease. Evaluation by the gynecologist will be equally meticulous and will attempt to rule out diverse physical etiologies, including vulvovaginitis, normal hormonal changes associated with menopause or perimenopause, endometriosis, and other pathologic conditions.

The field of gynecology has shown an increasing awareness of the need to assess sexual function, and most gynecologists recognize the need to collaborate with psychiatrists in this assessment. It is indeed the rare psychiatrist or gynecologist who is capable of independent assessment and treatment of the full spectrum of female sexual disorders. The requisite knowledge base crosses subspecialty boundaries and is still evolving. This chapter examines various topics at the interface of psychiatry and gynecology concerning female sexual response.

Nomenclature

*Sexual dysfunction due to a general medical condition* and *substance-induced sexual dysfunction* were added to the conditions defined in DSM-IV (American Psychiatric Association 1994). Other changes in DSM-IV included small changes in diagnostic criteria and in terminology. For example, *inhibited female orgasm* was changed to *female orgasm disorder* and *inhibited male orgasm* was changed to *male orgasm disorder.*

Reviewing the historical development of the nomenclature used to describe female sexual disorders will be helpful in highlighting the rapidly changing terminology in this area of psychiatry. Some consensus regarding terminology resulted from Masters and Johnson's (1966) description of four stages of sexual response (excitement, plateau, orgasm, and resolution) and definitions of three separate female psychosexual disorders: dyspareunia, vaginismus, and orgasmic dysfunction (primary and secondary). For approximately 10 years, the diagnostic system introduced by Masters and Johnson was used by most clinicians and clinical investigators. A major change in diagnostic nomenclature resulted from the work of two sex therapists: Lief (1977), who identified the phenomenon of low sexual desire, and Kaplan (1977), who introduced a three-stage model of sexual response—desire, excitement, and orgasm—and clearly influenced DSM-III (American Psychiatric Association 1980). In the revised manual, DSM-III-R (American Psychiatric Association 1987), a sexual aversion disorder was included; what previously had been diagnosed as frigidity or general sexual unresponsiveness might now be diagnosed as hypoactive sexual desire disorder. These rapid changes in terminology make it extremely difficult to combine findings from literature only 10–15 years old with findings of contemporary investigations.

Many investigators stress the importance of accurately diagnosing the impaired phase of the sexual response cycle. Kaplan (1983a) postulated that the earlier the impairment in the sexual response cycle occurred, the worse the psychopathology and prognosis. This hypothesis, however, has not been subjected to empirical investigation. Other investigators (K. B. Segraves and Segraves 1991a, 1991b; R. T. Segraves and Segraves 1991) have noted the large overlap between disorders of the various phases of the sexual response cycle. Because of the frequent overlap between organic and psychologic factors in sexual disorders, an international consensus conference recently proposed that the female sexual dysfunction nosology be modified to include both organic and psychologic factors in the same system (Basson et al. 2000b).

## Prevalence

It is difficult to obtain true estimates of the incidence and prevalence of female sexual disorders in the general population, because few studies have employed random sampling of the population, standardized sexual interviews, or operational definitions of syndromes (Nathan 1986). The changing nosology mentioned earlier also contributes to the difficulty in combining the available data base.

Several studies have indicated that female sexual disorders are quite common in general medical and gynecologic clinics (Burnap and Golden 1967; Catalan et al. 1981; Ende et al. 1984; Levine and Yost 1976). For example, Ende et al. (1984) reported that 27% of women attending a general medical practice reported lack of sexual desire, and 25% reported lack of orgasm. In a study of sexual problems in a gynecologic clinic, Levine and Yost (1976) found that 17% of the women reported difficulty achieving orgasm in partner-related activity.

Studies reporting the frequency with which different syndromes appear in treatment settings have reported high frequencies of orgasm disorders (Bancroft and Coles 1976; Renshaw 1988) and desire disorders (Hawton et al. 1986; Lief 1985; LoPiccollo 1980; Schover and LoPiccollo 1982). Most investigators have reported female arousal disorder to be somewhat rarely encountered in clinical practice (Nathan 1986). Vaginismus and dyspareunia each appear to have a prevalence rate close to 5% (Renshaw 1988).

The largest clinical study of the relative prevalence of female sexual disorders was of women seeking treatment as part of a large multisite pharmaceutical study (K. B. Segraves and Segraves 1991a, 1991b; R. T. Segraves and Segraves 1991). Of 532 women seeking treatment for sexual problems, 475 (89%) had a primary diagnosis of hypoactive sexual desire disorder; 40 had a primary diagnosis of female arousal disorder; and only 17 had orgasm disorders as a primary diagnosis. One of the most remarkable findings of this study was the frequency with which patients had multiple diagnoses. Of the women with a primary diagnosis of hypoactive sexual desire disorder, 41% had either an arousal or orgasm disorder as well, and 18% had disorders of all three phases of the sexual response cycle.

In a recent representative sample of adults in the United States who completed a sexual questionnaire (Laumann et al. 1994), women reported the following difficulties in the preceding 12 months: 1) inability to reach orgasm, 24%; 2) lack of interest in sex, 33%; and 3) trouble with lubrication, 18%. Another recent study involved a random selection of Icelanders between the ages of 55 and 57. This study found that 16% of women had inhibited sexual desire, 6% had inhibited sexual excitement, 3.5% had inhibited orgasm, and 3% had dyspareunia (Lindal and Stefansson 1993)

## Differential Diagnosis

It is important to emphasize that both biologic and psychologic factors may coexist in sexual disorders. Thus, rather than attempt to diagnose whether the problem is organic or psychogenic in etiology, the clinician should focus on which factor is the major contributor to the problems and which factor is correctable. In general, problems that are situational or partner-specific will be predominantly psychogenic in etiology (Moore 1989). Similarly, lifelong problems often have a large psychogenic component (Kaplan 1983b). In clinical practice, the presumption of a predominantly psychogenic etiology for a sexual problem is often made when a biologic etiology has been excluded in gynecologic examination. This is not an optimal strategy, however, because most sexual problems have a mixed organic/psychogenic etiology.

### Dyspareunia

Dyspareunia is a common complaint in gynecologic practice and often has a primary organic etiology. Various physical factors may cause dyspareunia (Kaufman 1983a; Moore 1989). Common organic causes are vaginitis, pelvic infections, vulvar vestibulitis, and senile vaginitis. The most common psychologic cause of dyspareunia is lack of sexual arousal (Rosen and Leiblum 1995), which may have numerous etiologies. The clinician must establish whether the dyspareunia is secondary to lack of lubrication. If the patient is postmenopausal, the possible diagnosis of atrophic vaginitis should be considered.

### Vaginismus

Vaginismus is caused by involuntary contractions of the perivaginal muscle. These involuntary contractions may result from any cause of pelvic pain, such as endometriosis or pelvic inflammatory disease, or from a psychologic fear of penetration (Kaplan 1983b). Some of these patients may have a history of sexual trauma or abuse (Becker et al. 1986; Kinzel et al. 1997). Although many forms of vaginismus occur with any attempt at vaginal penetration (e.g., coitus, pelvic examination, tampons), some cases may occur only with coitus and not during a pelvic examination. Thus, the absence of vaginal contractions during a pelvic examination does not rule out this diagnosis.

## Hypoactive Sexual Desire Disorder

Concern regarding disorders of sexual desire have assumed a position of increased importance in the field of sex therapy and are some of the most perplexing and prevalent of the sexual disorders (Rosen and Leiblum 1989; Spector and Carey 1990). One of the first steps in differential diagnosis is to determine whether the problem is primary or appears secondary to another disorder. For example, decreased sexual desire may be a response to other sexual dysfunction (Levine 1989), chronic illness (Schover and Jensen 1988), depressive illness (Levine 1989), or may be a side effect of medication (R. T. Segraves and Segraves 1993), fatigue, and external stressors. A second step in differential diagnosis is to determine whether the problem is global or situational. If a patient reports decreased sexual desire in her relationship but normal sexual fantasies and frequent masturbation, the clinician would suspect relationship deterioration as a probable etiology. Lifelong patterns of low sexual desire are generally assumed to be psychogenic, although it is quite possible that some patients have lifelong patterns of low sexual desire secondary to constitutional factors.

The role of hormonal influences in the genesis of hypoactive sexual desire disorders is unclear. Although some investigators have reported beneficial effects from androgen therapy in patients who have undergone surgical menopause (i.e., oophorectomy) (Alexander and Sherwin 1993), findings are inconsistent across studies (Andersen 1995; Beck 1995). Some clinicians use exogenous androgens in premenopausal women with hypoactive sexual desire disorder (Koehler 1998). Oral contraceptives frequently elevate serum hormone binding globulin, decreasing the amount of free testosterone and perhaps causing decreasing libido (Koehler 1998). A recent single-blind study suggested that bupropion may be effective in a subgroup of nondepressed women with hypoactive sexual desire disorder (Segraves et al. 2000).

## Female Sexual Arousal Disorder

Information concerning female arousal disorder is limited (Moore 1989; Nathan 1986; R. T. Segraves 1996), and this diagnosis is infrequently made in psychiatric practice. In one multisite study of 532 female patients with sexual disorder, only 8% had this diagnosis, and most also had problems with desire and/or orgasm; less than 2% had female sexual arousal disorder as a solitary diagnosis. However, this problem is found more commonly in gynecologic clinics (Rosen et al. 1993).

According to DSM-IV, the diagnosis of female arousal disorder can be made if vaginal lubrication fails. It is not uncommon for a discrepancy to exist between subjective and objective measures of sexual arousal and for some women to experience vaginal lubrication without conscious awareness of subjective sexual arousal (Hoon and Hoon 1978; Palace and Gorzalka 1992). In clinical practice, psychogenic arousal disorders usually present as a failure of subjective sexual arousal. A complaint of lubrication failure in the presence of increased subjective arousal is most often caused by estrogen deficiency (Bancroft 1983). Diabetes mellitus may also be associated with a decreased lubrication response to sexual stimulation (Kaufman 1983b). It is of note that a recent study did not find sildenafil to be effective in the treatment of idiopathic female arousal disorder (Basson et al. 2000a).

## Female Orgasmic Disorder

A careful sexual history is paramount in the differential diagnosis of inhibited female orgasm. First, it is necessary to establish whether the disorder is lifelong or acquired. Acquired inhibited female orgasm may be caused by various psychologic and biologic factors. If the problem is situational (e.g., anorgasmic with husband but easily orgasmic with masturbation or an alternative partner), the clinician should immediately suspect relationship deterioration. Global acquired inhibited female orgasm may be caused by affective disorder, anxiety disorder, or overwhelming transient stress (Kaplan 1992).

In most cases, sexual desire and arousal will also be affected. If the patient reports a decreased capacity to become orgasmic despite normal libido and normal sexual arousal, one should consider the possibility of organic etiologies. Various physical causes for anorgasmia exist (R.T. Segraves and Segraves 1993); correctable causes such as pharmacologic side effects should be ruled out first (R. T. Segraves 1995). Neurologic conditions such as spinal cord lesions (Berard 1989), multiple sclerosis (Lilius et al. 1976; Lundberg 1978), cancer, chemotherapy, and surgery injuring the neurologic innervation of the genitals (Poad and Arnold 1994) may result in the inability to reach orgasm. Current evidence suggests that anorgasmia may be a complication of diabetes mellitus in women (Kolodny 1971; Schreiner-Engel et al. 1987). Although it has been proposed that weak pubococcygeal muscles may decrease sexual responsivity (Kegel 1956), little evidence supports this contention (Chambless et al. 1984).

## Psychotherapeutic Treatment

Treatment for sexual complaints continues to evolve, ranging from a strict psychoanalytic intrapsychic approach, to a basic behavioral approach involving prescribing a "set" of homework exercises (regardless of the complaint), to the present approach, which relies on an individualized multiple perspective. Sexual functioning depends on multiple factors such as culture, values, beliefs, assumptions, and expectations as well as environmental factors. The biologic components (chronic health conditions, hormones, medication) and developmental events (menstruation, pregnancy, childbirth, and aging), although poorly understood in women, point to the complexity of sexual functioning. Today, therapists draw from multiple theoretic orientations when designing treatment approaches. Patients present with what appear to be more complicated complaints. One explanation for this is the way in which we now define sexual complaints. Another possible explanation is that most women now seeking treatment have tried various techniques suggested in self-help books and recommended by the popular press. Gone are the days when a woman would present with the problem of anorgasmia for which masturbation training would quickly reverse the problem.

A woman today may present with hypoactive sexual desire. When the therapist explores the problem, this woman reports no problem with arousal or orgasm. The interview reveals no medications or medical conditions that might help to explain the problem. The woman reports she is in a "good" and stable relationship and cannot identify any external stressors that might relate to her complaint. Another example is a woman with the complaint of secondary anorgasmia. The woman's history reveals that she was molested by an uncle when she was 10 years old. The woman is a computer analyst, has been married for the past 12 years, and has a 9-year-old daughter. She describes her marriage as stable and her husband as loving and nonabusive. Still another example is of a woman presenting with an unconsummated, 12-year, "stable and caring" relationship. Simply prescribing "sensate focus" exercises to these women would be a disservice. Indiscriminately assigning set exercises may exacerbate some sexual problems by emphasizing the negative associations to the behavior or may increase anxiety because of the performance component of the exercise. Such a treatment approach may diminish self-esteem or exacerbate partner conflict.

Therapists who treat the sexual complaints of women are made painfully aware of the paucity of available research concerning the sexual functioning of women. Women's sexual concerns necessitate both creative thinking and tenacity on the part of the therapist. A careful and comprehensive biopsychosocial assessment can aid in preparing effective treatment approaches. Identifying the predominant sexual phase involved in the complaint and the associated phases that may be secondarily affected is important in designing effective treatment plans. For example, a woman may report that she is unable to reach orgasm during extensive and what she determines to be adequate stimulation. Given the number of effective treatment approaches for anorgasmia, the therapist might be tempted to begin treatment. Further questioning, however, might reveal that this patient engages in sexual behavior when she experiences no sexual desire or drive. She reports the need to use artificial lubricant, as she reports being "dry" during foreplay. The woman denies having any pain during intercourse. When questioned, she reports that she is never conscious of "wanting" to engage in sexual activity of any kind. She is "willing and compliant" participant in sexual activity initiated by her partner because, by her report, she cares very much for her husband and for their relationship. Here, the presumptive diagnosis is anorgasmia secondary to hypoactive desire disorder. This condition is generally more difficult to reverse completely. Treatment would be tailored to the presumed contributing factors, with the realization that not much is known about the possible biologic contributing factors.

The therapist may want to interview the couple to determine how each perceives and explains the problem. The woman might be asked to become more aware of her sexual thoughts and level of sexual desire independent of her partner. Therapy might first focus on helping the woman to identify her internal dialogue, noting what is sexually enhancing and what is a sexual "turnoff." Attempting to build on any desire-enhancing thoughts and behaviors may provide a starting point from which an attempt can be made to increase the woman's sexual awareness. She might benefit from "fantasy training" exercises or increased exploratory exposure to romantic or erotic material (novels that are erotic and not necessarily explicit). These activities would be mutually arrived at (between therapist and patient) and carried out (without expectation of increased drive) so that the woman can "just experience" the activity. Thus, this is done more as awareness training rather than as the creation of a performance ideal. These activities might be followed by exploration of her internal dialogue during sexual activity or during exposure to sexual material and identification of her attitudes or feelings regarding her internal dialogue. The goal would be to make the woman more aware of her own drive, her sexual thoughts or fantasies, and her own comfort level for a range of sexual activities.

In time, the woman and her partner may benefit from "sensate-focus" exercises (pleasuring experiences) to help them learn what enhances or detracts from sexual arousal. During this treatment, the partner would benefit from knowing the treatment plan and being included in the process; the partner's cooperation and sensitivity would be important to the successful treatment of this problem. He/she might be asked to put his/her needs on hold temporarily in an effort to promote the woman's explorations into her sexuality.

Treatment approaches must be individualized to the patient/couple. Although sensate-focus exercises have a place in the treatment of certain sexual complaints, they are presented as a part of a more comprehensive approach to the woman's presenting problem. Treatment of sexual complaints might necessitate drawing from cumulative theories and techniques (e.g., psychodynamic, systems theory, cognitive-behavioral, marital, family, stress management, communication skills training, social skills training). It is hoped that identifying biologic determinants of female sexual functioning will help in the design of more effective and efficient treatment approaches to female sexual complaints.

## Effect of Pregnancy on Sexual Behavior

With a few exceptions (Masters and Johnson 1966), most investigators have reported a gradual decline in sexual interest as pregnancy progresses (Reamy et al. 1982) that is more pronounced in the third trimester and is accompanied by a decline in coital frequency and noncoital sexual activity (Cohen 1985; Perkins 1982). This decline in sexual activity is more marked in nulliparous than in multiparous women and is more marked in women who demonstrated minimal sexual interest prior to pregnancy (Cohen 1985). It should be noted that the decline in sexual activity during pregnancy has been found in multiple countries (Cohen 1985).

Various explanations have been advanced for this decline in sexual activity. Massive changes in hormone levels occur during pregnancy and the postpartum period; however, no evidence links these endocrine changes to changes in sexual activity. Cultural and psychologic factors are more likely to account for the change (Bancroft 1983). Religious and cultural taboos against sex during pregnancy are common (Bancroft 1983), and fears that sexual activity will cause miscarriage or complications of pregnancy, although unproven, are ingrained in many societies (Cohen 1985). Feelings of ambivalence and increased emotional lability are also common during pregnancy. In addition to affecting a woman's sense of body image, the somatic changes during pregnancy often require modification of sexual technique. Although sexual changes during pregnancy are common, psychiatric consultants are being used in rare cases.

# Effects of Gynecologic Conditions and Procedures on Sexual Behavior

## Involuntary Infertility

Diagnosis of infertility can result in a narcissistic crisis in one or both partners, depending on the level of personal investment in having a child. Given all of the factors involved in the discovery, evaluation, treatment, and aftermath of infertility, profound relationship changes, including changes in sexual function, should be expected.

Infertility may cause a series of emotions to surface within the couple. One or both partners may begin to feel alone, empty, anxious, depressed, ugly, sexually inadequate, unproductive, barren, and responsible for a break in the continuity of the family (Salzer 1986). Daily reminders of one's infertility, such as commercials and movies with cherub-like children cooing in their parents' faces, demonstrating the "perfect" family; announcements of the arrival or expectation of a baby among family and friends; and holidays that emphasize the family (Mother's Day and Father's Day often hit closest to the source of the pain) only enhance these emotions.

Sexual dysfunction may be the cause or the result of a couple experiencing infertility. A thorough psychosexual history is needed to determine whether the infertility is caused by a sexual problem, such as premature ejaculation, vaginismus, impotence, and retrograde ejaculation, that may rarely contribute to infertility.

When the male partner cannot penetrate the woman's vagina because of vaginismus, the couple may benefit from sex therapy. The woman is taught to begin to insert the smallest in a set of vaginal dilators. Once she is able to do this comfortably, her partner is instructed, under her guidance, to begin by inserting first one finger, then two, until the woman is mentally and physically ready to accommodate his penis. This process often requires a great deal of time and patience on the part of both couple and therapist. Treatment of infertility by artificial insemination with the man's sperm is an option during this process.

Although sexual dysfunction can be the cause of infertility, it is more often the result of both the evaluation and the ongoing treatment of infertility. Usually, it is the woman who seeks treatment first. In many cases, she is seen several times before her partner becomes involved. She may undergo physically invasive and painful diagnostic tests, and both partners may experience the evaluation and treatment of infertility as a major invasion of privacy. When the man is not involved in the work-up, his physician–patient relationship is limited, which may lead him to feel like an outsider or just a "producer of sperm." Involving both partners early in their fertility work-up can minimize some of these problems.

Vaginismus or erectile failure might occur only during the ovulatory period of the cycle (Leiblum 1993) or prior to specific tests. Stress imposed by the demand to engage in a completed intravaginal intromission can result in lack of lubrication or vaginismus in the woman and erectile failure in the man. The man may become impotent prior to certain tests (semen analysis, postcoital test, sperm penetration assay) for which he is asked to produce an erection and to ejaculate at a certain time of a specified day because he is aware that his sperm will be observed and graded within a couple of hours by a member of the treatment team.

During the process of trying to conceive, there may come a time when infertility becomes the final diagnosis. Even with all of the new techniques and advancements, treatment of infertility does not always lead to successful pregnancy and childbirth. A responsible treatment team should address this issue both among themselves and with the couple. Current practice often reinforces the couple's denial, delaying the reparative work needed to go beyond the infertility. Accepting the diagnosis of infertility may result in intense mourning, which may negatively impact whatever sexual functioning is left in the relationship. Sexual apathy may be predominant, along with sexual avoidance. During the struggle to conceive, sex becomes associated with reproduction. Accepting infertility often results in the couple not wanting to engage in intercourse because it reminds them of what can never be—"why bother?" Others may become promiscuous or want to engage in sex more frequently as a means of bolstering their sense of self-esteem or desirability.

Trying to recapture the active, spontaneous, mutually enjoyable sex life the couple experienced prior to the diagnosis of infertility is a difficult and sometimes impossible task. Some couples are never able to resume earlier pleasures. Infertility and its treatment may end in broken relationships. Other couples struggle to find new and different ways to be intimate and to engage in sexual relations that do not resonate with the times and positions that became routine during their attempts to conceive. Some couples need time to become intimate again before they can resume intercourse. The therapist must be sensitive to the wide variations in responses and the time needed to rebuild.

## Menopause

With menopause, a marked drop in estrogen production occurs that is often accompanied by vasomotor instability (hot flashes) and vaginal atrophy (Coop 1996). Some women report a decline in sexual activity associated with menopause (Pearce et al. 1995). Many factors may account for this decrease, including concomitant aging and decreased sexual ability in the partner (Coop 1984) as well as sociocultural expectations, psychologic distress associated with the symbolic meaning of menopause (Rinehart and Schiff 1985), and discomfort with menopausal symptoms (Bachmann et al. 1985). Estrogen replacement therapy may help alleviate the physical symptoms of menopause and thus contribute to an increase in coital frequency, although it is doubtful that estrogen has a direct effect on libido (Pearce et al. 1995).

Recent evidence suggests that androgens decline gradually with age and that the symptoms of androgen deficiency may develop insidiously. One of the major features of androgen deficiency is hypothesized to be loss of libido (Davis 1998; Kaplan 1977). Circulating testosterone levels in premenopausal women are approximately half that of women in their 20s. Most of the published evidence about the beneficial effects of androgen replacement have involved women who received this therapy after hysterectomy and/or oophorectomy (Young 1993). Davis (1998), however, has reported success using androgen replacement therapy in premenopausal women with androgen deficiency syndrome.

Two studies suggest that the reaction to erotic stimuli may undergo only minor changes with menopause. Morrell et al. (1984) found that postmenopausal women had decreased vaginal responses to erotic stimuli compared with premenopausal women. Differences in subjective arousal were also found. Myers and Morokoff (1985) did not find a difference in vaginal response to erotic stimuli (measured by photo plethysmography) between pre- and postmenopausal women. In view of the multiple influences on sexuality in the menopausal female, evaluation of a complaint of decreased sexual responsivity should involve close collaboration between the psychiatrist and the gynecologist.

## Hysterectomy

Evidence concerning the sexual consequences of hysterectomy combined with oophorectomy is unclear. Some investigators have found no evidence of harmful effects on sexual function (Coopen et al. 1981), whereas others have reported decreased libido after this procedure (Munday and Cox 1967). Clearly, research in this area is complicated by numerous factors, including the psychologic meaning to the patient, the partner's reaction, the degree of discomfort preceding the procedure, the presence or absence of postoperative complications, and whether the procedure includes bilateral oophorectomy (Farrell and Kieser 2000; R. T. Segraves and Segraves 1993). A recently published 2-year prospective study found that sexual functioning improved after hysterectomy (Rhodes et al. 1999).

Evidence indicates that estrogen-androgen preparations may be especially effective in restoring libido in women who have undergone surgical menopause. The first double-blind study was reported by Greenblatt et al. (1950). Postmenopausal women were randomly allocated to one of four groups taking diethylstilbestrol, methyltestosterone, a combination of both of these drugs, or placebo. The estrogen preparation relieved hot flashes, and the androgen preparation increased libido. Most women preferred the combination therapy. Similar findings have been reported by others.

## Surgery for Malignancy

In recent years, interest has focused on sexual functioning after treatment of gynecologic cancer (Andersen 1995, 1996; Schover et al. 1987). Research has documented considerable psychologic distress accompanied by sexual disinterest after disfiguring surgical procedures (Andersen 1996).

Pelvic exenteration involves surgical removal of the uterus, fallopian tubes, ovaries, urinary bladder, rectum, and vagina. Surgical reconstruction of a neovagina is often performed; however, many patients report a total cessation of sexual activity after this surgery (Andersen and Hacher 1983; Broun et al. 1972; Demsey et al. 1975).

Radical vulvectomy is often followed by loss of orgasmic capacity and blunting of genital sensation (Andersen and Hacher 1983; Andersen et al. 1988; DiSala et al. 1979). Schover and von Eschenbach (1985) reported that most women are able to resume normal sexual activity after radical cystectomy.

## Other Surgical Procedures

Certain surgical procedures such as sympathectomy, abdominoperitoneal resection, retroperitoneal lymphadenectomy, and aortoiliac surgery interrupt the sympathetic innervation of the genital organs and cause male sexual problems. It may be suspected that these procedures would also interfere with female sexual responsivity; however, minimal evidence exists concerning the sexual effects of these procedures in women (Schover and Jensen 1988). There have been reports that many women remain orgasmic after colectomy-proctomucusectomy and total misorectal excision (Havenga et al. 1996; Sjogren and Poppen 1995).

## Induced Abortion

An immediate negative response to therapeutic abortion is not uncommon (Friedman 1974); however, few women experience serious psychiatric complications or long-term adverse effects on sexual behavior (Gebhard et al. 1958).

## Oral Contraceptives and Sexual Behavior

Evidence of a relationship between oral contraceptive use and altered sexual behavior is inconclusive (R. T. Segraves and Segraves 1993). Although several investigators have reported an association between oral contraceptives and diminished libido (Leeton et al. 1978), available evidence does not suggest that oral contraceptive use has a direct effect on sexual desire (Bancroft 1983; Bardwick 1973; Cullberg 1972). Some women may experience diminished libido secondary to mild dysphoria or nausea during the first several months of oral contraceptive use. If a patient presents with a solitary complaint of diminished libido after beginning oral contraceptives and this does not appear to be related to the psychologic meaning of using birth control, a reasonable approach would be to confer with the gynecologist concerning whether a trial of a different agent is warranted.

## Psychiatric Drugs and Sexual Function

A fairly extensive body of literature documents the association of sexual dysfunction with the use of psychiatric drugs, especially antidepressants that inhibit serotonin reuptake) (Crenshaw and Goldberg 1996; Musher 1990; Rosen et al. 1999; R. T. Segraves 1995). All of the selective serotonin reuptake inhibitors (SSRIs) on the market in the United States, including fluoxetine, fluvoxamine, sertraline, and paroxetine, have been reported to cause anorgasmia (Ashton et al. 1997; Montejo et al. 1997) although fluvoxamine may have a lower incidence of drug-induced anorgasmia than the other SSRIs (Nemeroff et al. 1995; Waldinger 1998). Approximately 30%–50% of patients experience sexual difficulties while receiving SSRIs (R. T. Segraves 1996).

Cyclic antidepressants, such as imipramine, amitriptyline, desipramine, and nortriptyline, also appear to have a high incidence of drug-induced sexual dysfunction (Balon et al. 1993). Clomipramine, a tricyclic antidepressant in the world market but approved for the treatment of obsessive-compulsive disorder in the United States, probably has the highest incidence of drug-induced anorgasmia. One placebo-controlled, double-blind study of the efficacy of clomipramine for the treatment of obsessive-compulsive disorder found that more than 90% of patients experienced ejaculatory or orgasmic delay while receiving this drug (Monteiro et al. 1987). Sexual problems occurred in both men and women. Venlafaxine has multiple actions, including inhibition of sexual dysfunction similar to that of the SSRIs (Ashton et al. 1997).

The monoamine oxidase inhibitors are also associated with anorgasmia. A double-blind, placebo-controlled study by Harrison et al. (1986) found that both phenelzine and imipramine interfered with ejaculatory and orgasmic function.

Of the newer antidepressants, nefazodone (Feiger et al. 1996) and sustained-release bupropion (Hughes et al. 1996) have been shown to have minimal sexual side effects and a much lower incidence of such side effects than sertraline. The results of a questionnaire study by Modell et al. (1997) suggested that bupropion may augment sexual function beyond baseline, whereas the SSRIs depress sexual function. Mirtazapine may also have a very low incidence of sexual dysfunction.

Antidepressant-induced anorgasmia can be treated with drug substitution, lowering of dose, drug holidays, and the use of antidotes such as yohimbine or buspirone. We routinely combine SSRIs with bupropion to offset orgasmic delay induced by the SSRIs. Also, bupropion can be used on an as-needed basis (100 mg bupropion 1–2 hours prior to coitus). One recent controlled study found that high doses of buspirone were effective in reversing SSRI-induced sexual dysfunction, whereas another study found contradictory results (Landen et al. 1999; Michelson et al. 2000). Case reports suggest that sildenafil may reverse female anorgasmia induced by SSRIs (Fava et al. 1998; Schaller and Behar 1999).

A double-blind study by Riley and Riley (1986) demonstrated that diazepam delays orgasm attainment. Case reports suggest that alprazolam may have a similar effect (Sangal 1985). Anorgasmia has not been reported with buspirone. If a minor tranquilizer is required, buspirone would be the preferred choice.

There is minimal evidence concerning whether mood stabilizers affect sexual function in women. Carbamazepine could decrease libido because it causes an elevation of serum hormone binding globulin, thus decreasing the amount of free testosterone available (Isojarvi et al. 1995).

Orgasmic dysfunction has been reported with most of the antipsychotic drugs including thioridazine (Kotin et al. 1976), trifluoperazine (Degen 1982), and fluphenazine (Ghadirian et al. 1982). The new atypical antipsychotics may be associated with less sexual dysfunction than traditional antipsychotics, although futher research is necessary to establish this.

# Conclusions

This overview of sexual disorders at the boundary between obstetrics and gynecology and psychiatry is a reminder of how little definitive information is available and of the frequent need for a collaborative team approach to diagnosis and treatment planning. The field of human sexuality is an excellent opportunity for the psychiatrist, as a physician with training in both physical and psychologic medicine, to make a significant contribution to patient care.

# References

Alexander GM, Sherwin BB: Sex steroids, sexual behavior, and selective attention for erotic stimuli in women using oral contraceptives. Psychoneuroendocrinology 18:273–278, 1993

American Psychiatric Association: Diagnostic and Statistical Manual of Mental Disorders, 3rd Edition. Washington, DC, American Psychiatric Association, 1980

American Psychiatric Association: Diagnostic and Statistical Manual of Mental Disorders, 3rd Edition, Revised. Washington, DC, American Psychiatric Association, 1987

American Psychiatric Association: Diagnostic and Statistical Manual of Mental Disorders, 4th Edition. Washington, DC, American Psychiatric Association, 1994

Andersen BL: Quality of life for women with gynecological cancer. Curr Opin Obstet Gynecol 7:69–76, 1995

Andersen BL: Stress and quality of life following cervical cancer. J Natl Cancer Inst Monogr 21:61–70, 1996

Andersen BL, Hacher NF: Psychological adjustment following pelvic exenteration. Obstet Gynecol 61:331–338, 1983

Andersen BL, Turnquist D, LaPolla J, et al: Sexual functioning after treatment of in situ vulvar cancer: preliminary report. Obstet Gynecol 71:15–19, 1988

Ashton AK, Hamer R, Rosen RC: Serotonin reuptake inhibitor–induced sexual dysfunction and its treatments large scale retrospective study of 596 psychiatric outpatients. J Sex Marit Ther 23:165–175, 1997

Bachmann GA, Leiblum SR, Sandler B, et al: Correlates of sexual desire in postmenopausal women. Maturitas 7:211–216, 1985

Balon R, Yeragani UK, Pohl R, et al: Sexual dysfunction with antidepressant treatment. J Clin Psychiatry 54:209–212, 1993

Bancroft J: Human Sexuality and Its Problems. Edinburgh, UK, Churchill Livingstone, 1983

Bancroft J, Coles L: Three years' experience in a sexual problems clinic. BMJ 1:1575–1577, 1976

Bardwick J: Psychological factors in the acceptance and use of oral contraceptives, in Psychological Perspectives on Populations. Edited by Fawsett JT. New York, Basic Books, 1973, pp 133–152

Basson R, McInnes R, Smith MD, et al: Efficacy and safety of sildenafil in estrogenized women with sexual dysfunction associated with female sexual arousal disorder. Obstet Gynecol 95(suppl):S54, 2000a

Basson R, Berman J, Burnett A, et al: Report of the International Consensus Development Conference on Female Sexual Dysfunctions: definitions and classifications. J Urol 163:888–893, 2000b

Beck JG: Hypoactive sexual desire disorder: an overview. J Consult Clin Psychol 63:919–927, 1995

Becker JV, Skinner LJ, Abel GG, et al: Level of post-assault sexual functioning in rape and incest victims. Arch Sex Behav 15:37–49, 1986

Berard EJJ: The sexuality of spinal cord injured women: physiology and pathophysiology. A review. Paraplegia 27:99–112, 1989

Broun RS, Haddox J, Posada A, et al: Social and psychological adjustment following pelvic exenteration. Am J Obstet Gynecol 114:162–171, 1972

Burnap DW, Golden JS: Sexual problems in medical practice. J Med Educ 42:673–680, 1967

Catalan J, Bradley M, Gallwey J, et al: Sexual dysfunction and psychiatric morbidity in patients attending a clinic for sexually transmitted diseases. Br J Psychiatry 138:292–296, 1981

Chambless DL, Sultan FE, Stern TE: Effect of pubococcygeal exercise on coital orgasm in women. J Consult Clin Psychol 52:114–118, 1984

Cohen AW: Human sexuality during normal pregnancy, in Human Sexuality: Psychosexual Effects of Disease. Edited by Farber M. New York, Macmillan, 1985, pp 55–76

Coop J: Menopause: associated problems. BMJ 289:970, 1984

Coop J: Hormonal and non-hormonal intervention for menopausal symptoms. Maturitas 23:159–168, 1996

Coopen A, Bishop M, Beard RT, et al: Hysterectomy, hormones and behavior. Lancet 1:126–128, 1981

Crenshaw T, Goldberg JP: Sexual Pharmacology: Drugs that Affect Sexual Function. New York, WW Norton, 1996

Cullberg J: Mood changes and menstrual symptoms with different progestogen/estrogen combinations. Acta Psychiatr Scand Suppl 23:9–86, 1972

Davis SR: The clinical use of androgens in female sexual disorders. J Sex Marital Ther 24:153–163, 1998

Degen K: Sexual dysfunction in women using major tranquilizers. Psychosomatics 23:959–961, 1982

Demsey GM, Buchsbaum HJ, Morrison J: Psychosocial adjustment to pelvic exenteration. Gynecol Oncol 3:325–334, 1975

DiSala PJ, Creasman WT, Rich WM: An alternative approach to early cancer of the vulva. Am J Obstet Gynecol 133:825–829, 1979

Ende J, Rockwell S, Glasgow M: The sexual history in general medicine practice. Arch Intern Med 144:558–561, 1984

Farrell SA, Kieser K: Sexuality after hysterectomy. Obstet Gynecol 95:1045–1051, 2000

Fava M, Rankin MA, Alpert JE, et al: An open trial of oral sildenafil in antidepressant-induced sexual dysfunction. Psychother Psychosom 67:328–331, 1998

Feiger A, Kieva G, Shrivastava RK: Nefazodone versus sertraline in outpatients with major depression: focus on efficacy, tolerability and effects on sexual function and satisfaction. J Clin Psychiatr 57(suppl 1):1–11, 1996

Friedman CM: The decision-making process and the outcome of therapeutic abortion. Am J Psychiatry 131:1332–1337, 1974

Gebhard DH, Pomeroy WB, Martin CE, et al: Pregnancy, Birth, and Abortion. New York, Harper & Row, 1958

Ghadirian AM, Chouinard G, Annable L: Sexual dysfunction and plasma prolactin levels in neuroleptic-treated schizophrenia outpatients. J Nerv Ment Dis 170:463–467, 1982

Greenblatt RB, Barfield WE, Garner JF, et al: Evaluation of an estrogen, androgen, estrogen-androgen combination and a placebo in the treatment of the menopause. J Clin Endocrinol 10:1547–1558, 1950

Harrison WM, Rabkin JG, Ernhardt AA: Effects of antidepressant medication on sexual function: a controlled study. J Clin Psychopharmacol 6:144–149, 1986

Havenga K, Enker WE, McDermutt K, et al: Male and female sexual and urinary function after total mesorectal excision with autonomic nerve preservation for carcinoma of the rectum. J Am Coll Surg 182:495–502, 1996

Hawton K, Catalan J, Martin P, et al: Prognostic factors in sex therapy. Behav Res Ther 24:377–385, 1986

Hoon EF, Hoon PW: Styles of sexual expression in women: clinical implications of multi-variate analysis. Arch Sex Behav 7:105–116, 1978

Hughes A, Segraves RT, Kavoussi R, et al: Double-blind comparison of bupropion and sertraline in depressed outpatients: safety, efficacy, and sexual function. ACNP, San Juan, Puerto Rico, December 1996

Isojarvi JI, Pakarinen AJ, Ravtio A, et al: Serum sex hormone levels after replacing carbamazepine with oxcarbazepine. Eur J Clin Pharmacol 47:461–464, 1995

Kaplan HS: Hypoactive sexual desire. J Sex Marital Ther 3:3–9, 1977

Kaplan HS: The comprehensive evaluation of the psychosexual disorder, in The Evaluation of Sexual Disorders: Psychological and Medical Aspects. Edited by Kaplan HS. New York, Brunner/Mazel, 1983a

Kaplan HS: The data, in the Evaluation of Sexual Disorders: Psychological and Medical Aspects. Edited by Kaplan HS. New York, Brunner/Mazel, 1983b

Kaplan HS: Does the cat technique enhance female orgasm? J Sex Marit Ther 18:285–302, 1992

Kaufman SA: The gynecological evaluation of female dyspareunia and unconsummated marriage, in The Evaluation of Sexual Disorders: Psychological and Medical Aspects. Edited by Kaplan HS. New York, Brunner/Mazel, 1983a

Kaufman SA: The gynecological evaluation of female excitement disorders, in The Evaluation of Sexual Disorders: Psychological and Medical Aspects. Edited by Kaplan HS, New York, Brunner/Mazel, 1983b

Kegel AH: Sexual functions of the puboccygeous muscle. West J Surg 60:521–524, 1956

Kinzel FL, Mangweth B, Traweger C, et al: Sexuelle funktionsstorungen bei Mannern und Frauen. Psychother Psychosom Med Psychol 47:41–45, 1997

Koehler JD: Sexual dysfunction, in Primary Care in Obstetrics and Gynecology. Edited by Sanfilippo JS, Smith RP. New York, Springer, 1998, pp 485–524

Kolodny RC: Sexual dysfunction in diabetic females. Diabetes 20:557–559, 1971

Kotin J, Wilbert BE, Verburg D, et al: Thioridazine and sexual functioning. Am J Psychiatry 33:82–85, 1976

Laumann EO, Gagnon JM, Michael RT, et al (eds): The social organization of sexuality, in Sexual Practices in the United States. Chicago, University of Chicago, 1994

Leeton J, McMaster R, Worsley A: The effects on sexual response and mood after sterilization of women taking long term oral contraceptives: results of a double-blind crossover study. Aust N Z J Obstet Gynaecol 18:194–197, 1978

Leiblum SR: Impact of infertility on sexual and marital satisfaction. Ann Rev Sex Res 4:99–120, 1993

Levine SB: Hypoactive sexual desire and other problems of sexual desire, in Treatments of Psychiatric Disorders: A Task Force Report of the American Psychiatric Association, Vol 3. Washington, DC, American Psychiatric Association, 1989, pp 2264–2279

Levine SB, Yost MA: Frequency of sexual dysfunction in a general gynecological clinic: an epidemiological approach. Arch Sex Behav 5:229–238, 1976

Lief HI: Inhibited sexual desire. Medical Aspects of Human Sexuality 7:94–95, 1977

Lief HI: Evaluation of inhibited sexual desire: relationship aspects, in Comprehensive Evaluation of Disorders of Sexual Desire. Edited by Kaplan HS. Washington, DC, American Psychiatric Press, 1985, pp 59–76

Lilius HG, Valtonen EJ, Wikstrom J: Sexual problems in patients suffering from multiple sclerosis. J Chronic Dis 29:643–647, 1976

Lindal E, Stefansson JG: The lifetime prevalence of psychosexual dysfunction among 55–57 year olds in Iceland. Soc Psychiatry Psychiatr Epidemiol 28:91–95, 1993

LoPiccollo L: Low sexual desire, in Principles and Practice of Sex Therapy. Edited by Leiblum SR, Pervin LA. New York, Guilford, 1980, pp 29–64

Lundberg PO: Sexual dysfunction in patients with multiple sclerosis. Sexuality and Disability 1:218–222, 1978

Masters WH, Johnson VE: Human Sexual Response. Boston, MA, Little, Brown, 1966

Michelson D, Bancroft J, Targum S, et al: Female sexual dysfunction associated with antidepressant administration: a randomized, placebo-controlled study of pharmacological intervention. Am J Psychiatry 157:239–243, 2000

Modell JG, Katholi CR, Modell JD, et al: Comparative sexual side effects of bupropion, fluoxetine, paroxetine, and sertraline. Clin Pharmacol Ther 61:476–487, 1997

Monteiro WO, Noshirvani HF, Marks IM: Anorgasmia from clomipramine in obsessive-compulsive disorder: a controlled trial. Br J Psychiatry 151:107–112, 1987

Montejo AL, Lorca G, Izquierdo JA, et al: SSRI-induced sexual dysfunction: fluoxetine, paroxetine, sertraline, and fluvoxamine in a prospective multicenter and descriptive clinical study of 344 patients. J Sex Marital Ther 2:176–194, 1997

Moore C: Female sexual arousal disorder and inhibited female orgasm, in Treatments of Psychiatric Disorders: A Task Force Report of the American Psychiatric Association, Vol 3. Washington, DC, American Psychiatric Association, 1989, pp 2279–2290

Morrell MJ, Dixen JM, Carter SC, et al: The influence of age and cycling status on sexual arousability in women. Am J Obstet Gynecol 148:66–71, 1984

Munday RN, Cox LW: Hysterectomy for benign lesions. Med J Aust 2:759–763, 1967

Musher JS: Anorgasmia with the use of fluoxetine. Am J Psychiatry 147:948, 1990

Myers L, Morokoff P: Physiological and subjective sexual arousal in pre- and postmenopausal women. Poster presented at the annual meeting of the American Psychological Association, Los Angeles, CA, August 1985

Nathan SG: The epidemiology of the DSM-III psychosexual dysfunctions. J Sex Marital Ther 12:267–282, 1986

Nemeroff CB, Ninan PT, Ballenger J, et al: Double-blind comparison of fluvoxamine versus sertraline in the treatment of depressed outpatients. Depression 3:163–169, 1995

Palace EM, Gorzalka BB: Differential patterns of arousal in sexually functional and dysfunctional women: physiological and subjective components of sexual response. Arch Sex Behav 21:135–159, 1992

Pearce J, Hawton K, Blake F: Psychological and sexual symptoms associated with the menopause and the effects of hormone replacement. Br J Psychiatry 167:163–173, 1995

Perkins RP: Sexuality in pregnancy: what determines behavior? Obstet Gynecol 59:189–198, 1982

Poad D, Arnold EP: Sexual function after pelvic surgery in women. Aust N Z Obstet Gynecol 34:471–474, 1994

Reamy K, White S, Daniell W, et al: Sexuality and pregnancy. J Reprod Med 27:321–329, 1982

Renshaw DC: Profile of 2376 patients treated at the Loyola Sex Clinic between 1972 and 1987. J Sex Marital Ther 3:111–117, 1988

Rhodes JC, Kjerulff KH, Langenberg PW, et al: Hysterectomy and sexual functioning. JAMA 282:1934–1941, 1999

Riley AJ, Riley EJ: The effect of single dose diazepam on female sexual response induced by masturbation. Sexual and Marital Therapy 1:49–53, 1986

Rinehart JS, Schiff I: Sexuality and the menopause, in Human Sexuality: Psychosexual Effects of Disease. Edited by Farber M. New York, Macmillan, 1985, pp 77–84

Rosen RC, Leiblum SR: Assessment and treatment of desire disorders, in Principles and Practice of Sex Therapy. Edited by Leiblum SR, Rosen RC. New York, Guilford, 1989, pp 19–50

Rosen RC, Leiblum SR: Treatment of sexual disorders in the 1990's: an integrated approach. J Consult Clin Psychol 63:877–890, 1995

Rosen RC, Taylor JF, Leiblum SR, et al: Prevalence of sexual dysfunction in women: results of a survey study of 329 women in an outpatient gynecological clinic. J Sex Marital Ther 19:171–188, 1993

Rosen RC, Lane RM, Menza M: Effects of SSRIs on sexual function: a critical review. J Clin Psychopharmacol 19:67–84, 1999

Salzer LP: Infertility: How Couples Can Cope. Boston, MA, GK Hall, 1986

Sangal R: Inhibited female orgasm as a side effect of alprazolam. Am J Psychiatry 142:1223–1224, 1985

Schaller JL, Behar D: Sildenafil citrate for SSRI- induced sexual side effects. Am J Psychiatry 156:156–157, 1999

Schover LR, Jensen SB: Sexuality and Chronic Illness: A Comprehensive Approach. New York, Guilford, 1988

Schover LR, LoPiccollo J: Effectiveness of treatment for dysfunction of sexual desire. J Sex Marital Ther 8:179–197, 1982

Schover LR, von Eschenback AS: Sexual function and female radical cystectomy: a case series. J Urol 134:465–468, 1985

Schover LR, Evans RB, von Eschenback AC: Sexual rehabilitation in a cancer center: diagnosis and outcome in 384 consultations. Arch Sex Behav 16:445–461, 1987

Schreiner-Engel P, Schiavi RC, Vietrorisz D, et al: The differential impact of diabetes type on female sexuality. J Psychosom Res 31:23–33, 1987

Segraves KB, Segraves RT: Hypoactive sexual desire disorder: prevalence and comorbidity in 906 subjects. J Sex Marital Ther 17:55–58, 1991a

Segraves KB, Segraves RT: Multiple-phase sexual dysfunction. J Sex Educ Ther 17:154–156, 1991b

Segraves RT: Antidepressant induced orgasm disorder. J Sex Marital Ther 21:192–201, 1995

Segraves RT: Neuropsychiatric aspects of sexual dysfunction, in Neuropsychiatry. Edited by Fogel BS, Schiffer RB, Roa SM. Baltimore, MD, Williams and Wilkins, 1996, pp 757–770

Segraves RT, Segraves KB: Diagnosis of female arousal disorder. Sexual and Marital Therapy 6:9–14, 1991

Segraves RT, Segraves KB: Medical aspects of orgasm disorders, in Handbook on the Assessment and Treatment of Sexual Dysfunction. Edited by O'Donohue W, Geer JH. New York, Pergamon, 1993, pp 225–252

Segraves RT, Croft H, Kavousi R, et al: Bupropion sustained release for the treatment of hypoactive sexual desire in nondepressed women. Poster presentation, New Clinical Drug Evaluation Unit meeting, Boca Raton, FL, 2000

Sjogren B, Poppen B: Sexual life in women after colectomy-proctomucosectomy with S-pouch. Acta Obstet Gynecol Scand 74:51–55, 1995

Spector IP, Carey MP: Incidence and prevalence of the sexual dysfunctions: a critical review of the empirical literature. Arch Sex Behav 4:389–408, 1990

Waldinger MD, Hengeveld MW, Zwinderman AH, et al: Effect of SSRI antidepressants on ejaculation: a double-blind, randomized, placebo-controlled study with fluoxetine, fluvoxamine, paroxetine, and sertraline. J Clin Psychopharmacol 18:274–281, 1998

Young RL: Androgens in postmenopausal women. Menopause Management 2:21–24, 1993

# Psychopharmacology in Women

OLGA BRAWMAN-MINTZER, M.D.
KIMBERLY A. YONKERS, M.D.

## Introduction

For many years, pharmacologic treatment for women was based on the assumption that women and men metabolize and respond to drugs in a similar manner. This assumption was reinforced by a lack of research data due to the exclusion of women from the pharmacologic clinical treatment trials that determined therapeutic doses of drugs. Recently, however, the U.S. Food and Drug Administration revised the guidelines that excluded women of childbearing potential from clinical trials, and the National Institutes of Health introduced similar changes for government-sponsored studies (U.S. Food and Drug Administration 1993).

Despite these limitations, data from available studies suggest that considerable gender differences may exist in the pharmacokinetics (i.e., absorption, distribution, biotransformation, and elimination) and the pharmacodynamics (i.e., biochemical and physiologic effects) of many pharmacologic agents. It has also become clear that certain gender-specific events such as menstruation, oral contraceptive (OC) use, and pregnancy can affect drug metabolism and even end-organ receptor sensitivity.

As with other pharmacologic agents, the pharmacokinetics and pharmacodynamics of many psychotropic agents may be affected by these factors. Unfortunately, although women are prescribed psychotropic agents more frequently than are men, available data on gender-related variation in the effects of these agents are limited. This chapter highlights recent data on gender differences in the pharmacokinetics and pharmacodynamics of drugs and the effects of menstruation and OC use on the administration of psychotropic agents. It should be noted that issues such as use of psychotropic agents during pregnancy and breastfeeding are important topics as well, but are beyond the scope of this chapter.

## Gender Differences in Pharmacokinetics

### Absorption and Bioavailability

The amount of drug absorbed by the gastrointestinal tract depends on the acid base and lipophilic properties of the medication as well as the physiology of the gastrointestinal tract. The degree to which a drug is ionized affects its solubility. It has been suggested that women may secrete less gastric acid than do men, leading to potential gender differences in absorption (Grossman et al. 1963). This decrease in gastric acid secretion may decrease both enzymatic action and the absorption of weak acids but may increase absorption of weak bases.

Several studies suggest gender differences in gastric emptying and gastrointestinal transit time. For example, Wald et al. (1981) reported that gastrointestinal transit time was significantly prolonged in women during the luteal phase of the menstrual cycle. Other researchers (Datz et al. 1987) demonstrated similar results (i.e., that women empty solids from their stomachs more slowly than do men). The mechanism for these differences is unknown, but researchers hypothesize that it may be due to the effects of progesterone and estradiol on the gastrointestinal tract. However, some studies have failed to demonstrate significant effects of menstrual hormones on gastrointestinal transit time (Degen and Phillips 1996).

Gender differences in the activity of various gastrointestinal enzymes may also affect drug metabolism. For example, the gut contains large levels of cytochrome P450 (CYP450) 3A4 isoenzyme (Kolars et al. 1991; Strobel et al. 1991), an important liver enzyme that appears to be more active in women than in men. It is unknown, however, whether increased activity of CYP450 3A4 in the liver also affects the gastrointestinal enzyme analogue.

It should be noted that, despite potential differences in gastric acid secretion, gastrointestinal transit time, and enzyme activity, no consistent differences in the absorption and the bioavailability of specific agents have been observed. Only a few cases of gender differences in the absorption of some drugs have been documented. For example, Aarons et al. (1989) observed that, after oral administration, aspirin was absorbed more rapidly in women than in men, and other researchers have found higher bioavailability of aspirin in women then men, indicating potential clinically relevant gender differences in the gastrointestinal tract (Ho et al. 1985).

## Distribution

Several factors may affect the distribution of a drug in the body, including acid base, water and lipid solubility, and the affinity of the drug for binding proteins (Riester et al. 1980) as well as differences in blood volume, cardiac output, and organ size (Gilman et al. 1990). The ratio of lean body mass to adipose tissue mass may also affect distribution. In general, women have a lower ratio of lean body mass to adipose tissue (Seeman 1989). Thus, drugs with high affinity for adipose tissue, such as diazepam, would be expected to demonstrate a greater volume of distribution in women.

Specifically, the half-life for these drugs may become prolonged and serum levels may be greater in patients with less lean body mass. This information may be critical to understanding patients' responses to treatment. Women patients with a higher percentage of fat at any given body weight may also require higher initial dose, but maintenance of the same dose over time will cause drug accumulation leading to potentially toxic effects. However, the effects of gender in relationship to specific drugs have not been specifically studied.

## Metabolism

Metabolic processes in the liver are divided into two types of reactions. Phase I reactions, including oxidation, hydroxylation, N-demethylation, reduction, and hydrolysis, are mediated through CYP450. Phase II reactions consist of glucoronidation, sulfation, methylation, and acetylation of parent molecules and phase I reaction products. Data have indicated that significant gender-related differences in hepatic enzyme activity may exist.

### Cytochrome P450

In 1971, O'Malley et al. reported that the metabolism of phenazone (antipyrine) is influenced by gender. At that time, antipyrine metabolism was thought to reflect total CYP450 activity. However, in recent years many isoenzymes of CYP450 have been identified, and data on potential gender differences in the activity of these various isoenzymes is increasing. Because most antidepressants and antipsychotic drugs are either metabolized by—or inhibit to varying degrees—one or more CYP450 isoenzymes, the potential gender differences in the activity of these isoenzymes may be of particular relevance to the clinician.

**Cytochrome P3A4.** Cytochrome P3A4 (CYP3A4) is considered clinically the most important CYP450 enzyme, constituting as much as 60% of the total P450 content of in vitro liver specimens (Guengerich 1990). CYP3A4 metabolizes a broad range of compounds, including alprazolam, midazolam, diazepam, terfenadine, astemizole, carbamazepine, sertraline, tricyclic antidepressants (TCAs), calcium channel blockers, erythromycin, steroids, quinidine, lidocaine, and others (Kerr et al. 1994; Murray 1992; Pollock 1994; D. A. Smith and Jones 1992).

In vitro evidence for varied inhibition of CYP3A3/4 by frequently prescribed antidepressants, such as the selective serotonin reuptake inhibitors (SSRIs) fluvoxamine, fluoxetine, and sertraline, is important (von Moltke et al. 1995). Plasma concentrations of some drugs metabolized by this isoenzyme have been observed to increase during concomitant therapy with fluvoxamine, nefazodone, fluoxetine, and sertraline but not with paroxetine (Andersen et al. 1991). Thus, potential gender differences in the activity of CYP3A4 may be of considerable clinical importance. Indeed, substantial data indicate that young women may have approximately 1.4 times the CYP3A4 activity of men. For example, erythromycin is metabolized 25% more rapidly by microsomes made from the human female liver than by microsomes made from the male liver (Hunt et al. 1992).

Other drugs showing similar gender differences in clearance include diazepam (Greenblatt et al. 1980a; Hulst et al. 1994), verapamil (Schwartz et al. 1994), and midazolam (Gilmore et al. 1992; Rugstad et al. 1986). It is possible that progesterone, which has been shown to activate CYP3A4 in vitro (Kerlan et al. 1992; Kerr et al. 1994), may be responsible for the observed gender differences in enzyme activity in vivo. However, it should be noted that other researchers have found no evidence for gender-related differences in CYP3A4-mediated drug metabolism, although these discrepancies may be caused by interindividual variations in CYP3A4 activity (Lobo et al. 1986; May et al. 1994; Schmucker et al. 1990; Shimada et al. 1994; Sitar et al. 1989; Yee et al. 1986).

**Cytochrome P2D6.** Cytochrome P2D6 (CYP2D6) is the most extensively studied of the CYP450 isoenzymes (Brosen 1990). Approximately 5%–

10% of Caucasians lack this isoenzyme as a result of an autosomal recessively transmitted defect in gene expression. Such "poor metabolizers" may exhibit greater bioavailability, higher plasma concentrations, prolonged elimination half-lives, and (possibly) exaggerated pharmacologic response from standard doses of drugs metabolized by CYP2D6. When drugs that inhibit CYP2D6 are administered with drugs metabolized by this enzyme, individuals who are extensive metabolizers will, in effect, be converted to "poor metabolizers."

CYP2D6 metabolizes many different classes of drugs, including anti-depressants, antipsychotics, β-adrenergic blockers, type 1C antiarrhythmics, dextromethorphan, and some chemotherapeutic agents. Codeine and ven-lafaxine are both O-demethylated by this enzyme (Brosen and Gram 1989; Otton et al. 1994). Nortriptyline, desipramine, and imipramine are hydroxy-lated by CYP2D6. Several different drugs potentially inhibit the CYP2D6 enzyme, including quinidine, fluphenazine, haloperidol, thioridazine, ami-triptyline, desipramine, and clomipramine. All SSRIs except fluvoxamine are potent inhibitors of CYP2D6 in vitro (Brosen 1990; Crewe et al. 1992; Otton et al. 1993; Pollock 1994).

Few studies to date have examined the influence of gender on CYP2D6-mediated metabolism. Gex-Fabry et al. (1990) have shown that the hydroxy-lation of clomipramine is higher in men than in women. Similarly, Abernethy et al. (1985) found that oral clearance of desipramine is greater in men than in women. However, the authors of these two studies did not account for dif-ferences in body weight. Similar results were also shown for propranolol (Gilmore et al. 1992; Walle et al. 1985, 1989, 1994) and ondansetron (Prit-chard et al. 1992); however, some data indicate that these two drugs may not be metabolized predominantly by the CYP2D6 system (Ashford et al. 1994; Walle et al. 1989).

Cytochrome P2C.    Cytochrome P2C (CYP2C) is a subfamily of en-zymes that includes 2C9, 2C10, 2C19, and others. Diazepam, clomipramine, amitriptyline, and imipramine are demethylated by CYP2C enzymes. In ad-dition, warfarin (Rettie et al. 1992), phenytoin (D. A. Smith and Jones 1992), tolbutamide (Knodell et al. 1987), and certain nonsteroidal anti-inflammatory agents (Newlands et al. 1992) are also believed to be metabolized by CYP2C enzymes. Based on observed increases in plasma concentrations of concomi-tantly administered drugs metabolized by this family of enzymes, it is be-lieved that the SSRIs fluvoxamine, fluoxetine, and sertraline may inhibit CYP2C isoenzymes (Jalil 1992; Skjelbo and Brosen 1992).

Research has shown that the activity of CYP2C19 may be higher in men than in women. Hooper and Qing (1990) have demonstrated that men clear methyl phenobarbital, a compound metabolized by CYP2C19, approximately 1.3 times faster than in women. The metabolism of piroxicam exhibited a similar gender effect (Rugstad et al. 1986). However, these differences were not seen by others when adjustments were made for weight (Richardson et al. 1985).

**Cytochrome P1A2.** Cytochrome P1A2 (CYP1A2) isoenzyme is involved in the metabolism of theophylline, caffeine (Wrighton and Stevens 1992), TCAs (Brosen et al. 1993; Pollock 1994), clozapine (Jerling et al. 1994), and possibly thiothixene (Ereshefsky et al. 1991). CYP1A2 is induced by cigarette smoke, charcoal-broiled foods, and cabbage (Brosen et al. 1993; Guengerich 1992; Pollock 1994). Furthermore, CYP1A2 shows potent inhibition by fluvoxamine in vitro (Brosen et al. 1993). However, other SSRIs do not appear to inhibit this isoenzyme.

Data regarding gender-related differences in the activity of CYP1A2 are scarce and conflicting. Using data from studies of caffeine and thiothixene metabolism, it appears that CYP1A2 activity may be higher in men than in women (Ereshefsky et al. 1991; Relling et al. 1992). In contrast, Nafziger and Bertino (1989) reported that theophylline is cleared significantly faster in young women than in men. Interestingly, gender differences in theophylline metabolism do not appear to be present in elderly patients, suggesting that this difference could be hormone dependent rather than caused by genetic differences (Cuzzolin et al. 1990). Furthermore, clomipramine demethylation, which may be performed by CYP1A2, is not influenced by gender (Gex-Fabry et al. 1990). Thus, given the available data, no definite conclusions on the effects of gender on CYP1A2 activity can be drawn at this point.

*Conjugation*

Many drugs are excreted by the kidneys after conjugation with sulfate or glucuronic acid. Frequently, conjugation reactions are the second metabolic step after the drug has been metabolized, involving relatively slower cytochrome-mediated hydroxylation. Because cytochrome-mediated metabolism is often the rate-limiting step, it may not be possible to detect any gender-related differences in conjugation reactions for these drugs. However, several drugs are metabolized solely by conjugation and appear to display gender-related differences in their elimination. For example, the benzodiazepines temazepam and oxazepam, which are eliminated by conjugation, are cleared faster by men than by women (Divoll et al. 1981; Greenblatt et al. 1980b). Faster elimination in men was also observed for the clearance of digoxin (Yukawa et al.

1992), although the observed differences may be related to differences in renal function. Clearance of paracetamol was also greater (22%) in young men compared with young women (Miners et al. 1983). However, other compounds that are cleared by glucoronidation, such as ibuprofen, are not influenced by gender (Greenblatt et al. 1984).

## Effects of the Menstrual Cycle

As mentioned earlier, several possible menstrual-phase–specific changes may have considerable impact on the metabolism of drugs in women. For example, gastrointestinal transit time varies during the menstrual cycle (McBurney 1991; Sweeting 1992). Subsequently, absorption in the small intestine may be increased during the luteal phase when the gastrointestinal transit time is prolonged. Other potential menstrual-phase–related changes that may affect drug metabolism include increases and decreases in the volume of distribution. Although empirical data are lacking, it can be hypothesized that increases in fluid retention that are related to the menstrual phase may dilute the concentration of medications, thus resulting in lower plasma levels and vice versa. One study also found evidence of menstrual-phase changes in transcapillary fluid dynamics that resulted in fluid shifts between intravascular and extravascular spaces (Pollan and Oian 1986).

A small number of reports have demonstrated a menstrual-phase influence on drug pharmacokinetics. Lew et al. (1993) found that the elimination of methylprednisolone is more variable in premenopausal women than in postmenopausal women or in men, suggesting a menstrual cycle effect. These authors could not, however, correlate the magnitude of drug elimination to the phase of the menstrual cycle. Furthermore, Lane et al. (1992) found that caffeine clearance is slower in the luteal than in the follicular phase of the menstrual cycle. In contrast, phenytoin elimination appears to be highest at the end of the menstrual cycle (Shavit et al. 1984). The menstrual cycle does not, however, appear to affect the metabolism of other compounds studied, such as alprazolam (Kirkwood et al. 1991), nitrazepam (Jochemsen et al. 1982), and phenobarbital (Backstrom and Jorpes 1979).

Finally, data indicate that monoamine oxidase activity may be decreased by estrogens and increased by progesterone, suggesting menstrual variations in a critical metabolic pathway for most psychotropic drugs (Banwick 1976; Klaiber et al. 1979). The clinical significance of these changes is unknown.

These data highlight the importance of establishing menstrual cycle phase when investigating pharmacodynamic as well as pharmacokinetic properties of psychotropic medications in women. Furthermore, it may be clinically relevant to explore the potential effects of menstrual cycle phase when adverse effects of medications occur or when there are fluctuations in drug efficacy.

## Oral Contraception

Oral contraceptives are among the most widely used drugs in the world. OCs influence the pharmacokinetics and pharmacodynamics of other compounds. For example, estrogen exerts a stimulatory effect on protein synthesis, which in turn may affect protein-binding of various drugs. OCs may also interfere with the elimination of other drugs through inhibition of various cytochrome P450 isoenzymes (phase I reactions), which leads to increased pharmacologic activity of drugs metabolized by the appropriate isoenzymes. Clearance of the benzodiazepines triazolam, alprazolam (Stoehr et al. 1984), and nitrazepam (Jochemsen et al. 1982), compounds that are metabolized by CYP450 isoenzymes, was reduced when OCs were taken concomitantly. The TCA imipramine is also affected by OCs. For example, Abernethy et al. (1984) found that OCs inhibited the metabolism of intravenous imipramine. When imipramine was given orally, this effect was counterbalanced by the change in oral availability and decreased apparent oral clearance. In contrast, clomipramine is not influenced by OCs, although its metabolic rate is enhanced by estrogens and inhibited by progesterone in animal models (Fletcher et al. 1965). OCs may also affect phase II reactions, such as conjugation with glucoronic and sulfuric acid, through enzyme induction. Thus, benzodiazepines that undergo conjugation, such as temazepam, show higher clearance in the presence of OCs (Stoehr et al. 1984).

The clinical significance of the effects of concomitant OC use in patients receiving psychotropic medications was demonstrated by Ellinwood et al. (1984). They found impairment in cognitive and psychomotor tasks in women taking diazepam and OCs during the week that the subjects did not take hormones, because benzodiazepine levels peaked more quickly. They postulated that OCs decrease the rate of absorption of diazepam, and during the week off of hormones the plasma levels quickly rose to intoxicating levels. Contrasting findings were reported by Kroboth et al. (1985) for other benzodiazepines such as alprazolam, triazolam, and lorazepam. In this study, psychomotor changes were most marked in women who received OCs. However, in both cases plasma levels did not correlate with the observed clinical effect. Finally, although no data are available, changes in protein synthesis can affect end-organ response to drugs at the cellular level.

In summary, it appears that, given the potential interaction between exogenous hormones and various psychotropic medications, it may be important to assess OC use prior to any psychopharmacologic intervention.

# Gender Differences in Psychotropic Agents

## Antipsychotic Agents

The literature analyzing pharmacokinetics, pharmacodynamics, and side effects of psychotropic agents by gender is the most substantial for antipsychotic drugs. Most studies have found that women treated with antipsychotic medications experienced greater improvement than did men. For example, Chouinard and Annable (1982) found that women had greater improvement than did men after treatment with pimozide and chlorpromazine. Similarly, Szymanski et al. (1995) reported that female schizophrenic patients had a better treatment response to antipsychotics than did men, whereas plasma drug levels did not differ significantly between men and women. However, some reports have indicated a lack of gender differences in neuroleptic treatment response in men and women when subjects were matched for clinical, treatment, and demographic characteristics (Pinals et al. 1996).

Researchers have hypothesized that the generally greater efficacy of neuroleptics in young women may be caused by the presumed antidopaminergic effects of estrogen (Fields and Gordon 1982; Villeneuve et al. 1978). Estrogen has been thought to play a protective (i.e., neuroleptic-like) role in the disease protection process of schizophrenia, leading to the delay of illness development (Seeman 1996; Seeman and Lang 1990) and a better response to neuroleptics. Interestingly, Kulkarni et al. (1996) found that schizophrenic women who received estradiol in addition to neuroleptic treatment improved more rapidly compared with the group that received neuroleptics only. However, this difference was not sustained for the entire duration of the trial.

Clinicians have also noted that women may require lower doses of neuroleptics than men despite similarities in weight and age. It appears that women may achieve higher plasma levels of antipsychotics than men (Chouinard et al. 1986; Simpson et al. 1990). Simpson et al. (1990) found higher fluphenazine levels in women despite comparable dosing and similar age and weight characteristics. Chouinard et al. (1986) investigated fluspirilene, a long-acting injectable neuroleptic, and found that women required roughly half the dosage required by men despite similar weight and age characteristics. In this trial, the prescribed doses were titrated to therapeutic efficacy, but serum levels were not available. Another study found that men had significantly higher oral clearance of thiothixene than did women and that clearance did not necessarily correlate with body weight (Ereshefsky et al. 1991). The authors also found a reduction in clearance for subjects over the age of 50. Centorrino et al. (1994) reported that, despite a 60% lower milligram per kilogram dose in women, the levels of clozapine were 40% higher in nonsmoking women than men and did not vary by diagnosis or age in the study sample.

Gender-related differences were also observed in the expression of antipsychotic-induced side effects. For example, the incidence of tardive dyskinesia (TD) has been reported as greater in women than in men in several studies (Chouinard et al. 1979; J. M. Smith and Dunn 1979). Women have also been reported to suffer more severe TD symptoms. J. M. Smith and Dunn (1979) reported that the severity of TD increased significantly in women older than 67 years. Yassar and Jeste (1992) combined data from independent studies on prevalence, age, and gender differences in TD and found that TD is more prevalent in older women. Chouinard et al. (1980) noted that young men reported a higher prevalence of severe dyskinesias than did women; they explained this discrepancy by suggesting that postmenopausal status and loss of estrogen-induced supersensitivity may favor the development of TD in postmenopausal women.

Data on the impact of gender on the development of Parkinsonism are limited. Jeste (1995) reported that women who take lower doses of neuroleptic medications have similar or lower risks of Parkinsonism compared with men.

In summary, the available literature indicates that several clinically significant gender-related differences in the effects of neuroleptic medications may exist. However, further well-controlled research is clearly indicated.

## Benzodiazepines

In contrast to the research on antipsychotic agents, relatively few studies have evaluated the therapeutic effects and side effects of benzodiazepines in women. Available studies focus primarily on potential gender-related differences in the pharmacokinetics of benzodiazepines. For example, Greenblatt et al. (1980a) found that diazepam, which is oxidatively metabolized, has a higher clearance in younger women than in men. This difference disappeared in women 62–84 years of age. MacLeod et al. (1979) found that women metabolized diazepam more slowly than did men, regardless of age. Nitrazepam, a benzodiazepine metabolized by reduction, was not found to have gender-related differences in clearance (Jochemsen et al. 1982). Metabolism of alprazolam, a benzodiazepine that undergoes oxidation, was not influenced significantly by gender or menstrual cycle phase (Greenblatt and Wright 1993). However, temazepam and oxazepam, benzodiazepines that undergo conjugation, had slower clearance rates among women patients compared with men in several studies (Divoll et al. 1981; Greenblatt et al. 1980b; R. B. Smith et al. 1983). This difference was present regardless of age (R. B. Smith et al. 1983).

As mentioned, data regarding gender differences in the effects as well as the side effects of benzodiazepines are limited. Ellinwood et al. (1984) found that cognitive and psychomotor tasks performed by women taking diazepam and OCs were more impaired during the week off hormones because benzodiazepine levels peaked more quickly. Interestingly, van Haaren et al. (1997) observed that high doses of chlordiazepoxide increased response efficiency in male rats, but decreased response efficiency in female rats in animal models. Finally, Pesce et al. (1994) found that the incidence of benzodiazepine withdrawal seizures produced by the administration of flumazenil was significantly lower in male than in female diazepam-treated mice.

In summary, it appears that despite varied methodology in the available studies, current data suggest gender-related differences in the metabolism and potentially in the effects and side effects of the various benzodiazepines.

## Antidepressant Agents

Although mood disorders are more prevalent in women than in men (Kessler et al. 1996), little attention has been devoted to the research of antidepressant effects in women. This is not surprising in light of the exclusion of women from many pharmacologic trials, a policy that, as mentioned earlier, has only recently been revised.

Several gender-related differences in the pharmacokinetics of antidepressants have been reported, however. For example, higher plasma levels of certain TCAs were observed in women compared with those observed in men. Moody et al. (1967) found that women had higher plasma levels of imipramine than did men. Similarly, Preskorn and Mac (1985) reported that women and older subjects had higher plasma levels of amitriptyline than did young men. Gex-Fabry et al. (1990) found that the hydroxylation clearance of clomipramine is lower in women than in men, whereas Abernethy et al. (1985) reported greater oral clearance of desipramine in men than in women.

However, neither the Abernethy nor the Gex-Fabry studies normalized for body weight. In contrast, Ziegler and Biggs (1977) found no significant gender differences in plasma levels of amitriptyline and nortriptyline. Finally, Greenblatt et al. (1987) found that the volume of distribution of trazodone was greater in women and the elderly, but clearance was significantly reduced only in older men.

In recent years data have also emerged on potential gender differences in the pharmacokinetics of SSRIs and other new antidepressants. In fact, several researchers have observed that plasma concentrations of sertraline were approximately 35%–40% lower in young men than in women and elderly men (Ronfeld et al. 1997; Warrington 1991). Similarly, plasma concentrations of fluvoxamine have been shown to be 40%–50% lower in men than in women, with the magnitude of effect possibly greater at lower medication doses (Hartter et al. 1993). Of the other antidepressants, the levels of nefazodone were found to be higher in elderly women compared with younger subjects and elderly men (Barbhaiya et al. 1996). In contrast, Klamerus et al. (1996) reported that gender did not substantially alter the disposition or the tolerance of venlafaxine.

As mentioned, data regarding gender-related differences in treatment response to antidepressants are scarce. Several available studies indicate that women may respond less to TCAs than do men, but may respond better to SSRIs and monoamine oxidase inhibitors (MAOIs). A study by Davidson and Pelton (1986) evaluated the efficacy of TCAs and MAOIs by gender in three types of atypical depression. They found that depressed women who also had panic attacks had a more favorable response to MAOIs than to TCAs, whereas men who were depressed and had panic attacks responded more favorably to TCAs. Similarly, Raskin (1974) found that young women (younger than 40 years) responded less well to imipramine than did older women and men. Finally, Steiner et al. (1993) compared the effects of paroxetine, imipramine, and placebo in outpatients with major depression and found that women responded better to paroxetine than to imipramine.

Thus, it appears that some clinically meaningful gender-specific differences may exist in the efficacy and tolerability of the antidepressant medications.

## Conclusions

This chapter reviews the available literature on the potential gender-related differences in the pharmacokinetics and pharmacodynamics of psychotropic medications. The surprising outcome of this review is that significant gaps exist in the experimental data addressing these issues. Nevertheless, available evidence suggests certain potentially meaningful gender-related variations in the pharmacokinetics of various compounds. Furthermore, the menstrual cycle phase and the use of OCs may also affect the metabolism, distribution, and clearance of certain drugs. Examination of specific psychotropic agents indicates that 1) the effects of benzodiazepines are influenced by gender, menstrual cycle phase and concurrent use of OCs; 2) antipsychotic agents may be more effective in women, although women are more likely to experience adverse drug reactions; and 3) women may respond better to different classes of antidepressant agents than men, specifically the SSRIs and the MAOIs. These data also indicate the need for further well-controlled research in this field.

# References

Aarons L, Hopkins K, Rowland M, et al: Route of administration and sex differences in the pharmacokinetics of aspirin administered as its lysine sal. Pharm Res 6:660–666, 1989

Abernethy DR, Greenblatt DJ, Shader RI: Imipramine disposition in users of oral contraceptive steroids. Clin Pharmacol Ther 35:792–797, 1984

Abernethy DR, Greenblatt DJ, Shader RI: Imipramine and desipramine disposition in the elderly. J Pharmacol Exp Ther 232:183–188, 1985

Anderson BB, Mikkelsen M, Vesterager A, et al: No influence of the antidepressant paroxetine on carbamazepine, valproate, and phenytoin. Epilepsy Res 10:201–204, 1991

Ashford EI, Palmer JL, Bye A, et al: The pharmacokinetics of ondansetron after intravenous injection in healthy volunteers phenotyped as poor or extensive metabolisers of debrisoquine. Br J Clin Pharmacol 37:389–391, 1994

Backstrom P, Jorpes P: Serum phenytoin, phenobarbital, carbamazepine, albumin, and plasma estradiol progesterone concentrations during the menstrual cycle in women with epilepsy. Neurol Scand 58:63–71, 1979

Banwick JH: Psychological correlates of the menstrual cycle and oral contraceptive medications, in Hormones, Behavior, and Psychopathology. Edited by Sacher E. New York, Raven Press, 1976

Barbhaiya RH, Buch AB, Greene DS: A study of the effect of age and gender on the pharmacokinetics of nefazodone after single and multiple doses. J Clin Psychopharmacol 16:19–25, 1996

Brosen K: Recent developments in hepatic drug oxidation: implications for clinical pharmacokinetics. Clin Pharmacokinet 18:220–239, 1990

Brosen K, Gram LF: Clinical significance of the sparteine/debrisoquine oxidation polymorphism. Eur J Clin Pharmacol 36:537–547, 1989

Brosen K, Skjelbo E, Rasmussen BB, et al: Fluvoxamine is a potent inhibitor of cytochrome P4501A2. Biochem Pharmacol 45:1211–1214, 1993

Centorrino F, Baldessarini RJ, Kando JC, et al: Clozapine and metabolites: concentrations in serum and clinical findings during treatment of chronically psychotic patients. J Clin Psychopharmacol 14:119–125, 1994

Chouinard G, Annable L: Pimozide in the treatment of newly admitted schizophrenic patients. Psychopharmacology (Berl) 76:13–19, 1982

Chouinard G, Annable I, Ross-Chouinard A, et al: Factors related to tardive dyskinesia. Am J Psychiatry 136:79–83, 1979

Chouinard G, Jones BD, Annable I, et al: Sex differences and tardive dyskinesia (letter). Am J Psychiatry 137:507, 1980

Chouinard G, Annable L, Steinberg S: A controlled clinical trial of fluspirilene, a long-acting injectable neuroleptic, in schizophrenia patients with acute exacerbation. J Clin Psychopharmacol 6:21–26, 1986

Crewe HK, Kennard MS, Tucker GT, et al: The effect of selective serotonin reuptake inhibitors on cytochrome P4502D6 (CYP2D6) activity in human liver microsomes. Br J Clin Pharmacol 34:262–265, 1992

Cuzzolin L, Schinella M, Tellini U, et al: The effect of sex and cardiac failure on the pharmacokinetics of a slow-release theophylline formulation in the elderly. Pharmacol Res 22:137–138, 1990

Datz FL, Christian PE, Moore J: Gender-related differences in gastric emptying. J Nucl Med 28:1204–1207, 1987

Davidson J, Pelton S: Forms of atypical depression and their response to antidepressant drugs. Psychiatry Res 17:87–95, 1986

Degen LP, Phillips SF: Variability of gastrointestinal transit in healthy women and men. Gut 39:299–305, 1996

Divoll M, Greenblatt DJ, Harmatz JS, et al: Effects of age and gender on disposition of temazepam. J Pharm Sci 70:1104–1107, 1981

Ellinwood EH, Easler ME, Linnoila M, et al: Effects of oral contraceptives on diazepam-induced psychomotor impairment. Clin Pharmacol Ther 35:360–366, 1984

Ereshefsky L, Saklad SR, Watanabe MD, et al: Thiothixene pharmacokinetic interactions: a study of hepatic enzyme inducers, clearance inhibitors, and demographic variables. J Clin Psychopharmacol 11:296–301, 1991

Fields JZ, Gordon JH: Estrogen inhibits the dopaminergic super-sensitivity induced by neuroleptics. Life Sci 30:229–234, 1982

Fletcher HP, Miya TS, Bousquet WF: Influence of estradiol on the disposition of chlorpromazine in the rat. J Pharm Sci 54:1007–1009, 1965

Gex-Fabry M, Balanta-Gorgia AE, Balant LP, et al: Clomipramine metabolism: Model-based analysis of variability factors from drug monitoring data. Clin Pharmacokinet 19:241–255, 1990

Gilman AG, Rall TW, Nies AS, et al: The Pharmacological Basis of Therapeutics, 8th Edition. New York, Pergamon Press, 1990

Gilmore DA, Gal J, Gerber JG, et al: Age and gender influence of the stereoselective pharmacokinetics of propranolol. J Pharmacol Exp Ther 261:1181–1186, 1992

Greenblatt DJ, Wright CE: Clinical pharmacokinetics of alprazolam: therapeutic implications. Clin Pharmacokinet 24:453–471, 1993

Greenblatt DJ, Allen MD, Harmatz JS, et al: Diazepam disposition determinants. Clin Pharmacol Ther 27:301–312, 1980a

Greenblatt DJ, Divoll M, Harmatz JS, et al: Oxazepam kinetics: effects of age and sex. J Pharmacol Exp Ther 215:86–91, 1980b

Greenblatt DJ, Abernethy DA, Matlis R, et al: Absorption and distribution of ibuprofen in the elderly. Arthritis Rheum 27:1066–1069, 1984

Greenblatt DJ, Freidman H, Burstein ES, et al: Trazodone kinetics: effects of age, gender and obesity. Clin Pharmacol Ther 42:193–200, 1987

Grossman MI, Kirsner JB, Gillespie IA: Basal and histalog stimulated gastric secretion in control subjects and in patients with peptic ulcer or gastric cancer. Gastroenterology 45:14–26, 1963

Guengerich FP: Mechanism-based inactivation of human liver microsomal cytochrome P450 IIIA4 by gestodene. Chem Res Toxicol 3:363–371, 1990

Guengerich FP: Human cytochrome P450 enzymes. Life Sci 50:1471–1478, 1992

Hartter S, Wetzel H, Hammes E, et al: Inhibition of antidepressant demethylation and hydroxylation by fluvoxamine in depressed patients. Psychopharmacology 110:302–308, 1993

Ho PC, Triggs EJ, Bourn DWA, et al: The effects of age and sex on the disposition of acetylsalicylic acid and its metabolites. Br J Clin Pharmacol 19:675–684, 1985

Hooper WD, Qing M-S: The influence of age and gender on the stereoselective metabolism and pharmacokinetics of mephobarbital in humans. Clin Pharmacol Ther 48:633–640, 1990

Hulst LK, Fleishaker JC, Peters GR, et al: Effect of age and gender on tirilazad pharmacokinetics in humans. Clin Pharmacol Ther 55:378–384, 1994

Hunt CM, Westerkam WR, Stave GM: Effect of age and gender on the activity of human hepatic CYP3A. Biochem Pharmacol 44:275–283, 1992

Jalil P: Toxic reaction following the combined administration of fluoxetine and phenytoin: two case reports (letter). J Neurol Neurosurg Psychiatry 55:412–413, 1992

Jerling M, Lindstrom L, Bondesson U, et al: Fluvoxamine inhibition and carbamazepine induction of the metabolism of clozapine: evidence from a therapeutic drug monitoring service. Ther Drug Monit 16:368–374, 1994

Jeste DV: Gender and ethnicity differences in pharmacology of neuroleptics. Presented at the annual meeting of American Psychiatric Association, Miami, FL, 1995

Jochemsen R, Van der Graaf M, Boeijinga JK, et al: Influence of sex, menstrual cycle and oral contraception on the disposition of nitrazepam. Br J Clin Pharmacol 13:319–324, 1982

Kerlan V, Dreano Y, Bercovici JP, et al: Nature of cytochromes P450 involved in the 2-/4-hydroxylations of estradiol in human liver microsomes. Biochem Pharmacol 44:1745–1756, 1992

Kerr BM, Thummel KE, Wurden CJ, et al: Human liver carbamazepine metabolism: role of CYP3A4 and CYP2C8 in 10,11-epoxide formation. Biochem Pharmacol 47:1969–1979, 1994

Kessler RC, Nelson CB, McGonagle KA, et al: Comorbidity of DSM-III-R major depressive disorder in the general population: results from the US National Comorbidity Survey. Br J Psychiatry Suppl 30:17–30, 1996

Kirkwood C, Moore A, Hayes P, et al: Influence of menstrual cycle and gender on alprazolam pharmacokinetics. Clin Pharmacol Ther 50:404–409, 1991

Klaiber El, Broverman DM, Vogel W, et al: Estrogen therapy for severe persistent depressions in women. Arch Gen Psychiatry 36:550–554, 1979

Klamerus KJ, Parker VD, Rudolph RL, et al: Effects of age and gender on venlafaxine and O-desmethyl venlafaxine pharmacokinetics. Pharmacotherapy 16:915–923, 1996

Knodell RG, Hall SD, Wilkinson GR, et al: hepatic metabolism of tolbutamide: characterization of the form of cytochrome P450 involved in methyl hydroxylation and relationship to in vivo disposition. J Pharmacol Exp Ther 241:1112–1119, 1987

Kolars JC, Awni WM, Merion RM, et al: first-pass metabolism of cyclosporin by the gut. Lancet 338:1488–1490, 1991

Kroboth PD, Smith RB, Stoehr GP, et al: Pharmacodynamic evaluation of the benzodiazepine–oral contraceptive interaction. Clin Pharmacol Ther 38:525–532, 1985

Kulkarni J, de Castella A, Smith D: A clinical trial of the effects of estrogen in acutely psychotic women. Schizophr Res 20:247–252, 1996

Lane JD, Steege JF, Rupp SL, et al: Menstrual cycle effects on caffeine elimination in the human female. Eur J Clin Pharmacol 43:543–546, 1992

Lew KH, Ludwig EA, Milad MA, et al: Gender-based effects on methylprednisolone pharmacokinetics and pharmacodynamics. Clin Pharmacol Ther 54:402–414, 1993

Lobo J, Kack DB, Kendall MJ: The intra- and inter-subject variability of nifedipine pharmacokinetics in young volunteers. Eur J Clin Pharmacol 30:57–60, 1986

MacLeod SM, Giles HG, Bengert B, et al: Age and gender-related differences in diazepam pharmacokinetics. J Clin Pharmacol 19:15–19, 1979

May DG, Porter J, Wilkinson GR, et al: Frequency distribution of dapsone N-hydroxylase, a putative probe for P4503A4 activity in a white population. Clin Pharmacol Ther 55:492–500, 1994

McBurney M: Starch malabsorption and stool excretion are influenced by the menstrual cycle in women consuming low fiber western diets. Scand J Gastroenterol 28:880–886, 1991

Miners JO, Attwood J, Birkett DJ: Influence of sex and oral contraceptive steroids on paracetamol metabolism. Br J Clin Pharmacol 16:503–509, 1983

Moody JP, Tait AC, Todrick A: Plasma levels of imipramine and desmethyl imipramine during therapy. Br J Psychiatry 113:183–193, 1967

Murray M: P450 enzymes: Inhibition mechanisms, genetic regulation and effects of liver disease. Clin Pharmacokinet 23;132–146, 1992

Nafziger AN, Bertino JS Jr: Sex-related differences in theophylline pharmacokinetics. Eur J Clin Pharmacol 37:97–100, 1989

Newlands AJ, Smith DA, Jones BC, et al: Metabolism of nonsteroidal, antiinflammatory drugs by cytochrome P450 2C (abstract). Br J Clin Pharmacol 34:152P, 1992

O'Malley K, Crooks J, Duke E, et al: Effects of age and sex on human drug metabolism. BMJ 3:607–609, 1971

Otton SV, Wu D, Joffe RT, et al: Inhibition by fluoxetine of cytochrome P4502D6 activity. Clin Pharmacol Ther 53:401–409, 1993

Otton SV, Ball Se, Cheung SW, et al: Comparative inhibition of the polymorphic enzyme CYP2D6 by venlafaxine (VF) and other 5HT uptake inhibitors (abstract PI-71). Clin Pharmacol Ther 55:141, 1994

Pesce ME, Acevedo X, Pinardi G, et al: Gender differences in diazepam withdrawal syndrome in mice. Pharmacol Toxicol 75:353–355, 1994

Pinals DA, Malhotra AK, Missar CD, et al: Lack of gender differences in neuroleptic response in patients with schizophrenia. Schizophr Res 22:215–222, 1996

Pollan A, Oian P: Changes in transcapillary fluid dynamics—a possible explanation of the fluid retention in the premenstrual phase, in Hormones and Behavior. Edited by Dennerstein L, Fraser I. New York, Elsevier, 1986

Pollock BG: Recent developments in drug metabolism of relevance to psychiatrists. Harv Rev Psychiatry 2:204–213, 1994

Preskorn SH, Mac DS: Plasma level of amitriptyline: effect of age and sex. J Clin Psychiatry 46:276–277, 1985

Pritchard JF, Bryson JC, Kernodle AE, et al: Age and gender effects on ondansetron pharmacokinetics: evaluation of healthy aged volunteers. Clin Pharmacol Ther 51:51–55, 1992

Raskin A: Age-sex differences in response to antidepressant drugs. J Nerv Ment Dis 159:120–130, 1974

Relling MV, Lin JS, Ayers GD, et al: Racial and gender differences in N-acetyltrans-ferase, xanthine oxidase, and CYP1A2 activities. Clin Pharmacol Ther 52:643–658, 1992

Rettie AE, Korzekwa KR, Kunze KL, et al: Hydroxylation of warfarin by human cDNA-expressed cytochrome P450: a role for P4502C9 in the etiology of (S)-warfarin drug interactions. Chem Res Toxicol 5:54–59, 1992

Richardson CJ, Blocka KLN, Ross SG, et al: Effects of age and sex on piroxicam disposition. Clin Pharmacol Ther 37:13–18, 1985

Riester EF, Pantuck EJ, Pantuck CB, et al: Antipyrine metabolism during the menstrual cycle. Clin Pharmacol Ther 28:384–391, 1980

Ronfeld RA, Tremaine LM, Wilner KD: Pharmacokinetics of sertraline and its N-dimethyl metabolite in elderly and young male and female volunteers. Clin Pharmacokinet 32(suppl 1):22–30, 1997

Rugstad HE, Hundal O, Holme I, et al: Piroxicam and naproxen plasma concentrations in patients with osteoarthritis: relation to age, sex, efficacy and adverse events. Clin Rheumatol 5:389–398, 1986

Schmucker DL, Woodhouse KW, Wang RK, et al: Effects of age and gender on in vitro properties of human liver microsomal monoxygenases. Clin Pharmacol Ther 48:365–374, 1990

Schwartz J, Capili H, Daugherty J: Aging of women alters S-verapamil pharmacokinetics and pharmacodynamics. Clin Pharmacol Ther 55:509–517, 1994

Seeman MV: Neuroleptic prescription for men and women. Soc Pharmacol 3:219–236, 1989

Seeman MV: The role of estrogen in schizophrenia. J Psychiatry Neurosci 21:123–127, 1996

Seeman MV, Lang M: The role of estrogens in schizophrenia gender differences. Schizophr Bull 16:185–194, 1990

Shavit G, Lerman P, Koresyn A: Phenytoin pharmacokinetics in catamenial epilepsy. Neurology 34:959–961, 1984

Shimada T, Yamazaki H, Mimura M, et al: Interindividual variations in human liver cytochrome P-450 enzymes involved in the oxidation of drugs, carcinogens and toxic chemicals: studies with liver microsomes of 30 Japanese and 30 Caucasians. J Pharmacol Exp Ther 270:414–423, 1994

Simpson GM, Yadalam KG, Levinson DF, et al: Single dose pharmacokinetics of fluphenazine after fluphenazine decanoate administration. J Clin Psychopharmacol 10:417–421, 1990

Sitar D, Duke PC, Benthuysen JL, et al: Aging and alfentanil disposition in healthy volunteers and surgical patients. Can J Anaesth 36:149–154, 1989

Skjelbo E, Brosen K: Inhibitors of imipramine metabolism by human liver microsomes. Br J Clin Pharmacol 34:256–261, 1992

Smith DA, Jones BC: Speculations on the substrate structure-activity relationship (SSAR) of cytochrome P450 enzymes. Biochem Pharmacol 44:2089–2098, 1992

Smith JM, Dunn DD: Sex differences in the prevalence of severe tardive dyskinesia. Am J Psychiatry 136:1081–1082, 1979

Smith RB, Divoll M, Gillespie WR, et al: Effect of subject age and gender on the pharmacokinetics of oral triazolam and temazepam. J Clin Psychopharmacol 3:172–176, 1983

Steiner M, Wheadon DE, Kreider MS, et al: Antidepressant response to paroxetine by gender. Presented at the 146th annual meeting of the American Psychiatric Association, San Francisco, CA, May 22–27, 1993

Stoehr GP, Kroboth PD, Juhl RP, et al: Effect of oral contraceptives on triazolam, temazepam, alprazolam, and lorazepam kinetics. Clin Pharmacol Ther 36:683–690, 1984

Strobel HW, Hammond DK, White TB, et al: Identification and localization of cytochromes P450 in gut. Methods in Enzymology 206:648–655, 1991

Sweeting J: Does the time of the month affect the function of the gut? Gastroenterology 102:1084–1085, 1992

Szymanski S, Lieberman JA, Alvir JM, et al: Gender differences in onset of illness, treatment response, course, and biologic indexes in first-episode schizophrenic patients. Am J Psychiatry 152:698–703, 1995

U. S. Food and Drug Administration: Guideline for the study and evaluation of gender differences in the clinic evaluation of drugs. Federal Register 58(139):39406–39416, 1993

van Haaren F, Katon E, Anderson KG: The effects of chlordiazepoxide on low-rate behavior are gender dependent. Pharmacol Biochem Behav 58:1037–1043, 1997

Villeneuve A, Langlier P, Bedard P: Estrogens, dopamine, and dyskinesias. Can Psychiatr Assoc J 23:68–70, 1978

von Moltke LL, Greenblatt DJ, Court MH, et al: Inhibition of alprazolam and desipramine hydroxylation in vitro by paroxetine and fluvoxamine: comparison with other selective serotonin reuptake inhibitor antidepressants. J Clin Psychopharmacol 15:125–131, 1995

Wald A, Van Thiel DH, Hoechstetter L, et al: Gastrointestinal transit: the effect of the menstrual cycle. Gastroenterology 80:1497–1500, 1981

Walle T, Byington RP, Furberg CD, et al: Biologic determinants of propranolol disposition: results from 1308 patients in the beta-blocker heart attack trial. Clin Pharmacol Ther 38:509–518, 1985

Walle T, Walle UK, Cowart TD, et al: Pathway-selective sex differences in the metabolic clearance of propranolol in human subjects. Clin Pharmacol Ther 45:257–263, 1989

Walle T, Walle UK, Mathur RS, et al: Propranolol metabolism in normal subjects: association with sex steroid hormones. Clin Pharmacol Ther 56:127–132, 1994

Warrington SJ: Clinical implications of the pharmacology of sertraline. Int Clin Psychopharmacol 6:11–21, 1991

Wrighton SA, Stevens JC: The human hepatic cytochromes P450 involved in drug metabolism. Crit Rev Toxicol 22:1–21, 1992

Yassar J, Jeste DV: Gender differences in tardive dyskinesia: a critical review of the literature. Psychol Bull 1814:701–715, 1992

Yee GC, Lennon TP, Gmur DJ, et al: Age-dependent cyclosporine: pharmacokinetics in marrow transplant recipients. Clin Pharmacol Ther 40:438–443, 1986

Yukawa E, Mine H, Higuchi S, et al: Digoxin population pharmacokinetics from routine clinical data: role of patient characteristics for estimating dosing regimes. J Pharm Pharmacol 44:761–765, 1992

Ziegler VE, Biggs JT: Tricyclic plasma levels: effect of age, race, sex, and smoking. JAMA 238:2167–2169, 1977

# Alcohol and Substance Abuse in Obstetrics and Gynecology Practice

SHEILA B. BLUME, M.D., C.A.C.
MARCIA RUSSELL, PH.D.

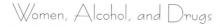

## Women, Alcohol, and Drugs

### Historical and Social Factors

Abuse of alcohol and other psychoactive drugs predates recorded history. Although the types of drugs used and abused in different cultures have varied over time, nearly all societies that have permitted substance use have had separate rules for each gender. These rules have been based on deeply ingrained cultural stereotypes of the differential effects of these drugs on men and women.

Western thought, dating back as far as the ancient Romans and Israelites (Gomberg 1986; McKinlay 1959), has held that alcohol is a sexual stimulant that makes women promiscuous. Although careful studies of women in the United States have not substantiated this idea (Klassen and Wilsnack 1986), the stereotype is widely accepted and has led to a destructive stigma applied to all chemically dependent women. This stigma characterizes them as both generally and sexually immoral (i.e., "fallen women"), and in turn simultaneously enhances denial and leads to underrecognition of chemical dependence in middle-class and professional women (Moore et al. 1989). It further results in the social acceptance of physical and sexual victimization of chemically dependent women (Blume 1991). Rapists are considered less responsible for their acts if intoxicated at the time of the rape, whereas victims are held more to blame if intoxicated (D. Richardson and Campbell 1982). It is hardly surprising, therefore, that women suffering from addictive diseases are often the victims of violence, both at home and in society (B.A. Miller et al. 1989; Testa and Parks 1996).

Social customs related to the use and abuse of substances affect women in various ways. Drinking norms that dictate lower levels of intake by women protect them from developing alcoholism (Klee and Ames 1987; Kubicka et al. 1995). The evolution of social custom has produced a convergence of use patterns for some drugs among male and female teenagers; more girls are now initiating smoking than are boys (Center on Addiction and Substance Abuse 1996). The tendency of physicians to prescribe more psychoactive drugs for women than for men (Cooperstock 1978) puts women at a higher risk for becoming dependent on prescription drugs and puts alcoholic women at increased risk for mixed addictions. Wives, daughters, and mothers of alcoholics or addicts often assume the social role of caretaker. In their efforts to cope with familial dysfunction, they may display maladaptive behavior characterized as *codependency* (Cermak 1986). Depression, somatic complaints, eating disorders and alcohol or drug abuse are often seen in this group.

## Epidemiology

Women's alcohol use has increased over the past half-century. Although no dramatic overall changes have occurred in the past few years, heavy drinking has continued to rise among younger cohorts. For the year 1992, Grant et al. (1994) found that 4.5 million American women suffered from alcohol abuse or dependence. A general population study of Americans aged 15–54 years yielded the following lifetime prevalence rates for women: any substance abuse or dependence 17.9% (versus 35.4% for men); alcohol abuse or dependence 14.6% (versus 32.6% for men); and other drug abuse/dependence, excluding nicotine, 9.4% (versus 14.6% for men). Among women, 12-month rates of abuse or dependence were any substance 6.6% (versus 16.1% for men); alcohol 5.3% (versus 14.1% for men); and other drugs 2.2% (versus 5.1% for men) (Warner et al. 1995). In evaluating epidemiologic surveys, the possible influence of social stigma on the accuracy of reporting by women should be considered. It is not known if women underestimate their substance use more than men.

In 1993 approximately 4.1% of women in the United States (4.4 million) admitted to some illicit drug use (including nonmedical use of prescription drugs) during the month prior to a household survey (Substance Abuse and Mental Health Services Administration 1994). Women of childbearing age reported a higher prevalence of 8.1% (1.2 million) for ages 18–25 and 5.9% (1.1 million) for ages 26–34.

High-risk groups for alcohol and drug problems among women include inner-city and criminal justice populations, women in the military, and lesbian women (Wilsnack 1984). A family history of alcoholism increases the risk of alcohol abuse or dependence in women (Russell et al. 1990).

Studies of gynecologic populations reveal higher prevalence rates than are found in the general public. For example, of 147 women visiting two private gynecologic practices for routine care, 12% met criteria for alcohol abuse or dependence. Of 95 women treated in the same locations for premenstrual syndrome, 21% were also alcoholic (Halliday et al. 1986). In a similar study of 1,967 gynecologic patients, 17% were heavy drinkers and 14% regularly used psychoactive drugs with the potential for nonmedical use (Russell and Coviello 1988). Data from 21 states participating from 1985 to 1988 in the Behavioral Risk Factor Surveillance System indicated that alcohol use by pregnant women declined from 32% to 20% over this period; binge drinking was reported by 2.8% (Serdula et al. 1991). No declines in alcohol use were observed among pregnant women who were less educated or under age 25 years, and rates of use were highest among smokers and unmarried women.

Positive urine toxicology screening tests have been reported in 13.1% of 335 women in private and 16.3% of 380 women in public obstetric care (Chasnoff 1990) and in 29.5% of 200 women admitted in active labor to an inner-city hospital (Parente et al. 1990).

## Psychologic Aspects

Longitudinal studies of girls who later developed drinking problems have revealed feelings of low self-esteem and impaired ability to cope (Jones 1971) and drinking to relieve shyness, get along better on dates, and get "high" (Fillmore et al. 1979). Additional risk factors have been identified in retrospective studies. In a large general-population sample of adult women, a history of sexual assault increased the risk for a lifetime diagnosis of alcohol abuse or dependence (3.5 times more likely) and drug abuse or dependence (four times more likely) (Winfield et al. 1990). In addition, women who develop chemical dependency are more likely than men to satisfy diagnostic criteria for an additional psychiatric diagnosis, especially major depression (Helzer and Pryzbeck 1988; Hesselbrock et al. 1985). Alcoholic women are also at risk for suicide (Gomberg 1986). When alcoholism and major depression occur in the same woman, the depression predates the onset of alcoholism two-thirds of the time. Such "dual-diagnosis" patients have a favorable prognosis if they receive adequate treatment for both disorders (Rounsaville et al. 1987), whereas efforts to relieve chemical dependence by treating "underlying" disorders alone have usually been unsuccessful.

## Physiologic Factors

Women have been found to be more sensitive to alcohol than are men. When given equal doses of alcohol per pound of body weight under standard conditions, women attain higher blood alcohol levels than do men. This is partly due to the lower average water content in the bodies of women, because alcohol is distributed in total body water. It may also be a result of more complete absorption of alcohol in women, which results from lower levels of the metabolic enzyme of alcohol, alcohol dehydrogenase, in gastric tissue (Frezza et al. 1990). Women also show more variable peak blood alcohol levels, which some, but not other, investigators have found to correlate with the menstrual cycle. Although little evidence exists that patterns of drug use vary with the menstrual cycle in normal women, those who suffer from premenstrual dysphoria tend to increase the use of alcohol and marijuana during the premenstruum (Mello 1986).

Gender differences in relative body water and fat content also lead to longer half-lives for lipid-soluble psychoactive drugs, such as diazepam and oxazepam, in women (Barry 1986). Aging further exaggerates this trend.

## Effects on Sexuality and Reproduction

In examining the effects of psychoactive substance use on women's sexuality, the strong influence of socially conditioned expectation must be considered (Wilsnack 1984). Because alcohol is thought to be sexually stimulating, women report more subjective sexual arousal when they have consumed alcohol, even when physiologic measurements show otherwise. In physiologic experiments, alcohol has been shown objectively to have a dose-related depressant effect on sexual arousal (Wilson and Lawson 1976) and orgasm (Malatesta et al. 1982) in women. Alcoholic women report a wide variety of sexual dysfunctions, including premenstrual dysphoria, lack of sexual interest, anorgasmia, vaginismus, and dyspareunia. At the same time, these women believe that alcohol arouses them and fear they will not enjoy sex if they are sober. Physicians can help these women by explaining alcohol's depressant effects and reassuring them that abstinence from alcohol and other drugs is likely to improve their sexual functioning in the long run (Gavaler et al. 1993).

Another commonly held expectation is that cocaine and amphetamines function as enhancers of sexual functioning. In fact, chronic use of either drug can cause impotence and ejaculatory failure in men, inhibition of orgasm in women, and loss of sexual desire in both sexes (Washton 1989).

Heroin dependence has been reported to depress sexual desire and suppress ovulation (Gaulden et al. 1964). Menstrual periods often return to normal within a few months after the institution of methadone maintenance treatment (Wallach et al. 1969). Methadone itself, however, depresses sexual activity in a dose-related fashion (Crowley and Simpson 1978). Abuse of sedative drugs and minor tranquilizers such as diazepam may also depress both sexual desire and orgasm in women.

Alcoholic women commonly experience amenorrhea, anovulatory cycles, luteal phase dysfunction, and early menopause (Mello et al. 1989). They may therefore seek help for infertility, unaware that their alcohol or sedative intake might play an etiologic role. In addition, even at levels of social drinking, alcohol has also been shown to increase the risk of spontaneous abortion, especially in the midtrimester (Mello et al. 1989).

Adverse effects of alcohol and drug abuse on pregnancy and the developing fetus are produced by a complex interaction of pharmacologic, lifestyle, and nutritional factors, including absent or insufficient prenatal care. Although some women use only one drug, multiple drug use, including heavy smoking, is common (Mello et al. 1989). Premature labor, abruptio placentae, stillbirth, and a wide variety of other obstetric complications have been reported to be associated with maternal abuse of alcohol and other chemicals (Levy and Koren 1990). Alcohol is also known to suppress uterine contractions and in the past was employed in the treatment of threatened preterm labor (Fadel and Hadi 1982).

Cocaine, because of its acute stimulant, vasoconstrictive, and cardiac arrythmia–producing properties, has been linked to sudden death in the pregnant woman (Burkett et al. 1990) as well as to premature rupture of the membranes, preterm labor, and fetal distress (Mastrogiannis et al. 1990). Unfortunately, the association between acute ingestion of cocaine and premature labor has led to a mistaken belief among young women that cocaine can shorten their labor while making it less painful (Skolnick 1990). This misconception may actually lead to an increase in the use of cocaine in late pregnancy. Investigations of additional specific adverse effects resulting from prenatal cocaine exposure, including structural birth defects, growth and developmental retardation, childhood behavior problems, and an increased incidence of sudden infant death syndrome, have produced contradictory and equivocal results (Center on Addiction and Substance Abuse 1996; G. A. Richardson and Day 1994). A full understanding of the long-term results of cocaine use in pregnancy awaits further research.

Cigarette smoking has been associated with an increased risk of spontaneous abortion, placenta previa, and abruptio placentae (Levy and Koren 1990). Studies of the influence of marijuana use on the course of pregnancy have been equivocal; some studies suggest an increased incidence of protracted labor and precipitate labor (Levy and Koren 1990).

Adverse effects of drugs of abuse on the fetus include both general and substance-specific influences. Table 20–1 summarizes these effects. In addition to those listed, an increased incidence of sudden infant death syndrome or neonatal apnea has been correlated with prenatal exposure to both cocaine and nicotine. Heroin dependence has been linked to a range of obstetric complications. On the other hand, women who are maintained on stable doses of methadone and are provided with adequate prenatal care and nutrition have an improved course of pregnancy and may produce offspring of normal size and weight (Blinick et al. 1973). Postnatal abstinence syndrome is common in such infants but can be managed (Hoegerman et al. 1990).

Evidence for long-term neurobehavioral abnormalities caused by methadone exposure is equivocal (Rosen and Johnson 1985). Fetal alcohol syndrome (FAS), first described and named in 1973, consists of the following signs and symptoms (Institute of Medicine 1996): 1) prenatal and postnatal growth retardation; 2) central nervous system dysfunction (including any combination of reduced head circumference, mental retardation, hyperactivity, and disordered learning, coordination, or balance); 3) a characteristic facial dysmorphism, with shortened palpebral fissures, epicanthic folds, and a shortened, depressed nose bridge, elongated, flattened upper lip, and displaced, deformed ears; and 4) additional birth defects ranging from mild (birthmarks, single palmar crease) to severe (cardiac, joint, eye, and ear abnormalities).

The term *alcohol-related birth defects* (ARBD) refers to abnormalities that are presumed or suspected to be related to maternal drinking during pregnancy and that do not meet the criteria for FAS. Although it has been established through both human and animal studies that heavy drinking throughout

**TABLE 20–1.** Commonly reported teratogenic effects of abused drugs

| Specific fetal effects | Opiates | Alcohol | Other sedative | Cocaine | Other stimulant | Hallucinogens | Marijuana | Nicotine |
|---|---|---|---|---|---|---|---|---|
| Structural nonspecific growth retardation | X | X | – | X | – | – | X | X |
| Specific dysmorphic effects | – | X | – | X | – | – | – | – |
| Behavioral | X | X | X | X | X | X | X | X |
| Neurobiochemical (abstinence syndrome) | X | X | X | – | – | – | – | – |
| Increased fetal and perinatal mortality | X | X | – | X | – | – | – | X |
| Women reporting use in pregnancy*, % | 5 | >50 | <5 | <20 | <5 | <5 | 5–34 | >50 |

*(varies with population)

*Source.* This table was first published in the *Western Journal of Medicine* (G. Hoegermann, C. A. Wilson, E. Thurmond, et al. Drug-exposed neonates. *West J Med* 1990; 152:559–564) and is reproduced by permission of wjm western journal of medicine.

most of pregnancy produces both FAS and ARBD, the relative risks of various amounts and patterns of drinking are still in question. Experiments in animals indicate that alcohol consumed in a binge pattern may produce more severe damage than an equal quantity consumed over a longer period.

Although no absolutely safe level of alcohol intake during pregnancy has been established, negative effects of light, moderate, or social drinking have been subtle and more difficult to document than the effects of heavier drinking (Institute of Medicine 1996; Russell 1991). Nevertheless, most authorities recommend abstinence, following the advice of the U.S. Surgeon General, who issued the following statement in 1981: "The Surgeon General advises women who are pregnant (or considering pregnancy) not drink alcoholic beverages and to be aware of the alcoholic content of foods and drugs" (p. 1).

Most drugs of abuse pass freely into breast milk and can cause harm to the nursing infant. Even small quantities of alcohol consumed during lactation may cause measurable differences in motor development (Little et al. 1989). Several available references address the treatment of the chemically dependent pregnant woman (Center for Substance Abuse Treatment 1993; L. J. Miller 1994; Mitchell 1994). Alcohol use may also be associated with an increased risk of breast cancer in women in a dose–response relationship (Longnecker et al. 1988).

## Other Physical Complications of Alcohol and Drug Use

Alcoholism has been found to progress more rapidly in women than in men. This is also true for the physical complications of alcoholism, including fatty liver, hypertension, obesity, anemia, malnutrition, peptic ulcer, cirrhosis of the liver (Ashley et al. 1977; Gavaler 1982), and both peripheral myopathy and cardiomyopathy (Urbano-Marquez et al. 1995). These conditions may in turn cause further obstetric and gynecologic morbidity (Blume 1986).

Another important set of complications of alcohol and drug dependence are sexually transmitted diseases. The proportion of women among all newly reported cases of AIDS has grown steadily over the past decade. Of AIDS cases in women, 79% are related to the use of drugs. Of these women, 50% have been users of intravenous drugs and 25% have been nonusing sexual partners of male intravenous drug users (Center on Addiction and Substance Abuse 1996). Studies of HIV-positive women participating in a methadone maintenance program showed no differences in fertility when compared with HIV-negative control subjects, and very few differences in the course of pregnancy were found between the two groups (Selwyn et al. 1989). About one-third of infants born to HIV-positive women will be HIV positive themselves at 18 months of age (Blanche et al. 1989).

A sharp rise in the incidence of both primary and secondary syphilis was reported during the 1980s, especially among women (Rolfs and Nakashima 1990). Seropositivity for syphilis in American women has been linked to drug use, including cocaine (Minkoff et al. 1990). However, analysis of a large, general-population sample showed problem drinking to be a predictor of sexually transmitted diseases in both genders, and a greater risk factor than illegal drug use (Ericksen and Trocki 1994).

## Identification and Treatment of Psychoactive Substance Abuse in Obstetric/Gynecologic Practice

### Screening

As discussed, the prevalence of heavy drinking and drug use is elevated in gynecologic patients, and maternal substance use increases pregnancy risk. Therefore, screening for substance use in obstetric and gynecologic settings is an important aspect of care. Currently, brief questionnaires are the most cost-effective and sensitive method of identifying risk drinking and risk for substance abuse. The TWEAK (Russell 1994) and TACE (Sokol et al. 1989) were developed in obstetric and gynecologic patients to detect risk drinking in pregnancy, and they also detect alcohol problems. A self-administered questionnaire that includes questions on smoking, alcohol, and other drug use and on risk factors for substance abuse (Figure 20–1) can be conveniently administered in the patient waiting room and then reviewed by the clinician with the patient. Elevated levels of mean corpuscular volume and/or $\gamma$-glutamyltransferase observed in routine blood tests, although less sensitive than questionnaires, may be helpful in detecting heavy alcohol use that is predictive of ARBD in obstetric patients  (Ylikorkala et al. 1987). Laboratory tests for drugs in maternal and newborn blood or urine are used to screen for substance use in some perinatal clinics, but this remains controversial because of the potential for false-positive results, problems of confidentiality, and the threat of legal sanctions that can complicate the delivery of prenatal care (Birchfield et al. 1995; Blume 1997).

Positive screening results should be followed in all cases by a careful diagnosis in which accepted criteria are used; a positive laboratory test should not be used as a substitute for a clinical assessment. Criteria for diagnoses of

Please check answers below.

| | Very Helpful | Not Helpful | Never tried |
|---|---|---|---|
| 1. When you are depressed or nervous, do you find any of the following helpful to feel better or to relax? | | | |
| a. Smoking cigarettes | ❑ | ❑ | ❑ |
| b. Working harder than usual at home or job | ❑ | ❑ | ❑ |
| c. Taking a tranquilizer | ❑ | ❑ | ❑ |
| d. Taking some other kind of pill or medication | ❑ | ❑ | ❑ |
| e. Having a drink | ❑ | ❑ | ❑ |
| f. Talking it over with friends or relatives | ❑ | ❑ | ❑ |

| | Yes | No |
|---|---|---|
| 2. Think of the times you have been most depressed; at those times did you: | | |
| a. Lose or gain weight | _____ | _____ |
| b. Lose interest in things that usually interest you | _____ | _____ |
| c. Have spells when you couldn't seem to stop crying | _____ | _____ |
| d. Suffer from insomnia | _____ | _____ |
| 3. Have you ever gone to a doctor, psychologist, social worker, counselor or clergyman for help with an emotional problem? | _____ | _____ |

4. How many cigarettes a day do you smoke?  Check one.

❑ More than 2 packs    ❑ 1–2 packs    ❑ Less than 1 pack    ❑ None

5. How often do you have a drink of wine, beer, or a beverage containing alcohol?

❑ 3 or more times a day ❑ Twice a day        ❑ Almost every day

❑ Once or twice a week ❑ Once or twice a month ❑ Less than once a month

❑ Never

**FIGURE 20–1.**  Health Questionnaire

6. a. If you drink wine, beer, or beverages containing alcohol, how often do you have four or more drinks?

   ❑ Almost always     ❑ Frequently     ❑ Sometimes     ❑ Never

   b. If you drink wine, beer, or beverages containing alcohol, how often do you have one or two?

   ❑ Almost always     ❑ Frequently     ❑ Sometimes     ❑ Never

7. What prescribed medications do you take? _____

_____

8. What other drugs or medications do you use? _____

_____

|  | Yes | No |
|---|---|---|
| 9. Does your drinking or taking other drugs sometimes lead to problems between you and your family, that is, wife, husband, children, parent, or close relative? | ____ | ____ |
| 10. During the past year, have close relatives or friends worried or complained about your drinking or taking other drugs? | ____ | ____ |
| 11. Has a friend or family member ever told you about things you said or did while you were drinking or using other drugs that you do not remember? | ____ | ____ |
| 12. Have you, within the past year, started to drink alcohol and found it difficult to stop before becoming intoxicated? | ____ | ____ |
| 13. Has your father or mother ever had problems with alcohol or other drugs? | ____ | ____ |

**FIGURE 20–1.** Health Questionnaire *(continued)*

alcohol and drug abuse or dependence have been published by the American Psychiatric Association (1994). In addition, women may drink excessively or use drugs without meeting criteria for a diagnosis of alcohol or drug abuse or dependence. However, they should be counseled about the potential risks to their health, especially as it relates to their reproductive health, and those who are unable or unwilling to moderate their substance use should be encouraged to use reliable methods of contraception if they are at risk of becoming pregnant. Heavy drinkers or drug users planning to become pregnant should be advised to attain abstinence before conceiving to avoid damage to the fetus early during gestation.

## Treatment Considerations

The most important factors in approaching the chemically dependent woman identified in obstetric/gynecologic practice are a nonjudgmental, helping attitude; a thorough knowledge of available specialist practitioners and treatment resources in the community; and the involvement of family members or significant others in carrying out the referral to treatment for chemical dependency. Education or warnings about the need for abstinence are not sufficient for alcohol- or drug-dependent pregnant women. Although some are able to abstain during pregnancy without treatment, most relapse after delivery, to the detriment of their health, family life, and future pregnancies. These women need rehabilitative treatment, sometimes preceded by detoxification, to recover. Sample protocols are available to assist in detoxification of the pregnant woman who is dependent on alcohol or sedatives. Opiate-dependent pregnant women may be either detoxified or shifted to a methadone maintenance regimen (Center for Substance Abuse Treatment 1993). Self-help fellowships such as Alcoholics Anonymous, Narcotics Anonymous, and Women for Sobriety are widely available and play an essential role in long-term recovery.

Both self-help (e.g., Al-Anon Family Groups, Naranon, Adult Children of Alcoholics groups) and professional services are indicated for those obstetric/gynecologic patients whose lives have been adversely affected by the chemical dependence of a family member. At times a structured intervention can be arranged in which family and friends confront the alcohol- or drug-dependent person with the assistance of a trained professional (Johnson Institute 1983). Structured intervention should be considered as an approach if the chemically dependent obstetric/gynecologic patient is initially unwilling to accept the need for alcohol or drug treatment concomitant with her obstetric/gynecologic care.

## Barriers to Treatment

Women are seriously underrepresented in alcoholism treatment in the United States. Although they constitute approximately one-third of alcoholics, only one-fourth to one-fifth of patients in treatment are female. Likewise, there is a serious shortage of treatment for other drug dependence, especially for the pregnant patient. A study by the U.S. General Accounting Office (1990) found that approximately 280,000 pregnant women needed drug abuse treatment in 1989, but less than 11% of this number received it.

Many women who are in need of care are single parents and unemployed or underemployed, which makes them less likely to have adequate insurance coverage. Furthermore, the lack of available child care often prevents them from entering inpatient or residential programs. Although a few programs admit both mothers and children, such facilities are rare.

An additional barrier to treatment is the fear of losing child custody. Women who must rely on a public agency for child care in order to enter treatment are often reluctant to do so because of the risk of being found guilty of neglect (Blume 1997). Pregnant patients also fear criminal prosecution for prenatal child abuse or for the delivery of controlled substances to a minor (via the umbilical cord). Publicized cases of prosecution and incarceration of pregnant or newly delivered women have further eroded the fragile trust of chemically dependent women in the health care system and will lead to more births to mothers lacking prenatal care. In some jurisdictions, the removal of newborn infants from their mothers solely on the basis of a positive drug test, without any effort at assessment, diagnosis, intervention, or treatment, has created a reluctance among both professionals and patients to make use of this important diagnostic tool. The ensuing policy debate has led to proposed legislation in several states to protect the rights of women and encourage chemical dependency treatment rather than prosecution (Blume 1997).

## Educating Obstetrician/Gynecologists About Psychoactive Substance Abuse

Programs aimed at the prevention of chemical dependency in women and chemical-related birth defects in children have taken two related approaches: public and professional education. Both aim at acquainting young people and adults with the teratogenicity of alcohol and other drugs and with the concept of chemical dependencies as treatable diseases. Both also depend on enhancing the health care professional's recognition of these diseases in women and successful referral of these patients to treatment.

The evaluations of efforts at professional education have shown that obstetrician/gynecologists will read and respond to a state-sponsored FAS information packet (Russell et al. 1983) or a community education program (Little et al. 1983). To sustain appropriate screening and referral patterns in obstetric practice, however, ongoing educational efforts are necessary (Weiner et al. 1983). Primary care workers and health educators must also be involved, especially in high-risk populations such as Native Americans and Alaska Natives, but preliminary evidence indicates that such prevention programs can be effective (May and Hymbaugh 1989).

Psychiatrists have an important role in these prevention activities. The training of all obstetrician/gynecologists should include methods of identifying, motivating, and referring women who have chemical dependencies. This training can be provided by psychiatrists who have skills and experience in this area. Other opportunities arise in consultation and continuing-education programs for physicians and other health professionals. Psychiatrists can also help improve the procedures for screening and intervention in obstetric/gynecologic practice.

The goals of prevention through social change include education to remove the inaccurate social stigma attached to chemically dependent women. At the same time, they stress the promotion of supportive networks that preserve women's social protections from the expectation that they drink or take drugs "like men." Finally, they provide psychosocial support for women undergoing stressful transitions, such as separation, divorce, and bereavement, to help them cope with these changes without developing dependence on chemicals of abuse. Psychiatrists can participate by helping to organize such support systems and by acting as consultants to community-based prevention programs. Finally, all concerned citizens can advocate enlightened public policies that offer appropriate and accessible help to women in need rather than punitive and stigmatizing measures.

# References

American Psychiatric Association: Diagnostic and Statistical Manual of Mental Disorders, 4th Edition. Washington, DC, American Psychiatric Association, 1994

Ashley MJ, Olin JS, LeRiche WH, et al: Morbidity in alcoholics: evidence for accelerated development of physical disease in women. Arch Intern Med 137:883–887, 1977

Barry PP: Gender as a factor in treating the elderly, in Women and Drugs: A New Era for Research (NIDA Research Monograph 65). Edited by Ray BA, Braude MC. Washington, DC, U.S. Department of Health and Human Services, 1986, pp 65–69

Birchfield M, Scully J, Handler A: Perinatal screening for illicit drugs: policies in hospitals in a large metropolitan area. J Perinat 15:208–214, 1995

Blanche S, Rouzious C, Moscato ML, et al: A prospective study of infants born to women seropositive for HIV type 1. N Engl J Med 32:1643–1648, 1989

Blinick G, Jerez E, Wallach RC: Methadone maintenance, pregnancy, and progeny. JAMA 225:477–479, 1973

Blume SB: Women and alcohol: a review. JAMA 256:1467–1470, 1986

Blume SB: Sexuality and stigma: the alcoholic woman. Alcohol Health and Research World 15:139–146, 1991

Blume SB: Women and alcohol: issues in social policy, in Gender and Alcohol: Individual and Social Perspectives. Edited by Wilsnack R, Wilsnack S. New Brunswick, NJ, Rutgers Center of Alcohol Studies, 1997, pp 462–489

Burkett G, Bandstra ES, Cohen J, et al: Cocaine-related maternal death. Am J Obstet Gynecol 163:40–41, 1990

Center on Addiction and Substance Abuse: Substance Abuse and American Women. New York, Center on Addiction and Substance Abuse, 1996

Center for Substance Abuse Treatment: Pregnant, Substance-Using Women: Treatment Improvement Protocol Series (Publication No. (SMA) 93-1998). Washington, DC, Department of Health and Human Services, 1993

Cermak TL: Diagnosing and Ttreating Codependence. Minneapolis, MN, Johnson Institute, 1986

Chasnoff IJ: The prevalence of illicit drug or alcohol use during pregnancy and discrepancies in mandatory reporting in Pinellas Co. Florida. N Engl J Med 322:1202–1206, 1990

Cooperstock R: Sex differences in psychotropic drug use. Soc Sci Med 12:179–186, 1978

Crowley TJ, Simpson R: Methadone dose and human sexual behavior. Int J Addict 13:285–295, 1978

Ericksen KP, Trocki KF: Sex, alcohol, and sexually transmitted diseases: a national survey. Family Plan Perspect 26:257–263, 1994

Fadel HE, Hadi HA: Alcohol effects on the reproductive function, in Encyclopedic Handbook of Alcoholism. Edited by Pattison EM, Kaufman E. New York, Gardner Press, 1982, pp 293–300

Fillmore KM, Bacon SD, Hyman M: The 27-year longitudinal panel study of drinking by students in college: report 1979 to National Institute of Alcoholism and Alcohol Abuse (DHHS Publ No ADM 281-76-0015). Washington, DC, U.S. Government Printing Office, 1979

Frezza M, diPadova C, Pozzato G, et al: High blood alcohol levels in women. N Engl J Med 322:95–99, 1990

Gaulden EC, Littlefield DC, Putoff OE, et al: Menstrual abnormalities associated with heroin addiction. Am J Obstet Gynecol 90:155–160, 1964

Gavaler JS: Sex-related differences in ethanol-induced liver disease: artifactual or real? Alcohol Clin Exp Res 6:186–196, 1982

Gavaler JS, Rizzo A, Rossaro L: Sexuality of alcoholic women with menstrual cycle function: effects of duration of alcohol abstinence. Alcohol Clin Exp Res 17:778–781, 1993

Gomberg ESL: Women: alcohol and other drugs, in Perspectives on Drug Use in the United States. Edited by Segal B. New York, Haworth Press, 1986, pp 75–110

Grant BF, Harford TC, Dawson DA, et al: Prevalence of DSM-IV alcohol abuse and dependence. Alcohol Health and Research World 18:243–248, 1994

Halliday A, Bush B, Cleary P, et al: Alcohol abuse in women seeking gynecologic care. Obstet Gynecol 68:322–326, 1986

Helzer JE, Pryzbeck TR: The co-occurrence of alcoholism with other psychiatric disorders in the general population and its impact on treatment. J Stud Alcohol 249:219–224, 1988

Hesselbrock MJ, Meyer RE, Keener JJ: Psychopathology in hospitalized alcoholics. Arch Gen Psychiatry 49:1050–1055, 1985

Hoegerman G, Wilson CA, Thurmond E, et al: Drug-exposed neonates. Western J Med 152:559–564, 1990

Institute of Medicine: Fetal alcohol syndrome: research base for diagnostic criteria, epidemiology, prevention, and treatment. Washington, DC, National Academy Press, 1996

Johnson Institute: Intervention: A Professional's Guide. Minneapolis, MN, Johnson Institute, 1983

Jones MC: Personality antecedents and correlates of drinking patterns in women. J Consult Clin Psychol 36:61–69, 1971

Klassen AD, Wilsnack SC: Sexual experiences and drinking among women in a US national survey. Arch Sex Behav 15:363–392, 1986

Klee L, Ames G: Reevaluating risk factors for women's drinking: a study of blue collar wives. Am J Prev Med 3:31–41, 1987

Kubicka L, Csemy L, Kozeny J: Prague women's drinking before and after the "velvet revolution" of 1989: a longitudinal study. Addiction 90:1471–1478, 1995

Levy M, Koren G: Obstetric and neonatal effects of drug abuse. Emerg Med Clin North Am 8:633–652, 1990

Little RE, Streissguth AP, Guzinski GM, et al: Change in obstetrician advice following a two-year community educational program on alcohol use and pregnancy. Am J Obstet Gynecol 146:23–28, 1983

Little RE, Anderson KW, Ervin CH, et al: Maternal alcohol use during breast-feeding and infant mental and motor development at one year. N Engl J Med 321:425–430, 1989

Longnecker MP, Berlin JA, Orza MJ, et al: A meta-analysis of alcohol consumption in relation to risk of breast cancer. JAMA 260:652–656, 1988

Malatesta MV, Pollack RH, Crotty TD, et al: Acute alcohol intoxication and female orgasmic response. J Sex Res 18:1–17, 1982

Mastrogiannis DS, Decavalas GO, Verma U, et al: Perinatal outcome after recent cocaine usage. Obstet Gynecol 76:8–11, 1990

May PA, Hymbaugh KJ: A macro-level FAS prevention program for Native Americans and Alaskan Natives: description and evaluation. J Stud Alcohol 50:508–518, 1989

McKinlay AP: The roman attitude toward women's drinking, in Drinking and Intoxication. Edited by McCarthy RG, New Haven, CT, College and University Press, 1959, pp 58–61

Mello NK: Drug use patterns and premenstrual dysphoria, in Women and Drugs: A New Era for Research (NIDA Research Monograph 65). Edited by Ray BA, Braude MC, Washington DC, U.S. Department of Health and Human Services, 1986, pp 31–48

Mello NK, Mendelson JH, Teoh SK: Neuroendocrine consequences of alcohol abuse in women. Ann NY Acad Sci 562:211–240, 1989

Miller BA, Downs WR, Gondoli DM: Spousal violence among alcoholic women as compared to a random household sample of women. J Stud Alcohol 50:533–540, 1989

Miller LJ: Detoxification of the addicted woman in pregnancy, Chapter XVI-3, in American Society of Addiction Medicine Principles of Addiction Medicine. Chevy Chase, MD, American Society of Addiction Medicine, 1994, pp 1–10

Minkoff HL, McCalla S, Delke I, et al: The relationship of cocaine use to syphilis and HIV infections among inner city parturient women. Am J Obstet Gynecol 163:521–526, 1990

Mitchell JL: Treatment of the addicted woman in pregnancy, Chapter XVI-4, in American Society of Addiction Medicine Principles of Addiction Medicine. Chevy Chase, MD, American Society of Addiction Medicine, 1994, pp 1–4

Moore RD, Bone LR, Geller G, et al: Prevalence, detection, and treatment of alcoholism in hospitalized patients. JAMA 261:403–408, 1989

Parente JT, Gaines B, Lockridge R, et al: Substance abuse during pregnancy. NY State J Med 90:336–337, 1990

Richardson D, Campbell J: The effect of alcohol on attributions of blame for rape. Personality and Social Psychology Bulletin 8:468–476, 1982

Richardson GA, Day NL: Detrimental effects of prenatal cocaine exposure: illusion or reality? J Am Acad Child Adolesc Psychiatry 33:28–34, 1994

Rolfs RT, Nakishima AK: Epidemiology of primary and secondary syphilis in the U.S. 1981 through 1989. JAMA 246:1432–1437, 1990

Rosen TS, Johnson HL: Long-term effects of prenatal methadone maintenance, in Consequences of Maternal Drug Abuse (NIDA Research Monograph 59). Edited by Pinkert TM. Washington, DC, U.S. Department of Health and Human Services, 1985, pp 73–83

Rounsaville BJ, Dolinsky ZS, Babor TF, et al: Psychopathology as a predictor of treatment outcome in alcoholics. Arch Gen Psychiatry 44:505–513, 1987

Russell M: Clinical implications of recent research on the fetal alcohol syndrome. Bull NY Acad Med 67:207–222, 1991

Russell M: New assessment tools for risk drinking during pregnancy: TACE, TWEAK, and others. Alcohol Health and Research World 18:55–61, 1994

Russell M, Coviello D: Heavy drinking and regular psychoactive drug use among gynecological outpatients. Alcohol Clin Exp Res 12:400–406, 1988

Russell M, Kang GE, Uhteg L: Evaluation of an educational program on FAS for health professionals. J Alcohol Drug Educ 29:48–61, 1983

Russell M, Cooper, ML, Frone MR: The influence of sociodemographic characteristics on familial alcohol problems: data from a community sample. Alcohol Clin Exp Res 14:221–226, 1990

Selwyn PA, Schoenbaum EE, Davenny K et al: Prospective study of human immunodeficiency virus and pregnancy outcomes in intravenous drug users. JAMA 261:1289–1294, 1989

Serdula M, Williamson DF, Kendrick JS, et al: Trends in alcohol consumption by pregnant women: 1985 through 1988. JAMA 265:876–879, 1991

Skolnick A: Cocaine use in pregnancy: physicians urged to look for problem where they least expect it. JAMA 264:306–309, 1990

Sokol RJ, Martier SS, Ager JW: The TACE questions: practical prenatal detection of risk-drinking. Am J Obstet Gynecol 160:863–870, 1989

Substance Abuse and Mental Health Services Administration: National household survey on drug abuse: population estimates 1993 (Publication No. [SMA] 94-3017). Washington, DC, Department of Health and Human Services, 1994

Testa M, Parks KA: The role of women's alcohol consumption in sexual victimization. Aggression and Violent Behavior 1:217–234, 1996

U. S. General Accounting Office: Drug-exposed infants: a generation at risk (Publication No. GAO/HRD 90-138). Washington, DC, General Accounting Office, 1990

U.S. Surgeon General: Surgeon General's advisory and alcohol and pregnancy. FDA Drug Bulletin 11:1, 1981

Urbano-Marquez A, Rubin E, Fernandez-Sola J, et al: The greater risk of alcoholic cardiomyopathy and myopathy in women compared with men. JAMA 274:149–154, 1995

Wallach RC, Jerez E, Blinick G: Pregnancy and menstrual function in narcotics addicts treated with methadone: the Methadone Maintenance Treatment Program. Am J Obstet Gynecol 105:1226–1229, 1969

Warner LA, Kessler RC, Hughes M, et al: Prevalence and correlates of drug use and dependence in the United States. Arch Gen Psychiatry 52:219–228, 1995

Washton AM: Cocaine Addiction. New York, Norton, 1989

Weiner L, Rosett HL, Edelin KC: Behavioral evaluation of fetal alcohol education for physicians. Alcohol Clin Exp Res 6:230–233, 1983

Wilsnack SC: Drinking sexuality and sexual dysfunction in women, in Alcohol Problems in Women. Edited by Wilsnack SC, Beckman LJ. New York, Guilford, 1984, pp 189–227

Wilson GT, Lawson DM: Effects of alcohol on sexual arousal in women. J Abnorm Psychol 85:489–497, 1976

Winfield I, George LK, Swartz M, et al: Sexual assault and psychiatric disorders among a community sample of women. Am J Psychiatry 147:335-341, 1990

Ylikorkala O, Stenman U, Halmesmaki E: Gammaglutamyl transferase and mean cell volume reveal maternal alcohol abuse and fetal alcohol effects. Am J Obstet Gynecol 157:344–348, 1987

# Eating Disorders and Reproduction

Donna E. Stewart, M.D., D.Psych., F.R.C.P.C.
Gail Erlick Robinson, M.D., D.Psych., F.R.C.P.C.

The social and medical construction of the term *eating disorders* is in itself a paradox. Although obesity affects approximately 30% of North American adult women, resulting in greatly increased morbidity, mortality, health care costs, and social stigma (Carek et al. 1997; Rosenbaum et al. 1997), *eating disorders* has usually been restricted to anorexia nervosa, bulimia nervosa, and variants of these disorders, which affect about 5% of young North American women. In addition, the epidemic of malnutrition prevalent throughout the world, including among poor North American families, has been largely ignored by eating disorder interest groups other than as a point of reference for the effects of starvation. One might well wonder how this construction of eating disorders has evolved.

The study of eating disorders, involving (as it usually does) relatively attractive middle-class teenagers and young women, appears to be of much greater interest to the (largely male) experts than the study of predominantly older, relatively less attractive, lower social class, high-risk obese and overweight middle-aged and older women. The problems of malnutrition receive less attention in the developed world, probably because they are seen to have socioeconomic causes and solutions and are thought to be geographically remote. In fact, caloric restriction, overconsumption, and under supply are all critically important issues in women's physical, psychologic, and sociocultural health. This chapter narrowly focuses on the topics traditionally included in eating disorders (caloric restriction) as they affect one specific aspect of women's lives—reproduction.

Social pressures for thinness in women escalated greatly during the twentieth century as a result of remarkable shifts in attitudes concerning women's attractiveness. After centuries of admiration for curvaceous women, thinness became idealized. One paradoxic aspect of this quest for thinness is that, as nutrition has improved, the average weight of women in industrialized societies has increased by five pounds (Polivy et al. 1986). These factors have led to a greatly increased pressure to diet.

Various theories have been proposed to explain this emphasis on thinness. One factor may be the tendency of modern society to idealize youthfulness (Shainess 1979). Prepubescent girls acting as fashion models promote the belief that the ideal shape is that of a child. Excessive thinness eliminates the curves suggestive of adulthood. Moreover, throughout history, upper-class women have served as role models for fashion. In contradistinction to the past, being overweight no longer denotes wealth. Rather, in today's industrialized society, it is lower-class women with inadequate diets and insufficient exercise who are the most likely to be overweight (Polivy et al. 1986).

The devotion to thinness that began in the upper classes has now spread throughout society. Preoccupation with weight may also reflect the new pressures on women to compete with men; eliminating the feminine figure may be an attempt to reinforce the move away from traditional female stereotypes (Orbach 1978). Because dieting may be regarded as a sign of internal control, slim women may be viewed as more disciplined and in control.

Pressures for thinness have resulted in a general increase in body consciousness that is much more marked for women than for men. Surveys of high school students indicate that girls usually want to weigh less than their current weight (Jakobovits et al. 1977), whereas most boys want to gain weight. National surveys of adults conclude that a woman's self-esteem often relates to her feeling pretty and slim (Berscheid et al. 1973). Surveys of college-age women have found dieting and disordered eating to be widespread (Herman and Polivy 1980).

One way that young women may control body weight is through excessive exercising. The athletic triad of amenorrhea, osteopenia, and eating disorders has received increasing attention in the past decade. Adolescents may seek care for amenorrhea or other menstrual problems without disclosing an eating disorder. Rome et al. (1996) found 18.9% of adolescents attending a reproductive endocrinology clinic to have elevated Eating Attitudes Test (EAT)-26 scores suggestive of an eating disorder.

Many women with eating disorders are secretive about them, and problems in diagnosis are compounded by the fact that some women with eating disorders appear to be of normal weight by actuarial or population mean standards. Careful examination of their longitudinal weight histories, however, may reveal premorbid obesity that led to highly restrictive dieting coupled with bulimic behaviors. Relative starvation and nutritional chaos may thus be obscured. Eating disorders result in a mortality rate of approximately 5% and lead to significant morbidity secondary to weight loss, vomiting, electrolyte disturbances, gastrointestinal problems, osteoporosis, psychiatric sequelae, and reproductive complications (Garfinkel 1982). Although the medical effects have been described for many years, the reproductive aspects of eating disorders have been inadequately studied (Stewart and Robinson 1989).

It is known that many patients with eating disorders develop amenorrhea, and over the past decade more attention has been paid to infertility in these women (Abraham et al. 1990; Allison et al. 1988; Stewart et al. 1990). As more effective treatment of eating disorders and infertility evolves, more women with eating disorders eventually become pregnant. Little is known about the course of their pregnancies or the health of their infants. Many psychologic conflicts that are common in patients with eating disorders, such as body image, autonomy, sexuality, dependency, and relationships to parents, are highlighted during normal pregnancy. It is therefore likely that pregnancy is an especially stressful time for women with eating disorders (Jenkin and Tiggemann 1997; Stewart et al. 1987). This chapter examines what is currently known about the effects of eating disorders on menstruation, sexuality and fertility, pregnancy, the fetus and newborn, and infant feeding. Several studies have shown that the postpartum period and breastfeeding are also important risk periods for eating disorders (Foster et al. 1996; Jenkin and Tiggemann 1997; Stein and Fairburn 1996).

## Definition of Eating Disorders

### Anorexia Nervosa

*Anorexia nervosa* is a psychiatric disorder characterized by refusal to maintain body weight at or above a minimally normal weight for age and height (e.g., weight loss leading to maintenance of a body weight less than 85% of that expected or failure to achieve expected weight gain during a period of growth, leading to body weight less than 85% of that expected); intense fear of gaining weight or of becoming fat even though underweight; disturbance in the way in which one's body weight or shape is experienced, undue influence of body weight or shape on self-evaluation, or denial of the seriousness of the current low body weight; and, in postmenarcheal females, amenorrhea (i.e., the absence of at least three consecutive menstrual cycles—a woman is considered to have amenorrhea if her periods occur only following hormone administration) (American Psychiatric Association 1994). This self-imposed starvation triggered by the relentless pursuit of thinness and fear of fatness occurs in serious form in about 1% of adolescent and young adult women (Garfinkel and Garner 1982).

## Bulimia Nervosa

A related disorder, bulimia nervosa, has several key characteristics: 1) Recurrent episodes of binge eating occur—that is, eating, in a discrete period of time (e.g., within any 2-hour period), an amount of food that is definitely larger than most people would eat during a similar period of time and under similar circumstances. These binges are usually accompanied by a sense of lack of control over eating during the episode (e.g., a feeling that one cannot stop eating or control what or how much one is eating). 2) To prevent weight gain from binge eating, recurrent inappropriate compensatory behaviors are employed, such as self-induced vomiting; misuse of laxatives, diuretics, enemas, or other medications; fasting; or excessive exercise. 3) This binge/purge cycle occurs, on average, at least twice a week for 3 months. 4) Self-evaluation is unduly influenced by body shape and weight. 5) The disturbance does not occur exclusively during episodes of anorexia nervosa (American Psychiatric Association 1994). Bulimia nervosa may occur within the context of anorexia nervosa or as a separate syndrome with little weight loss. Its prevalence in serious form is 1.7% among adolescent and young women (Ben-Tovim 1988).

## Eating Disorder Not Otherwise Specified

The eating disorder not otherwise specified (EDNOS) category is for disorders of eating that do not meet criteria for a specific eating disorder: 1) For females, all of the criteria for anorexia nervosa are met except that the individual has regular menses. 2) All of the criteria for anorexia nervosa are met except that, despite significant weight loss, the individual's current weight is in the normal range. 3) All of the criteria for bulimia nervosa are met except that the binge eating and inappropriate compensatory mechanisms occur at a frequency of less than twice a week or for a duration of less than 3 months. 4) Inappropriate compensatory behaviors are used by an individual of normal body weight after eating small amounts of food (e.g., self-induced vomiting after the consumption of two cookies). 5) Large amounts of food are repeatedly chewed and spit out but not swallowed. 6) Recurrent episodes of binge eating occur without regular use of inappropriate compensatory behaviors (binge eating disorder) (American Psychiatric Association 1994). ED-NOS occurs in an additional 5% of the female population (Button and Whitehouse 1981; King 1986).

## Effects on Menstruation

It has long been known that women with anorexia nervosa may suffer from primary or secondary amenorrhea (Gull 1974). Indeed, one of the criteria for the diagnosis of anorexia nervosa includes absence of periods for three cycles. Pirke et al. (1985) have shown that 50% of patients with bulimia nervosa also suffer from amenorrhea. It is therefore prudent for clinicians to inquire about eating and dieting behaviors in women who report absent or irregular menstrual cycles.

Starkey and Lee (1969) observed the menstruation cycles of 58 patients with a previous diagnosis of anorexia nervosa and found that all patients had established menstrual patterns prior to the onset of the disorder, but most became amenorrheic concurrent with the onset of the eating disorder. Most reported improved weight gain with treatment but, in the group who did not gain weight, none experienced the return of menses. Nillius (1978) reported that 34% of 287 amenorrheic women had amenorrhea caused by self-induced weight loss. Fries (1974) found a high proportion of women with eating disorders among 30 Scandinavian women with secondary amenorrhea caused by self-induced weight loss.

Copeland and Herzog (1987) and Devlin et al. (1989) described endocrine findings associated with menstrual cycle abnormalities in women with anorexia nervosa and bulimia nervosa. In general, these women tended to have fewer secretory spikes of luteinizing hormone (LH) and a trend toward lower mean 24-hour LH levels than did control subjects. Stimulation with gonadotropin-releasing hormone produced elevated LH responses in women with bulimia nervosa and blunted LH responses in those with anorexia. Estradiol levels were uniformly lower in women with anorexia nervosa, and stimulation with estradiol revealed diminished LH augmentative responses and a trend toward diminished follicle-stimulating hormone (FSH) augmentative responses in patients with anorexia nervosa and bulimia nervosa compared with control subjects. Pirke et al. (1985, 1988) have shown that approximately 50% of normal-weight women who have bulimia nervosa have menstrual abnormalities with impaired follicle maturation caused by impaired gonadotropin secretion. These authors have also shown that in normal young women of normal body weight who diet for 6 weeks (800–1,000 kcal/day), various changes in endocrine function develop and, in about 20% of these women, menstrual cycle disruption occurs for 3–6 months after dieting.

Kreipe et al. (1989) have shown that women with EDNOS also frequently have menstrual dysfunction. Because this disorder occurs more frequently than criteria-confirmed anorexia or bulimia nervosa, the full extent of the contribution of eating disorders to the clinical symptom of disordered menstruation is still unknown. However, it is likely to be substantial in developed countries (see also Rome et al. 1996).

## Effects on Sexuality and Fertility

Psychologic theory has postulated that eating disorders may be a defense against sexuality in young women. Eating disorder patients show delays in several aspects of psychosexual development including age at first kiss, masturbation, genital fondling, and first intercourse (Schmidt et al. 1995). Morgan et al. (1999) reported that unplanned pregnancies were the norm in women with bulimia nervosa, especially resulting from mistaken beliefs about fertility.

Of all couples having regular, unprotected intercourse in the childbearing years, 15%–18% are unable to conceive within 1 year (Menning 1980). It has been assumed that among women with eating disorders, only those with anorexia nervosa accompanied by amenorrhea contributed to the overall rates of infertility. Recent studies, however, have shown that unexplained infertility may sometimes be due to an undisclosed eating disorder or severe weight control. At the other end of the spectrum, obesity may also interfere with sexuality and fertility (Clark et al. 1998; Galletly et al. 1996).

Bates et al. (1982) found that 47 women with unexplained infertility or menstrual dysfunction who were referred to a reproductive endocrinology clinic had practiced weight control by caloric restriction to maintain a fashionable body habitus. When 36 of the women followed a dietary regimen designed to increase their weight to predicted ideal body weight, 73% conceived spontaneously and 90% with secondary amenorrhea resumed menstruation. It is of interest that 97% of these "infertile" women and their husbands had been previously evaluated for infertility with various diagnostic gynecologic studies without any cause being discovered.

In infertility patients with amenorrhea, Nillius (1978) found that a number of costly and complicated gynecologic and endocrinologic investigations, and sometimes hormonal induction of ovulation, were carried out without the patients' inadequate dietary intake ever coming to light. Allison et al. (1988) found an increased prevalence of abnormal eating attitudes in a small sample of infertility clinic patients. Stewart et al. (1990) reported a 17% prevalence of eating disorders in 66 consecutive patients attending a reproductive biology unit for infertility investigations. The patients were prospectively screened with the EAT-26 item (Garner et al. 1982), and women with positive screening tests then underwent a standardized interview to confirm or refute the diagnosis of an eating disorder. Of these women, 7.6% had anorexia nervosa or bulimia nervosa and 9.1% had EDNOS. Among infertile women with amenorrhea or oligomenorrhea, 58% had eating disorders. It is of interest that none of these patients had previously disclosed her eating disorder to the infertility specialist. The similarity of this finding to that of Rome et al. (1996), who found a prevalence of 18.9% of elevated EAT-26 scores in adolescents attending a reproductive endocrine clinic, is striking.

Abraham et al. (1990) raised the question of whether ovulation should be induced in women suffering or recovering from an eating disorder in view of their poorer prognosis in pregnancy. They found that 13 of 14 consecutive women in whom ovulation had been induced met the criteria for an eating disorder at some time in the past, with five women currently fulfilling these criteria.

Several investigators have recommended that infertility specialists routinely ask questions about a women's eating and dieting behavior, history of eating disorders, exercising habits, and past and present body weight before proceeding with infertility investigations (Abraham et al. 1990; Stewart and MacDonald 1987; Stewart et al. 1990). Patients usually fail to volunteer information about eating disorders to their gynecologists and may appear to be of normal weight. An awareness of the frequency of eating disorders in infertility patients, however, followed by careful clinical inquiry, should correctly identify most cases. It has become more common for infertility clinics to provide psychologic support services for couples who are distressed by the diagnosis, investigation, and management of infertility problems (Stewart et al. 1992). Psychiatrists working with infertility patients can provide useful resources in the early identification and treatment of concurrent eating disorders or disordered eating that fails to meet full eating-disorder diagnostic criteria.

## Prevalence of Eating Disorders in Pregnancy

The best data on the prevalence of eating disorders in pregnancy derives from a study of 530 pregnant women screened with the Eating Attitudes Test. Test results indicated that 4.9% of the women scored above the recommended threshold (Turton et al. 1999). Eating disorder symptomatology was associated with younger age, previous symptomatology, lower education, poorer housing, lack of employment, and previous miscarriage.

## Effects on Pregnancy

### Hyperemesis Gravidarum

*Hyperemesis gravidarum* is intractable vomiting during pregnancy that requires hospitalization and is accompanied by dehydration, electrolyte imbalance, ketonuria, and weight loss. In a study of patients with hyperemesis gravidarum who were referred for psychiatric consultation (Stewart and MacDonald 1987), it was found that several had had an eating disorder before conception but had not revealed this initially. A comparison with women who had hyperemesis gravidarum without a history of eating disorders found that those with eating disorders responded less favorably to treatment and spent twice as many days in the hospital during pregnancy. Approximately half of the hyperemesis patients with eating disorders had presented to an infertility clinic for induction of ovulation. Lingam and McCluskey (1996) also draw attention to this issue. Although hyperemesis gravidarum may be caused by various psychologic, social, physical, and physiologic problems, it is wise for obstetricians and consulting psychiatrists to remember that an eating disorder may also play an important role in some women. Further studies are required to investigate the true prevalence of eating disorders in women with hyperemesis gravidarum.

Food aversions, cravings, and pica are common occurrences in pregnancy. Their association, if any, to eating disorders is unknown. These phenomena may accompany hyperemesis gravidarum but often present in the absence of vomiting. Most food aversions and cravings are considered normal in pregnancy.

### Low Maternal Weight Gain

Low maternal weight before pregnancy and poor weight gain during pregnancy correlate significantly with an increase in intrauterine growth retardation, low birth weight, congenital anomalies, and perinatal mortality (Abrams and Laros 1986). Although many of the data were collected during famines or in concentration camps, eating disorders are also a cause of low prepregnancy weight and failure to gain weight in pregnancy because of inadequate nutrition. Stewart et al. (1987) described 15 women who had previously suffered from anorexia nervosa or bulimia nervosa and who later conceived a total of 23 pregnancies. Compared with women whose eating disorders were in remission, women who had an active eating disorder throughout pregnancy gained less weight and had more pregnancy complications. Lacey and Smith (1987) examined the impact of pregnancy in a report on eating behavior in 20 patients who had untreated bulimia nervosa and who were of normal weight. They found that although the frequency of bulimic behavior generally diminished as pregnancy advanced, symptoms tended to return in the puerperium. In nearly half of the study sample, eating patterns were more disturbed after delivery than before conception.

Careful nutritional, weight, and psychosocial histories should be obtained in women who fail to gain weight adequately in pregnancy. Early psychiatric referral is indicated in women with psychiatric diagnoses or eating disorders.

## Effects on the Fetus and Newborn

Several investigators (Brinch et al. 1988; Lacey and Smith 1987; Stewart et al. 1987; Strimling 1984; Treasure and Russell 1988) have described fetal problems associated with a maternal eating disorder. More recently, Blais et al. (2000) reported elevated therapeutic abortion rates in women with eating disorders. These difficulties may include intrauterine growth retardation, prematurity, low birth weight, low Apgar scores, increased risk of congenital anomalies, and higher perinatal mortality. Intrauterine growth retardation from any cause may have considerable consequences including fetal antenatal or intrapartum asphyxia, which may lead to fetal death or an increase in fetal distress and damage (Van der Spuy 1985). Once delivered, these small infants are at increased risk for hypothermia, hypoglycemia, and infection and have increased perinatal mortality (Van der Spuy 1985). Stewart et al. (1987) found that babies born to women with active eating disorders during their pregnancies were smaller and had lower 5-minute Apgar scores than did babies of mothers whose eating disorders were in remission. Lacey and Smith (1987) described higher incidences of fetal abnormalities, including cleft lip and palate; multiple gestation; obstetric complications, including breech presentation; and surgical intervention in 20 untreated bulimic women of normal weight. Brinch et al. (1988) followed-up with 50 women with histories of eating disorders and found double the rate of premature births in their offspring and six times the expected rate of perinatal mortality. Treasure and Russell (1988) described the outcome of seven pregnancies in women with anorexia nervosa who conceived despite low weight. The abdominal circumference of all seven babies was well below the third percentile at birth. Conti et al. (1998) found that women with disordered eating were at greater risk of delivering a small-for-gestational-age term infant. Bulik et al. (1999) found that women with anorexia nervosa had more miscarriages and cesarean sections, premature births, and low birth weight infants. These studies all suffer from small sample sizes, and further work is required to replicate their findings and assess effective interventions in large, controlled studies.

## Effects in the Postpartum Period

Investigators have described a postpartum exacerbation of clinical eating disorders (Lacey and Smith 1987; Stewart et al. 1987). Eating disorder symptoms may also increase markedly in the 3 months postpartum and then plateau over the next 6 months. Weight concerns and concern about residual weight after the birth of the child were found by Stein and Fairburn (1996) to be particularly distressing to many women and served to precipitate a clinical eating disorder in a few cases. Moreover, women with eating disorders have been shown to be at risk of depression and anxiety in the postpartum period (Stewart et al. 1987). Morgan et al. (1999) reported postnatal depression in one-third of women with bulimia nervosa. They also found that although bulimic symptoms improved during pregnancy, 57% of women had worse symptoms after delivery but 34% were no longer bulimic. Blais et al. (2000) found that women with bulimia nervosa showed a decrease in eating disorder severity during pregnancy and postpartum, whereas women with anorexia nervosa returned to prepregnancy levels by 6 months postpartum.

## Effects on the Infant and Feeding

In general, low birth weight infants who survive the early weeks of life are at risk for long-term developmental consequences with continued delays in physical and neurologic development and impaired intellectual ability, particularly when associated with low intrauterine growth before 26 weeks of gestation (Van der Spuy 1985). No work has yet been reported on the long-term follow-up of low birth weight infants born to mothers with eating disorders. It is hoped that, in view of the prevalence of eating disorders in young women, this work will soon be undertaken.

An additional problem in some mothers with eating disorders results from the worry that their infants will become obese, a concern that leads to early nutritional deprivation or caloric restriction. Lacey and Smith (1987) found that 15% of bulimic mothers reported restricting calories in their child before 1 year of age. Stewart et al. (1987) found a decreased rate of breast-feeding in women with active eating disorders and more difficulties with postpartum adjustment. Brinch et al. (1988) reported a 17% rate of failure to thrive in the first year of life in the infants of mothers with eating disorders. Stein et al. (1996) found that although the infants were smaller (length and weight for age), little evidence showed that these mothers preferred smaller children, were dissatisfied with their child's shape, or misperceived the child's size. They concluded that the growth disturbance did not appear to be a direct extension of the maternal psychopathology to the infant. Treasure and Russell (1988) reported that the children of four patients attending their eating disorders clinic had been investigated for poor growth attributed to inadequate feeding. They also reported that five of six mothers with anorexia nervosa had difficulty in breastfeeding and introduced bottle-feeds in the first few months of life. Foster et al. (1996) reported that body shape dissatisfaction and low maternal fetal attachment may account for why some women chose to bottle feed. Stein and Fairburn (1989), Fahy and Treasure (1989), and Van Wezel-Meijler and Wit (1989) also found poor nutrition, concerns about the mother–child relationship, and developmental concerns while assessing the infants of eating disordered women. McCann et al. (1994) found the eating habits and attitudes toward body shape and weight in 26 mothers of children with nonorganic failure to thrive had higher levels of dieting restraint than in 26 matched mothers of normal weight infants. Despite their children's low weight, 50% of index mothers restricted "sweet" foods and 30% restricted "fattening or unhealthy" foods. Stein et al. (1995) also found abnormal eating habits and attitudes in mothers of children with feeding disorders, and Waugh and Bulik (1999) found that mothers with eating disorder had more difficulty with breastfeeding and made fewer positive comments about food and eating than did other mothers of toddlers.

Pediatricians (Pugliese et al. 1987) have also reported failure to thrive in infants whose parents had been restricting calories in their children because of fears that they might become overweight, although it is not clear that these parents actually had eating disorders themselves (as opposed to overconcern about obesity). Further investigations are required to establish the role of maternal eating disorders in nutritionally deprived children in wealthy developed countries.

## Conclusions

Currently available information suggests that a history of eating disorders or weight-reducing behavior should be part of the routine assessment of patients with amenorrhea, oligomenorrhea, and infertility as well as in prenatal patients with hyperemesis gravidarum, those who fail to gain weight adequately in pregnancy, and those who have babies who are small for gestational date. Women in whom eating disorders are discovered before conception should be counseled to delay pregnancy until the eating disorder is adequately treated and truly in remission. If the woman has already conceived, the earliest possible diagnosis of an eating disorder should be made so that proper psychiatric treatment, dietary advice, and weight monitoring can be implemented to reduce the risk of maternal and fetal complications. Follow-up after delivery should be vigilant for postpartum exacerbations of eating disorders and depression. Infants of mothers with eating disorders should also be carefully observed for failure to thrive so that early corrective measures can be implemented. Similarly, the parents of infants who fail to thrive should be assessed for eating disorders, overconcern about obesity, or abnormal eating behaviors. Franko and Spurrell (2000) recommended a team approach that emphasizes communication and clear goal setting for pregnant women with eating disorder. Study of the reproductive effects of eating disorders offers many rich opportunities for psychiatrists to collaborate with obstetricians and gynecologists, nutritionists, nurses, and perinatologists in primary and secondary prevention programs directed toward mother and infant.

## References

Abraham S, Mira M, Llewellyn-Jones D: Should ovulation be induced in women recovering from an eating disorder or who are compulsive exercisers? Fertil Steril 52:566–568, 1990

Abrams BF, Laros RK: Pregnancy weight, weight gain, and birth weight. Am J Obstet Gynecol 154:503–509, 1986

Allison S, Kalucy R, Gilchrist P, et al: Weight preoccupation among infertile women. Int J Eat Disord 7:743–748, 1988

American Psychiatric Association: Diagnostic and Statistical Manual of Mental Disorders, 4th Edition. Washington, DC, American Psychiatric Association, 1994

Bates GW, Bates SR, Whitworth NS: Reproductive failure in women who practice weight control. Fertil Steril 37:373–378, 1982

Ben-Tovim DI: DSM-III, draft DSM-III-R, and the diagnosis and prevalence of bulimia in Australia. Am J Psychiatry 145:1000–1002, 1988

Berscheid E, Walster E, Bohrnstedt GW: The happy American body: a survey report. Psychology Today 7:119–131, 1973

Blais MA, Becker AE, Burwell RA, et al: Pregnancy: outcome and impact on symptomatology in a cohort of eating-disordered women. Int J Eat Disord 27:140–149, 2000

Brinch M, Isager T, Tolstrup K: Anorexia nervosa and motherhood: reproductional pattern and mothering behaviour of 50 women. Acta Psychiatr Scand 77:98–104, 1988

Bulik CM, Sullivan PF, Fear JL, et al: Fertility and reproduction in women with anorexia nervosa: a controlled study. J Clin Psychiatry 60:130–135, 1999

Button EJ, Whitehouse A: Subclinical anorexia nervosa. Psychol Med 11:509–516, 1981

Carek PJ, Sherer J, Stier Carson D: Management of obesity: medical treatment options. American Family Physician 55:551–558, 1997

Clark AM, Thornley B, Tomlinson L, et al: Weight loss in obese infertile women results in improvement in reproductive outcome for all forms of fertility treatment. Hum Reprod 13:1502–1505, 1998

Conti J, Abraham S, Taylor A: Eating behavior and pregnancy outcome. J Psychosom Res 44:465–477, 1998

Copeland PM, Herzog DB: Menstrual abnormalities, in the Psychobiology of Bulimia. Edited by Hudson JI, Pipe HG. Washington, DC, American Psychiatric Press, 1987, pp 31–54

Devlin MJ, Walsh BT, Katz JL, et al: Hypothalamic–pituitary–gonadal function in anorexia nervosa and bulimia. Psychiatry Res 28:11–24, 1989

Fahy T, Treasure J: Children of the mothers with bulimia nervosa. BMJ 299:1031, 1989

Foster SF, Wilson K, Slade P: Body image, maternal fetal attachment and breast-feeding. J Psychosom Res 41:181–184, 1996

Franko DL, Spurrell EB: Detection and management of eating disorders during pregnancy. Obstet Gynecol 95:942–946, 2000

Fries H: Secondary amenorrhea, self-induced weight reduction, and anorexia nervosa. Acta Psychiatr Scand 248(suppl):1–69, 1974

Galletly C, Clark A, Tomlinson L, et al: Improved pregnancy rates for obese, infertile women following a group treatment program: an open pilot study. Gen Hosp Psychiatry 18:192–195, 1996

Garfinkel PE, Garner D: Anorexia Nervosa: A Multidimensional Perspective. New York, Brunner/Mazel, 1982, pp 307–326

Garner DM, Olmsted MP, Bohr Y, et al: The Eating Attitudes Test: psychometric features and clinical correlates. Psychol Med 12:871–878, 1982

Gull WW: Anorexia nervosa. Transactions of the Clinical Society of London 7:22–28, 1974

Herman CP, Polivy J: Restrained Eating in Obesity. Edited by Stunkard A. Philadelphia, WB Saunders, 1980, pp 208–239

Jakobovits C, Halstead P, Kelley L, et al: Eating habits and nutritional intakes of college women over a thirty-year period. J Am Diet Assoc 71:405–411, 1977

Jenkin W, Tiggemann M: Psychological effects of weight retained after pregnancy. Women Health 25:89–98, 1997

King MB: Eating disorders in general practice. BMJ 293:1412–1414, 1986

Kreipe RE, Strauss J, Hodgman CH, et al: Menstrual cycle abnormalities and subclinical eating disorders: a preliminary report. Psychosom Med 51:1–86, 1989

Lacey JH, Smith G: Bulimia nervosa: the impact of pregnancy on mother and baby. Br J Psychiatry 150:777–781, 1987

Lingam R, McCluskey S: Eating disorders associated with hyperemesis gravidarum. J Psychosom Res 40:231–234, 1996

McCann JB, Stein A, Fairburn CG, et al: Eating habits and attitudes of mothers of children with nonorganic failure to thrive. Arch Dis Childhood 70:234–236, 1994

Menning BE: The emotional needs of infertile couples. Fertil Steril 34:313–319, 1980

Morgan JF, Lacey JH, Sedgwick PM: Impact of pregnancy on bulimia nervosa. Br J Psychiatry 174:135–140, 1999

Nillius SJ: Psychopathology of weight-related amenorrhea, in Advances in Gynaecological Endocrinology. Edited by Jacobs HS. London, England: Royal College of Obstetricians and Gynaecologists, 1978, pp 118–130

Orbach S: Fat is a Feminist Issue: The Anti-Diet Guide to Permanent Weight Loss. New York, Paddington, 1978

Pirke KM, Ulrich S, Lemmel W, et al: The influence of dieting on the menstrual cycle of healthy young women. J Clin Endocrinol Metab 60:1174–1179, 1985

Pirke KM, Dogs M, Fichter MM, et al: Gonadotrophins, oestradiol, and progesterone during the menstrual cycle in bulimia nervosa. Clin Endocrinol 29:265–270, 1988

Polivy J, Garner DM, Garfinkel PE: Causes and consequences of the current preference for thin female physiques, in Physical Appearance: Stigma and Social Behavior. Edited by Herman CP, Zanna MP, Higgins ET. Hillsdale, NJ, Lawrence Erlbaum, 1986, pp 89–112

Pugliese MT, Weyman-Daum M, Moses M, et al: Parental health beliefs as a cause of nonorganic failure to thrive. Pediatrics 80:175–182, 1987

Rome ES, Gidwani G, Rybicki LA, et al: Prevalence of abnormal eating attitudes and behaviors in hospital-bases primary and tertiary care clinics: a window of opportunity? J Pediatr Adolesc Gynecol 9:133–138, 1996

Rosenbaum M, Leibel R, Hirsch J: Obesity. N Engl J Med 337:396–405, 1997

Schmidt U, Treasure J, Tiller J, et al: Puberty, sexual milestones, and abuse: how are they related in eating disorder patients? Psychol Med 25:413–417, 1995

Shainess N: The swing of the pendulum: from anorexia to obesity. Am J Psychoanal 39:225–234, 1979

Starkey TA, Lee RA: Menstruation and fertility in anorexia nervosa. Am J Obstet Gynecol 105:374–379, 1969

Stein A, Fairburn CG: Children of mothers with bulimia nervosa. BMJ 299:777–778, 1989

Stein A, Fairburn CG: Eating habits and attitudes in the postpartum period. Psychosom Med 58:321–325, 1996

Stein A, Stein J, Walters EA, et al: Eating habits and attitudes among mothers of children with feeding disorders. BMJ 310:228, 1995

Stein A, Murray L, Cooper P, et al: Infant growth in the context of maternal eating disorders and maternal depression: a comparative study. Psychol Med 26:569–574, 1996

Stewart DE, MacDonald OL: Hyperemesis gravidarum and eating disorders in pregnancy, in Eating Disorders and Disordered Eating. Edited by Abraham S, Llewellyn-Jones D. Sydney, Australia, Ashwood House, 1987, pp 52–55

Stewart DE, Robinson GE: Pregnancy and eating disorders, in The Free Woman. Edited by Van Hall E. Carnforth, UK, Parthenon, 1989, pp 812–817

Stewart DE, Raskin J, Garfinkel PE, et al: Anorexia nervosa, bulimia, and pregnancy. Am J Obstet Gynecol 157:1194–1198, 1987

Stewart DE, Robinson GE, Goldbloom DS, et al: Infertility and eating disorders. Am J Obstet Gynecol 163:1196–1199, 1990

Stewart DE, Boydell KM, McCarthy K, et al: A prospective study of the effectiveness of brief professionally led support groups for infertility patients. Int J Psychiatry Med 22:173–182, 1992

Strimling BS: Infant of a pregnancy complicated by anorexia nervosa. Am J Dis Child 138:68–69, 1984

Treasure JL, Russell GFM: Intrauterine growth and neonatal weight gain in babies of women with anorexia nervosa. BMJ 296:1038, 1988

Turton P, Hughes P, Bolton H, et al: Incidence and demographic correlates of eating disorder symptoms in a pregnant population. Int J Eat Disord 26:448–452, 1999

Van der Spuy Z: Nutrition and reproduction. Clin Obstet Gynecol 12:579–604, 1985

Van Wezel-Meijler G, Wit JM: The off-spring of mothers with anorexia nervosa: a high-risk group for undernutrition and stunting? Eur J Pediatr 149:130–135, 1989

Waugh E, Bulik CM: Offspring of women with eating disorders. Int J Eat Disord 25:123–133, 1999

# Breast Disorders and Breast Cancer

Barbara L. Andersen, Ph.D.
William B. Farrar, M.D.

## Introduction

Although the diagnosis of cancer is a devastating experience, most women cope successfully. In fact, many report renewed vigor in their approach to life, stronger interpersonal relationships, and a "survivor" adaptation. These outcomes do not, however, describe the process of adjustment, which may include feelings of an emotional crisis at diagnosis, fears of cancer treatment and changes it may bring, and a dread of life changes or adjustments. For decades the understanding of the psychologic processes and outcomes was largely clinical, consisting of detailed case studies of patients and clinical descriptions of difficult treatment experiences (e.g., Sutherland et al. 1952). The message from these reports was that the psychologic trajectory for women treated for breast cancer was guarded at best.

More recently, controlled research on the behavioral and psychologic aspects of cancer has described the specific difficulties that cancer patients may face, the proposed etiologic mechanisms for these processes, and the tested psychologic interventions to enhance coping (see Andersen 1992 for a review). In much of this research women with breast cancer have been the study participants, although those with disease at other sites have received study as well (e.g., Fawzy et al. 1990).

This chapter provides a scholarly overview of the psychologic processes

This research was supported by grant No. DAMD17-96-1-6294 from the United States Army Medical Research and Development Command and grant No. 1 RO1 MH51487 from the National Institute of Mental Health (NIMH).

of adjustment to breast cancer from symptom appearance to cure or death. We also include discussion of the biobehavioral factors that may influence the course of the disease and brief discussions of intervention strategies for the consulting psychiatrist. In preface we briefly review benign breast disorders because many produce symptoms or signs closely resembling those of breast cancer.

## Benign Breast Disorders

Benign breast disorders are common. Fibrocystic disease, the most frequent condition, is clinically apparent in about 50% of women. This disease is characterized by hyperplastic changes that may involve any or all of the breast tissues. Changes may be hormonally mediated and caused by a relative or absolute decline in progesterone or, by contrast, an increase in estrogen. When hyperplastic changes are also accompanied by cellular atypia, the risk for malignancy is increased. The clinical picture is usually one of multiple bilateral lesions that may become painful and/or tender, particularly premenstrually. The disease is often diagnosed and problematic during the young adult years, with the end of symptoms after menopause (unless, of course, exogenous estrogens are taken). Treatment decisions are moderated by the age of the woman, symptom severity, and the relative risk for breast malignancy. Particularly troublesome cysts are aspirated to relieve pain (and to determine the absence of malignancy), but in severe circumstances subcutaneous mastectomies may be considered.

Several other types of benign breast growths may be found. Fibroadenoma is the most common benign tumor. Clinically, these neoplasms are circumscribed, solitary, and freely movable; they are found most commonly in women younger than 30 years. These tumors require pathologic evaluation for definitive diagnosis. Other benign growths include intraductal papilloma, mammary duct ectasia, and galactocele. In diagnosing these conditions, mammography or cytologic examination of the fluids is required.

## Breast Cancer

### Epidemiology, Clinical Features, and Disease Description

Breast cancer accounts for 30% of all cancers and 17% of all cancer deaths in women (Parker et al. 1997). Incidence rates are lower for black and Asian females than for white, Hispanic, and Native American females. Relative survival rates have fluctuated over the years but have remained basically unchanged. Despite the lower incidence of disease, survival rates have remained consistently lower for black women. Similarly, fewer black women are initially diagnosed with localized disease (48%) than are white women (60%) (Parker et al. 1997).

Several variables have been identified as correlates (risk factors) of breast cancer. The demographic factors of age (age increases risk), race (as discussed above), ethnicity (Jewish women, particularly Askenazi Jews, have higher rates than non-Jewish women), and socioeconomic status (women in the highest group have a risk almost twice as great as those in the lowest group) have been noted. Reproductive variables are important; nulligravida women and women who have their first child after the age of 30 have almost a threefold increase in risk compared with those giving birth the first time at age 20 or younger. Much of the above findings of increased risk among women with nulliparity, late first birth, and other factors, such those associated with late menopause, have led to varying hormonal hypotheses. Finally, the role of diet in breast cancer is controversial, although it has led to recommendations such as reducing fat intake.

One important factor for breast cancer may be familial or genetic risk. Women who have had a mother or sister diagnosed with breast cancer are at almost three times the risk. Not all women with such profiles, however, actually have either of the BRCA1 or BRCA2 gene mutations that have been identified for breast cancer. In fact, the latter mutations account for no more than 5%–10% of all breast cancers in the United States. Since the identification of the genes, researchers have struggled to catch up with the many psychologic issues that surround the choice to pursue genetic testing and subsequent cancer-prevention follow-up measures that a woman may elect (e.g., watchful waiting, prophylactic mastectomy). Early psychosocial research suggests that women who are eligible for but decline genetic testing may be those who are, indeed, experiencing the greatest psychologic distress surrounding these issues. Perhaps even more importantly, even those women tested and found to be carriers of the gene mutations show low rates of mammogram adherence—only 24% of carriers versus 21% of testing decliners report having followed through with a mammogram at regularly scheduled 6-month intervals (Nelson 1998). Thus, although women who receive adequate genetic counseling and testing may not experience the negative emotional sequelae feared, this information may not lead to reductions in cancer morbidity and mortality.

Despite the emphasis on mammography as a screening device, carcinoma of the breast is usually first discovered as a lump (usually in the upper outer quadrant) by the woman or her physician. Usually, it is painless and freely mobile, but with progressive growth the tumor may become fixed to the chest wall. A less common sign is a serous or bloody nipple discharge. Extension to the skin may cause retraction and dimpling, whereas ductal involvement may cause nipple retraction. Blockage of skin lymphatics may cause lymphedema and thickening of the skin, a change referred to as *peu d'orange*. Inflammatory signs may also appear, such as warmth and redness of the overlying skin and swelling of the surrounding breast tissues.

Definitive diagnosis requires either tissue cytology (open breast biopsy) or a fluid biopsy (fine needle aspiration). Malignant tumor types vary greatly. Approximately 90% of cases arise in the ducts, and the remainder originate in the lobules. About 70% of all breast cancers are infiltrating duct carcinomas. Less common types include medullary, invasive lobular, mucinous, tubular, and papillary; in many tumors, several patterns exist.

Breast cancer spreads by local infiltration, moving directly into the surrounding breast tissue and eventually involving the overlying skin or the underlying muscle. When it occurs, lymphatic spread is mainly to the axillary nodes, with 40%–50% of patients having progressed to nodal involvement at diagnosis. Nodal status (both axillary and internal mammary) and tumor size are among the most important prognostic factors (Donegan 1997). In the National Surgical Adjuvant Breast Project studies (a federally funded cancer clinical trial cooperative group), women with negative lymph nodes had an actuarial 5-year survival rate of 83% compared with 73% for patients with one to three positive nodes, 45% for those with four or more positive nodes, and 28% for those with more than 13 positive nodes (Fisher et al. 1983).

In 1894 radical mastectomy was described by Halsted and Meyer. This procedure consisted of an en bloc dissection of the entire breast, the pectoralis major and minor muscles, and the axilla. By 1970, however, controversy surrounding surgical management was apparent and a prospective randomized clinical trial was begun by the National Surgical Adjuvant Breast Project. More than 1,700 women with clinically negative axillary nodes were enrolled and received radical mastectomy, total (simple) mastectomy followed by local-regional radiation, or total mastectomy alone. Results indicated that in node-negative as well as surgically determined node-positive women, no differences occurred between groups in survival times, indicating that the less radical surgery could provide superior functional and cosmetic results without compromising mortality. Also, breast reconstruction performed at mastectomy or later was possible. Most women treated with lumpectomy are those with small primary tumors (less than 2 cm in diameter); whether such women then go on to receive adjuvant radiation therapy is usually determined by the presence, if any, of nodal disease. Radiation therapy for women with positive axillary nodes significantly reduces local-regional relapse (e.g., surgical site, chest wall), but its effect on survival remains controversial.

Because breast cancer is often a systemic disease, adjuvant chemotherapy or hormonal therapy is standard. In fact, data now suggest that chemotherapy will benefit nearly all early stage breast cancer patients (McNeil 1997), including the previously untreated node-negative and/or postmenopausal estrogen receptor–positive women who received tomoxifan alone. The four most commonly used chemotherapy agents are cyclophosphamide, methotrexate, 5-fluorouracil, and adriamycin; newer studies also include paclitaxel (Taxol). Used alone, each of these agents can induce responses in 25%–45% of patients; when combined (typically as either cyclophosphamide–methotrexate–5-fluorouracil or as cyclophosphamide–adriamycin–5-fluorouracil), they are even more effective. Hormonal therapy with tomoxifen is often given for upwards of 5 years after diagnosis. Response is correlated with the incidence of estrogen and progesterone receptors. For example, the response rate to progesterone treatment in estrogen receptor–positive tumors is 50%–60%, whereas it is less than 10% in estrogen receptor–negative tumors.

For women with metastatic disease, symptoms may be palliated with combination chemotherapy. Partial responses are obtained in 50%–75% of patients, but complete clinical responses are seen infrequently (5%–10%), with the mean survival time following recurrence diagnosis being 18 months. Because of these discouraging data and the similarly difficult prognosis for those initially diagnosed with multiple positive nodes (e.g., more than 8), bone marrow transplant with autologous stem cell rescue is being considered as an option. However, the differential effectiveness of this procedure is as yet unknown (Zujewski et al. 1998).

## Detection

Development of malignancy and appearance of symptoms can be protracted. The psychologic and behavioral aspects of illness representation (Leventhal et al. 1980) and symptom interpretation (Andersen et al. 1995) have been offered as theoretic frameworks for understanding illness interpretations and patient delay. Studies indicate that the lion's share of cancer delay (i.e., from symptom/sign awareness to seeking a physician consultation) is accounted for by the time necessary for the patient to decide the symptoms indicate "illness" rather than a normal and/or nonserious health condition (e.g., a breast lump is thought to be a cyst or fibrocystic disease rather than a cancerous lump) (Andersen et al. 1995). This delay in accepting symptoms as serious also occurs among physicians who postpone cancer-diagnostic testing (e.g., Howson 1950; Mommsen et al. 1983).

## Diagnosis

Diagnosis of cancer, whether initial or recurrence, is the period of greatest acute stress for the patient. This crisis is defined by sadness (depression), fear (anxiety), confusion, and occasionally anger (Andersen et al. 1989b). The cognitive coping responses prompted by diagnosis include positive/confronting strategies, fatalistic responses, hopelessness/helplessness, and denial/avoidance (Burgess et al. 1988).

To examine the emotional responses at diagnosis, we assessed the moods of 65 women with cancer (clinical stage I or II gynecologic cancer) within 5–10 days of learning their diagnosis and prior to treatment (Andersen et al. 1989b). Their responses on a self-report mood questionnaire (Profile of Mood States [POMS]; McNair et al. 1971) were compared with those of women from two age-matched comparison groups, a group of women with recently diagnosed benign gynecologic disease and gynecologically healthy women receiving routine examinations. The cancer patients were followed-up for approximately 4 years. During that time a subset of the women experienced cancer recurrence, and moods were reassessed at this second diagnosis.

Depression was significantly elevated for the cancer patients only at the time of the initial diagnosis; a further, significant increment in distress occurred at cancer recurrence. Anxiety was a common affective experience for women who were anticipating medical treatment, whether for benign or malignant disease, but no further elevations were found at recurrence. This pattern suggests that the anxiety may be prompted, in part, by treatment-related fears. Anger was present to a significant degree for the cancer patients only at the time of recurrence, but levels at the initial diagnosis were not elevated. These data indicate that initial diagnosis is characterized by significant depressed affect, whereas recurrence may be characterized by anger and more significant depressed affect. Anxiety is also present during both diagnostic periods.

### Depression

Depression is the most prevalent affective problem for cancer patients (Derogatis et al. 1983; Lansky et al. 1985). When major depression and adjustment disorder with depressed mood are considered, prevalence rates are on the order of 15% (Derogatis et al. 1983). In general, higher rates of depression are found for patients in active treatment than for those who are in follow-up, who are receiving palliative rather than curative treatment, who have pain or other disturbing symptoms, and who have a history of affective disorder. Among individuals who do not have these characteristics, the base rate of major depression is likely to be on the order of 6%, comparable with that of the general population.

It can be difficult to make a diagnosis of depression in cancer patients, as it is for patients with other serious illnesses, although we note some salient considerations. Vegetative symptoms—that is, poor appetite or actual weight loss, sleep disturbance (e.g., insomnia, hypersomnia), loss of energy or fatigue, and loss of sexual desire or interest—must be determined to be representative of depression, disease-related events, or some combination of factors.

Depression for most cancer patients is reactive—it occurs soon after the diagnosis, and the content of the depressive ruminations reflect the diagnostic event (Noyes and Kathol 1986). When depressive symptoms are present at the time of diagnosis, they tend to be intermittent and rarely persist once treatment has begun or is concluded. Emotional "rebound" following treatment appears to occur, particularly for anxiety-related symptoms (van't Spijker et al. 1997). Finally, because cancer is a realistic health stressor, patients and physicians alike regard a depressive reaction to the diagnosis as normal. As such, patients may not feel comfortable (or able) to complain about their feelings, even when the feelings are extreme. Similarly, physicians or nurses may not recognize severe depressive reactions because of their infrequent occurrence and because of the normality of less severe reactions. These circumstances lead to the underrecognition and undertreatment of major depression among cancer patients (Derogatis et al. 1979). However, the effect of depressive symptoms and medical conditions on adjustment and well-being is additive; individuals experiencing depression in the context of cancer report twice the reduction in social functioning than would, for example, be associated with either condition alone (Wells et al. 1989).

When depression does occur, some symptoms are more or less characteristic for the patient. In addition to dysphoric mood, other common symptoms may include loss of interest or pleasure, loss of energy or fatigue, and difficulty thinking or concentrating (e.g., feeling confused or bewildered). Other common feelings include intermittent anxiety, helplessness, and concern about the future (Lansky et al. 1985). Endicott (1984) suggested other possible but less common reactions, including fearful or depressed appearance, social withdrawal or decreased talkativeness, brooding or pessimism, and mood that is not reactive (i.e., the patient cannot be cheered up, does not smile, and/or does not react to good news). Reactions such as these can be considered as symptoms or signs of major depression in medical patients. In contrast, psychologic characteristics of depressed psychiatric patients that are uncommon for cancer patients include feelings of low self-esteem and guilt; it is also rare for cancer patients to be melancholic, psychotic, or suicidal (Bukberg et al. 1984; Saunders and Valente 1988).

## Anxiety Disorders

Anxiety disorder is the psychiatric problem second in frequency among cancer patients. Derogatis et al. (1979) estimated the prevalence to be 7% among cancer outpatients undergoing treatment. In a study of 44 breast cancer patients interviewed at diagnosis, Hughes (1981) estimated that 25% had severe anxiety reactions. Anxiety-related problems are typically manifest by symptoms of generalized anxiety: the classic fear, worry, and rumination. Other symptoms include motor tension (e.g., shaky feeling, muscle tension, restless, and easy fatigability), autonomic hyperactivity (e.g., abdominal distress, frequent urination), and/or indications of vigilance and scanning (e.g., difficulty concentrating, trouble falling or staying asleep, feeling on edge). Much of the anxiety-provoking thought content is focused on medical examinations and cancer treatments (e.g., fear of pain or disfigurement) and the short- and long-term disruption they may produce. Other targets include the life disruption and change that may occur because of the cancer; the most common spheres of worry include family, money, work, and illness (e.g., who will care for the children when I am in the hospital? What if our insurance does not cover the bills? Will I be able to go back to work? Will my life ever be the same?).

The suggestion that responses to life-threatening diseases such as cancer could meet the criteria for posttraumatic stress disorder (PTSD) is an interesting development in the study of the anxiety-related problems of cancer patients (American Psychiatric Association 1994). Early studies have suggested that although anxiety responses of this magnitude may indeed occur, they are not prevalent. Alter et al. (1996) assessed 27 women at least 3 years after their cancer diagnosis and reported that 4% of the women had current PTSD symptoms whereas 22% met criteria for lifetime cancer-related PTSD. Cordova et al. (1995) assessed 55 women and reported a 5%–10% rate of symptoms. Current data suggest that the incidence of these responses may be directly related to the rigor of cancer therapy and/or the occurrence of significant morbidities.

## *Anger*

Anger has occupied a special role in theorizing. It has been hypothesized that anger is relevant to the etiology and/or progression of cancer (e.g., Morris et al. 1981), but empirical evidence is weak. As discussed previously, we have not found any evidence of elevated anger at initial diagnosis; however, higher levels may be reported at cancer recurrence. The foci for the anger at recurrence include frustration with the failure of presumably curative treatments.

## *Biobehavioral Responses*

Various data indicate that adults undergoing chronic stressors experience high rates of adjustment difficulties and important biologic effects, including effects on the immune system. For individuals with cancer—particularly women with breast cancer—the immune system may be relevant to host resistance against progression and metastatic spread. Andersen et al. (1998) examined the relationship between stress and several aspects of the cellular immune response in the context breast cancer diagnosis and the postsurgery period. Women ($n = 116$) newly diagnosed and surgically treated for stage II (70%) or III (30%) invasive breast cancer participated in the study. Before beginning adjuvant therapy, all patients completed a validated questionnaire assessing stress about the cancer experience and provided a blood sample for a panel of natural killer cell and T-cell assays. The researchers hypothesized a negative relationship between stress and immunity. All data analyses controlled for variables that might also be expected to exert short- or long-term effects on these responses, such as age, stage of disease, and length of time of surgical recovery, and ruled out other potentially confounding variables (e.g., nutritional status). Significant effects were found and replicated between and within assays, including the finding that stress significantly ($P < 0.05$) predicted natural killer cell lysis, a measure of the capacity of the women's immune systems to find and kill target (cancer) cells. Data showed that the physiologic effects of stress inhibited a panel of cellular immune responses, including cancer-relevant natural killer cell cytotoxicity and T-cell responses. Further studies will need to determine whether health consequences emerge for individuals who report high levels of stress with the diagnosis and surgical treatment of their tumors and will also need to clarify the biobehavioral mechanisms proposed for such adverse effects (Andersen et al. 1994).

## Treatment

Anticipation of difficult treatment is a component of the emotional distress occurring at diagnosis. Current therapies include surgery, radiotherapy, chemotherapy, hormonal therapy, and, for some, bone marrow transplant. These treatments are significant stressors, and supporting data consistently portray more distress (particularly fear and anxiety), slower rates of emotional recovery, and perhaps additional behavioral difficulties (e.g., conditioned anxiety reactions) among patients receiving these therapies compared with reactions in relatively healthy women undergoing medical treatment for benign conditions.

Few investigations of the psychologic reactions to cancer surgery have been performed. For breast cancer patients, part of the fear surrounding surgery is responding to the loss of all or part of the breast. In addition, women are fearful of surgery in general. Studies indicate that postoperative anxiety is predictive of recovery—patients with lower levels of postoperative anxiety recover more quickly (e.g., get out of bed, complain less) than do those with higher levels of anxiety. What may distinguish cancer surgery patients, however, are higher overall levels of distress and slower emotional rebound. Gottesman and Lewis (1982), for example, found greater and more lasting feelings of crisis and helplessness among cancer patients in comparison with benign surgery patients for as long as 2 months following discharge.

Considering the latter data, findings on the interaction patterns of physicians and cancer patients on morning surgical rounds is disturbing. Blanchard et al. (1987) found attending physicians on a cancer unit to be less likely to engage in supportive behaviors and to address patients' needs than were physicians treating general medical patients. The heavier volume and more seriously ill patients common to cancer units may account for this unfortunate finding. Oncology nurses may find their job significantly more stressful than other assignments (e.g., cardiac, intensive care, or operating room nursing) (Stewart et al. 1982). Taken together, these data suggest that the interactions between oncologists, oncology nurses, and cancer inpatients may influence adjustment more than is commonly acknowledged.

For empirical understanding of radiation fears, the surgical anxiety studies described above have been used as a paradigm. Here, again, high levels of anticipatory anxiety are found, and if interventions to reduce distress are not conducted (Rainey 1985), heightened posttreatment anxiety is also found (Andersen and Tewfik 1985; Andersen et al. 1984) and may be maintained for as long as 3 months after therapy (King et al. 1985). However, when acute treatment side effects (e.g., fatigue, skin reactions) resolve, no higher incidence of emotional difficulties is found for radiotherapy patients than for surgery patients (Hughson et al. 1987).

Of all cancer treatments, the behavioral and psychologic aspects are best understood for chemotherapy, particularly its side effects of nausea and vomiting. A classical conditioning conceptualization has been offered to explain anticipatory nausea and vomiting–that is, following at least one cycle of chemotherapy, patients may report nausea and/or vomiting prior to chemotherapy administration (usually on the first day) of the second or subsequent cycles. Treatments such as the use of hypnosis, progressive muscle relaxation with guided imagery, systematic desensitization, attentional diversion or redirection, and biofeedback can be helpful to patients (see Carey and Burish 1987 for a review). Research has also targeted individual differences among patients (e.g., high pretreatment anxiety or general distress, severity of posttreatment vomiting in the early cycles, age) and situational issues (e.g., more emetogenic regimens, higher dosages or greater amounts of chemotherapy) that increase risk of anticipatory reactions.

## Immediate Posttreatment Recovery

Despite the difficulties of cancer treatment, the crisis levels of emotional distress that occur at diagnosis lessen during treatment initiation, continuance, and early recovery (i.e., 2–12 months posttreatment) (Andersen et al. 1989b; Bloom 1987; Devlen et al. 1987). Bloom (1987) reported on the controlled prospective longitudinal study of women with stage I or II breast cancer treated with modified radical mastectomy. Comparisons were made with women receiving biopsy for benign disease, women receiving cholecystectomy for gall bladder disease, and healthy women. All women were seen within 3 months of surgery and again at 6, 9, and 12 months after treatment. Women with breast cancer showed greater psychologic distress related to social and interpersonal relationships. In addition, more distress was seen in women with stage II disease; these women also had more negative attitudes toward self and the future, more concern with physical symptoms, more anxiety, more strain, and more interpersonal difficulties. They did not, however, show any greater evidence of psychopathology warranting psychiatric intervention during the first posttreatment year.

Similar patterns of positive long-term adjustment have been found in other longitudinal studies of cancer patients (Andersen et al. 1989b; Devlen et al. 1987). Investigators have pursued these findings by testing mediators for adjustment and individual differences that might be related to outcomes. For example, women who approach the breast cancer experience with optimism rather than pessimism tend to fare better, coping with the experience with acceptance rather than denial or surrender (Carver et al. 1993).

Several investigations have been made into the psychologic counseling provided to breast cancer patients during the early recovery months. Interventions are typically provided as either individual or group therapy. Studies have varied in their methodologic sophistication; however, they have generally demonstrated more positive outcomes for women receiving intervention when compared with women not receiving intervention. For example, P. Maguire et al. (1983) provided individual counseling by a nurse specialist to women immediately following mastectomy. The 152 women who participated were assigned to either intervention or control conditions and followed-up for 12–18 months. Women receiving the intervention reported greater social recovery, were more likely to return to work, and had better adaptation to breast loss and use of a prothesis than did women in the comparison group.

The beneficial effects of another multimodal intervention were reported by Gordon et al. (1980). Three intervention components were included: education (providing information about cancer, its treatment, and its emotional effects); counseling (to provide support and clarification of feelings); and environmental efforts (e.g., advocacy for patients in the health care system). Outcome assessment continued for 6 months after treatment. Intervention patients reported a more rapid diminution of negative affect, such as anxiety and depression, a greater likelihood of returning to their previous vocation, and a more active resumption of activities.

Social support and participation in support groups are components of another intervention format. Social support may consist of emotional concern, physical aid, or information provision and may commonly be provided by friends and family. Various data indicate that social support can reduce psychologic distress and perhaps improve health outcomes. Perhaps the most well-known peer social support intervention is the American Cancer Society's Reach to Recovery patient visitation program for women with breast cancer. The effects of such a visitation program in the Netherlands was reported by van den Borne et al. (1987). In their study, regular contact between patients appeared to decrease negative affect and feelings of uncertainty and to increase self-esteem.

Telch and Telch (1986) compared supportive group therapy with a coping skills intervention offered to male and female cancer patients. Participants were randomly assigned to either of the interventions or a no-treatment control group. Analyses revealed a consistent superiority to the coping intervention, which provided relaxation and stress management; communication, assertion, and problem-solving skills; emotional management; and activity planning. Final assessment at 6 weeks after treatment indicated that patients receiving the coping intervention reported improvement across all outcome variables, including mood, self-efficacy, the number of problems experienced, and activity management.

## Long-Term Recovery and Survival

The long-term picture for those treated for breast cancer is clouded by the unpredictable course of this disease; even those with years of asymptomatic disease can recur with distant metastases and rapidly decline. Thus for the "cured" cancer patient (i.e., typically referring to individuals surviving at least 5 years), two broad classes of stressors have been suggested (Cella and Tross 1986). The first includes residual sequelae, including lingering emotional distress from the cancer experience and life threat. This might be manifest when patients dread follow-up physical examinations or ruminate about disease recurrence. The second class of stressors includes continuing sequelae, such as coping with the changes to one's premorbid life and making adjustments that require new behaviors or emotions.

The earliest writings (from the 1950s to the 1980s) suggested that the psychologic trajectory of cancer patients was troubled with somatic problems, psychologic distress (Bard and Sutherland 1952; G. P. Maguire et al. 1978), impaired relationships (Dyk and Sutherland 1956; Wortman and Dunkel-Schetter 1979), preoccupation with death (Gullo et al. 1974), and/or general life disruption such as reduced employment or career opportunities (Schonfield 1972). Many of these pioneering reports (of primarily breast cancer patients) were clinical in focus and generally uncontrolled on disease variables now recognized as moderators of adjustment. By the end of this same period, cancer had become more public, more survivable, and clinical trials were able to examine treatment toxicity following the establishment of effectiveness. Although little change has occurred in the age-adjusted death rate for breast cancer since the 1950s (American Cancer Society 1997), significant changes have been made in the standard therapy (as discussed above).

Data on the interpersonal relationships of cancer patients suggest that, in general, satisfaction predominates. Study of women treated for breast cancer indicates that most relationships remain intact, satisfactory, and on occasion become stronger (Lichtman and Taylor 1986; Tempelaar et al. 1989). The most important relationships are those within the family, and thus studies have focused on them. When problems do occur, they include the estrangement and distress originally hypothesized for most patients (Wortman and Dunkel-Schetter 1979). In one common scenario, the woman may be inclined to discuss her feelings and experiences in an attempt to cope with or understand the cancer stressor, but her partner may be more inclined to advise her to "put the experience behind you" and may not want to listen (Lichtman and Taylor 1986). It is clear that the level of distress in kin may approach that of the patient (B. R. Cassileth et al. 1985). Another common stressor for women with breast cancer is the subsequent risk of disease for their female children.

For many breast cancer patients, the one life area that is at some risk is sexual functioning, although the incidence of sexual problems has declined with the lesser surgeries. Lumpectomy patients report less alteration in body image, greater comfort with nudity and discussing sexuality with one's partner, no or few changes in intercourse frequency, and a lower incidence of sexual dysfunction than do patients receiving more extensive surgeries. Additionally, important individual differences in the extent of sexual morbidity may exist, such as how a woman views herself as a sexual person (Andersen et al. 1997). Even if sexual disruption occurs, however, it need not portend disturbance of other life areas, such as marital adjustment, as indicated in studies comparing breast cancer patients with healthy women (Andersen and Jochimsen 1985).

## Recurrence

Cancer recurrence is devastating. As noted earlier, the magnitude of distress is even greater than that found with the initial diagnosis. Studies in which cancer patients with no evidence of disease are contrasted with those receiving palliative treatment (e.g., B. R. Cassileth et al. 1985) report the greatest distress for those with disseminated disease. Difficult decisions (e.g., beginning a regimen that offers little chance for cure and has side effects versus no treatment) are made in a context of extreme emotional distress and physical debilitation (P. A. Cassileth and Cassileth 1983).

We previously reviewed the psychologic interventions to assist coping with difficult treatments or the recovery process. Data also indicate that important gains can be achieved during terminal stages (e.g., Linn et al. 1982). Group support interventions have been important because they can serve various purposes not offered by individual therapy (Taylor et al. 1986). Group members can serve as role models for each other in their coping efforts and in confronting the possibility of decline and death, and they can also provide altruistic support to one another. Spiegel et al. (1981) have provided two important reports on the emotional and survival benefits of such an intervention. Using a randomized, prospective design, women with metastatic breast cancer were assigned to group therapy or no-treatment conditions. The study assessments occurred at the beginning and at 4, 8, and 12 months later, although the groups continued to meet for 2 years. Women participating in the support groups reported less emotional distress and fewer maladaptive coping responses, such as overeating, smoking, or drinking. A later report provided data on 10-year survival differences between the groups (Spiegel et al. 1989). At that time, only three of the 86 patients were alive and death records were obtained on all other participants. Survival from time of randomization and onset of intervention was a mean of 36.6 months in the intervention group compared with 18.9 months in the control group, a significant difference. Survival plots indicated that divergence in survival began at 20 months after entry, or 8 months after the formal intervention study ended. Hypotheses for this important effect include the additional provision of social support from the therapy sessions or enhanced self-care (e.g., better treatment compliance, improved diet, hypnosis for pain control, more exercise), among others. Future studies will examine the reliability and the mechanisms for these remarkable findings.

## Reducing Psychologic Distress Throughout the Cancer Experience: Roles for the Psychiatrist

Suggestions have been made regarding the management of emotional distress in the cancer patient (Massie and Holland 1990). An often overlooked strategy is the continuing emotional support of the patient by the oncologist. Psychiatrists are in a unique position to assist their physician colleagues with such supportive efforts. Supplementary psychiatric consultation may be considered when severe affective symptoms last more than 2 weeks, when they worsen, or when they interfere with the patient's ability to function or cooperate with treatment. Brief crisis-oriented therapy may be particularly useful at time of diagnosis (initial or recurrent), and may help the woman regain a sense of self in this difficult circumstance, correct misconceptions regarding diagnosis or treatment, and integrate the illness experience into prior life experiences. Other therapeutic efforts may be to include family members in the intervention sessions or to suggest participation in patient support groups.

When medication is considered, surveys of current psychotropic medications indicate that hypnotics (43% of all prescriptions), antipsychotics (28%), anxiolytics (27%), and antidepressants (3%) are typically chosen for psychologic and physical symptom management (e.g., hypnotics and antipsychotics are often prescribed for nausea and vomiting rather than for affective distress) (Stiefel et al. 1990). For depression and anxiety, the tricyclic or selective serotonin reuptake inhibitor antidepressants can be safely and effectively prescribed and should be used (Massie and Holland 1990). Severe depression in advanced disease can be effectively treated with psychostimulants, such as methylphenidate, to improve mood and energy levels.

# References

Alter CL, Pelcovitz E, Axelrod A, et al: Identification of PTSD in cancer survivors. Psychosomatics 37:137–143, 1996

American Cancer Society: Cancer Facts and Figures: 1997. Atlanta, GA, American Cancer Society, 1997

American Psychiatric Association: Diagnostic and Statistical Manual of Mental Disorders, 4th Edition. Washington, DC, American Psychiatric Association, 1994

Andersen BL: Psychological interventions for cancer patients to enhance the quality of life. J Consult Clin Psychol 60:552–568, 1992

Andersen BL, Jochimsen PR: Sexual adjustment among breast cancer, gynecologic cancer, and healthy women. J Consult Clin Psychol 53:25–32, 1985

Andersen BL, Tewfik HH: Psychological reactions to radiation therapy: reconsideration of the adaptive aspects of anxiety. J Pers Soc Psychol 48:1024–1032, 1985

Andersen BL, Karlsson JA, Anderson B, et al: Anxiety and cancer treatment: response to stressful radiotherapy. Health Psychol 3:535–551, 1984

Andersen BL, Anderson B, deProsse C: Controlled prospective longitudinal study of women with cancer, II: psychological outcomes. J Consult Clin Psychol 57:692–697, 1989b

Andersen BL, Kiecolt-Glaser JK, Glaser R: A biobehavioral model of cancer stress and disease course. American Psychologist 49:389–404, 1994

Andersen BL, Cacioppo JT, Roberts DC: Delay in seeking a cancer diagnosis: delay stages and psychophysiological comparison processes. Br J Soc Psychol 34:33–52, 1995

Andersen BL, Woods XA, Copeland LJ: Sexual self schema and sexual morbidity among gynecologic cancer survivors. J Consult Clin Psychol 65:221–229, 1997

Andersen BL, Farrar WB, Golden-Kreutz D, et al: Stress and immune responses following surgical treatment of regional breast cancer. J Natl Cancer Inst 90:30–36, 1998

Bard M, Sutherland AM: Adaptation to radical mastectomy. Cancer 8:656–671, 1952

Blanchard CG, Ruckdeschel JC, Labrecque MS, et al: The impact of a designated cancer unit on house staff behaviors toward patients. Cancer 60:2348–2354, 1987

Bloom JR: Psychological aspects of breast cancer study group: psychological response to mastectomy. Cancer 59:189–196, 1987

Bukberg J, Penman D, Holland JC: Depression in hospitalized cancer patients. Psychosom Med 46:199–212, 1984

Burgess C, Morris T, Pettingale KW: Psychological response to cancer diagnosis, II: evidence for coping styles (coping styles and cancer diagnosis). J Psychosom Res 32:263–272, 1988

Carey MP, Burish TG: Etiology and treatment of the psychological side effects associated with cancer chemotherapy. Psychol Bull 104:307–325, 1987

Carver CS, Pozo C, Harris SD, et al: How coping mediates the effect of optimism on distress: a study of women with early stage breast cancer. J Consult Clin Psychol 65:375–390, 1993

Cassileth BR, Lusk EJ, Strouse TB, et al: A psychological analysis of cancer patients and their next-of-kin. Cancer 55:72–76, 1985

Cassileth PA, Cassileth BR: Clinical care of the terminal cancer patient: part I and II. Medical Times March:57S–66S, 1983

Cella DF, Tross S: Psychological adjustment to survival from Hodgkin's disease. J Consult Clin Psychol 54:616–622, 1986

Cordova MJ, Andrykowski MA, Kenady DE, et al: Frequency and correlates of post-traumatic-stress-disorder-like symptoms after treatment for breast cancer. J Consult Clin Psychol 63:981–986, 1995

Derogatis LR, Feldstein M, Morrow G, et al: A survey of psychotropic drug prescriptions in an oncology population. Cancer 44:1919–1929, 1979

Derogatis LR, Morrow GR, Fetting J, et al: The prevalence of psychiatric disorders among cancer patients. JAMA 249:751–757, 1983

Devlen J, Maguire P, Phillips P, et al: Psychological problems associated with diagnosis and treatment of lymphomas, I: retrospective study and II: prospective study. BMJ 295:953–957, 1987

Donegan WL: Tumor-related prognostic factors for breast cancer. CA Cancer J Clin 47:28–51, 1997

Dyk RB, Sutherland AM: Adaptation of the spouse and other family members to the colostomy patient. Cancer 9:123–138, 1956

Endicott J: Measurement of depression in patients with cancer. Cancer 53:2243–2248, 1984

Fawzy FI, Cousins N, Fawzy N, et al: A structured psychiatric intervention for cancer patients, I: changes over time in methods of coping and affective disturbance. Arch Gen Psychiatry 47:720–725, 1990

Fisher B, Bauer M, Wickerham DL, et al: Relation of number of positive axillary nodes to the prognosis of patients with primary breast cancer. Cancer 52:1551–1557, 1983

Gordon WA, Freidenbergs I, Diller L, et al: Efficacy of psychosocial intervention with cancer patients. J Consult Clin Psychol 48:743–759, 1980

Gottesman D, Lewis M: Differences in crisis reactions among cancer and surgery patients. J Consult Clin Psychol 50:381–388, 1982

Gullo V, Cherico J, Shadick R: Suggested stages and response styles in life threatening illness: a focus on the cancer patient, in Anticipatory Grief. Edited by Schoenberg E, Carr E, Kutscher G, et al. New York, Columbia University Press, 1974, 153–165

Howson JT: The procedures and results of the Philadelphia Committee for the study of pelvic cancer. The Wisconsin Medical Journal 3:215–219, 1950

Hughes J: Emotional reactions to the diagnosis and treatment of early breast cancer. J Psychosom Res 26:277–283, 1981

Hughson AVM, Cooper AF, McArdle CS, et al: Psychosocial effects of radiotherapy after mastectomy. BMJ 294:1515–1518, 1987

King KB, Nail LM, Kreamer K, et al: Patients' descriptions of the experience of receiving radiation therapy. Oncol Nurs Forum 12:55–61, 1985

Lansky SB, List MA, Herrmann CA, et al: Absence of major depressive disorders in female cancer patients. J Clin Oncol 3:1553–1560, 1985

Leventhal H, Meyer D, Nerenz D: The common sense representation of illness danger, in Contributions to Medical Psychology, Vol 2. Edited by Rachman S. Oxford, England, Pergamon, 1980, 7–30

Lichtman RR, Taylor SE: Close relationships and the female cancer patient, in Women with Cancer: Psychological Perspectives. Edited by Andersen BL. New York, Springer-Verlag, 1986, pp 233–256

Linn MW, Linn BS, Harris R: Effects of counseling for late stage cancer patients. Cancer 49:1048–1055, 1982

Maguire GP, Lee EG, Bevington DJ, et al: Psychiatric problems in the first year after mastectomy. BMJ 1:963–965, 1978

Maguire P, Brooke M, Tait A, et al: The effect of counselling on physical disability and social recovery after mastectomy. Clin Oncol 9:319–324, 1983

Massie MJ, Holland JC: Depression and the cancer patient. J Clin Psychiatry 51(suppl):12–17, 1990

McNair DM, Lorr M, Droppleman LF: Profile of Mood States. San Diego, CA, Educational Testing Service, 1971

McNeil C: Chemotherapy benefits nearly all early breast cancer patients. J Natl Cancer Inst 89:838–839, 1997

Mommsen S, Aagaard J, Sell A: Presenting symptoms, treatment delay and survival in bladder cancer. Scand J Urol Nephrol 17:163–167, 1983

Morris T, Greer S, Pettingale KW, et al: Patterns of expression of anger and their psychological correlates in women with breast cancer. J Psychosom Res 25:111–117, 1981

Nelson NJ: Another taxane takes center stage in San Antonio. J Natl Cancer Inst 90:189–190, 1998

Noyes R, Kathol RG: Depression and cancer. Psychiatr Dev 2:77–100, 1986

Parker SL, Tong T, Bolden S, et al: Cancer statistics, 1997. CA Cancer J Clin 47:5–27, 1997

Rainey LC: Effects of preparatory patient education for radiation oncology patients. Cancer 56:1056–1061, 1985

Saunders JM, Valente SM: Cancer and suicide. Oncol Nurs Forum 15:575–581, 1988

Schonfield J: Psychological factors related to delayed return to an earlier life-style in successfully treated cancer patients. J Psychosom Res 16:41–46, 1972

Spiegel D, Bloom JR, Yalom I: Group support for patients with metastatic cancer. Arch Gen Psychiatry 38:527–533, 1981

Spiegel D, Bloom JR, Kraemer HC, et al: Effect of psychosocial treatment on survival of patients with metastatic breast cancer. Lancet 888–891, 1989

Stewart BE, Meyerowitz BE, Jackson LE, et al: Psychological stress associated with outpatient oncology nursing. Cancer Nurs 5:383–387, 1982

Stiefel FC, Kornblith AB, Holland JC: Changes in the prescription patterns of psychotropic drugs for cancer patients during a 10 year period. Cancer 65:1048–1053, 1990

Sutherland AM, Orbach CF, Dyk RB, et al: The psychological impact of cancer and cancer surgery, I: adaptation to the dry colostomy. Cancer 5:857–872, 1952

Taylor SE, Falke RL, Shoptow SJ, et al: Social support, support groups, and the cancer patient. J Consult Clin Psychol 54:608–615, 1986

Telch CF, Telch MJ: Group coping skills instruction and supportive group therapy for cancer patients: a comparison of strategies. J Consult Clin Psychol 54:802–808, 1986

Tempelaar R, DeHaes JC, DeRuiter JH, et al: The social experiences of cancer patients under treatment: a comparative study. Soc Sci Med 29:635–642, 1989

van den Borne HW, Pruyn JFA, van den Heuvel WJA: Effects of contacts between cancer patients on their psychosocial problems. Patient Educ Couns 9:33–51, 1987

van't Spijker A, Trijsburg RW, Duivenvoorden HJ: Psychological sequelae of cancer diagnosis: a meta-analytical review of 58 studies after 1980. Psychosom Med 59:280–293, 1997

Wells KB, Steward A, Hays RD, et al: The functioning and well-being of depressed patients: results from the medical outcomes study. JAMA 262:914–919, 1989

Wortman CB, Dunkel-Schetter C: Interpersonal relationships and cancer: a theoretical analysis. J Soc Issues 35:120–155, 1979

Zujewski J, Nelson A, Abrams J: Much ado about not . . . enough data: high-dose chemotherapy with autologous stem cell rescue for breast cancer. J Natl Cancer Inst 90:200–209, 1998

# Women and Violence

CAROLE WARSHAW, M.D.

Violence against women constitutes a major social and public health problem—one that affects women of all ages, cultural backgrounds, and socio-economic levels (American Medical Association 1992; Crowell and Burgess 1996; Koss et al. 1994). Abuse and violence are common, often chronic social experiences rather than unusual events that occur among a small percentage of women. The greatest risk of sexual and physical violation will come from someone a woman knows and trusts—a parent, a caretaker, a person she is dating, or an intimate partner.

Over the past several decades, an overarching framework for understanding the impact of trauma on the human psyche has emerged through work with survivors of both civilian and combat trauma (Bloom 1997; Herman 1992b; Horowitz 1974, 1986; van der Kolk 1987). Information about specific forms of violence against women, such as childhood sexual abuse, sexual assault, and domestic violence, however, is often found in separate literatures, and knowledge about the cumulative effects of violence across the lifespan and experiences of women from diverse communities is still limited. Despite these limitations, research documenting the effects of violence against women and girls demonstrates that abuse, violence, and discrimination play a significant role in many of the mental health problems experienced by women in this country and throughout the world (Crowell and Burgess 1996; Felitti et al. 1998; Fischbach and Herbert 1997; Golding 1999; Heise et al. 1994; Koss et al. 1994; Marella et al. 1996).

While Veterans Administration (VA) hospitals were focusing almost exclusively on the combat-related trauma symptoms experienced by male Vietnam veterans, rape crisis workers and therapists were hearing about similar traumatic responses from women who were talking about sexual assault experiences for the first time. Recognition that many of these women were being raped by husbands or partners led to a burgeoning awareness of the pervasiveness of ongoing violence in women's lives and to the birth of the domestic violence advocacy movement. At the same time, large numbers of women were also being seen within the mental health system for symptoms associated with childhood sexual abuse that were not initially recognized as such. Initial pathologizing or victim-blaming responses on the part of mental health providers led to tensions between women's advocates and clinicians. Conscious of the need to create a public awareness that would "hold abusers accountable for their violence, not victims," advocates have been reluctant to frame women's responses to abuse in purely psychologic terms. These approaches have been instrumental in reconfiguring clinical paradigms and underscoring the importance of framing victimization as a societal problem rather than as an attribute of the victim. As Brown (1995) has pointed out, we do not look for characteristics of other crime victims to understand why they have been victimized. Misdiagnosis and retraumatization within the mental health system itself have not been uncommon experiences for abuse survivors (Ray and Rappaport 1995). Over the past 10 years, many of these practices have been changed (Carmen and Rieker 1998). In areas such as domestic violence, however, collaborative models integrating both treatment and advocacy approaches have been slower in developing.

This chapter summarizes what the past two decades of research and clinical work have taught us about the prevalence, impact, and treatment of different forms of violence against women. Although many similarities exist in the ways women experience abuse and violence and in the treatment of violence-related mental health issues, important differences can also be found. Some of these differences relate to issues surrounding the particular types of violence a woman has experienced; others involve factors unique to a woman's development, social context, and life experiences. Thus, the recommendations that follow must be tailored to the individual woman with whom one is working.

# Definitions

## Rape

*Rape* is commonly defined as a sexual act involving oral, anal, or vaginal penetration by a penis, other body parts, or objects accompanied by the use of threat, duress, physical force, intimidation, deception, or lack of ability to consent. Like other forms of violence, sexual assault may be experienced at any point during the lifespan. Sexual assault or coercion by a stranger, marital partner, acquaintance, or date are all considered to be rape. Women and girls are most likely to be raped by someone they know.

## Childhood Sexual Abuse

*Childhood sexual abuse* involves sexual contact and/or other sexual behaviors (e.g., genital exposure, involvement in pornography) by an adult or adults or, in some definitions, by a person or persons at least 5 years older than the victim (Wyatt and Peters 1986). Such abuse may be incestuous or not. Sexually abusive behaviors range from single perpetrator exhibitionism, fondling, or intercourse to child pornography and systematic assault by multiple perpetrators. Abuse may be accompanied by "loving" or seductive behaviors or may be brutal and sadistic. Although isolated abusive events do occur, sexual abuse is often chronic, with an average duration of 4 years (Courtois 1988). In addition, sexually abused children often face many other adversities in the course of their development that contribute to later difficulties (e.g., emotional abuse and neglect; parental substance abuse; and punitive, blaming, or dismissive responses if they reveal the abuse) (Goodwin 1996).

## Domestic Violence

*Domestic violence* is an ongoing pattern of domination and control perpetrated against a current or former intimate partner sustained by a combination of actual or threatened physical violence, sexual assault, and psychologic abuse. This occurs in adult and adolescent dating, in married or separating relationships, and among both homosexual and heterosexual couples. Physical violence is only one of many tactics batterers use to harm their victims, undermine their autonomy and sense of self, and keep them isolated and entrapped (American Medical Association 1992; Ganley 1995; Renzetti 1992).

Whenever physical or sexual abuse occurs, psychologic abuse is invariably present and may be quite severe. This often takes the form of verbal intimidation and threats, ridicule and humiliation, destruction of property, threats to significant others, stalking and monitoring a victim's activities, and controlling access to money, personal items, and contact with friends, family, and children (Browne 1987; Carmen 1995; Follingstad et al. 1990; L. E. Walker 1984, 1994). Accusations about sexual infidelity can be particularly humiliating. Emotional withdrawal, threats of abandonment, and threats to harm or take away children are also used as tactics of control.

Psychologic abuse is not only a significant component of domestic violence but is also more pervasive and often more damaging than physical abuse. Recent studies indicate that psychologic abuse is more predictive of low self-esteem, depression, and posttraumatic stress disorder (PTSD) than is physical abuse and in some couples predicts future physical and/or sexual violence (Arias and Pape 1999; Murphy and Cascardi 1993; O'Leary 1999). Women who are being abused describe the psychologic abuse as the worst aspect of their experiences. The combination of the abuser's use of these tactics and social conditions that limit options for freedom and safety is what keeps women trapped in abusive relationships (Warshaw 1996a).

## Prevalence of Gender-Based Violence in the United States

### Overall Rates

It has been well documented that women bear a disproportionate share of intimate violence in our society. Across studies, acute risk appears to be the highest for young women, particularly those between the ages of 12 and 18 years (Bachman and Saltzman 1995). Estimates of the lifetime prevalence of sexual assault among women averages between 13% and 25% (Brickman and Briere 1984; Crowell and Burgess 1996; Essock-Vitale and McGuire 1985; Kilpatrick et al. 1987, 1992; Koss and Oros 1982; Koss et al. 1987; Tjaden and Thoennes 1998; Wyatt 1992). Earlier retrospective studies of childhood sexual abuse suggested that between 8% and 62% of women have been sexually abused as children (Felitti 1998; Finkelhor et al. 1990; Russell 1982, 1984; Tjaden and Thoennes 1998; Wyatt 1985). Most current estimates fall in the 27%–28% range, but these may be low (Wyatt 1992). Longitudinal follow-up studies of adults with documented histories of childhood abuse indicate that respondents are likely to underestimate the occurrence of such events (Felitti et al. 1998; Femina et al. 1990; Williams 1995). Researchers conducting general population studies estimate the 1-year incidence of partner abuse among heterosexual women to be from 1.2% to 12% (Schulman 1979; Straus and Gelles 1990; Straus et al. 1980; Tjaden and Thoennes 1998). Lifetime prevalence ranges from 21% to 34% (Frieze et al. 1980; Russell 1982; Tjaden and Thoennes 1998).

## Cultural Differences

Data on violence against women across cultures are mixed. Studies that controlled for socioeconomic status have found similar rates of domestic violence and childhood sexual abuse among black, Hispanic, and Caucasian women (Centerwell 1984; Stark 1993; Torres 1991; Wyatt 1994). Rates of partner abuse also appear to be comparable between lesbian and heterosexual couples (Lie and Gentlewarrier 1991; Lie et al. 1991; Lockhart et al. 1994; Schilit et al. 1990; Waterman et al. 1989). In some studies, reports of sexual assault and partner abuse are lower among Latina women (Sorenson 1996) and Asian-American women, whereas Native American women report higher rates of domestic violence (Tjaden and Thoennes 1998). How women *experience* abuse may be influenced to some extent by race and ethnicity (Plichta 1995; Wyatt 1992, 1994).

## Revictimization

Up to 50%–65% of adult rape victims report histories of childhood sexual abuse (Russell 1982; Wyatt et al. 1992). Women who were sexually abused as children were often physically abused as well (Cloitre et al. 1997) and are at increased risk for later sexual (Fromuth 1986; Gidycz et al. 1993; Koss and Dinero 1989; Urquiza and Goodlin 1994; Wyatt and Riederle 1994; Wyatt et al. 1992) and physical assault (McCauley et al. 1997; Messman and Long 1996; Sappington et al. 1997; Schaaf and McCanne 1998). Recent epidemiologic data indicate, for example, that 18% of women who reported being raped before the age of 18 also report being raped as adults–twice the rate of women who have not been raped as children or adolescents (Tjaden and Thoennes 1998). Some authors have attributed this phenomenon to dissociative states associated with severe trauma that may impair a woman's ability to attend to danger signals (Cloitre et al. 1997), whereas others have attributed it to women not learning that they have a right to protect themselves from harm.

Low-income women appear to be at even greater risk for revictimization. In one study, the lifetime prevalence of severe physical or sexual assault among very-low-income women was found to be 84%; 63% of those studied had been physically assaulted as children, 40% had been sexually assaulted as children, and 60% had been physically assaulted by an intimate partner (Bassuk et al. 1998). Women living in extreme poverty face multiple sources of stress in addition to violence, including ongoing discrimination, lack of social and material necessities, and lack of access to resources–conditions that can adversely affect trauma recovery.

## Medical Consequences of Abuse

In recent years, attention to the impact of abuse and violence on women's health has grown. Prevalence studies indicate that 5%–27% of women seen in a range of clinical settings are currently being abused by their partners (Abbott et al. 1995; Dearwater et al. 1998; Gin et al. 1991; McCauley et al. 1995). Between 36.9% and 54.2% of women seen in emergency departments have reported physical or emotional abuse by a partner at some time in their lives, and in one study, 14.4% said they had experienced physical or sexual abuse during the past year (Dearwater et al. 1998).

Numerous studies have described the high prevalence of abuse histories among women seeking care for medical problems other than physical injuries (Koss 1993; Stark et al. 1979). Presentations associated with abuse include chronic pain (e.g., persistent headaches, chest pain, back pain, and pelvic pain) (Domino and Haber 1987; Karol et al. 1992; Rapkin et al. 1990; E. A. Walker et al. 1988) and complications of head and neck injuries such as seizures (Bowman 1993; Loewenstein 1991; Ross 1989) or difficulties with concentration, impulse control, and performance (L. S. Brown 1989). Positive correlations have also been found between a lifetime history of abuse and gastrointestinal illnesses (e.g., irritable bowel syndrome) (Drossman 1994; Drossman et al. 1995; Leserman and Drossman 1995; E. A. Walker et al. 1993, 1995) and autoimmune disorders (van der Kolk 1997). There appears to be a strong dose–response relationship between the degree of exposure to adverse childhood experiences (childhood abuse and household dysfunction), health risk factors (smoking, drug and alcohol abuse, obesity), and serious adult illnesses (ischemic heart disease, cancer, chronic lung disease, and liver disease) (Felitti et al. 1998). Complications of pregnancy, prolonged labor, preterm deliveries, low birth weight, and postpartum difficulties are also found at higher rates among women with histories of physical and sexual abuse (Boyer 1995; Jacobs 1992; McFarlane et al. 1992). Additionally, sexual abuse and assault increase women's risk for exposure to the complications of unprotected sex, such as HIV/AIDS, other sexually transmitted diseases, and unplanned pregnancies (Boyer 1995; Cohen et al. 2000; Zierler et al. 1995).

Women who have been abused frequently present with exacerbations or poor control of chronic medical conditions, such as diabetes, hypertension, asthma, or angina (Courtois 1988; Warshaw and Ganley 1995), or develop sleep and appetite disturbances, fatigue, dizziness, weight change, and other physical symptoms associated with depression, anxiety, or posttraumatic stress. Often the abusers prevent their partners from receiving medical care or restrict their access to sleep, exercise, proper diet, and medication. Additionally, avoidant posttraumatic stress responses associated with a history of sexual abuse or assault may interfere with taking medication, having regular Pap smears or mammograms, or agreeing to invasive medical procedures that may retrigger the experience of physical violation and loss of control (Courtois 1993; Goldman et al. 1995).

For some women, abuse increases during pregnancy, whereas for others pregnancy may be a protected time. Rates of intimate partner abuse during pregnancy range from 0.9% to 20% depending on when and how women are asked (Gazmararian et al. 1996; Parker et al. 1993). Pregnant adolescents appear to experience intimate partner abuse at higher rates than adults (Parker et al. 1993). Poverty also increases women's risk for abuse during pregnancy. One study of low-income women found that 65% of women experienced either verbal or physical abuse during pregnancy and 20% experienced either moderate or severe violence (O'Campo et al. 1994). Violence also appears to predict substance abuse during pregnancy (Amaro et al. 1990; J. Campbell and Kubb 1996; Bennett 1995; Martin et al. 1996).

Disabled women may be at even greater risk for physical and sexual violation (Gil et al. 1994). Although partner abuse among women with disabilities has not been systematically assessed, one case comparison study found the prevalence of partner abuse to be equal among women with and without physical disabilities. However, disabled women were more likely to be abused by attendants or health care providers and to be abused for a longer duration (Young et al. 1997). Women with physical disabilities or other chronic health conditions are also more likely to be sexually abused as children and sexually assaulted as adults (Golding 1994; Sobsey et al. 1995). In one small study, over 70% of disabled women had experienced violent sexual encounters at some time in their lives (Stimpson and Best 1991). Women who are hearing impaired (Melling 1984) or developmentally disabled (Doucette 1986; Hard 1986; Mansell et al. 1998; Sobsey and Varnhagen 1991) are particularly vulnerable to abuse.

## Mental Health Consequences of Abuse and Violence

In mental health settings the prevalence of abuse appears to be even higher. For example, individual studies have found that 81% of women psychiatric inpatients (Jacobson and Richardson 1987) and 68% of women outpatients (Jacobson 1989) had histories of abuse either as adults or children. In another study, 72% of women psychiatric inpatients reported childhood sexual or physical abuse or both (Bryer et al. 1987). Histories of childhood sexual abuse are reported by 30%–75% of the women who are seen in inpatient and outpatient psychiatric settings (Briere and Runtz 1988; Bryer et al. 1987; Chu and Dill 1990; Courtois 1993; Craine et al. 1988; Elvik et al. 1990; Goodwin 1989; Lombardo and Pohl 1997). In addition, approximately 50%–65% of the women who use public mental health services have been found to be survivors of childhood abuse (Carmen et al. 1984; Craine et al. 1988; Jacobson and Herald 1990; Muenzenmaier et al. 1993; Rose et al. 1991).

Specific psychiatric disorders associated with interpersonal violence include acute stress and posttraumatic stress disorders, other anxiety disorders such as panic and obsessive-compulsive disorders, somatization and eating disorders, major depression and dysthymia, dissociative disorders, and Axis II diagnoses such as borderline personality disorder as well as sexual dysfunction, self-mutilation, and substance abuse (Alpert et al. 1995; Astin et al. 1995; Briere and Runtz 1988; Burnam et al. 1988; J. C. Campbell and Alford 1989; Carnes 1991; Commonwealth Fund and Commission on Women's Health 1995; Craine et al. 1988; Crowell and Burgess 1996; Den Herder and Redner 1991; Gelles and Straus 1988; Golding et al. 1988; Hotaling and Sugarman 1986; Houskamp and Foy 1991; Kluft 1990; Maltz 1991; Resick 1987; Russo and Green 1993; Westerlund 1992; Winfield et al. 1990). Between 68% and 86% of hospitalized patients diagnosed with borderline personality disorder have been found to have histories of childhood physical and/or sexual abuse or to have witnessed severe violence (Bryer et al. 1987; Herman et al. 1986; Westen et al. 1990); similar findings have been reported for outpatients diagnosed with this disorder (Herman et al. 1989; Wagner et al. 1989). Survivors of more severe, long-standing childhood abuse are two to five times as likely to develop a psychiatric disorder (Briere and Elliott 1994) and may present with as many as six or seven discrete diagnoses as part of a more complex posttraumatic response (Turkus 1995).

## Posttraumatic Stress Disorder

Several authors have suggested that PTSD may be the most appropriate diagnosis for women suffering from the range of psychologic sequelae that follow sexual assault, battering, and childhood sexual abuse (Chalk and King 1998; Koss et al. 1994). Women who have been assaulted develop responses similar to those of victims of other types of trauma: shock, confusion, horror, and helplessness as well as dissociation, nightmares, flashbacks, numbing, avoidance, and hypervigilance (Crowell and Burgess 1996; Herman 1992b). Flashbacks can be visual, auditory, olfactory, tactile, or somatic and may be triggered by a range of stimuli: subsequent abuse, hearing about someone else being assaulted, media portrayals of violence, sensory stimuli associated with the original traumatic experience(s), invasive medical procedures, or anniversaries of the trauma. Flashbacks can also can also be cognitive (paranoid or suicidal thoughts), affective (feeling terrified or enraged), behavioral (cringing or fleeing), or interactional (Elliott and Briere 1995; Pearlman and Saakvitne 1995; Turkus 1995; van der Kolk et al. 1996).

The PTSD framework makes sense of the fluctuations that trauma survivors experience between being flooded and needing to dampen those feelings while remaining vigilant to potential new dangers. PTSD may present as an extension of acute stress disorder or may develop after a period of dormancy (delayed PTSD). It may resolve on its own or with treatment or may take on a chronic form. The relative intensity of PTSD symptoms may vary over time. Although flashbacks are more prominent initially, avoidant symptoms may predominate later in the course. This symptom progression may make trauma-engendered fears less accessible to change and thus painfully constrict women's lives, particularly in the areas of intimacy, sexuality, and the ability to move freely in the world (Blank 1993). The hypervigilance associated with PTSD can also constrain a woman's sense of freedom and safety. It is these adaptations that appear to have the most profound and potentially damaging effects (Carmen and Rieker 1998).

## Neurobiology of Trauma

The recent flood of research on the neurobiology of trauma has led to greater understanding of the links between biology, behavior, and psychologic distress. As van der Kolk (1997) has described, people with PTSD develop significant alterations in physiologic reactivity and stress hormone secretion, making it difficult to "properly evaluate sensory stimuli and respond with appropriate levels of physiologic and neurohormonal arousal." Several psychophysiologic models have been posited to explain PTSD (Davidson and van der Kolk 1996). These include noradrenergic dysregulation (increased sensitivity of the sympathetic nervous system under stress) (Southwick et al. 1999), disturbances of serotonergic activity (stress resilience, sleep regulation, impulse control, conditioned avoidance, and aggression), and kindling (lowering of the excitability threshold after repeated electrical stimulation). After traumatic exposure, limbic nuclei become sensitized, leading to excessive responsivity and increased startle and arousal responses–cores feature of PTSD that often persist after other symptoms resolve. Activation of the amygdala is postulated to mediate the autonomic stimulation resulting from exposure to trauma, thus transforming sensory input into physiologic signals that, in turn, produce and modulate emotional responses (van der Kolk 1997).

In addition, people with PTSD may exhibit enhanced reactivity and negative feedback inhibition of the hypothalamic–pituitary–adrenal (HPA) axis, a pattern that appears to be distinct from that found in depression and from acute and chronic stress among individuals who have not developed PTSD (Yehuda et al. 1991). Adaptations to chronic stress result in reduced resting glucocorticoid levels, decreased secretion in response to subsequent stress, and increased concentration of glucocorticoid receptors in the hippocampus (Resnick et al. 1995; Yehuda et al. 1993, 1995). This reduced cortisol response following assault has been associated with an increased likelihood of developing PTSD, leading to the hypothesis that elevated cortisol is important to the integration of traumatic experiences (van der Kolk 1997). Other studies have indicated that HPA axis hyperreactivity among women exposed to early childhood abuse causes increased adrenocorticotropic hormone and cortisol responses to lab-induced stress. These changes in corticotropin releasing factor activity may predispose women to the development of subsequent mood and anxiety disorders (Heim et al. 2000).

Recent data also indicate several neurologic differences among adults who were abused as children that affect the development of the limbic system and cerebral cortex, particularly the left hemisphere (Cicchetti and Carlson 1989) and the connecting structures used to process and interpret sensory data (van der Kolk 1997). Hippocampal volume, for example, may be reduced in women who have experienced severe childhood sexual abuse (Stein et al. 1997). These findings are similar to those of combat veterans with PTSD and may either represent a consequence of trauma exposure or a risk factor for the development of psychiatric complications following exposure. Stein et al. (1997) suggested that mesial temporal lobe dysfunction may directly mediate certain aspects of PTSD and dissociative disorder symptoms. Interestingly, they found no differences in memory testing between abused and nonabused groups. They speculate that these data may be better conceptualized as a dysfunction within the systems that monitor and regulate access to memory in emotionally charged contexts (Stein et al. 1997), potentially interfering with the processing of new stimuli (van der Kolk 1997). In addition, subjects with PTSD exposed to scripts of their traumatic experiences show decreased activity in the speech areas of the left hemisphere (Broca's area) necessary for the cognitive labeling and sequencing of experience, making it more difficult for trauma survivors to process the initial trauma and subsequent triggering events and to describe their experiences in a coherent narrative form (Marmar et al. 1994; Shalev et al. 1996; van der Kolk 1997).

## Trauma and Memory

Recent concerns about the possibility of therapists implanting false memories of childhood abuse have created considerable controversy within the mental health field (Hyman and Pentland 1996; Hyman et al. 1995). Research examining the nature of traumatic memory and recognition of the ubiquity of dissociation under conditions of extreme duress have expanded current understanding of these phenomena. Although much is still unknown (e.g., the mechanisms for forgetting and recovering memory for traumatic events), clear evidence has shown that childhood memories can be both forgotten and later recalled (see International Society of Trauma Stress Studies 1998 for critical review of these issues). Retrospective studies indicate that between 20% and 59% of those in treatment for childhood sexual abuse report prior memory deficits or total lack of recall for the abuse (Briere and Conte 1993; Elliott 1997; Herman and Schatzow 1987; Loftus et al. 1994). More compelling are the handful of prospective follow-up studies of young adults with documented childhood sexual abuse, which demonstrated that 32%–60% of female respondents did not recall the abuse on reinterview (Widom and Morris 1997; Williams 1995; Williams and Banyard 1997) and that previously forgotten memories of abuse can be recovered with reasonable accuracy (Scheflin and Brown 1996; Williams and Banyard 1997), although methodologic concerns have been raised about some of this research (Pope and Hudson 1995).

Considerable laboratory evidence also suggests that patients can, in fact, be induced to remember events inaccurately and to believe that they experienced events that they did not. Again, critiques of these studies focus on the artificial nature of the experiments, small sample sizes, and the fact that most subjects resist implantation. However, some individuals do appear to be more vulnerable to this type of manipulation (Schooler et al. 1997). Finally, some disagreement remains as to whether traumatic memories are qualitatively different than other memories. Several authors have posited that traumatic memories, although similar in many ways, are more accurate and less likely to deteriorate. Encoding may be enhanced by the increased levels of stress hormones and neuromodulators present during intense emotional arousal, and memories may be stored in sensory rather than narrative form (Shobe and Kihlstrom 1997; van der Kolk et al. 1996; Yehuda and McFarlane 1997). When trauma occurs during childhood, before the development of complex language capacities, memories may be even more fragmented and resurface as sounds (abuser's voice, family enjoying Thanksgiving dinner in the next room), bodily sensations (nausea, gagging, or pain), smells (alcohol, semen, or abuser's cologne), childhood affect states (feeling "icky"), or images (a window or door that was stared at, a large hovering belly). Positron emission tomography scans of PTSD patients have shown heightened brain activity in the parts of the limbic system connected with amygdala, which suggests that traumatized people "experience emotions as physical states rather than verbally encoded experiences" (van der Kolk et al. 1996, p. 233).

## Sexual Assault and Posttraumatic Stress Disorder

Adult victims of sexual assault (particularly of completed rape) represent the largest single group of trauma victims affected by PTSD (Foa et al. 1991; Kessler et al. 1995). Immediately following sexual assault, up to 95% of women develop symptoms of acute PTSD. Distress seems to reach its peak at 3 weeks after the assault for victims of single-episode sexual assault in adulthood and continue at this level for the next month (Crowell and Burgess 1996; Davidson and Foa 1991; Rothbaum et al. 1992). Although many symptoms may resolve after 3 months, residual fear, sexual difficulties, and problems with self-esteem can persist for 18 months or longer (Resick 1987), and nearly 25% of victims continue to be affected for several years (Hanson 1990). Other studies indicate that after 3 months, approximately one-half of adult sexual assault survivors will still meet criteria for PTSD; many will meet these criteria for a year or more (Foa et al. 1995; Resnick et al. 1993; Rothbaum and Foa 1993; Rothbaum et al. 1992). Postrape recovery appears to be more difficult when assault occurs an earlier age and when women experience greater fear of being injured or killed (Hanson 1990; Kilpatrick et al. 1987; Resick 1987). Sexual assault by a known assailant is at least as devastating as stranger rape (Katz 1991; Koss et al. 1987), but women are less likely to seek help or file police reports under those conditions (Golding et al. 1989).

## Domestic Violence and Posttraumatic Stress Disorder

Rates of PTSD among battered women are estimated to be between 33% and 58% (Astin et al. 1993, 1995; Dutton 1992; Houskamp and Foy 1991; Kemp et al. 1991; Kubany 1996). PTSD in victims of partner abuse has been corre-lated with the severity of the abuse, a history of repeated (Norris and Kani-asty 1994) and/or childhood victimization (Astin et al. 1995; O'Keefe 1998), the presence of sexual assault (Browne 1993a, 1993b; J. C. Campbell and Al-ford 1989; Shields and Hanneke 1988), and the degree of psychologic abuse (Arias and Pape 1999). Serious mental illness and disorders related to severe childhood abuse (e.g., dissociative identity disorder, disorders of extreme stress not otherwise specified [DESNOS], borderline personality disorder) not only leave women more vulnerable to adult victimization but also to symptoms that are exacerbated by the abuse.

For women who are still in danger, even if they have left the situation the stress is not "post"—the trauma is ongoing and symptoms may be an adaptive response to danger. Development of PTSD, however, can make it more diffi-cult to mobilize resources, putting women at even greater risk for being iso-lated and controlled by an abuser. Although it appears that many battered women do well without mental health intervention because their symptoms decrease or disappear once they are relatively safe, others need assistance in reducing their distress before they can mobilize the resources necessary to change their lives. For some women, the long-term posttraumatic sequelae of abuse do not appear until much later. In addition, many women continue to be traumatized even after they have left an abusive partner—through stalking, prolonged divorce or custody hearings, visitation, and revictimization by the legal system.

## Comorbidity and Posttraumatic Stress Disorder

Increased rates of psychiatric and medical comorbidity, service use, function-al impairment, and cost are also associated with PTSD (Solomon and David-son 1997). The prevalence of bulimia nervosa, particularly purging behavior, appears to be significantly higher among women with histories of sexual vic-timization and PTSD (Dansky et al. 1997; Kilpatrick 1997; Waller 1991). PTSD also influences the risk for first-onset major depression and alcohol de-pendence (Breslau et al. 1991, 1997).

## Depression

Depression is common among women who have been sexually (as well as physically) assaulted in childhood and/or adulthood. Several factors seem to increase a woman's risk for depression, including perpetrator behavior and a history of multiple sexual victimizations (Kilpatrick et al. 1987; Sorenson and Golding 1990). Women with histories of childhood sexual abuse and adult sexual assault show significantly higher rates of depression than do women in control groups (Bagle and Ramsey 1986; Brown and Root 1990; Ellis et al. 1982; Gidycz and Koss 1989; Jehu 1988). In fact, the lifetime prevalence of major depressive disorder among victims of sexual assault is more than twice that of nonassaulted women (Burnam et al. 1988; Sorenson and Golding 1990). This is particularly true for the women at greatest risk for revictimization—homeless women diagnosed with serious mental illness. The chronic and intense exposure to violence that such women face has been found to contribute to the severity of their psychiatric symptoms (Goodman et al. 1997). Depression associated with PTSD may be a distinct phenomenon. The numbing and feelings of deadness associated with PTSD are among the most difficult symptoms to eradicate, even when intrusion and hyperarousal have improved (van der Kolk et al. 1994).

Although symptoms of anxiety predominate immediately after sexual assault, early signs of depression can be seen within a few hours. Women report sadness, apathy, and suicidal thoughts (Ruch et al. 1991). Within a few weeks, moderate to severe depression may develop (43%–56%) (Frank et al. 1979) and last up to 3 months according to some studies (Ellis et al. 1982; Foa et al. 1989; Resick 1987). Other retrospective studies have found that postrape depression may persist for many years (Ellis et al. 1982; Resick 1987; Resick and Schnicke 1992).

Domestic violence also increases women's risk for depression. Prevalence rates for depression among women abused by an intimate partner range from 37% to 63% (J. Campbell and Kubb 1996; Gelles and Straus 1988; Gleason 1993; Hilberman 1980; Hilberman and Munson 1978; McGrath et al. 1990). Frequency and severity of violence (R. Campbell et al. 1995; Cascardi et al. 1999; Gelles and Straus 1988), psychologic abuse (Follingstad et al. 1990; O'Leary 1999) and lack of social support (R. Campbell et al. 1995) appear to be stronger predictors of depression than are cultural and demographic factors or prior history of mental illness (J. Campbell and Kubb 1996). In several studies, significant reductions in depression occurred among women who were able to end the violence (R. Campbell et al. 1995; Follingstad et al. 1991). Finally, the prevalence of suicidal ideation and suicide attempts are significantly higher among victims of sexual assault (Ellis et al 1982; Frank et al. 1979; Kilpatrick et al. 1985; Stepakoff 1998), women battered by their partners (Stark et al. 1979), and women who were sexually abused as children (Briere and Runtz 1986).

## Substance Abuse

Follette et al. (1996) reported that approximately one-third of previously abused women had lifetime alcohol problems compared with approximately 20% of women in the general population. Other studies confirm the relationship between childhood sexual abuse and subsequent alcohol and drug abuse by women (Briere and Runtz 1988; Bryer et al. 1987; Epstein et al. 1997; Langeland and Harters 1998; Najavits et al. 1997; Wilsnack et al. 1997). In one study, the risk of alcohol abuse was nine times greater among women who had been sexually abused as children (Briere and Runtz 1988).

Strong correlations have also been found between battering and substance abuse among both victims and perpetrators. This relationship is a complex one. Alcohol consumption may contribute to violent behavior in already abusive men, but there is no evidence that substance abuse actually causes violence against women and children (Bennett 1995; Bennett et al. 1994; Substance Abuse and Mental Health Services Administration 1998). Research also suggests that alcohol and drug use among abuse survivors is more likely to result from current or past victimization (e.g., self-medication or coercion into consuming alcohol and other drugs) (Collins et al. 1997), with the use of alcohol and drugs by battered women increasing dramatically after physical abuse begins (Hotaling and Sugarman 1986; Stark and Flitcraft 1988). A woman may be punished by an abusive partner for refusing to drink with him or for entering substance abuse treatment.

Alcohol consumption has also been cited as a risk factor for sexual assault among adolescent and college-age women. Again, this relationship is not straightforward. Alcohol may impair a woman's judgment about the safety of her situation. Drinking may also place women in environments in which they are more likely to encounter offenders, or it may be misperceived by men as a sign of sexual availability. It is important to remember that although high levels of drug or alcohol consumption may put a woman at risk, they do not cause the violence (Crowe and George 1989; Crowell and Burgess 1996; Fillmore 1985; W. H. George et al. 1992, 1995; Lasley 1989; Winfield et al. 1990).

## Dissociation

For those who experience the most extreme forms of childhood abuse (e.g., sadistic; systematic; multiple perpetrators; greater duration, intensity, frequency, and threats; infliction of injury and humiliation; forced witnessing or participation in abuse of others), dissociation is a common response (Chu et al. 1990). The degree of dissociation appears to vary with the severity of the abuse (Goodwin 1996; Putnam 1985). This may manifest as a component of DESNOS or in any of the dissociative spectrum disorders or states. In one study of individuals diagnosed with multiple personality disorder (now called dissociative identity disorder), 97% had experienced serious trauma in child-hood and 68% of those had been sexually abused (Putnam et al. 1986). Nu-merous reports have been made of women initially misdiagnosed with schizophrenia who were later found to have trauma-related dissociative dis-orders, all of which can manifest with transient psychotic states (Gabbard 1992; Goodwin 1996; Jennings 1994a).

## Complex Posttraumatic Stress Disorder or Disorders of Extreme Stress Not Otherwise Specified

Although the PTSD diagnosis adequately captures the psychophysiologic re-sponse to adult single-event sexual assault, important dimensions of the im-pact of ongoing abuse and violence are not addressed by this diagnostic construct. The frequency of comorbidity associated with PTSD, in fact, has led to the notion that *comorbidity* is a misnomer masking a more complex form of PTSD that develops in people who have been abused over long periods of time—one that includes both Axis I and Axis II sequelae of chronic abuse (Brady 1997; S. Roth et al. 1997; Zlotnick et al. 1996). Childhood sexual abuse and entrapment in an abusive partner relationship are qualitatively dif-ferent from many other types of trauma; according to several studies, they are premeditated, ongoing, and most often perpetrated by someone to whom the victim is attached and on whom she depends (Courtois 1995, 1997; Dutton 1992; Goodwin 1996; Herman 1992b; Hilberman and Munson 1978; Rieker and Carmen 1986; Stark et al. 1979). The abuser often denies and distorts the abuse, and the victim is coerced or threatened to maintain secrecy (Rieker and Carmen 1986). When abuse occurs during childhood, it has the potential to derail personal and social development (Putnam and Trickett 1993).

   *Complex posttraumatic stress disorder* (Herman 1992a, 1992b), or *disorders of extreme stress not otherwise specified*, is not officially listed as a diagnosis in DSM-IV (American Psychiatric Association 1994), although it is contained in the International Classifications of Disease (ICD)-9. The symptoms that make up DESNOS are listed as associated features of PTSD. DSM-IV field trials indicate that this construct is internally consistent and reliable (Peclovitz et al. 1997) and distinguishes early from late onset trauma (van der Kolk et al.

1996). Women who are severely abused by a partner may also experience more complex posttraumatic responses, particularly if they were abused in childhood as well.

Diagnostic criteria for DESNOS are consistent with developmental models (S. Roth et al. 1997) and involve alterations in the following domains: affect and impulse modulation (suicide attempts, high-risk behavior and self-mutilation) (Boudewyn and Liem 1995); states of consciousness (dissociation) (Waldinger et al. 1994); self-perception (self-loathing and shame); perceptions of the perpetrator (idealization); relations with others (e.g., traumatic reenactments, intense rage) (Kendall-Tackett et al. 1993); and systems of meanings (no one can be trusted) (Angel and Gronfein 1988; Johnson et al. 1997; Kleinman 1977; Pepitone and Triandis 1988; S. Roth et al. 1997). In addition, women's sexuality is often affected, manifesting as compulsive sexual behavior, dissociation during sex, or sexual avoidance (Turkus 1995). These responses reflect some of the complex ways women attempt to regain a sense of control over feelings of violation and betrayal. Symptoms may also develop in response to triggering life events (a woman's daughter reaching the same age she was when she was abused) or therapy-related events (real or perceived abandonment by therapist) (Harvey and Harney 1995; Turkus 1995).

## Developing a More Complex Trauma Framework

The developmental impact of prolonged exposure to abuse by a caretaker or of sexual assault on a woman's sense of herself goes far beyond what is described by current psychiatric nosology, even by diagnoses that specifically address traumatic events. For example, although a PTSD diagnosis may explain the terrifying flashbacks many women have when they attempt to resume sexual activity after an assault and *sexual dysfunction* may describe their symptoms, neither diagnosis captures the complex ways in which women reconfigure their experience of themselves as sexual beings following rape. The effects of abuse in childhood and/or adulthood affect women's experiences of themselves and others throughout their lives (Browne 1993a; Campbell and Kubb 1996; Carmen et al. 1984; Den Herder and Redner 1991; Herman 1992b). Many women who have been victimized do not develop psychiatric disorders, but few are unaffected by those experiences (Courtois 1997).

Over time, the experiences of trauma survivors and the mental health professionals working with them have challenged traditional symptom-driven models of behavior that pathologize victims but fail to examine the circumstances that have caused symptoms to emerge. Trauma theory provides a framework for understanding symptoms as psychophysiologic survival strategies used to adapt to potentially life-shattering situations. It also allows for a more balanced approach to treatment—one that focuses on resilience and strength as well as on psychologic harm (Briere 1997; Dutton 1992, 1996; Gondolf and Browne 1998; Herman 1992b; McCann and Pearlman 1990).

For example, trauma theory has reframed borderline symptoms as both reenactments of abusive or neglectful interactions with caretakers and as efforts to protect the self and others from potentially annihilating psychic assaults (Goodwin 1996). Without a trauma framework, it is difficult to make therapeutic sense of the feelings and behaviors (e.g., rageful feelings and self-destructive behaviors) that can make life so stormy for survivors of severe abuse.

Work with battered women has led to similar perspectives. Many women initially attempt to remedy their situations themselves by talking, seeking help, fighting back, or trying to change the conditions that they either perceive or are told caused the abuse. When those attempts fail, they may retreat into a mode that appears more passive and compliant but may actually reflect how they have learned to reduce their immediate danger. When those tactics no longer work, they may learn to dissociate from feelings that have become unbearable, perceiving that if they cannot change what is happening outside of them—or if they face near-certain death if they try to leave—they can at least try to change their own responses and "leave the situation" emotionally. For some women, substance abuse becomes another way of either coping with or leaving the situation. For those who become increasingly isolated from outside resources, suicide or homicide may seem like the only way to end the abuse (Dutton 1992; Warshaw 1996a).

Nor do women experience these events in isolation. A body of clinical literature describes the retraumatizing effects of more subtle forms of social and cultural victimization (e.g., microtraumatization due to gender, race, ethnicity, sexual orientation, disability, and/or socioeconomic status or what Root [1996] describes as "insidious trauma") and the ramifications of living in societies that tolerate the pervasive disregard of the human rights of women and children (L. Brown 1995; Hamilton 1989; Kanuha 1994; Root 1996). Other authors stress the importance of understanding how gender discrimination and other forms of oppression affect women's experience of violence (G. R. Brown and Anderson 1991; Espin and Gawalek 1992; Greene 1994; Joseph and Lewis 1981). Greene (1994), for example, noted that "internalized racism and discrimination" based on one's race, ethnicity, gender, or sexual orientation "create a range of overlapping psychological realities that may facilitate, challenge, or undermine optimal development" (p. 344) as well as recovery from trauma. It is not just the experience of discrimination or victimization that influences women's psychologic development; it is also their complex responses to those experiences and the social contexts in which they occur. As Weskott (1986) describes, female development is a process in which "devaluation is both internalized and struggled against" (p. 4). These struggles are clearly compounded by abuse. It is those very strategies of resistance, however, that subsequently become both growth-limiting adaptations and important sources of strength (Krieger 1996; Root 1996; Weskott 1986).

## Limitations of Mental Health Models

Even a trauma framework defines an overwhelming response to minor stimuli as being part of a disorder. Viewing this heightened sensitivity as pathologic rather than as a reflection of acute social awareness is risky because it discounts the experience that allows women to recognize potentially dangerous behaviors and attitudes before they reach more serious levels (Warshaw 1992). It defines the problem as being "in the woman" and she, rather than a society that tolerates this type of abuse, becomes the focus of intervention (Warshaw 1992).

Clinicians who work within a purely biologic or disorder-specific framework run risks similar to those of their medical and surgical colleagues of failing to recognize and respond to the continuing violence in a patient's life. They may see abuse as being caused by a particular woman's vulnerability or as only a secondary problem—a social stressor affecting the course of her primary biologic or developmental disorder.

Traditional psychoanalytic theory presents a different set of limitations. The context of ongoing violence and danger that creates and perpetuates a woman's symptoms may not be addressed or may be regarded as symptomatic rather than etiologic. In addition, a clinician bound by the constraints of remaining true to the neutrality of a psychodynamic framework may find it difficult to play a more active role in advocating for safety and in helping women gain access to community resources. There are, of course, more recent models that recognize the importance of social and relational contexts (Atwood and Stolorow 1984; L. S. Brown and Root 1990; Dutton 1992; Kleinman 1977; Koss and Harvey 1991; Triandis 1972).

When domestic violence is framed solely under the rubric of "family violence," it obscures the gendered aspects of this problem and is more likely to be seen in terms of dysfunctional couple or family dynamics. In doing so, clinicians can lose sight of the larger social dynamics that shape gendered behaviors in families and are thus less able to help women to gain perspective or mobilize necessary resources. Family systems approaches can, in fact, present even greater dangers to battered women. Assuming equal power within and responsibility for relationship dynamics, it inadvertently holds a battered woman responsible for her partner's criminal behavior and keeps her engaged in the countertherapeutic task of trying to change herself in order to change him. In addition, couples sessions often precipitate further threats or violence. The dynamics of battering have been described as a form of domestic terrorism, more akin to hostage situations than to dysfunctional couples (Andersen et al. 1991; L. E. Walker 1988). In that kind of setting, particularly when her partner continues to engage in violent, controlling behavior or threats, it is not safe for a woman to be honest or to assert herself. Nor is she likely to be free to make her own choices (Gondolf and Fisher 1988; Krueger 1988). Again, newer models of family and couples therapy are being developed that specifically address domestic violence (Goldner 1999; Hansen 1993). However, little data exist on the effectiveness or safety of these treatment modalities, and they have been studied in couples in which the level of violence is low (O'Leary 1999).

# Clinical Interventions: Assessment, Treatment, and Collaboration

Over the past 25 years, principles and practices for working with survivors of abuse and violence have evolved to form current standards of care. These apply to all types of gender-based trauma and can be easily integrated into clinical practice.

## Recognizing Safety as a Priority

For all victims of abuse and violence, the issue of safety is paramount. The traditional focus of mental health interventions has been on safety from self-harm. However, ongoing danger from a current or former perpetrator and prevention of victimization by others are also critical safety issues.

## Attending to Issues of Respect and Collaboration

The experience of being treated with respect, feeling free to make one's own choices, and participating in straightforward, caring, give-and-take relationships can be therapeutic in itself and provides an opportunity to counter internalized abuse-related dynamics. Because victims of abuse are often more vulnerable to reinjury and exquisitely attuned to relationship dynamics, the power imbalances inherent to clinical interactions must be consciously attended to. This is of particular concern when using more directive treatment modalities.

Actively communicating that the perpetrator alone is responsible for his (or her) abusive behavior and that he (or she) is the one responsible for stopping it counters the abuser's power to convince the victim that the abuse is or was her fault. Therapies that focus on helping women understand why they unconsciously chose an abusive partner or seduced a caretaker or that labels them as codependent or enabling are not only ineffective but harmful as well (Koss et al. 1994). Addressing the influence of earlier abusive relationships on women's ability to find safe, mutually honoring relationships as adults can be taken up in the later phases of treatment, when they are no longer being bullied by a partner, being revictimized by the courts, or blaming themselves for experiences that were beyond their control. Although experiencing or witnessing abuse in childhood appears to increase a woman's risk of being abused as an adult, the major risk factor for partner abuse is being a woman in a society that tolerates domestic violence. Using a trauma framework to address coping strategies such as substance abuse, self-cutting, or seeming passivity in the face of ongoing threats not only provides perspective for women on behaviors they may experience as shameful but also reduces the likelihood that clinicians will respond in ways that are inadvertently judgmental or pathologizing (Dutton 1992).

## Advocating for Women and for System Change

Advocacy on the victim's behalf adds another dimension to traditional clinical interactions. It facilitates rather than directs change by actively helping women become aware of their options, gain access to community resources, make their own choices about how best to end ongoing violence, and mitigate the impact of the abuse on their lives. It is important for clinicians to acknowledge the barriers women face in ending and recovering from abuse and to advocate for change in those systems using the vehicles available to them. This could involve advocating with insurance companies to reimburse an individual patient for long-term trauma therapy, working through professional organizations to influence reimbursement policies on a larger scale, incorporating issues of abuse and violence into clinical training curricula, or working with other systems to increase their understanding of the psychologic effects of trauma.

## Assessing for Trauma

Anyone seen in a clinical setting should be asked specifically about past and current abuse. It is important to let women know that

- Abuse experiences are common.
- You are willing to listen.
- You believe her and are concerned.
- The abuse is not her fault and no one deserves to be treated that way.
- Resources are available to help her if she is currently in danger.
- She will not be judged or stigmatized as a result of what she has said to you.
- All information will be kept confidential within the confines of subpoenas and mandatory reporting laws (inform women about the limitations of confidentiality in your state; this information can usually be obtained through state professional organizations).

Routine inquiry is essential to avoid misdiagnosis and misinterpretation of symptoms and to provide appropriate intervention (Dutton 1996). It helps reduce the isolation that abusers use to establish control over their victims. Although assessment is often the initial phase of treatment, it is also an ongoing process. Many survivors have concrete reasons for not initially disclosing abuse. A woman could lose custody of her children if she is given a psychiatric diagnosis or if it is discovered that she lives in a violent household. Her partner may have told her that he will kill her or her children if she reports the abuse or tries to leave. Survivors may also experience intense guilt and shame, particularly about sexual assault and abuse; this can make it difficult for them to raise or discuss these issues until they feel safe in the therapeutic relationship or more secure in their own lives (Harvey and Harney 1995). For women who have been sexually abused as children, memories may be absent or incomplete at the time they enter treatment (Briere 1992a).

Inquiries about abuse should not be made in the presence of a possible perpetrator or another person whom the woman has not privately identified as someone she can trust with that information. Such questions should not be asked during a couple's therapy session, through an untrained translator, with a personal assistant or guardian in the room, or in the presence of a person providing additional information, even if a woman is acutely psychotic or unable to provide it herself. These questions should not be asked on questionnaires sent to the woman's home. Patients should be told that the information they give is confidential and, within the confines of the law, will not be revealed to the batterer or anyone else without their permission. For those clinicians who practice in states with mandatory reporting laws, it is essential to inform the patient of this requirement at the beginning of the evaluation, preferably before he or she has discussed the abuse. It is also important to discuss reporting obligations before inquiring about child abuse. In addition, strategies should be developed for safely separating patients from abusers should that become necessary. If there appears to be an immediate threat from the abuser, the clinician should be prepared to notify the police or security and to outline any potential risk (e.g., abuser is in the waiting room intimidating staff). Once initial safety is established, however, a patient's wish to have another person present should be respected.

It sometimes feels awkward to suddenly introduce the subject of abuse, particularly if there are no obvious indications that the woman has been victimized. Abuse-related questions can be framed in many ways that let women know their experiences are common and that you are comfortable with and interested in knowing (e.g., "I don't know if this has happened to you, but because so many women experience abuse and violence in their lives, it's something I always ask about" or "Tell me about your relationship"). It is, however, important to ask explicit questions about specific abusive experiences. Simply asking a woman "Have you ever been abused?" places her in the doubly difficult position of having to evaluate her assailant's behavior as well as report it (Table 23–1).

Several trauma screening tools are available, such as the Trauma Symptoms Inventory (Briere 1995; Briere et al. 1995), the Clinician Administered PTSD Scale (CAPS) (Blake et al. 1995), the Structured Interview for Disorders of Extreme Stress (SIDES) (Peclovitz et al. 1997), and the Dissociative Experiences Scale (DES) (Bernstein and Putnam 1986), to name a few. These can usually be obtained by contacting the authors (Briere 1997; E. B. Carlson 1997; Tolman 1988, 1999; J. P. Wilson and Keane 1997). Questions can easily be adapted from instruments such as these and integrated into standard

---

**TABLE 23–1.** Asking about abuse

---

**Partner abuse**

Has your partner ever physically hurt you? Has he (or she) ever threatened to hurt you or someone you care about? (Give examples of specific acts)

Do you feel safe in your current relationship? Are you ever afraid of your partner?

What kinds of things does he or she do that make you afraid?

Has your partner ever humiliated you, controlled you, or tried to keep you from doing things you want to do? When you are with your partner, do you feel like you are walking on eggshells?

Has your partner ever forced or pressured you into engaging in sexual activities that made you uncomfortable or into having sex when you didn't want to?

Do you feel you can say no if you don't want to have sex?

**Childhood sexual abuse and sexual assault**

Were you ever told by an adult to keep a secret and threatened if you did not?

Were you ever touched in a way you didn't like?

How old were you when you first had sex (including anal, vaginal, and oral penetration)?

How old was the person you had sex with?

Were you ever forced or pressured into engaging in sexual activity when you were a child? At any other time in your life?

Did you tell anyone about what happened to you?

How did they respond? What happened as a result of your telling?

---

assessments (see Norris and Riad 1997).

If a woman discloses a history of current or past victimization, a more in-depth assessment of her situation is required. More information is needed about the nature of her traumatic experiences and the scope of their impact on her life; her current safety status; how the abuse has affected her and her children and how she protects them and herself; the presence of medical illnesses and psychiatric symptoms (disorders known to be related to trauma, including suicidality, self-cutting, and high-risk sexual behavior, as well as co-existing health, mental health, or substance abuse problems); the coping strategies she uses and how they affect her daily life (currently and at the time of trauma); her developmental context (e.g., family dynamics, quality of other relationships, events surrounding childhood abuse, response of others, feelings at the time and currently, self-organization); her degree of isolation versus support; what she has tried in the past and how that did or did not work for her; and her own assessment of the situation—what she would like to see happen and what issues she faces in achieving those goals.

## Specific Assessment Issues

Women seeking help for a recent sexual assault or rape-related PTSD may have already been asked to provide detailed accounts of their experience to emergency room personnel and to the police. It is important to assess the nature of the trauma that precipitated treatment. Acquisition of more detailed information should be paced to the patient's needs.

For women currently being abused by an intimate partner, the same caveats apply. Asking about the details of the abuse (e.g., pattern of abuse, tactics of control and intimidation, level of fear and entrapment, sexual coercion or assault, and the abuse's impact on the woman and her children) can serve several important functions. It allows providers to document critical information for women seeking legal protection, redress, or custody and provides a safe opportunity to examine the ongoing nature of the abuse and its impact. In addition, asking a woman what she has done to try to remedy her situation and how her efforts have been received creates a chance to explore new options and to acknowledge the resourcefulness she has exhibited in coping with her situation.

It is important to remember that although the symptoms or issues that emerge during an assessment may seem to point to a history of trauma, the woman before you may not see it that way. Although some women may seek treatment for symptoms or issues explicitly related to a particular traumatic experience, not everyone will link their current distress to such events. Many will not recall earlier traumas until later in the course of therapy. Therefore, it is incumbent on therapists to keep an open mind about the potential presence of trauma in a woman's history, to attend to abuse-related information as it arises, and to validate those perceptions without "digging" for memories or assuming that because a woman has a particular constellation of symptoms she has been sexually abused as a child. It is also important to document women's descriptions of abusive experiences in their own words, particularly when there is the potential for legal action. Guidelines have been developed by several responsible professional organizations to help clinicians negotiate this complex terrain (American Psychiatric Association [1993], American Psychological Association, International Society for Traumatic Stress Studies, American Medical Association [see Goldman et al. 1995]).

### Race, Ethnicity, Culture, and Religion

Women of color may be reluctant to discuss abuse if they perceive this as betraying their community or likely to invoke discriminatory criminal justice actions toward the perpetrator. Cultural or religious constraints may make it difficult for a woman to discuss the abuse with someone outside her community. Alternatively, women may be afraid to discuss these issues with someone from the same cultural background. Issues of privacy, shame, safety, and confidentiality all affect a woman's decision to reveal that she is being abused. Mental health treatment may be stigmatized, making it more difficult for women to seek help for trauma-related symptoms. Women may face social isolation and ostracism if they attempt to leave an abusive spouse, making it harder for them to consider this as a possibility. The idea of breaking marriage vows may create serious spiritual conflicts for some women as well.

Immigrant women also face obstacles to treatment. Those who are undocumented may find it even more difficult to reveal a history of partner abuse, in part because they are afraid of bringing attention to their situation, and in part because batterers threaten to have them deported if they tell and to leave them without resources or support. Some batterers control their wives by deliberately failing to file their petitions for permanent residency. State domestic violence coalitions are usually aware of services that specifically address these issues

### Lesbian Women

Discussing partner abuse may also be difficult for women in lesbian relationships who have experienced homophobic responses outside the gay and lesbian community and denial about domestic violence within. It may be more difficult for lesbians to find confidential sources of help, particularly when their abusive partner is involved in organizations that provide services to battered women. Not uncommonly, a lesbian batterer will attempt to control her partner by threatening to "out" her if she reveals the abuse or tries to leave (homophobic control; Hard 1986) or by defining the woman's efforts to defend herself as "mutual combat," undermining her efforts to get help (Hard 1986; Renzetti 1992; West 1998). Internalized responses to homophobia and violence in a woman's family of origin may contribute both to perpetration and to an increased vulnerability to victimization once it occurs. Although there are couples in which the abuse or violence is mutual or in which one partner initiates and the other fights back, for many women the pattern of one partner systematically controlling the other is no different from that in abusive heterosexual relationships (Marrujo and Kreger 1996). It is important to ask for explicit examples of what actually happens in the relationship when these questions arise. Abusers typically use tactics of denial and distortion and do not take responsibility for their behaviors. Any therapist working with lesbian couples must interview each partner separately to ask about abuse.

Therapists should also be aware that lesbian survivors of childhood sexual abuse may have some unique concerns about the therapeutic relationship. They may be grappling, for example, with their sense of safety as a lesbian within the therapy. This may manifest as a need to know about a therapist's view of lesbianism or familiarity and comfort in working with lesbians. A client's sense of safety may be undermined by a therapist's refusal to disclose his or her own views and experiences; by a therapist's interpretation of lesbianism as a response to the incest; or by a therapist's inability to identify the homophobia faced by the client as a potential cause of trauma-related disorders (T. Pintzuk, personal communication, 1998).

## Women with Disabilities or Other Mental Health Problems

Women already diagnosed with mental health or substance abuse problems contend with an additional set of concerns. They may fear not being taken seriously because of previous experiences with helping professionals or because abusers have convinced them this is so. These issues may affect a woman's ability to process information and sort out options and may limit her access to shelter. In addition, women with serious physical disabilities or medical problems, some of which have been caused by the abuse, may find it even more difficult to leave a partner or family member on whom she depends for access to services and basic care.

Disabled women are even more likely to feel trapped in abusive relationships, particularly when jobs and transportation are limited or when their only alternative is to live in an institution or return to an abusive family (Asch and Fine 1992). Personal assistants may also turn out to be abusers, further decreasing women's options for living independently. In addition, women with disabilities are often perceived as asexual and de-gendered, reducing the likelihood that partner abuse will be recognized. These relationships—harder won—may also be harder to give up (Gil et al. 1994). Therapists can learn more about the specific needs of women with nonpsychiatric disabilities and find ways to make their own practice settings more accessible by contacting a disability rights advocacy group such as the Disabled Women's Network (DAWN) in Canada or the Health Resource Center for Women with Disabilities in Chicago.

Treatment and Intervention

## Overview

Recognition of the impact of abuse and violence against women has led to the emergence of a number of treatment approaches. Although few have been tested empirically, there is growing consensus about the types of interventions that are most helpful to survivors of abuse. Published studies have focused on interventions following single-event sexual assaults. These have shown considerable success in preventing or reducing the severity of PTSD and, to some extent, depression and anxiety. Focal short-term psychodynamic therapies have also demonstrated some efficacy in treating PTSD (Marmar 1991). There is less research on which treatment modalities will be most helpful for individual women (Chalk and King 1998; Crowell and Burgess 1996). Few outcome studies have been completed that assess treatment for women sexually abused as children or women abused by intimate partners. Most reports are descriptive, feature nonstandardized approaches to care, or demonstrate relatively modest positive results (Barnett et al. 1997). The dearth of studies in this area is not surprising given that treatment for the chronic effects of abuse is often multimodal and long-term.

As clinicians come to recognize the distinct developmental affects of chronic abuse, more complex treatment models have begun to evolve. These approaches combine trauma theory with developmental psychodynamic perspectives (self-psychology and object relations) and a feminist-based emphasis on empowerment and social context. They often involve nontraditional, body-centered therapies as well. Feminist theory explicitly addresses the role of power dynamics both within a woman's life and within therapeutic encounters. Advocacy models attend to the social reality of ongoing danger and entrapment and the impact of social institutions and communities on a woman's ability to change her life. These flexible client-responsive treatment approaches are more difficult to study than short-term protocol-driven models but nonetheless reflect current expert opinion in this area.

There are also several promising studies of group treatment modalities (Courtois 1988; Lubin and Johnson 1997; Talbot et al. 1998; Winick et al. 1992; Zlotnick et al. 1997) and interventions designed specifically for managing the symptoms and self-harming behavior of women diagnosed with borderline personality disorder, a high percentage of whom have experienced abuse in childhood (Linehan 1993; Simpson et al. 1998). Many of those techniques have been adapted into more complex treatment programs designed specifically for women with severe trauma histories and DESNOS (e.g., Bloom 1997; Courtois 1997) or SMI (Harris 1998). More recently, eye movement desensitization and reprocessing has been shown to be effective as an adjunctive tool for treating PTSD (Shapiro 1995).

Although many techniques are available for treating PTSD, dissociative identity disorder, and DESNOS, they generally are geared toward addressing specific sets of symptoms. Healing from the interpersonal and developmental effects of abuse and violence requires the safety, consistency, caring, and respect of an ongoing therapeutic relationship. Although some women respond to short-term interventions, others may need many years to recover from the traumatic effects of longstanding abuse. Often, therapists are trained to value specific intervention techniques or particular theoretic orientations, which may lead them to dismiss other forms of treatment that might be helpful. Although the issues unique to sexual assault, sexual abuse, and domestic violence are described in separate sections, many of these also overlap. Trauma must be addressed within the context of who a woman is and where she is in her life and must acknowledge her particular strengths, vulnerabilities, resilience, defenses, and support.

The following section describes a phase model for treatment that reflects the growing consensus among clinicians and researchers working with survivors of sexual abuse and other forms of chronic severe trauma (Courtois 1997; Harvey and Harney 1995; Herman 1992b). The emphasis is on establishing stability and safety and on building a therapeutic relationship (early phase) before proceeding to the trauma-focused work (middle phase) that can be painful and disruptive to both the therapist and the client. The final phase involves the integration of memories, development of new capacities, reconnection to others, and rebuilding of one's life (Dutton 1992). This process is not linear, of course, but rather provides a framework for conceptualizing and conducting this often challenging work.

## Building Collaborative Alliances: The Centrality of the Client–Therapist Relationship in the Early Phase of Treatment

For many women, recovering from the sequelae of abuse is an ongoing struggle fraught with relationship difficulties and symptoms that fluctuate over time. In some situations, a woman and her therapist may be able to navigate through these difficulties without additional intervention. In other circumstances, debilitating symptoms, work instability, ongoing danger, coexisting substance abuse or eating disorders, and other harmful behaviors often require a wider range of interventions than can be addressed by an individual therapist alone.

For someone who has experienced severe, chronic abuse, particularly as a child, the work involved in building therapeutic alliances cannot be overestimated. As Elliott and Briere (1995) noted, "therapy is a powerful re-stimulator of abuse-era related feelings, perceptions, and experiences." It can take years to create an environment in which a woman can reframe her relationship to the traumatic events she has endured and reconstruct her beliefs about how relationships can function in the absence of coercion and violence. This outcome is possible only if the relationship between client and therapist is collaborative (Briere 1996; Courtois 1997; Dutton 1992; Herman 1992b; Schechter 1996; Warshaw 1996b). Providing information about trauma and other related issues is strongly encouraged, and treatment plans should be jointly conceived, evaluated, and redesigned on a regular basis.

## Challenges of Collaboration:
## Transference, Countertransference, and Ethics

The process of constructing a collaborative relationship poses challenges to both client and therapist. Survivors of abuse may, for example, express thoughts or feelings or engage in behaviors that represent conscious or dissociated reenactments of or strategies to protect themselves from traumatic interpersonal experiences. Therapists unaware of transference dynamics may respond in complementary ways (e.g., react angrily to being accused of acting like a perpetrator) instead of realizing that a component of the clinical interaction or a concurrent life event is reminiscent of a past negative event or relationship (Rieker and Carmen 1986). On the other hand, abuse may be occurring in the present and such reactions must not be attributed to earlier experiences or transference when that is not the case.

The therapist is vulnerable to reactions such as distancing from clients and avoiding issues that seem overwhelming. Listening to women talk about their experiences of abuse can evoke a range of painful responses that can be traumatizing in themselves. This phenomenon of secondary or vicarious traumatization has been increasingly recognized within the trauma field (Dutton 1992; Elliott and Briere 1995; Pearlman and Saakvitne 1995). In addition, many therapists have experienced some form of gender-based trauma themselves and are at risk for having their own feelings triggered when working with other survivors.

It is important for therapists to discuss the parameters of treatment with clients so they will know what they can and cannot expect from a therapeutic relationship and to create the opportunity for clients to discuss their own concerns. It is easy to perceive clients as "too needy" or "demanding" when they exceed the capacity of the therapist or of an ethical treatment to meet needs that should have been met at an earlier time. It is important to protect both the client and the therapist from unrealistic expectations and disappointments that can re-create dynamics of earlier abusive interactions. There will be disappointments or times when a client may feel rejected, abandoned, or not seen; agreeing on parameters at the outset helps create a safe and mutually respectful atmosphere in which to explore these issues when they arise.

Overinvolvement on the part of the therapist, whether it be exploitive (meeting one's own needs at the expense of the patient) or well intentioned but naïve (overidentifying with the client or wanting to "cure" her through unlimited caring and availability) is problematic. Women who have been sexually abused in the past are more likely to be subjected to boundary violations by mental health providers (Gabbard 1994; Gartrell et al. 1986). Any form of exploitation, including sexual involvement, is clearly unacceptable and if therapists become aware of those dynamics, immediate consultation should be sought. Therapists who extend themselves beyond their capacities may find themselves becoming depleted and unable to respond appropriately and protecting themselves in ways that ultimately abandon the patient. This type of overinvolvement can curtail a client's autonomy, disrupt her ability to experience rage (including rage at the therapist), and interfere with opportunities to grieve irreparable losses—crucial issues for many survivors. Fears of being overwhelmed by a patient's demands, fears for the patient's safety, concerns about liability, or fears of invoking the "boundary police" may also cause therapists to become overly rigid and to distance themselves from patients. These behaviors, although protective of the therapist, are in fact diminishing and disrespectful to patients, who in turn may experience them as punitive, rejecting, and abandoning.

With patients for whom abuse has severely disrupted their capacity to trust, relate to others, and protect themselves; who may be more volatile and who have not internalized mechanisms for managing intolerable feelings; and who engage others in roller coaster–like attempts to manage themselves, it is important to understand not only the context of these behaviors but our own responses as well. This is notoriously difficult when patients are chronically suicidal and the therapist feels responsible for their survival. Without adequate support, therapists may distance themselves from their patients, hospitalize them either too soon or too late, become punitive, or make themselves continuously available in ways that disrupt their own lives.

On the other hand, providing genuine care, respect, and kindness; going out of one's way during crises (e.g., scheduling additional contact, visiting a client in the hospital, mutually determining the best way to handle emergencies); or facilitating access to necessary resources should not be cause for concern. A fine line exists between continual and consistent availability; it is the therapist's consistency that helps clients create the internal sense of security necessary to weather emotional storms. Therapists cannot undo what was done in the past nor should they attempt to protect patients from their own knowledge, feelings, and experiences. Outside perspective, support, and consultation are vital for therapists doing this type of work to reduce their own isolation, depletion, and traumatization.

These dynamics are not limited to one-on-one clinical interactions. Survivors of abuse can experience retraumatization as a result of interactions with the health and mental health systems as well. The distortion of meaning and denial of experience that are used as tactics of psychologic control in abusive relationships can be inadvertently repeated in clinical/medical encounters if clinicians are unable to recognize and validate the traumatic contexts in which a person's symptoms are developed and maintained.

### Co-Creating Safety and Stability

While the therapeutic relationship is being built, the therapist works with the client to ensure her safety, manage stress, and perform daily tasks. Helping a client stabilize her life may include working with her to initiate or maintain a regular day and evening schedule, engage in some form of exercise, receive medical care, learn and practice grounding and self-soothing techniques, and create or strengthen a support network that values and nurtures her in this process. In addition to these activities, the therapist and client can work together to discover what kinds of events or interactions trigger dissociation and flashbacks so that the client can begin restructuring her responses to these triggers and thus reduce their negative impact on her life. This process of restructuring can be aided by various relaxation and other de-escalation techniques. Medication may also be helpful, provided that the woman is educated about it and that the medication does not interfere with her ability to protect herself (Bloom 1997; Courtois 1997; Turkus 1995). Benzodiazepine use, for example, can compromise a woman's ability to protect herself or to leave an abusive relationship. For women with symptoms that may necessitate hospitalization, reviewing preferred de-escalation strategies (e.g., finding alternatives to or more tolerable forms of restraint and seclusion) before or at admission can reduce the risk of retraumatization and can enhance a woman's sense of choice and empowerment. Several individual states and institutions have begun to modify their seclusion and restraint policies accordingly and model policies are available (Carmen and Rieker 1998; Jennings 1994b).

## Special Considerations When Abuse is Ongoing: Domestic Violence–Specific Issues

Many abused women are still in danger at the time they seek help and are at greater risk when they try to leave or seek outside help to end the violence. Inquire about perpetrator risk factors such as suicide attempts; depression; past violence; violence toward others; types of substance abuse; threats of further violence, suicide, or homicide; escalation of threats or actual violence; availability of weapons; obsession with or access to his/her partner or signs of stalking; abuse during pregnancy; or violent sexual assault. Exposure to other dangerous environments should also be assessed. After reviewing all of these risk factors, a woman should be asked to consider whether she thinks she is in danger of being seriously injured or killed. If she says yes, this should be taken very seriously. If she says no but the clinician still has concerns about her safety, these should be discussed frankly and efforts should be made to help her think through her options. If she is at risk and is planning to leave the relationship, the clinician should advise her to seriously consider leaving without informing her partner and should assist her in finding a safe place to go.

Women currently in danger should be encouraged to develop safety and escape plans if they are staying with an abusive partner or the abuser has access to them and to explore their options if leaving. It is helpful for women to rehearse their plans so they will be in place when needed. Women can do a number of things in addition to calling the police or a crisis line or getting a protective order from the courts. They can review previous episodes for information that identifies predictable patterns and locations that may be dangerous; think about how to anticipate and reduce danger if possible; make provisions for children (rehearse escape strategies, places to stay, numbers to call, how to make credit card calls); locate (in advance) a safe place to go in an emergency; make provisions for leaving quickly; and have necessary items and papers packed, accessible, and if at all possible hidden from the abuser. Police can escort a woman back to her home if she needs to gather belongings, but if an abuser suspects his/her partner is leaving he/she may destroy valuable items and papers. A woman can also develop and rehearse an escape plan and develop a plan for getting help when she cannot escape (e.g., signal to neighbors, teach the children to dial 911)

## Clinical Issues

Women trapped in abusive relationships may be immobilized by depression, panic attacks, or severe stress responses such as brief reactive psychoses, acute stress disorder, or PTSD. In such situations, treatment is clearly warranted to enhance a woman's capacity to function and make choices that will ultimately lead her to safety. However, reframing these disorders as understandable responses to terror and entrapment will lead to intervention strategies that both provide perspective to the woman and focus on the dangers she is facing.

Battering appears to be a risk factor for suicide attempts (Stark and Flitcraft 1995). Some women do not feel they have any other options for ending the abuse and the pain they are experiencing. They may have made multiple unsuccessful attempts to protect themselves, stop the abuse, or leave. For other women, the risk of suicide may increase after they have left the relationship, before they have had a chance to recover their sense of self-worth and their ability to function on their own. Whether the separation is by choice or because the batterer has left them for another woman, the experience of abandonment and loss may become too painful to tolerate (Dutton 1992).

Homicidal ideation also warrants emergency psychiatric evaluation. In most cases, women who kill their partners have been severely abused for long periods of time and see no other way out. They believe they need to kill to prevent the murder or serious injury of themselves or their children. Experienced clinicians have found it very rare for battered women to premeditate the murder of an abusive partner. Rather, they develop self-defense strategies (e.g., carrying a weapon) that have potentially lethal outcomes both for the victim and her partner. Assessing a woman's level of danger and discussing the risk of lethality, the likelihood of incarceration, and the range of other alternatives can help diffuse the immediate danger. Discussing the possibility of measures such as being transported to out-of-state shelters, relocation, witness protection plans, and hospitalization provides the victim with alternatives to homicide when her own danger is high (Dutton 1992). The therapist should try to assess if such circumstances reflect her current situation by asking her to describe how she perceives her options for safety; if homicide is a possible scenario, she should be asked directly whether she has plans to kill or harm her partner and, if so, whether she has a weapon or plan for carrying out that action. If she has a plan, duty-to-warn considerations come into play.

If a clinician is aware of a patient's intent to harm a third party, such as the patient's spouse or partner, the practitioner may have a legal duty to breach the patient's confidentiality and warn the third party of the impending danger. The Tarasoff (1976) decision enjoins clinicians to take reasonable steps to protect a third party from harm. This may include hospitalization or sheltering of a victim who sees homicide as the only way to be safe.

## Confidentiality and Documentation Issues

Any information that becomes available to the batterer can increase a woman's danger and can be used to control her or used against her in court with regard to custody issues. It is important to be sensitive to nuances of documentation. Any symptoms that result from or are aggravated by abuse should be documented, and the potential for the symptoms to subside once the victim is safe should be discussed. Diagnoses and medications should be used with caution (consider using *acute stress disorder* or *adjustment disorder not otherwise specified* rather than PTSD if a woman is still being abused). Discussion should be framed around the relationship of symptoms to the abuse; the woman's strengths, coping strategies, ability to care for her children, and efforts made to protect them should be described. For therapists involved in custody evaluations, it is important to recognize the appropriateness of a woman's anger toward the abuser and her reluctance to expose her children to a violent, abusive parent. Women are often penalized in these situations for being the less cooperative parent. Therapists must take care not to be fooled by the seeming health of an abuser whose partner may look more symptomatic (Koss et al. 1994). Abusers frequently use custody battles and visitation as ways to control a partner who is attempting to leave.

## Providing Information About Domestic Violence

Many battered women are either numb or in a state of terror and confusion at the time they seek help and have not had room to do more than survive. Providing information about the dynamics of abuse; typical battering tactics; common sequelae; the pattern of abuse and the likelihood that it will continue; the impact of abuse on children; risks, danger, and safety planning; and available options and resources is also a powerful intervention tool. It helps decrease isolation and shame, helps women gain perspective, aids in decreasing psychologic entrapment, and offers a sense of hope and connection.

Abusers control and intimidate their partners to make themselves feel powerful. The typical controlling behaviors used by perpetrators should be described. It is important to convey the message that despite a partner's promises, most violence continues and escalates over time and has serious medical, psychologic, and social consequences; even if the violence is infrequent, it still has a powerful effect. A single violent incident paired with threats, intimidation, and psychologic abuse will continue to undermine a woman's freedom and self-confidence, thus increasing the feelings of fear, isolation, and entrapment that will keep her at risk for future assault.

If a woman is seeking help for her abusive partner, discuss what is known about perpetrators, about the limits of treatment programs, the possibility of his continued controlling behavior even if he stops his violence, and his need for long-term commitment to counseling and change. The importance of a genuine commitment to change cannot be overestimated. When a woman's abusive partner is in counseling, she may stay with him longer in the hope that he will stop the abuse. Many batterers enter counseling solely to keep their partners from leaving. It may be necessary to revisit these issues during the course of therapy to ensure her safety.

Recent outcomes research indicates that cognitive-behavioral, gender-based intervention programs for batterers can be effective in reducing assault recurrences, particularly for men who complete the programs (Gondolf 1997). Men who were court-ordered into treatment programs were more likely to complete them. Within the 15-month follow-up period of this study (Gondolf 1997), only one-third of the men were still physically violent toward their partners. Counter to the initial hypotheses, batterer personality profile did not predict outcome. Being intoxicated during the follow-up period increased the likelihood of recidivism (Gondolf and Browne 1998). Treatments for batterers that do not directly address their abusive behavior are ineffective and may actually increase the violence (Substance Abuse and Mental Health Services Administration 1998).

Because of the ongoing dangers battered women face, it is important to be aware of interventions that can potentially increase their risk of harm, such as confronting the batterer with the intention of getting him to change. In some cases, violence may escalate during treatment; therefore, programs for batterers without supports for battered women should not begin until women have access to adequate shelter and advocacy. In addition, many agencies offer anger control groups that fail to confront the underlying issues of power and control. A batterer may then feel entitled to "lose control" and reprimand or punish his partner. Anger management alone is a potentially ill-fated intervention unless it also challenges the batterer's need to control his partner and his right to use violence against her (Schechter 1987). According to the Substance Abuse and Mental Health Services Administration (1998),

> Batterers' treatment can be effective if programs place a premium on survivor safety (even though the batterer is the client), insist that batterers take personal responsibility for their behavior, mandate "no-violence contracts," impart emotional regulation techniques, follow up on treatment completers and dropouts, and evaluate program outcomes regularly. (p. 54)

Referral to couples counseling in situations of ongoing violence, threats, or intimidation is another potentially harmful intervention. Schechter (1987) and Dutton (1992) outlined clear parameters for addressing the issue of couples therapy in the context of domestic violence. Some women may request a referral for couples therapy because they feel this is the only way to get "help" for their partner. However, couples counseling is indicated only when violence and coercive tactics have ceased for longer than the longest period for which the abuse stopped in the past, after the batterer has successfully completed a treatment program, and when both parties request this form of treatment. The abuser must take exclusive responsibility for his or her assaults and acknowledge that family reunification is not the goal of treatment. Working to rebuild the relationship and repair the damage will only be helpful if that dynamic has truly changed (Dutton 1992; Schechter 1987). Stopping the abuser's violence and controlling behavior should not be the focus of couples therapy. If a woman does pursue couples therapy, however, these behaviors do need to be addressed.

Court mediation is also not an appropriate intervention in cases of domestic violence. It assumes the presence of two equal parties who can negotiate in good faith and solve problems together. Abusers, however, manipulate, intimidate, and bully their partners and cannot negotiate responsibly. Because of this, battered women should be encouraged to seek legal assistance before discussing divorce, child custody, visitation, and other issues with their partners (Schechter 1987).

Many batterers check the odometers on their partners' cars and go through their partners' purses, briefcases, pockets, and drawers. Insurance information sent to the home may also put her in danger. The therapist and the victim should discuss what written material will be safe for her to take home and whether precautions should be taken to avoid written information about the abuse on materials he may see. She may need to write important phone numbers on scraps of paper or memorize them, or she may be able to leave the information at work or with a friend.

## Providing Access to Community Resources: Role of Domestic Violence Advocacy Programs

Domestic violence advocacy programs and shelters provide various services for battered women and their children as well as public education and training for service providers. They are the major source of support for many women. Others may feel most safe when connected to a mental health provider (with advocacy playing an important but adjunctive role) or in peer support groups. Most battered women do not stay in shelters, either because of insufficient resources or because they have other options, but they do use a wide range of services available through domestic violence programs. Clinicians should find out about the nearest domestic violence programs in their communities. Typical services include a 24-hour hotline and crisis intervention counseling; assistance in evaluating options, resources, safety planning, and referrals; information about legal remedies and legal and court advocacy (such as assistance with protective orders); emergency shelter, hotel vouchers, or safe homes; counseling, support groups, and referrals for therapy; immigrant rights information; advocacy with child protective services; literacy programs, job training, and transitional housing; and appropriate referrals for perpetrators/abusers. It is important to note that some of these services may not be available in the victim's community.

## Rape-Specific Treatment

Sexual assault hotlines and advocacy groups provide a framework for addressing women's needs in the immediate aftermath of an assault. They address issues of safety and stabilization, assist women in negotiating the medical and legal systems, help women deal with other people's reactions to the assault, inform women about the range of posttraumatic responses they might experience, and provide a supportive place for women to process their experiences.

Outcomes-based research on sexual assault has focused primarily on crisis intervention of a different sort—the reduction and/or prevention of PTSD symptoms. These interventions have used treatment modalities that are amenable to this type of empirical research, such as limited numbers of sessions, cognitive or behavioral techniques, and protocol- rather than client-centered approaches to session content and pace. Although it is not possible to generalize about the efficacy of these approaches for women who experience more chronic forms of trauma, several recent studies have demonstrated promising results for victims of violence in general.

Sexual assault, even as a single event, must be responded to in context, addressing feelings of shame, guilt, responsibility, anger, and despair as well as posttraumatic fears that may arise. The time in a woman's life (e.g., first sexual experience), the circumstances surrounding the assault, and her relationship to the perpetrator affect her experience and must be attended to in therapy, regardless of techniques used to address symptoms.

## Techniques

*Stress inoculation training* was adapted by Kilpatrick et al. (1982) and Veronen and Kilpatrick (1983) from learning theory concepts (Meichenbaum 1974) to treat the fear and anxiety experienced by rape victims. Over the course of treatment, participants identify cues that trigger fear, develop coping skills through the use of deep breathing, thought stopping, and role playing, and apply these techniques when engaging in feared behaviors (Kilpatrick et al. 1982; Resick et al. 1988; Resnick and Newton 1992).

*Cognitive processing therapy* provides victims with exposure to traumatic memories and trains them to challenge maladaptive cognitions (i.e., meanings and lessons one has taken from the traumatic experience) that cause unnecessary pain and constrict women's lives. Participants are encouraged to write about the traumatic event and are taught how to reconfigure their thinking about the trauma in ways that modify its impact on daily functioning. This technique has been effective in reducing PTSD and depression (Resick and Schnicke 1992). In comparison with control subjects, patients receiving this intervention had a significantly greater reduction in symptoms 3 months after the training.

Two other studies examined the effectiveness of these treatments for rape victims suffering from PTSD immediately after an assault. Foa et al. (1991) compared the effectiveness of stress inoculation training with the use of prolonged exposure techniques (i.e., repetitive descriptions of the rape and its aftermath within a highly structured, intensive treatment program), and supportive counseling. They found that all three led to posttreatment improvement; stress inoculation training was most effective in reducing fear, anxiety, and depression, but exposure was most effective for reducing PTSD at 3 months. Any contact with a therapist was found to reduce many forms of rape-induced distress (Koss et al. 1994), but active treatment seems to be necessary to reduce PTSD.

Although exposure therapy appears to be highly successful for selected individuals, negative effects have also been reported. These treatment modalities appear to be more appropriate for women who do not have dissociative symptoms, who are not primarily depressed, and who are physically safe (Ehlers et al. 1998; Pitman et al. 1991). In one study, participants exhibited a poorer response if they felt defeated during a traumatic experience, alienated following the event, and had developed a sense that their lives would never be the same. Because this pattern of responses is common for trauma survivors, further investigation is necessary to determine which women would and would not benefit from these techniques. For survivors of chronic childhood abuse who have not yet developed the internal capacity to modulate affect and arousal, symptoms may be exacerbated by exposure.

Many clinicians see group interventions as the modality of choice for survivors of rape. Groups uniquely undermine rape-induced isolation, validate feelings, confirm experiences, counteract self-blame, and empower survivors by offering them an opportunity to work through issues in a nonhierarchical setting (Koss and Harvey 1991).

Women who have been raped may seek treatment for other reasons and only later in therapy address issues specifically related to the assault. For example, a woman may have accommodated her posttraumatic sexual avoidance, which may emerge later as a concern in a new relationship, or a woman may have previous assault experiences triggered by current life events (harassment at work) that make those experiences more available for working through. In addition, a woman may be raped during the course of therapy, raising issues for the non–cognitive-behavioral therapist about how best to prevent chronic PTSD. Developing relationships with local sexual assault programs and clinicians who are skilled in some of the above techniques can provide useful adjuncts to ongoing treatment (Foa 1997; Foa and Rothbaum 1998).

## Working Through the Trauma: Acknowledgment, Grieving, Acceptance, and Integration in the Middle Phase of Treatment

Additional work involving the traumatic material that exacerbates symptoms generally begins once safety and a collaborative therapeutic relationship have been established, but this is not always the case. The therapeutic process is generally more fluid than linear, flowing back and forth between phases as the circumstances of the client's life change. In any case, if involuntary intrusions continue to interfere with a client's functioning, controlled and predictable exposure to traumatic material can help her to further integrate this material and contain its impact.

The goal of the middle phase of treatment is to gradually help a woman reexperience the trauma in a safe and tolerable way that allows her to acknowledge and come to terms with what has happened in her life. For a survivor of childhood sexual abuse, this might involve helping her slowly reconstruct her story and struggle with the doubts she may entertain about abusive incidents and her role in them. Helping women reduce their sense of shame, addressing the anger and rage that may or may not be directed toward the abuser, and processing the grief or noncompensable losses (Dutton [1992]) that one could not previously afford to feel are also important tasks during this time.

For women recovering from the traumatic effects of an abusive partner relationship, freedom from violence is an ongoing goal. Taking cues from each woman about her sense of pacing and timing is crucial. Sometimes women may be overzealous about discovering what happened and may become traumatized if therapists do not provide perspective to these patients on the importance of pacing their uncovering and taking care of themselves in the process.

A range of techniques may be used to assist the patient in this process, including writing, drawing, music, movement, body work, and other expressive therapies. As with rape survivors, groups can help to reduce isolation, expand support networks, and destigmatize events experienced as shameful. Time-limited groups have also been useful, allowing women to tell their stories in a safe and structured way in the presence of others who have had similar experiences and to address issues of grief and mourning. Many survivors find 12-step and other peer support groups helpful as well, depending on the needs of the woman and the style of the group.

Another modality that appears to be helpful is eye movement desensitization and reprocessing therapy (Shapiro 1989, 1995; Vaughan et al. 1994; S. A. Wilson et al. 1995, 1997), which involves the deconditioning of anxiety through reactivation and reexposure to traumatic memories and the transformation of pervasive abuse-related beliefs about one's self and one's world into more adaptive cognitions (van der Kolk et al. 1996). In this treatment, exposure is under the control of the patient, which often engenders an increased sense of mastery in the face of the traumatic experience. Some studies have suggested unusually rapid therapeutic responses using three to four sessions of therapy to treat isolated trauma. Although the body of research supporting the efficacy of this modality is growing (Boudewyns and Hyer 1996; J. Carlson et al. 1998; Marcus et al. 1997; Rothbaum 1997; Scheck et al. 1998), some reports have questioned these findings, citing studies that suggest that the eye movements do not contribute to the therapeutic effects (Lohr et al. 1995, 1998). The technique should be used after initial stabilization, and at present is perhaps best considered a trauma-focused modality to be used in the context of comprehensive treatment by practitioners well versed in trauma-focused therapy.

## Cultivating Self and Relational Development, Reconnecting, and Rebuilding: Late Phase of Treatment

The client and therapist face additional challenges in the late stage of treatment, including restructuring the relationships that need to change to reflect the woman's growing sense of empowerment and mourning the loss of relationships that cannot survive this transition. Other issues that may not have received priority at stages in which crisis was more common can now be more easily addressed, including concerns about sexuality, non–life-threatening eating disorders, and addictions that have not responded to earlier interventions. Additional work on boundary and other interpersonal communication issues at home and in the workplace may also be done during this time. Eventually the process of terminating therapy will emerge as an appropriate next step. This is significant and restorative work. It provides an opportunity for the client and therapist to jointly explore and work through the feelings of abandonment, grief, and fear that are nothing new to individuals whose most significant relationships have been characterized by betrayal and violence (Briere 1992a; Courtois 1997; Dutton 1992; Herman 1992b; Harvey and Harney 1995).

Spiritual needs may also emerge during this phase if not earlier. Women may find themselves reclaiming a spiritual dimension that was lost in the face of the abuse. For many women, reconnecting to a former religious practice or discovering new forms of spirituality can reflect an opening to life beyond the abuse and may provide connections to others who have been on similar healing journeys. Spiritual endeavors/work/practices can also provide a framework for women to make sense of their experiences and to recognize the strength and wisdom they have gained during this difficult process. The transition from experiencing life as a continuous state of seige to creating a community and reclaiming one's capacity for compassion and generosity can be important aspects of healing. Some women may emerge from this process with deep commitments to help others who have had similar experiences or to change conditions that perpetuate violence and abuse.

## Medication

Although there is currently no psychopharmacology of abuse, treatment recommendations are based on a limited number of randomized clinical trials for PTSD treatment conducted with combat veterans and assault survivors and a small but growing number of open drug trials for civilian PTSD. Despite the dearth of controlled-trial research, clinicians have been able to draw on treatment literature for associated disorders (depression, anxiety, panic, and borderline personality disorder) and the ongoing treatment experience of PTSD/trauma centers. Existing studies have not examined response differences for victims of single versus multiple traumas or acute versus chronic PTSD, nor have they examined gender differences in treatment response.

Medication should be used in the context of ongoing trauma therapy and offered in ways that enhance a woman's sense of control over her life. This can be done by discussing options and encouraging choices. Women should be encouraged to discuss the pros, cons, and possible impact of taking medication, and clinicians should make efforts to ensure that women will not be defined by or controlled by their use of it. By taking psychotropic medication within the context of an abusive relationship, the victim can provide ammunition for the abuser, who might use this information to reinforce the idea that she (the victim) is the one with problems, not him. For example, an abuser may use a prescription for psychotropic medication as "evidence" that his/her partner is "crazy" and/or incapable of caring for their children. Discussing these issues directly can help a woman counter those perceptions and reduce an abusive partner's ability to define her reality.

Medications can, however, be a valuable part of treatment for PTSD and can be used to achieve the following goals (Davidson 1997): reduction of core PTSD symptoms of intrusiveness, avoidance, psychic numbing and hyperarousal; reduction of associated disability and vulnerability to stress; treatment of comorbid symptoms (e.g., depression, anxiety, panic); reduction of psychotic and dissociative symptoms; and improved impulse control and reduction of self-destructive behavior.

Options for treatment include antidepressants, anxiolytics, anticonvulsants, opioid antagonists, and mood stabilizers. Data emerging from double-blind, placebo-controlled clinical trials support the use of antidepressants, particularly selective serotonin reuptake inhibitors (SSRIs) and tricyclic antidepressants for treatment of PTSD. In some studies (Dow and Kline 1997) both tricylics and SSRIs were found to be useful in patients with depression plus PTSD, but those agents predominantly affecting serotonin reuptake were associated with better outcomes than were those affecting norepineph-rine reuptake. The magnitude and type of trauma may also influence an individual's response (Davidson 1997). Although heightened anxiety is characteristic of PTSD, benzodiazepines have not proved useful in controlled trials and may be associated with rebound anxiety when discontinued. Small open studies of anticonvulsants have demonstrated moderate to good improvement of PTSD.

## Monoamine Oxidase Inhibitors

Results of studies using irreversible monoamine oxidase inhibitors (MAOIs) have been mixed. In general, MAOIs have led to improvement in intrusive symptoms and insomnia but not in avoidance and numbing, hyperarousal, depression, or panic (Southwick et al. 1994). Side effects (e.g., sexual dysfunction, dizziness, sleep disruption, weight gain) and dietary restrictions tend to limit use of these drugs. Reversible MAOIs do show some promise for broader reduction of PTSD symptoms. Moclobemide significantly reduced both intrusive and avoidant symptoms in one open trial and may prove useful once it is available in the United States.

## Tricyclic Antidepressants

Imipramine (Frank et al. 1988) and amitryptiline (Davidson et al. 1990) also reduce symptoms of PTSD, depression, and anxiety as compared with placebo. They appear to be more effective for intrusive symptoms and less effective in reducing numbing and avoidance (Layton and Dager 1998). In addition, they appear to be more effective in patients with less severe symptoms, more stability, and fewer panic attacks. As Layton and Dager (1998) have pointed out, dosages used in these studies were high and caused intolerable side effects for many patients. Desipramine, however, did not demonstrate significant effectiveness. SSRIs appear to be more effective and have a more tolerable side effect profile. Tricyclic antidepressants have been tested mainly in veterans with severe and chronic PTSD, whereas SSRIs have been tested on civilians as well.

## Selective Serotonin Reuptake Inhibitors

The SSRIs have been effective in reducing PTSD symptoms in open trials (Layton and Dager 1998). In the only double-blinded, placebo-controlled study (van der Kolk et al. 1994), fluoxetine provided significant reduction in overall PTSD symptoms (all three clusters), particularly numbing and arousal. Interestingly, these findings are more robust in civilian trauma than in combat trauma. Sertaline, paroxetine, and fluvoxamine also have shown efficacy in open trials. In one small ($n = 5$) open 12-week clinical trial, Rothbaum et al. (1992) found that sertraline significantly reduced PTSD among women who had been raped. A more recent randomized controlled trial confirmed these results (Brady et al. 2000).

Treatment of depression does not necessarily reduce psychic numbing, which appears to be a distinct phenomenon. SSRIs, unlike other drugs that have been studied for PTSD, seem to address both (Friedman 1997; van der Kolk et al. 1994). They may provide additional efficacy for reducing alcohol consumption (Brady et al. 1994) and a range of possible serotonergically mediated symptoms associated with PTSD such as rage, impulsivity, suicidal intent, depression, panic, and obsessional thinking (Friedman 1997).

## Trazodone and Nefazodone

In another open trial, nefazodone (a 5-HT$_2$ antagonist with SSRI properties) showed promise in reducing all three symptom clusters among civilians with chronic PTSD who completed the trial (Davidson et al. 1998). The dropout rate in this study, however, was greater than 50%. Trazodone has also shown some efficacy in reducing combat PTSD symptoms, particularly reexperiencing and arousal (open trial) (Davis et al. 2000). Trazodone is frequently used to treat the sleep disturbance associated with PTSD and with some of the SSRIs.

## Buspirone and Cyproheptadine

Buspirone, a nonsedating anxiolytic that acts as 5-HT$_{1A}$ partial agonist, has been reported to reduce anxiety, depression, insomnia, and flashbacks. Cyproheptadine, a 5-HT antagonist, appears to reduce nightmares in some patients with PTSD.

## Anticonvulsants

Anticonvulsants have also been shown to have some beneficial effects in people with chronic PTSD (Lipper et al. 1986; Wolf et al. 1988). In open trials valproic acid (Fesler 1991) and carbemazepine were found to reduce reexperiencing and arousal, and valproate reduced avoidance, numbing, and arousal. Carbemazepine may also be useful in reducing some of the self-injurious behaviors associated with borderline personality disorder or DESNOS (Layton and Dager 1998). Gabapentin, a newer anticonvulsant, has shown promise for treating PTSD with dissociation.

## β-Adrenergic Blockers

High-dose β-blockers were found to be effective in two open studies for reducing explosiveness, nightmares, intrusive recollections, sleep disturbance, hyperalertness, and startle responses among veterans of the Vietnam War (Kolb et al. 1984). They also improved self-esteem and psychosocial functioning. In another study, β-blockers produced some improvement in hypervigilance and hyperarousal among abused children (Famularo et al. 1988). They were not successful in one open trial with Cambodian refugees (Friedman 1997).

## $\alpha_2$ Agonists

$\alpha_2$ Agonists reduce $\alpha_2$-adrenergic receptor activity in the locus caeruleus, thus decreasing adrenergic tone. There have been positive findings at 0.2–0.4 mg/day in Vietnam War veterans, including reductions in self-mutilation, intrusive symptoms, insomnia, startle responses, and angry outbursts as well as improvement in mood and concentration (Kolb et al. 1984; van der Kolk 1987). For some, clonidine appears to lose efficacy over time.

## Benzodiazepines

Recommendations for the use of benzodiazepines to treat acute and chronic PTSD remain unclear and studies have yielded mixed results. Benzodiazepines appear to reduce anxiety, arousal, irritability, and insomnia in people with PTSD and in a small number of those with dissociative identity disorder. They have not been found to be effective for intrusive symptoms or for avoidance and numbing. Davidson et al. (1997) have posited that a reduction in startle response and hyperarousal during the acute phase may prevent the development of chronic PTSD and may thus make these agents useful in conjunction with other medications, such as antidepressants or anticonvulsants (Friedman 1997). Several authors, however, have voiced concerns about the potential exacerbation of hyperarousal symptoms on withdrawal, particularly from shorter-acting agents such as alprazolam, and about the risks associated with concomitant substance abuse. Recently, observations with temazepam have been promising. Clonazepam and buspirone have also demonstrated some efficacy in reducing PTSD symptoms (Ryan et al. 1992; Shalev et al. 1993).

## Narcotic Antagonists

Use of narcotic antagonists, studied because they should theoretically reduce endogenous opioid-induced numbing, has met with mixed results, showing improvement in some studies and worsening in others. One open-label trial found naltrexone to be useful in reducing self-injurious behavior among a small sample ($n = 7$) of women, presumably by blocking postcutting opioid elevations (A. S. Roth et al. 1996).

## Antipsychotics

Few studies are available on the use of antipsychotics for PTSD, dissociative identity disorder, or DESNOS. They have not proven to be useful in those contexts and are currently only recommended for treatment of concomitant psychotic symptoms or disorders. Dissociative symptoms can sometimes be relieved with low doses of antipsychotic agents (Saporta and Case 1991). The auditory hallucinations, thought withdrawal, and delusions of passive influence sometimes seen in people with dissociative identity disorder (Kluft 1985), however, do not appear to respond to these medications (Loewenstein et al. 1988; Putnam 1989).

In summary, SSRIs are the most effective medications for PTSD after assault or abuse and, among civilian trauma survivors, appear to have the fewest side effects. If symptoms only partially resolve after a few weeks, clinicians should consider using a second drug such as an anticonvulsant or β-blocker. Associated insomnia can be treated with low-dose trazodone at bedtime, and acute or persistent agitation can be treated with clonidine or small regular doses of a benzodiazepine such as clonazepam. Mood stabilizers can also be useful in treating agitation. For acute trauma, reduction of autonomic arousal with a benzodiazepine or clonidine might theoretically prevent the development of chronic PTSD.

## Addressing Systemic Barriers to Care

Clinicians face several structural barriers that may interfere with their ability to respond to women who have been abused. For example, increasing time constraints and capitation agreements that restrict referral for social and psychologic services make it harder for clinicians to integrate routine inquiry about abuse. Policies that can potentially place women in jeopardy if they do receive services, such as mandatory reporting and discriminatory insurance practices, have made some clinicians and patients reluctant to discuss these issues. Mental health reimbursement policies that make diagnosis a prerequisite for treatment place women with a history of past or current abuse in the position of having to choose between receiving mental health services and risking having these diagnoses used against them by the abuser or child protective services to obtain custody of their children.

Micromanagement strategies, used by insurance companies to reduce "unnecessary" mental health care use, can be disruptive and traumatic in themselves. They create an environment in which short-term medication management or potentially retraumatizing directive treatments focused on symptom reduction rather than healing have become the standard of care. In many settings, the consistency and safety required for long-term trauma recovery are no longer reimbursable.

It is unfortunate that just when an expanding body of research is clearly delineating the impact of trauma on the human psyche and the need for more intensive treatment for many survivors (Smith et al. 1995; Straus et al. 1996), market forces are decreasing the likelihood that these kinds of services will be available. This becomes increasingly true as managed care further erodes the possibility of choosing one's provider and type of treatment, removing even the consumer-based economic power from individuals seeking care. For low-income women whose only access to services has been through the public mental health system, this lack of choice has been the norm (Carmen 1995).

Thus, clinicians are often in the predicament of responding to new practice expectations without necessarily having the skills, supports, or resources to do so and are faced with policies that place their own economic and professional needs in conflict with the needs of their patients. Although these developments can certainly increase provider frustration, they are also leading to new partnerships between the mental health, legal, and advocacy communities to generate awareness and to prevent these types of systemic revictimization (Warshaw 1997).

In addition to the larger systemic issues, mental health providers may also be isolated in their practice settings and lack the necessary supports to sustain this important and challenging work. Cultivating sources of personal renewal and professional support (e.g., consultation, peer supervision, individual therapy, diversification, social action) can be invaluable to therapists in both creating balance in their own lives and sustaining the empathic presence so necessary to this work.

It can be useful to find other clinicians who do trauma-related therapy and to develop referral networks and participate in cross-consultations with those providers. Some domestic violence programs have identified mental health providers who are experienced in working with battered women and/ or addressing the overlap between mental health, legal, and safety issues. State sexual assault coalitions can also provide those resources. In addition, there are networks of therapists who specialize in working with trauma survivors and who may conduct peer consultation groups or know of trauma-related list servers. State or national domestic violence and sexual assault coalitions or professional organizations, such as the International Society of Traumatic Stress Studies, American Psychiatric Association, American Psychological Association, or the National Association of Social Workers, may provide additional resources. In addition, each state has a federally funded protection and advocacy office and a state-sponsored office of consumer affairs that may know of peer support resources for clients receiving publicly funded mental health services. Some of these services are available through not-forprofit organizations under contract to provide services for state-system clients.

## Conclusion

Working collaboratively with other systems to create the kind of society that will stop violence against women and prevent its traumatic sequelae is also important. Mental health providers have a significant role to play in voicing concerns about the impact of abuse and violence on the lives of the women they work with clinically and in not allowing those concerns to be dwarfed by the current emphasis on neuroscience and limited mental health reimbursement policies. Working with women who have survived unthinkable trauma teaches us about the complexity and unpredictability of human life; of the intersections among individual biology, human development, social and cultural contexts, and larger societal norms; and of the importance of caring, respectful human interactions. When we do not address the denial of intolerable feelings at a personal level we are in danger of re-creating them not only in individual relationships but also on a social and political level as well, and when we do not acknowledge the impact of social forms of abuse of power, they are often internalized and reproduced through individual interactions. Mental health providers can play a critical role in preventing violence against women in addition to treating its consequences by beginning to address the social as well as psychologic conditions that create and support this kind of violence in our society.

# References

Abbott J, Johnson R, Koziol-McLain J, et al: Domestic violence against women: incidence and prevalence in an emergency room population. JAMA 273:1763, 1995

Alpert JL, Brown LS, Courtois CA: Symptomatic clients and memories of childhood abuse: what the trauma and child sexual abuse literature tells us, in Working Group on Investigation of Memories of Childhood Abuse: Final Report. Washington, DC, American Psychological Association, 1995, p 15

Amaro H, Fried LE, Cabral H, et al: Violence during pregnancy and substance abuse. Am J Public Health 80:575–579, 1990

American Medical Association: Memories of Childhood Abuse: Report of the Council on Scientific Affairs. Chicago, IL, American Medical Association, 1992

American Psychiatric Association: Statement on Memories of Sexual Abuse: APA Board of Trustees. Washington, DC, American Psychiatric Association, 1993

American Psychiatric Association: Diagnostic and Statistical Manual of Mental Disorders, 4th Edition. Washington, DC, American Psychiatric Association, 1994

Andersen SM, Boulette TR, Schwartz AH: Psychological maltreatment of spouses, in Case Studies in Family Violence. Edited by Ammerman RT, Hersen M. New York, Plenum, 1991, pp 293–328

Angel R, Gronfein W: The use of subjective information in statistical models. American Sociological Review 53:464–473, 1988

Arias I, Pape KT: Psychological abuse: implications for adjustment and commitment to leave violent partners. Violence and Victims 14:55–67, 1999

Asch A, Fine M: Beyond Pedestals: Women with Disabilities. Essays in Psychology, Culture, and Politics. Philadelphia, PA, Temple University, 1988

Astin MC, Lawrence KJ, Foy DW: Posttraumatic stress disorder among battered women: risk and resiliency factors. Violence and Victims 8:17–28, 1993

Astin MC, Ogland-Hand SM, Foy DW, et al: Posttraumatic stress disorder and childhood abuse in battered women: comparisons with maritally distressed women. J Consult Clin Psychol 63:308–312, 1995

Atwood G. Stolorow R: Structures of Subjectivity: Explorations in Psychoanalytic Phenomenology. Hillsdale, NJ, Analytic Press, 1984

Bachman R, Saltzman LE: Violence Against Women: Estimates from the Redesigned Survey NCJ-1 54348. Washington, DC, Bureau of Justice Statistics, US Department of Justice, 1995

Bagle and Ramsey 1986

Barnett OW, Miller-Perrin CL, Perrin RD: Family Violence Across the Lifespan: An Introduction. Thousand Oaks, CA, Sage Publications, 1997

Bassuk EL, Melnick S, Browne A: Responding to the needs of low-income and homeless women who are survivors of family violence. JAMWA 53:57–64, 1998

Bennett LW: Substance abuse and the domestic assault of women. Social Work 40:760–772, 1995

Bennett L, Tolman R, Rogalski C, et al: Domestic abuse by male alcohol and drug addicts. Violence and Victims 65:157–167, 1994

Bernstein EM, Putnam FW: Development, reliability and validity of a dissociation scale. J Nerv Ment Dis 174:727–735, 1986

Blake DD, Weathers FW, Nagy LM, et al: The development of a clinician-administered PTSD scale. J Trauma Stress 8:75–90, 1995

Blank AS: The longitudinal course of posttraumatic stress disorder, in Posttraumatic Stress Disorder: DSM-IV and Beyond. Edited by Davidson JRT, Foa EB. Washington, DC, American Psychiatric Press, 1993, pp 3–12

Bloom S: Creating Sanctuary: Toward an Evolution of Sane Societies. New York, Routledge, 1997

Boudewyn AC, Liem JH: Psychological, interpersonal, and behavioral correlates of chronic self-destructiveness: an exploratory study. Psychol Rep 77:1283–1297, 1995

Boudewyns PA, Hyer LA: Eye movement desensitization and reprocessing (EMDR) as treatment of posttraumatic stress disorder (PTSD). Clin Psychol Psychother 3:185–195, 1996

Bowman ES: Etiology and clinical course of pseudo-seizures: relationship to trauma, depression, and dissociation. Psychosomatics 34:333, 1993

Boyer D: Adolescent pregnancy: the role of sexual abuse. NRCCSA News 4:1–8, 1995

Brady KT, Killeen T, Saladin ME: Comorbid substance abuse and posttraumatic stress disorder. Am J Addict 3:160–164, 1994

Brady KT: Posttraumatic stress disorder and comorbidity: recognizing the many faces of PTSD. J Clin Psychiatry 9(suppl):12–15, 1997

Brady K, Pearlstein T, Baher D, et al: Efficacy and safety of sertraline treatment of posttraumatic stress disorder: a randomized controlled trial. JAMA 283:1827–1844, 2000

Breslau N, Davis C, Andreski P, et al: Traumatic events and posttraumatic stress disorder in an urban population of young adults. Arch Gen Psychiatry 48:216–222, 1991

Breslau N, Davis GC, Peterson EL, et al: Psychiatric sequelae of posttraumatic stress disorder in women. Arch Gen Psychiatry 54:81–87, 1997

Brickman J, Briere J: Incidence of rape and sexual assault in an urban Canadian population. International Journal of Women's Studies 7:195–206, 1984

Briere J: Child Abuse Trauma: Theory and Treatment of the Lasting Effects. Newbury Park, CA, Sage Publications, 1992a

Briere J: Medical symptoms, health risk, and history of childhood sexual abuse. Mayo Clin Proc 67:603, 1992b

Briere J: Trauma Symptom Inventory Professional Manual. Odessa, FL, Psychological Assessment Resources, 1995

Briere J: Therapy for Adults Molested as Children. New York, Springer, 1996

Briere J: Psychological Assessment of Adult Posttraumatic States. Washington, DC, American Psychological Association Books, 1997

Briere J, Conte J: Self-reported amnesia for abuse in adults molested as children. J Trauma Stress 6:21–31, 1993

Briere J, Elliott D: Immediate and long-term impacts of child sexual abuse. The Future of Children 4:54–69, 1994

Briere J, Runtz M: Suicidal thoughts and behaviors in former sexual abuse victims. Can J Behav Sci 18:413–423, 1986

Briere J, Runtz M: Sympomatology associated with childhood sexual victimization in a nonclinical sample. Child Abuse and Neglect 12:51, 1988

Briere J, Elliott DM, Harris K, et al: Trauma Symptom Inventory: Psychometrics and association with childhood and adult trauma in clinical samples. Journal of Interpersonal Violence 10:387–401, 1995

Brown GR, Anderson B: Psychiatric morbidity in adult patients with childhood histories of sexual and physical abuse. Am J Psychiatry 148:55–61, 1991

Brown LS: The contribution of victimization as a risk factor for the development of depressive symptomatology in women. Paper presented at the 97th annual convention of the American Psychological Association, New Orleans, LA, August, 1989

Brown L: Not outside the range: one feminist perspective on psychic trauma, in Trauma: Explorations in Memory. Edited by Caruth C. Baltimore, MD, Johns Hopkins University Press, 1995, pp 100–112

Brown LS, Root MPP (eds): Diversity and Complexity in Feminist Therapy. New York, Haworth, 1990

Browne A: When Battered Women Kill. New York, The Free Press, 1987

Browne A: Family violence and homelessness: the relevance of trauma histories in the lives of homeless women. Am J Orthopsychiatry 63:370–384, 1993a

Browne A: Violence against women by male partners: prevalence, outcomes, and policy implications. American Psychologist 48:1077–1087, 1993b

Bryer JB, Nelson BA, Miller JB, et al: Childhood sexual and physical abuse as factors in adult psychiatric illness. Am J Psychiatry 144:1426, 1987

Burnam MA, Stein JA, Golding JM, et al: Sexual assault and mental disorders in a community population. J Consult Clin Psychol 56:843, 1988

Campbell JC, Alford P: The dark consequences of marital rape. Am J Nurs 89:946, 1989

Campbell J, Kubb J: Depression in battered women. JAMWA 51:101–110, 1996

Campbell R, Sullivan CM, Davidson WS: Depression in women who use domestic violence shelters: changes in depression over time. Psychol Women Q 19:237–255, 1995

Carlson EB: Trauma Assessments: A Clinician's Guide. New York, Guilford Press, 1997

Carlson J, Chemtob CM, Rusnak K, et al: Eye movement desensitization and reprocessing for combat-related posttraumatic stress disorder. J Trauma Stress 11:3–24, 1998

Carmen E: Inner city community mental health: the interplay of abuse and race in chronically mentally ill women, in Mental Health, Racism, and Sexism. Edited by Willie C, Rieker P, Kramer B, et al. Pittsburgh, PA, University of Pittsburgh Press, 1995

Carmen E, Rieker PP: Rethinking the use of restraint and seclusion for mentally ill women with abuse histories. JAMWA 53:192–197, 1998

Carmen E, Rieker PP, Mills T: Victims of violence and psychiatric illness. Am J Psychiatry 141:378–383, 1984

Carnes PJ: Don't Call It Love. New York, Bantam Books, 1991

Cascardi M, O'Leary AD, Schlee KA: Co-occurrence and correlates of posttraumatic stress disorder and major depression in physically abused women. Journal of Family Violence VOL:227–249, 1999

Centerwell B: Race, socioeconomic status, and domestic homicide: Atlanta, 1971. Am J Public Health 74:813, 1984

Chalk R, King P (eds): Violence in Families: Assessing Prevention and Treatment Programs. Washington, DC, National Academy Press, 1998

Chu JA, Dill DL: Dissociative symptoms in relation to childhood physical and sexual abuse. Am J Psychiatry 147:887–892, 1990

Cicchetti D, Carlson V: Child Maltreatment: Theory and Research on the Causes and Consequences of Child Abuse and Neglect. New York, Cambridge University Press, 1989

Cloitre M, Scarvalohne P, Difede J: Posttraumatic stress disorder: self and interpersonal dysfunction among sexually retraumatized women. Journal of Traumatic Stress Studies 10:437–452, 1997

Cohen M, Deamant C, Barkan S, et al: Domestic violence and childhood sexual abuse in HIV-infected women and women at risk for HIV. Am J Public Health 90:560–565, 2000

Collins J, Kroutil L, Roland J, et al: Issues in the Linkage of Alcohol and Domestic Violence, Vol 13: Recent Developments in Alcoholism. Edited by Galanter M. New York, Plenum, 1997

Commonwealth Fund, Commission on Women's Health: Violence Against Women in the United States: A Comprehensive Background Paper. New York, Commonwealth Fund, 1995

Courtois CA: Healing the Incest Wound: Adult Survivors in Therapy. New York, WW Norton, 1988

Courtois CA: Adult survivors of sexual abuse, in Primary Care Clinics of North America: Special Issue on Family Violence and Abusive Relationships. Edited by Elliott BA, Halverson KC, Hendricks-Matthews M. Philadelphia, PA, WB Saunders, 1993, pp 433–446

Courtois CA: Assessment and diagnosis, in Treating Women Molested in Childhood. Edited by Classen C, Yalom I. San Francisco, CA, Josey-Bass, 1995, pp 1–34

Courtois CA: Healing the incest wound: a treatment update with attention to recovered-memory issues. Am J Psychother 51:464–496, 1997

Craine LS, Henson CE, Colliver JA, et al: Prevalence of a history of sexual abuse among female psychiatric patients in a state hospital system. Hospital and Community Psychiatry 39:300, 1988

Crowe LC, George WH: Alcohol and human sexuality: review and integration. Psychol Bull 105:374–386, 1989

Crowell NA, Burgess AW: Understanding Violence Against Women. Washington, DC, National Academy Press, 1996

Dansky BS, Brewerton TD, Kilpatrick DG, et al: The National Women's Study: relationship of victimization and posttraumatic stress disorder to bulimia nervosa. Int J Eat Disord 21:213–228, 1997

Davidson J: Biological therapies for posttraumatic stress disorder: an overview. J Clin Psychiatry 9(suppl):29–32, 1997

Davidson JR, Foa EB: Diagnostic issues in posttraumatic stress disorder: considerations for the DSM-IV. J Abnorm Psychol 100:346–365, 1991

Davidson JR, van der Kolk BA: The psychopharmacological treatment of posttraumatic stress disorder, in Traumatic Stress: The Effects of Overwhelming Experience on Mind, Body, and Society. Edited by van der Kolk BA, McFarlane AC, Weisaeth L. New York, Guilford, 1996, pp 510–524

Davidson J, Kudler H, Smith R, et al: Treatment of posttraumatic stress disorder with amitryptiline and placebo. Arch Gen Psychiatry 47:259–266, 1990

Davidson JR, Malik ML, Sutherland SN: Response characteristics to antidepressants and placebo in posttraumatic stress disorder. Int Clin Psychopharmacol 12:291–296, 1997

Davidson JR, Weisler RH, Malik ML, et al: Treatment of posttraumatic stress disorder with nefazodone. Int Clin Psychopharmacol 13:111–113, 1998

Davis LL, Nugent AL, Murray J, et al: Nefazodone treatment for chronic posttraumatic stress disorder: an open trial. J Clin Psychopharmacol 20:159–164, 2000

Dearwater SR, Coben JH, Campbell JC, et al: Prevalence of intimate partner abuse in women treated at community hospital emergency departments. JAMA 280:433–438, 1998

Den Herder D, Redner L: The treatment of childhood sexual trauma in chronically mentally ill adults. Health Social Work 16:50, 1991

Domino JV, Haber JD: Prior physical and sexual abuse in women with chronic headache: clinical correlates. Headache 27:310, 1987

Doucette J: Violent Acts Against Disabled Women. Toronto, Canada, Disabled Women's Network, 1986

Dow B, Kline N: Antidepressant treatment of posttraumatic stress disorder and major depression in veterans. Ann Clin Psychiatry 9:1–5, 1997

Drossman DA: Physical and sexual abuse and gastrointestinal illness: what is the link? Am J Med 97:108, 1994

Drossman DA, Talley NJ, Leserman J, et al: Sexual and physical abuse and gastrointestinal illness: review and recommendations. Ann Intern Med 123:774, 1995

Dutton MA: Empowering and Healing the Battered Woman: A Model for Assessment and Intervention. New York, Springer, 1992

Dutton MA: Battered women's strategic response to violence: the role of context, in Future Interventions with Battered Women and Their Families (Sage Series on Violence Against Women, Vol 3). Edited by Edleson JL, Eisikovits ZC. Thousand Oaks, CA, Sage Publications, 1996, pp 201–215

Ehlers A, Clark DM, Dunmore E, et al: Predicting response to exposure treatment in PTSD: the role of mental defeat and alienation. J Trauma Stress 11:457–471, 1998

Elliott DM: Traumatic events: prevalence and delayed recall in the general population. J Consult Clin Psychol 65:811–820, 1997

Elliott DM, Briere J: Transference and countertransference, in Treating Women Molested in Childhood. Edited by Classen C, Yalom I. San Francisco, CA, Josey-Bass, 1995, pp 187–226

Ellis EM, Atkeson BM, Calhoun KS: An examination of differences between multiple- and single-incident victims of sexual assault. J Abnorm Psychol 91:221–224, 1982

Elvik S, Berkowitz C, Nicholas E, et al: Sexual abuse in the developmentally disabled: dilemmas of diagnosis. Child Abuse and Neglect 14:497, 1990

Epstein JN, Saunders BE, Kilpatrick DG: Predicting PTSD in women with a history of childhood rape. J Trauma Stress 10:573–588, 1997

Espin OM, Gawalek MA: Women's diversity: ethnicity, race, class, and gender in theories of feminist psychology, in Personality and Psychopathology: Feminist

Reappraisals. Edited by Ballou M, Brown LS. New York, Guilford, 1992, pp 88–107

Essock-Vitale SM, McGuire MT: Women's lives viewed from an evolutionary perspective: sexual histories, reproductive success, and demographic characteristics of a random sample of American women. Ethnology and Sociobiology 6:137, 1985

Famularo R, Kinscherf R, Fenton T: Propanolol treatment for childhood posttraumatic stress disorder, acute type: a pilot study. Am J Dis Child 142:1244–1247, 1988

Felitti VJ, Anda R, Nordenberg D, et al: Relationship of childhood abuse and household dysfunction to many of the leading causes of death in adults: the Adverse Childhood Experiences (ACE) Study. Am J Prev Med 13:245–258, 1998

Femina DD, Yeager CA, Lewis DO: Child abuse: adolescent records vs. adult recall. Child Abuse and Neglect 14:227–231, 1990

Fesler FA: Valproate in combat-related posttraumatic stress disorder. J Clin Psychiatry 152:361–364, 1991

Fillmore KM: The Social Victims of Drinking. Br J Addict 80:307–314, 1985

Finkelhor D, Hotaling GT, Lewis IA, et al: Sexual abuse in a national survey of adult men and women: prevalence, characteristics, and risk factors. Child Abuse and Neglect 14:19, 1990

Fischbach RL, Herbert B: Domestic violence and mental health: correlates and conundrums within and across cultures. Soc Sci Med 45:1161–1176, 1997

Foa EB: Trauma and women: course, predictors, and treatment. J Clin Psychiatry 58(suppl):25–28, 1997

Foa EB, Rothbaum BO: Treating the Trauma of Rape: Cognitive-Behavioral Therapy for PTSD. New York, Guilford Press, 1998

Foa EB, Steketee GS, Rothbaum BO: Behavioral/cognitive conceptualizations of posttraumatic stress disorder. Behavior Therapy 20:155–176, 1989

Foa EB, Rothbaum BO, Riggs DS, et al: Treatment of posttraumatic stress disorder in rape victims: a comparison between cognitive procedures and counseling. J Consult Clin Psychol 59:715, 1991

Foa EB, Hearst-Ikeda DE, Perr KJ: Evaluation of a brief cognitive-behavioral program for the prevention of chronic PTSD in recent assault victims. J Consult Clin Psychol 63:948–955, 1995

Follette VM, Polusny MA, Bechtle AE, et al: Cumulative trauma: the impact of child sexual abuse, adult sexual assault, and spouse abuse. J Trauma Stress 9:25–35, 1996

Follingstad DR, Rutledge LL, Berg BJ, et al: The role of emotional abuse in physically abusive relationships. Journal of Family Violence 5:107–120, 1990

Follingstad DR, Brennan AF, Hause ES, et al: Factors moderating physical and psychological symptoms of battered women. Journal of Family Violence 6:81–95, 1991

Frank E, Turner SM, Duffy B: Depressive symptoms in rape victims. J Affect Disord 1:269–277, 1979

Frank JB, Kosten TR, Giller EL, et al: A randomized clinical trial of phenelzine and imipramine for posttraumatic stress disorder. Am J Psychiatry 145:1289–1291, 1988

Friedman MJ: Posttraumatic stress disorder. J Clin Psychiatry 58(suppl):33–36, 1997

Frieze IH, Knoble J, Washburn C, et al: Types of battered women. Paper presented at the meeting of the Annual Research Conference of the Association for Women in Psychology, Santa Monica, CA, March 1980

Fromuth ME: The relationship of child sexual abuse with later psychological adjustment in a sample of college women. Child Abuse and Neglect 10:5–15, 1986

Gabbard G: Commentary on Dissociative Processes and Transference–Countertransference Paradigms by Messler J and Frawley MG. Psychoanalytic Dialogues 2:37–49, 1992

Gabbard G: Psychotherapists who transgress sexual boundaries with patients. Bull Menninger Clin 58:124–135, 1994

Ganley AL: Understanding domestic violence, in Improving the Health Care Response to Domestic Violence: A Resource Manual for Health Care Providers. Edited by Warshaw C, Ganley AL, Salber PR. San Francisco, CA, Family Violence Prevention Fund, Pennsylvania Coalition Against Domestic Violence, 1995

Gartrell N, Herman J, Olarte S, et al: Psychiatrist–patient sexual contact: results of a national survey. I: Prevalence. Am J Psychiatry 143:1126–1131, 1986

Gazmararian JA, Lazorick S, Spitz AM, et al: Prevalence of violence against pregnant women. JAMA 275:1915–1920, 1996

Gelles RJ, Straus MA: Intimate Violence. New York, Simon & Schuster, 1988

George L, Winfield L: Sexual Assault: Prevalence and Mental Health Consequences. Final Report. Rockville, MD, National Institute of Mental Health, 1986

George LK, Winfield I, Blazer DG: Sociocultural factors in sexual assault: comparison of two representative samples of women. Journal of Social Issues 48:105–126, 1992

George WH, Cue KL, Lopez PA, et al: Self-reported alcohol expectancies and post-drinking sexual inferences about women. J Appl Soc Psychol 25:164–186, 1995

Gidycz CA, Koss MP: The impact of adolescent sexual victimization: standardized measures of anxiety, depression, and behavioral deviancy. Violence and Victims 4:139–149, 1989

Gidycz CA, Coble CN, Latham L, et al: Sexual assault experience in adulthood and prior victimization experiences: a prospective analysis. Psychol Women Q 17:151–168, 1993

Gil CJ, Kirschner KL, Reis JP, et al: Health services for women with disabilities: barriers and portals, in Reframing Women's Health: Multidisciplinary Research and Practice. Thousand Oaks, CA, Sage Publications, 1994, pp 357–366

Gin NE, Rucker L, Frayne S, et al: Prevalence of domestic violence among patients in three ambulatory care internal medicine clinics. J Gen Intern Med 6:317, 1991

Gleason WJ: Mental disorders in battered women: an empirical study. Violence and Victims 8:53–68, 1993

Golding JM: Sexual assault history and physical health in randomly selected Los Angeles women. Health Promotion 13:130–138, 1994

Golding JM: Intimate partner violence as a risk factor for mental disorders: a meta-analysis. Journal of Family Violence 14:99–132, 1999

Golding JM, Stein JA, Siegal JM, et al: Sexual assault history and use of health and mental health services. Am J Community Psychol 16:625, 1988

Golding JM, Stein JA, Siegal JM, et al: Social support sources following sexual assault. Journal of Community Psychology 19:92–107, 1989

Goldman L, Horan D, Warshaw C, et al: Diagnostic and Treatment Guidelines on Mental Health Effects of Family Violence. Chicago, IL, American Medical Association, 1995

Goldner V: Morality and multiplicity: perspectives on the treatment of violence in intimate life. Journal of Marital and Family Therapy 25:325–336, 1999

Gondolf EW: Patterns of reassault in batterer's programs. Violence and Victims 12:373–387, 1997

Gondolf E, Browne A: Recognizing the strengths of battered women, in Assessing Woman Battering in Mental Health Services. Edited by Gondolf E. Thousand Oaks, CA, Sage Publications, 1998, pp 95–112

Gondolf EW, Fisher ER: Battered Women as Survivors: An Alternate to Treating Learned Helplessness. Lexington, MA, Lexington Books, 1988

Goodman L, Dutton MA, Harris M: The relationship between violence dimensions and symptom severity among homeless, mentally ill women. J Trauma Stress 10:51–70, 1997

Goodwin J: Sexual Abuse: Incest Victims and Their Families. Chicago, IL, CV Mosby, 1989

Goodwin J: Adult survivors of child abuse and neglect, in Family Violence: A Clinical and Legal Guide. Edited by Kaplan SJ. Washington, DC, American Psychiatric Press, 1996

Greene B: African-American women, in Women of Color: Integrating Ethnic and Gender Identities in Psychotherapy. Edited by Comas-Diaz L, Greene B. New York, Guilford, 1994, pp 10–29

Hall ER, Flannery PJ: Prevalence and correlates of sexual assault experiences in adolescents. Victimology 9:398, 1984

Hamilton JA: Emotional consequences of victimization and discrimination in special populations of women. Psychiatr Clin North Am 12:35–51, 1989

Hansen M: Feminism and family therapy: a review of feminist critiques of approaches to family violence, in Battering and Family Therapy: A Feminist Perspective.

Edited by Hansen M, Harway M. Thousand Oaks, CA, Sage Publications, 1993, pp 69–81

Hanson RK: The psychological impact of sexual assault on women and children: a review. Ann Sex Res 3:187–232, 1990

Hard S: Sexual abuse of the developmentally disabled: a case study. Presented at the national conference of Executives of Associations for Retarded Citizens, Omaha, NE, October, 1986

Harris M: Trauma Recovery and Empowerment: A Clinician's Guide for Working in Groups. New York, The Free Press, 1998

Harvey MR, Harney PA: Individual psychotherapy, in Treating Women Molested in Childhood. Edited by Classen C, Yalom I. San Francisco, CA, Josey-Bass, 1995, pp 63–94

Heim C, Newport J, Heit S, et al: Pituitary-adrenal and autonomic responses to stress in women after sexual and physical abuse in childhood. JAMA 284:592–597, 2000

Heise LL, Pitanguy J, Germain A: Violence Against Women: The Hidden Health Burden. World Bank Discussion Paper No. 255. Washington, DC, World Bank, 1994

Herman J: Complex PTSD: a syndrome in survivors of prolonged and repeated trauma. J Traumatic Stress 5:377–391, 1992a

Herman JL: Trauma and Recovery: The Aftermath of Violence. Domestic Abuse to Political Terror. New York, Basic Books, 1992b

Herman JL, Schatzow E: Recovery and verification of memories of childhood sexual trauma. Psychoanalytic Psychology 4:1–14, 1987

Herman J, Russell D, Trocke K: Long-term effects of incestuous abuse in childhood. Am J Psychiatry 143:123–129, 1986

Herman JL, Perry JC, van der Kolk BA: Childhood trauma in borderline personality disorder. Am J Psychiatry 146:490–495, 1989

Hilberman E: Overview: the "wifebeater's wife" reconsidered. Am J Psychiatry 137:1337–1347, 1980

Hilberman E, Munson K: Sixty battered women. Victimology 2:460, 1978

Horowitz MJ: Stress response syndromes: character style and dynamic psychotherapy. Arch Gen Psychiatry 31:768–781, 1974

Horowitz MJ: Stress Response Syndromes, 2nd Edition. Northvale, NJ, Jason Aronson, 1986

Hotaling GT, Sugarman DB: An analysis of risk markers in husband to wife violence: the current state of knowledge. Violence and Victims 1:101, 1986

Houskamp BM, Foy D: The assessment of posttraumatic stress disorder in battered women. Journal of Interpersonal Violence 6:367, 1991

Hyman L, Pentland J: The role of mental imagery in the creation of false childhood memories. Journal of Memory and Language 35:101–117, 1996

Hyman L, Husband TH, Billins FJ: False memories of childhood experiences. Applied Cognitive Psychology 9:181–197, 1995

International Society of Traumatic Stress Studies: Childhood Trauma Remembered: A Report on the Current Scientific Knowledge Base and Its Applications. Northbrook, IL, International Society of Traumatic Stress Studies, 1998

Jacobs JL: Child sexual abuse victimization and later sequelae during pregnancy and childbirth. Journal of Child Sexual Abuse 1:103, 1992

Jacobson A: Physical and sexual assault histories among psychiatric outpatients. Am J Psychiatry 146:755–758, 1989

Jacobson A, Herald C: The relevance of childhood sexual abuse to adult psychiatric inpatient care. Hospital and Community Psychiatry 41:154–158, 1990

Jacobson A, Richardson B: Assault experiences of 100 psychiatric inpatients: evidence of the need for routine inquiry. Am J Psychiatry 144:908–913, 1987

Jehu D: Beyond Sexual Abuse: Therapy with Women Who Were Childhood Victims. New York, Wiley, 1988

Jennings A: On being invisible in the mental health system. J Ment Health Admin 21:374–387, 1994a

Jennings A: Retraumatizing the victim. Resources: Newsletter of the Human Resource Association of the Northeast 6:11, 1994b

Johnson T, O'Rourke D, Chavez N, et al: Social cognition and responses to survey questions among culturally diverse populations, in Survey Measurement and Process Quality. Edited by Lyberg L, Biemer P, Collins M, et al. New York, John Wiley & Sons, 1997, pp 87–113

Joseph GI, Lewis J (eds): Common Differences: Conflict in Black and White Feminist Perspectives. New York, Anchor, 1981

Kanuha V: Women of color in battering relationships, in Women of Color: Integrating Ethnic and Gender Identities in Psychotherapy. Edited by Comas-Diaz L, Greene B. New York, Guilford, 1994, pp 428–454

Karol RL, Micka RG, Kuskowski M: Physical, emotional, and sexual abuse among pain patients and health care providers: implications for psychologists in multidisciplinary pain treatment centers. Professional Psychology: Research and Practice 23:480, 1992

Katz B: The psychological impact of stranger versus nonstranger rape on victim's recovery, in Acquaintance Rape: The Hidden Crime. Edited by Parrot A, Bechhofer L. New York, Wiley, 1991, pp 251–269

Kemp A, Rawlings EI, Green BL: Posttraumatic stress disorder in battered women: a shelter sample. J Trauma Stress 4:137–148, 1991

Kendall-Tackett KA, Williams LM, Fineklhor D: Impact of sexual abuse on children: a review and synthesis of recent empirical studies. Psychol Bull 113:164–180, 1993

Kessler R, Sonnea A, Bromet F, et al: Posttraumatic stress disorder in the National Comorbidity Survey. Arch Gen Psychiatry 52:1048–1060, 1995

Kilpatrick DG: National Women's Study: relationship of victimization and PTSD to bulimia nervosa. Int J Eat Disord 21:213–228, 1997

Kilpatrick DG, Veronen LJ, Resick PA: Psychological sequelae to rape: assessment and treatment strategies, in Behavioral Medicine: Assessment and Treatment Strategies. Edited by Dolays DM, Meredith RL. New York, Plenum, 1982, pp 473–497

Kilpatrick DG, Best CL, Veronen LJ, et al: Mental health correlates of criminal victimization: a random community sample. J Consult Clin Psychol 53:866–873, 1985

Kilpatrick DG, Saunders BE, Veronen LJ, et al: Criminal victimization: lifetime prevalence, reporting to police, and psychological impact. Crime and Delinquency 33:479, 1987

Kilpatrick DG, Edmunds CN, Seymour AK: Rape in America: A Report to the Nation. Arlington, VA, National Victim Center, 1992

Kleinman A: Depression, somatization, and the "new cross-cultural psychiatry." Soc Sci Med 11:3–10, 1977

Kluft RP: Childhood Antecedents of Multiple Personality Disorder. Washington, DC, American Psychiatric Press, 1985

Kluft RP: Incest and subsequent revictimization: the case of therapist–patient sexual exploitation with a description of the sitting duck syndrome, in Incest-Related Syndromes of Adult Psychopathology. Edited by Kluft RP. Washington, DC, American Psychiatric Press, 1990, pp 263–287

Kolb LC, Burris BC, Griffiths S: Propanolol and clonidine in the treatment of post-traumatic stress disorders of war, in Posttraumatic Stress Disorder: Psychological and Biological Sequelae. Edited by van der Kolk BA. Washington, DC, American Psychiatric Press, 1984, pp 98–105

Koss MP: The impact of crime victimization on women's medical use. J Women Health 2:67, 1993

Koss MP, Dinero TE: Discriminant analysis of risk factors for sexual victimization among a national sample of college women. J Consult Clin Psychol 57:242–250, 1989

Koss MP, Harvey MP: The Rape Victim: Clinical and Community Interventions. Newbury Park, CA, Sage, 1991

Koss MP, Oros C: The sexual experiences survey: a research instrument investigating sexual aggression and victimization. J Consult Clin Psychol 50:455–457, 1982

Koss MP, Gidcyz CA, Wisniewski N: The scope of rape: incidence and prevalence of sexual aggression and victimization in a national sample of higher education students. J Consult Clin Psychol 42:162–170, 1987

Koss MP, Woodruff WJ, Koss PG: Criminal victimization among primary care medical patients: prevalence, incidence, and physician usage. Behav Sci Law 9:85, 1991a

Koss MP, Koss P, Woodruff J: Deleterious effects of criminal victimization on women's health and medical utilization. Arch Intern Med 151:342–347, 1991b

Koss M, Goodman A, Browne L, et al: No Safe Haven: Male Violence Against Women at Home, at Work, and in the Community. Washington, DC, American Psychological Association, 1994

Krieger N: Inequality, diversity, and health: thoughts on "race/ethnicity" and "gender." JAMWA 51:133–136, 1996

Krueger RA: Focus Groups: A Practical Guide for Applied Research. Newbury Park, CA, Sage Publications, 1988

Kubany ES, McKenzie WF, Owens JA, et al: PTSD among women survivors of domestic violence in Hawaii. Hawaii Med J 55:164–165, 1996

Langeland W, Harters C: Child sexual and physical abuse and alcoholism: a review. J Studies Alcohol 59:336–348, 1998

Lasley JR: Drinking routines, lifestyles, and predatory victimization: a causal analysis. Justice Quarterly 6:529–542, 1989

Layton ME, Dager SR: Treatment of anxiety disorders, in The Psychiatric Clinics of North America Annual of Drug Therapy. Edited by Dunner DL, Rosenbaum JF. Philadelphia, PA, WB Saunders, 1998, pp 183–209

Leserman J, Drossman DA: Sexual and physical abuse history and medical practice. Gen Hosp Psychiatry 17:85, 1995

Lie GY, Gentlewarrier S: Intimate violence in lesbian relationships: discussion of survey findings and practice implications. Journal of Social Service Research 149:41–59, 1991

Lie GY, Schilit R, Bush J, et al: Lesbians in currently aggressive relationships: how frequently do they report aggressive past relationships? Violence and Victims 6:121–135, 1991

Linehan MM: Cognitive-Behavioral Treatment of Borderline Personality Disorder. New York, Guilford, 1993

Lipper S, Davidson JRT, Grady TA, et al: Preliminary study of carbamazepine in posttraumatic stress disorder. Psychosomatics 27:849–854, 1986

Lockhart LL, White BW, Causby V, et al: Letting out the secret: violence in lesbian relationships. Journal of Interpersonal Violence 9:469–492, 1994

Loewenstein RJ: Rational psychopharmacology in the treatment of multiple personality disorder. Psychiatr Clin North Am 14:721–740, 1991

Loewenstein RJ, Hornstein H, Farber B: Open trial of clonazepam in the treatment of posttraumatic stress symptoms in multiple personality disorder. Dissociation 1:3–12, 1988

Loftus E, Polonsky S, Fullilove MT: Memories of childhood sexual abuse: remembering and repressing. Psychol Women Q 18:67–84, 1994

Lohr JM, Kleinknecht RA, Tolin DF, et al: The empirical status of the clinical application of eye movement desensitization and reprocessing. J Behav Ther Exp Psychiatry 26:285–302, 1995

Lohr JM, Tolin DF, Lillienfeld SO: Efficacy of eye movement desensitization and reprocessing: implications for behavior therapy. Behavior Therapy 29:123–156, 1998

Lombardo S, Pohl R: Sexual abuse history of women treated in a psychiatric outpatient clinic. Psychiatric Services 48:534–538, 1997

Lubin H, Johnson DR: Interactive psychoeducational group therapy for traumatized women. Int J Group Psychother 47:271–290, 1997

Maltz W: The Sexual Healing Journey. New York, Harper Collins, 1991

Mansell S, Sobsey D, Moskal R: Clinical findings among sexually abused children with and without developmental disabilities. Ment Retard 36:12–22, 1998

Marcus S. Marquis P, Sakai C: Controlled study of treatment of PTSD using EMDR in an HMO setting. Psychotherapy 34:307–315, 1997

Marella A, Friedman M, Gerrity E, et al: Ethnocultural Aspects of Posttraumatic Stress Disorder: Issues, Research, and Clinical Applications. Washington, DC, American Psychological Association, 1996

Marmar CR: Brief dynamic psychotherapy of posttraumatic stress disorder. Psychiatr Ann 21:405–414, 1991

Marmar CR, Weiss DS, Schlener WE, et al: Peritraumatic dissociation and posttraumatic stress in male Vietnam theater veterans. Am J Psychiatry 151:902–907, 1994

Marrujo B, Kreger M: Definition of roles in abusive lesbian relationships. Journal of Gay and Lesbian Social Services 4:22–32, 1996

Martin SL, English KT, Clark KA, et al: Violence and substance abuse among North Carolina pregnant women. Am J Public Health 86:873–998, 1996

McCann IL, Pearlman LA: Psychological Trauma and the Adult Survivor: Theory, Therapy, and Transformation. New York, Brunner/Mazel, 1990

McCauley JM, Kern DE, Kolodner K, et al: The battering syndrome: prevalence and clinical characteristics of domestic violence in primary care internal medicine practices. Ann Intern Med 123:737–746, 1995

McCauley J, Kern DE, Kolodner K, et al: Clinical characteristics of women with a history of childhood abuse: unhealed wounds. JAMA 277:1362–1368, 1997

McFarlane J, Parker B, Soeken K, et al: Assessing for abuse during pregnancy. JAMA 267:31–76, 1992

McGrath E, Keita BP, Strickland BR, et al (eds): Women and Depression: Risk Factors and Treatment Issues. Washington, DC, American Psychological Association, 1990

Meichenbaum D: Cognitive Behavior Modification. Morristown, NH, General Learning Press, 1974

Melling L: Wife abuse in the deaf community: response to violence in the family and sexual assault. Response to Violence in the Family and Sexual Assault 7:1–2, 12, 1984

Messman TL, Long PJ: Child sexual abuse and its relationship to revictimization in adult women: a review. Clin Psychol Rev 16:397–420, 1996

Moore KA, Nord CW, Peterson JL: Nonvoluntary sexual activity among adolescents. Family Plan Perspect 21:110–114, 1989

Muenzenmaier K, Meyer I, Streuning E, et al: Childhood abuse and neglect among women outpatients with chronic mental illness. Hospital and Community Psychiatry 44:666–670, 1993

Murphy M, Cascardi M: Psychological aggression and abuse in marriage, in Family Violence: Prevention and Treatment. Edited by Hampton R, Gulotta T, Adams G, et al. Newbury Park, CA, Sage Publications, 1993

Najavits LM, Weiss RD, Shaw SR: The link between substance abuse and posttraumatic stress disorder in women: a research review. Am J Addict 6:273–283, 1997

Norris FH, Kaniasty K: Psychological distress following criminal victimization in the general population: cross-sectional, longitudinal, and prospective analyses. J Consult Clin Psychol 62:111–123, 1994

Norris FH, Riad JK: Standardized self-report measures of civilian trauma and posttraumatic stress disorder, in Assessing Psychological Trauma and PTSD. Edited by Wilson JP, Keane TM. New York, Guilford, 1997

O'Campo P, Gielen AC, Faen RR, et al: Verbal abuse and physical violence among a cohort of low-income pregnant women. Women's Health Issues 4:29–37, 1994

O'Keefe M: Posttraumatic stress disorder among incarcerated battered women: a comparison of battered women who killed their abusers and those incarcerated for other offenses. J Trauma Stress 11:71–85, 1998

O'Leary KD: Psychological abuse: a variable deserving critical attention in domestic violence. Violence and Victims 14:3–23, 1999

Parker B, McFarlane J, Soeken K, et al: Physical and emotional abuse in pregnancy: a comparison of adult and teenage women. Nurs Res 42:173–178, 1993

Pearlman LA, Saakvitne KW: Trauma and the Therapist: Countertransference and Vicarious Traumatization in Psychotherapy with Incest Survivors. New York, WW Norton, 1995

Peclovitz D, van der Kolk B, Roth S, et al: Development of a criteria set and a structured interview for disorders of extreme stress (SIDES). J Trauma Stress 10:3–16, 1997

Pepitone A, Triandis HC: On the universality of social psychological theories. Journal of Cross-cultural Psychology 18:471–497, 1988

Pitman RK, Altman B, Greenwald E, et al: Psychiatric complications during flooding therapy for posttraumatic stress disorder. J Clin Psychiatry 52:12–20, 1991

Plichta SB: Domestic violence: building paths for women to travel to freedom and safety. Paper presented at the Symposium on Domestic Violence and Women's Health: Broadening the Conversation, New York, September, 1995

Pope HG, Hudson JI: Can memories of childhood sexual abuse be repressed? Psychol Med 25:121–126, 1995

Putnam FW: Dissociation as a response to extreme trauma, in Childhood Antecedents Washington, DC, American Psychiatric Press, 1985, pp 65–97

Putnam FW: Diagnosis and Treatment of Multiple Personality Disorder. New York, Guilford, 1989

Putnam FW, Trickett PK: Child sexual abuse: a model of chronic trauma. Psychiatry 56:82–95, 1993

Putnam FW, Guroff JJ, Silberman EK, et al: The clinical phenomenology of multiple personality disorder: review of 100 recent cases. J Clin Psychiatry 47:285–293, 1986

Rapkin AJ, Kames LD, Darke LL, et al: History of physical and sexual abuse in women with chronic pelvic pain. Obstet Gynecol 76:92, 1990

Ray ND, Rappaport ME: Use of restraint and seclusion in psychiatric settings in New York state. Psychiatric Services 46:1032–1037, 1995

Renzetti C: Violent Betrayal: Partner Abuse in Lesbian Relationships. Newbury Park, CA, Sage Publications, 1992

Resick PA: Psychological effects of victimization: implications for the criminal justice system. Crime and Delinquency 33:468, 1987

Resick PA, Schnicke MK: Cognitive processing therapy for sexual assault victims. J Consult Clin Psychol 60:748, 1992

Resick PA, Jordan CG, Girelli SA, et al: A comparative outcome study of behavioral group therapy for sexual assault victims. Behavior Therapy 19:385–401, 1988

Resnick HS, Newton T: Assessment and treatment of posttraumatic stress disorder in adult survivors of sexual assault, in Treating PTSD: Cognitive-Behavioral Strategies. New York, Guilford, 1992, pp 99–126

Resnick HS, Kilpatrick DG, Dansky BS, et al: Prevalence of civilian trauma and posttraumatic stress disorder in a representative national sample of women. J Consult Clin Psychol 61:984–991, 1993

Resnick H, Yehuda R, Pitman RK, et al: Effect of previous trauma on acute plasma cortisol level following rape. Am J Psychiatry 152:1675–1677, 1995

Rieker PP, Carmen E: The victim-to-patient process: the disconfirmation and transformation of abuse. Am J Orthopsychiatry 5:360–370, 1986

Root M: Women of color and traumatic stress in domestic captivity: gender and race as disempowering statuses, in Ethnocultural Aspects of Posttraumatic Stress Disorder: Issues, Research, and Clinical Applications. Edited by Marella A, Friedman M, Gerrity E, et al. Washington, DC, American Psychological Association, 1996

Rose SM, Peabody CG, Stratieas B: Responding to hidden abuse: a role for social work in reforming mental health systems. Social Work 36:408–413, 1991

Ross CA: Multiple Personality Disorder: Diagnosis, Clinical Features, and Treatment. New York, Wiley, 1989

Roth AS, Ostroff RB, Hoffman RE: Naltrexone as a treatment for repetitive self-injurious behavior: an open-label trial. J Clin Psychiatry 57:233–237, 1996

Roth S, Newman E, Peclovitz D, et al: Complex PTSD in victims exposed to sexual and physical abuse: results from the DSM-IV Field Trial for Posttraumatic Stress Disorder. J Trauma Stress 10:539–555, 1997

Rothbaum BO: A controlled study of eye movement desensitization and reprocessing in the treatment of posttraumatic stress disordered sexual assault victims. Bull Menninger Clin 61:317–334, 1997

Rothbaum BO, Foa EB: Symptoms of posttraumatic stress disorder and duration of symptoms, in Posttraumatic Stress Disorder: DSM-IV and Beyond. Edited by Davidson JRT, Foa EB. Washington, DC, American Psychiatric Press, 1993, pp 23–26

Rothbaum BO, Foa EB, Riggs DS, et al: A prospective examination of posttraumatic stress disorder in rape victims. J Trauma Stress 5:455–475, 1992

Ruch LO, Amedeo SR, Leon JJ, et al: Repeated sexual victimization and trauma change during the acute phase of the sexual assault trauma syndrome. Women Health 17:1–19, 1991

Russell D: The prevalence and incidence of forcible rape and attempted rape of females. Victimology 7:81–93, 1982

Russell D: Sexual Exploitation. Newbury Park, CA, Sage Publications, 1984

Russo NF, Green BL: Women and mental health, in Psychology of Women. Edited by Denmark EL, Paludi MA. Westport, CT, Greenwood Press, 1993, pp 379–436

Ryan SG, Sherman SL, Terry JC, et al: Startle disease or hyperekplexia: response to clonazepam and assignment of the gene (STHE) to chromosome 5q by image analysis. Ann Neurol 3:663–668, 1992

Saporta JA Jr, Case J: The role of medication in treating adult survivors of childhood trauma, in Treating Adult Survivors of Incest. Edited by Paddison P. Washington, DC, American Psychiatric Press, 1991, pp 101–134

Sappington AA, Pharr R, Tunstall A, et al: Relationships among child abuse, date abuse, and psychological problems. J Clin Psychol 53:319–329, 1997

Schaaf KK, McCanne TR: Relationship of childhood sexual, physical, and combined sexual and physical abuse to adult victimization and posttraumatic stress disorder. Child Abuse and Neglect 22:1119–1133, 1998

Schechter S: Domestic Violence Guidelines for Mental Health Practitioners. Washington, DC, National Coalition Against Domestic Violence, 1987

Schechter S: Improving the Response to Domestic Violence: Recommendations to Federal Agencies. Washington, DC, U.S. Department of Health and Human Services and Centers for Disease Control and Prevention, 1996

Scheck MM, Schaeffer JA, Gillette C: Brief psychological intervention with traumatized young women: the efficacy of eye movement desensitization and reprocessing. J Trauma Stress 11:25–44, 1998

Scheflin AW, Brown D: Repressed memory of dissociative amnesia: what the science says. J Psychiatry Law 24:143–188, 1996

Schilit R, Lie GY, Montagne M: Substance use as a correlate of violence in intimate lesbian relationships. Journal of Homosexuality 19:51–65, 1990

Schooler JW, Bendiksen M, Ambadar Z: Taking the middle line: can we accommodate both fabricated and recovered memories of sexual abuse? in False and Recovered Memories. Edited by Conway M. Oxford, England, Oxford University Press, 1997, pp 251–292

Schulman M: A Survey of Spousal Violence Against Women in Kentucky. Washington, DC, U.S. Department of Justice, Law Enforcement Administration, 1979

Shalev AY, Galai T, Eth S: Levels of trauma: a multidimensional approach to the treatment of PTSD. Psychiatry 56:166–177, 1993

Shalev AY, Peri T, Caneti L, et al: Predictors of PTSD in injured trauma survivors: a propsective study. Am J Psychiatry 153:219–225, 1996

Shapiro F: Eye movement desensitization: a new treatment for posttraumatic stress disorder. J Behav Ther Exp Psychiatry 20:211–217, 1989

Shapiro F: Eye Movement Desensitization and Reprocessing: Basic Principles, Protocols, and Procedures. New York, Guildford, 1995

Shields NM, Hanneke CR: Multiple sexual victimization: the case of incest and marital rape, in Family Violence and Its Consequences: New Directions in Research. Edited by Hotaling GT, Finkelhor D, Kirkpatrick JT, et al. Newbury Park, CA, Sage, 1988, pp 255–269

Shobe KK, Kihlstrom JF: Is traumatic memory Special? Current Directions in Psychological Science 6:70–74, 1997

Simpson EB, Pistorello J, Begin A, et al: Use of dialectical behavior therapy in a partial hospital program for women with borderline personality disorder. Psychiatric Services 49:669–673, 1998

Smith PH, Earp JA, DeVellis R: Measuring battering: development of the Women's Experience With Battering (WEB) Scale. Women's Health: Research on Gender, Behavior, and Policy 1:273–288, 1995

Sobsey D, Varnhagen C: Sexual abuse, assault, and exploitation of Canadians with disabilities, in Preventing Child Sexual Abuse. Edited by Bagley C. Toronto, Canada, Wall and Emerson, 1991, pp 203–216

Sobsey D, Wells D, Lucardie R, et al: Violence and Disability: An Annotated Bibliography. Baltimore, MD, Paul H. Brookes, 1995

Solomon SD, Davidson JRT: Trauma: prevalence, impairment, service use, and cost. J Clin Psychiatry 58(suppl):5–11, 1997

Sorenson SB: Violence against women: examining ethnic differences and commonalities. Evaluation Review 20:123, 1996

Sorenson S, Golding J: Depressive sequelae for recent criminal victimization. J Trauma Stress 3:337–350, 1990

Southwick SM, Yehuda R, Giller EL, et al: use of tricyclics and monoamine oxidase inhibitors in the treatment of PTSD: a quantitative review, in Catecholamine

Function in Posttraumatic Stress Disorder: Emerging Concepts. Washington, DC, American Psychiatric Press, 1994, pp 293–305

Southwick SM, Bremner JD, Rasmusson A, et al: Role of norepinephrine in the pathophysiology and treatment of posttraumatic stress disorder. Biol Psychiatry 46:1192–1204, 1999

Stark E: The myth of black violence. Social Work 38:485, 1993

Stark E, Flitcraft A: Violence among intimates: an epidemiological review, in Handbook of Family Violence. Edited by Van Hasselt VB, Morrison RL, Bellack AS, et al. New York, Plenum, 1988, pp 293–318

Stark E, Flitcraft A: Killing the beast within: woman battering and female suicidality. Int J Health Serv 25:43–64, 1995

Stark E, Flitcraft A, Frazier W: Medicine and patriarchal violence: the social construction of a private event. Int J Health Serv 9:461, 1979

Stein MB, Koverola C, Hanna AC, et al: Hippocampal volume in women victimized by child sexual abuse. Psychol Med 27:951–959, 1997

Stepakoff S: Effects of sexual victimization on suicidal ideation and behavior in U.S. college women. Suicide Life Threat Behav 28:107–126, 1998

Stimpson L, Best MC: Courage Above All: Sexual Assault Against Women with Disabilities. Toronto, Canada, Disabled Women's Network, 1991

Straus MA, Gelles RJ: Physical Violence in American Families: Risk Factors and Adaptation to Violence in 8,145 families. New Brunswick, NJ, Transaction, 1990

Straus MA, Gelles RJ, Steinmetz S: Behind Closed Doors: Violence in the American Family. Garden City, NY, Anchor Press, 1980

Straus MA, Hamby SL, Boney-McCoy S, et al: The revised Conflict Tactics Scales (CTS2): development and preliminary psychometric data. Journal of Family Issues 17:283–316, 1996

Substance Abuse and Mental Health Services Administration: Substance Abuse Treatment and Domestic Violence Treatment Improvement Protocol (TIP), Series 25. Rockville, MD, Department of Health and Human Services, Public Health Service, Substance Abuse and Mental Health Services Administration, Center for Substance Abuse Treatment, 1998

Talbot N, Houghtalen R, Cyrulik S, et al: Women's safety in recovery: group therapy for patients with a history of childhood sexual abuse. Psychiatric Services 49:213–217, 1998

Tarasoff v. Regents of the University of California. 17 Col 425, 131CAL Rptr 14, 551 P2d

Tjaden P, Thoennes N: Prevalence, Incidence, and Consequences of Violence Against Women: Findings from the National Violence Against Women Survey. Washington, DC, U.S. Department of Justice, National Institute of Justice, and Centers for Disease Control, 1998

Tolman RM: The initial development of a measure of psychological maltreatment of women by their male partners. Violence and Victims 4:159–178, 1988

Tolman RM: The Psychological Maltreatment of Women Inventory. Violence and Victims 14:25–37, 1999

Torres S: A comparison of wife abuse between two cultures: perception, attitudes, nature, and extent. Issues in Mental Health Nursing 12:113–131, 1991

Triandis HC: The Analysis of Subjective Culture. New York, Wiley-Interscience, 1972

Turkus J: Crisis intervention, in Treating Women Molested in Childhood. Edited by Classen C, Yalom I. San Francisco, CA, Josey-Bass, 1995, pp 35–62

Urquiza A, Goodlin BL: Child sexual abuse and adult revictimization with women of color. Violence and Victims 9:223, 1994

van der Kolk BA: Psychological Trauma. Washington, DC, American Psychiatric Association, 1987

van der Kolk BA: The psychobiology of posttraumatic stress disorder. J Clin Psychiatry 58(suppl):16–24, 1997

van der Kolk BA, Dreyfuss D, Michaels MJ, et al: Fluoxetine in posttraumatic stress disorder. J Clin Psychiatry 55:517–522, 1994

van der Kolk BA, McFarlane AC, Weisaeth L (eds): Traumatic Stress: The Effects of Overwhelming Experience on Mind, Body, and Society. New York, Guilford, 1996

Vaughan K, Wiese M, Gold R, et al: Eye-movement desensitization: symptom change in posttraumatic stress disorder. Br J Psychiatry 164:533–541, 1994

Veronen LJ, Kilpatrick DG: Stress management for rape victims, in Stress Reduction and Prevention. Edited by Meichenbaum D, Jaremko ME. New York, Plenum, 1983, pp 341–374

Waldinger RJ, Swett C, Frank A, et al: Levels of dissociation and histories of reported abuse among women outpatients. J Nerv Ment Dis 182:625–630, 1994

Walker EA, Katon WJ, Harrop-Griffiths J, et al: Relationship of chronic pelvic pain to psychiatric diagnoses and childhood sexual abuse. Am J Psychiatry 147:75, 1988

Walker EA, Katon WJ, Roy-Byrne PP, et al: Histories of sexual victimization in patients with irritable bowel syndrome or inflammatory bowel disease. Am J Psychiatry 150:1502, 1993

Walker EA, Gelfand AN, Gelfand MD, et al: Medical and Psychiatric symptoms in female gastroenterology clinic patients with histories of sexual victimization. Gen Hosp Psychiatry 17:85, 1995

Walker LE: The Battered Woman Syndrome. New York, Springer, 1984

Walker LE: The battered woman syndrome, in Family Abuse and its Consequences. Edited by Hotalin GT, Finkelhor D, Kirkpatrick JT, et al. Beverly Hills, CA, Sage Publications, 1988, pp 139–148

Walker LE: Abused Women and Survivor Therapy. Washington, DC, American Psychological Association, 1994

Waller G: Sexual abuse as a factor in eating disorders. Br J Psychiatry 159:664–671, 1991

Warshaw C: Domestic violence: challenges to medical practice. J Womens Health 2:73–80, 1992

Warshaw C: Domestic violence: changing theory, changing practice. JAMWA 51:87–91, 1996a

Warshaw C: Domestic Violence: Treatment vs. Advocacy: Developing Collaborative Models for Meeting the Mental Health Needs of Battered Women. Commissioned Report. Harrisburg, PA, National Resource Center on Domestic Violence, 1996b

Warshaw C: Domestic violence and medical education: creating a framework for change. Academic Medicine 72:526–537, 1997

Warshaw C, Ganley AL: Improving the Health Care Response to Domestic Violence: a Resource Manual for Health Care Providers. San Francisco, CA, Family Violence Prevention Fund, Pennsylvania Coalition Against Domestic Violence, 1995

Waterman CK, Dawson LJ, Bologna MJ: Sexual coercion in gay male and lesbian relationships: predictors and implications for support services. J Sex Res 26:118–124, 1989

Weskott M: The Feminist Legacy of Karen Horney. New Haven, CT, Yale University Press, 1986

West CM: Leaving a second closet: outing partner violence in same-sex couples, in Partner Violence: A Comprehensive Review of 20 Years of Research. Edited by Jasinksi JL, Williams LM. Thousand Oaks, CA, Sage Publications, 1998, pp 163–183

Westen D, Ludolph P, Misle B, et al: Physical and sexual abuse in adolescent girls with borderline personality disorder. Am J Orthopsychiatry 60:55–66, 1990

Westerlund E: Women's Sexuality After Childhood Incest. New York, WW Norton, 1992

Widom CS, Morris S: Accuracy of adult recollections of childhood victimization, part 2: childhood sexual abuse. Psychological Assessment 9:34–36, 1997

Williams LM: Recovered memories of abuse in women with documented child sexual victimization histories. J Trauma Stress 8:649–673, 1995

Williams LM, Banyard VL: Gender and recall of child sexual abuse: a prospective study, in Recollections of Trauma: Scientific Evidence and Clinical Practices. Edited by Read JD, Lindsay DS. New York: Plenum, 1997, pp 371–377

Wilsnack SC, Vogeltanz ND, Klassen AD, et al: Childhood sexual abuse and women's substance abuse: national survey findings. J Stud Alcohol 58:264–271, 1997

Wilson JP, Keane TM: Assessing Psychological Trauma and PTSD. New York, Guildford, 1997

Wilson SA, Becker LA, Tinker RH: Eye movement desensitization and reprocessing (EMDR) treatment for psychologically traumatized individuals. J Consult Clin Psychol 63:928–937, 1995

Wilson SA, Becker LA, Tinker RH, Fifteen-month follow-up of eye movement desensitization and reprocessing (EMDR) treatment for posttraumatic stress disorder and psychological trauma. J Consult Clin Psychol 65:1047–1056, 1997

Winfield I, George LK, Swartz M, et al: Sexual assault and psychiatric disorders among a community sample of women. Am J Psychiatry 147:335, 1990

Winick C, Levine A, Stone WA: An incest survivors' therapy group. Journal of Substance Abuse Treatment 9:311–318, 1992

Wolf ME, Alavi A, Mosnaim AD: Posttraumatic stress disorder in Vietnam veterans' clinical and EEG findings: possible therapeutic effects of carbemazepine. Biol Psychiatry 23:642–644, 1988

Wyatt GE: The sexual abuse of Afro-American and white American women in childhood. Child Abuse and Neglect 9:507–519, 1985

Wyatt GE: The sociocultural context of African American and white American women's rape. Journal of Social Issues 48:77–91, 1992

Wyatt G: Sociocultural and epidemiological issues in the assessment of domestic violence. Social Distress and the Homeless 1:7–21, 1994

Wyatt GE, Peters SD: Issues in the definition of child sexual abuse in prevalence research. Child Abuse and Neglect 10:231, 1986

Wyatt GE, Riederle M: Sexual harassment and prior sexual trauma among African-American and white American women. Violence and Victims 9:233–247, 1994

Wyatt GE, Guthrie D, Notgrass CM: Differential effects of women's child sexual abuse and subsequent sexual victimization. J Consult Clin Psychol 60:167, 1992

Yehuda R, McFarlane AC (eds): Psychobiology of Posttraumatic Stress Disorder: Annals of the New York Academy of Sciences, Vol 821. New York, Academy of Sciences, 1997

Yehuda R, Giller EL, Southwick SM, et al: Hypothalamic-pituitary-adrenal dysfunction in posttraumatic stress disorder. Biol Psychiatry 30:1031–1048, 1991

Yehuda R, Southwick SM, Krystal JH, et al: Enhanced suppression of cortisol following dexamethasone administration in posttraumatic stress disorder. Am J Psychiatry 150:83–86, 1993

Yehuda R, Kahana B, Binder-Byrnes K, et al: Low urinary cortisol excretion in Holocaust survivors with posttraumatic stress disorder. Am J Psychiatry 152:982–986, 1995

Young ME, Nosek MA, Howland C, et al: Prevalence of abuse of women with physical disabilities. Arch Phys Med Rehabil 78(suppl):S34–S38, 1997

Zierler S, Feingold L, Laufer D, et al: Adult survivors of childhood sexual abuse and subsequent risk of HIV infection. Am J Public Health 81:572–575, 1995

Zlotnick C, Zakriski AL, Shea MT, et al: The long-term sequelae of sexual abuse: support for a complex posttraumatic stress disorder. J Trauma Stress 9:195–205, 1996

Zlotnick C, Shea T, Rosen K, et al: An affect-management group for women with posttraumatic stress disorder and histories of childhood sexual abuse. J Trauma Stress 10:425–436, 1997

# Psychological Aspects of Lesbian Health Care

MARGERY S. SVED, M.D.

A study of excellent care for women that is mindful of the complex interface between medical and psychologic issues must examine this interface as it relates to all women. The needs and issues of both majority and minority women should be included. This text seeks to ameliorate the troubled relationship between women and the providers of their obstetric and gynecologic care. In their introduction, Drs. Stewart and Stotland discuss the difficult relationship that has arisen between women and their physicians. This relationship, often fraught with adversarial undertones, leaves some women preferring to not seek health care services. Training programs are cited as deficient in attention to the development of interpersonal skills, the understanding of psychodynamics, and other psychologic aspects of health care. The way medical care is currently administered—complicated by the access issues of the managed care environment—stands as an impediment to the evolution of a healthy doctor–patient relationship.

Into this relationship (or lack thereof) comes the lesbian patient. The same barriers to good care that have complicated the relationship between all physicians and women are evident in the relationship between a lesbian patient and a physician. Other complex barriers are also frequently in place. This chapter defines the barriers to care that exist for lesbian women and suggests ways to remove those barriers. It attempts to address the question of which medical and psychologic issues must be considered when providing primary or obstetric/gynecologic care to lesbian women. The ultimate goal of this book is the development of professionals who are knowledgable not only about female sexual organs but also about female sexual feelings and behaviors; who are dedicated to understanding not only the familiar majority but also the often-invisible minorities; and who are invested not only in the delivery of mechanical medical services, but also in the delivery of sensitive and humane medical care.

## Definitions

In the context of health care, lesbians have been an invisible minority (Robertson 1992). Although somewhere between 2% and 10% of North American women are lesbian, they have been a marginalized and ignored element of the population (Michaels 1996). Hepburn and Gutierrez (1988) surveyed heterosexuals and found that only 25% reported knowing an individual who is homosexual. In an earlier study, Johnson et al. (1981) found that of 110 gynecologists surveyed, 50% were sure that they had never treated a lesbian patient.

A *lesbian* is a woman whose sexual and affectional orientation is directed toward other women. An individual's behavior may range from celibate to exclusively homosexual, bisexual, or situationally heterosexual. Any number of factors can influence or direct an individual's behavior. These include economic status, cultural milieu, genetics, sexual desire, family pressures, personal awareness, and various internally and externally generated factors. Not all women who partner with women consider themselves to be lesbians; similarly, not all women who partner with men consider themselves to be heterosexuals. Labeling or defining oneself as lesbian, bisexual, or heterosexual is a highly individualized phenomenon. Such self-definition may change over time. A practitioner should be interested in both an individual's self-generated label and in her history of behavior.

Lesbians are as diverse a group as the population at large, including individuals from all geographic, economic, racial, religious, ethnic, age, and occupational groups. The spectrum includes women who may be actively involved in gay and lesbian politics and/or culture, women who may be "closeted" and isolated from the supports and resources available within the lesbian community, and women who view their sexual orientation as only a minor part of their personal identity.

Lesbian sexual behavior has the same potential diversity as all human behavior. Lesbian sexual activity includes a full range of human sexual expression, including (but not limited to) kissing, breast stimulation, fantasy, masturbation, digital or manual penetration of the vagina, penetration of the anus, and use of sex toys including vibrators. Types of contact may include genital/genital, oral/genital, and oral/anal. Some women may be celibate, either by choice or circumstance. Other women may have male sexual partners, again by choice or by circumstance. Some women may engage in sadomasochistic activity and some women may be professional sex workers with male and/or female clients.

## Barriers to Health Care for Lesbians

Many women find themselves forced to hide their relationships with other women from their employers, medical providers, family of origin, or religious community for fear of being ostracized or rejected because of their sexual orientation. A medical provider dedicated to providing good quality medical care must be attuned to these kinds of fears and work to create an environment of trust and confidentiality in which patients can freely discuss all of the issues that affect their health and well-being. Several researchers have published work suggesting that lesbian women are likely to avoid seeking both routine health care and care for medical problems (Banks and Gartrell 1996; Bradford and Ryan 1988; Deevey 1990; Hume 1983; Stevens and Hall 1988; Trippet and Bain 1992; J. C. White and Dull 1997; Zeidenstein 1990). Chafetz et al. (1974), Saunders et al. (1988), and J. C. White and Dull (1997) wrote that lesbian women were often more inclined to seek advice and help for medical issues from their circle of friends or nonallopathic practitioners than from medical physicians. Several factors have been identified as barriers to health care for lesbians. These include previous negative experiences with health care providers; previous negative experiences with legal, social, or other services; incorrect assumptions on the part of both lesbian women and medical practitioners regarding the need for routine health screening for lesbian women; the decreased likelihood among many lesbian women that contraceptive issues or perinatal care will serve as an entree into medical care; financial constraints, made worse because lesbian partners are rarely eligible for insurance coverage on their partner's policy; and aspects of some lesbian communities that may encourage self-care or nonallopathic health care (Rankow 1995c).

A great deal of research has revealed institutionalized heterosexism within the medical establishment. Numerous researchers (Chaimowitz 1991; Douglas et al. 1985; Garfinkle and Morin 1978; Mathews et al. 1986; Randall 1989; Townsend 1997; Wallick 1997; T. A. White 1979) have documented aspects of this negative attitude toward homosexuals by health care providers including nurses, psychologists, medical students, and physicians. Some of these researchers revealed that significant percentages of health care workers have an aversion to homosexual clients, considering them repulsive, immoral, and generally less healthy than heterosexual clients. A survey of gay and lesbian physicians documented that 67% of respondents knew of gay, lesbian, or bisexual individuals who received substandard care because of their sexual orientation (Shatz and O'Hanlan 1994). Neither medical school curricula nor residency training programs have been found to adequately deal with issues of homosexuality. Of 86 medical school curricula studied by Wallick et al. in 1992, the mean class time devoted to teaching about homosexuality (out of a total of 4 years of study) was 3 hours, 26 minutes. However, exposure to a curriculum focused on cultural competency and homosexuality may help improve attitudes (Muller and White 1997; Olsen and Mann 1997; Rankow 1997b; Townsend and Wallick 1996).

When a lesbian woman does seek medical care, the same factors outlined above may affect her ability to reveal her sexual orientation to her health care provider (Johnson and Guenter 1987). As a result of the well-documented homophobia among both the general population and among health care providers, lesbians are often understandably hesitant to reveal their sexual orientation. Fear of rough treatment during physical examination, fear of hostility, fear of inadequate or denied medical care, and fear that a breach of confidentiality may jeopardize her employment, her home, her standing in the community at large, her family relationships, or the legal custody of her children may all affect a woman's likelihood to seek medical care or to disclose her sexual orientation. In fact, the fears associated with involvement in the traditional medical community often greatly outweigh the fears associated with potential illness, even though delays in screening and treatment have the potential to increase both morbidity and mortality. Furthermore, Stevens and Hall (1988) listed these possible problems when the patient feels unable to disclose that she is lesbian: 1) "invisibility" within the health care system; 2) the assumption by practitioners that all patients are heterosexual; 3) missed opportunities for health education and irrelevant health education; 4) offensive and often heterosexist lines of questioning and comments; and 5) faulty diagnosis and treatment.

## Decreasing Barriers to Care for Lesbian Women

Barriers will truly be lowered only when society at large ceases to discriminate on the basis of gender or sexual orientation. Medical training will then be more likely to include information on the needs of lesbian clients, which will help practitioners foster a supportive practice environment for all patients. In the meantime, however, a health care provider can attempt to create a practice open to anyone regardless of sexual orientation, beginning with members of the phone staff (e.g., receptionists, nurses) who are usually the patient's first contact with a medical practice and continuing with modification of the various intake forms a patient fills out and of the attitudes expressed both overtly and covertly by all staff members with whom a patient comes into contact (e.g., nurses, physician extenders, laboratory technicians, and physicians).

One of the most important factors in the care of lesbians and all women involves avoiding language that implies assumptions. Female patients should not be assumed to be "Mrs." Smith, and when asking about health insurance, questions such as "is the policy under your husband's name?" should be avoided. It also should not be assumed that the woman needs to use or is using contraception. When the initial interactions of a relationship include such assumptions, the patient may feel that the questioner has a bias in favor of patients who fit an assumed profile. Assertively correcting the questioner ("Call me Ms. Smith"; "No, I'm not married"; "No, I don't need any birth control") can feel extremely risky.

An individual patient's sexual orientation should not be assumed based on appearance, marital status, or whether an individual has ever been pregnant. Furthermore, an individual who states that she is lesbian should not be assumed to have no sexual contact with men. Abandoning assumptions means asking very basic, nonjudgmental, open-ended questions, such as "Are you involved in a significant relationship?"; "Tell me about your living situation. Who shares the household with you?"; "Tell me about the people who are important to you. Where do you get the most support?"; "Are your relationships satisfying or are there any concerns you'd like to discuss?"; "Are you sexually active? With men, with women, or with both?"; "Do you have any need to discuss birth control?"; "How are you dealing with issues of 'safer sex?'"; "Are there any other questions or concerns that you would like to discuss?" (Rankow 1995c).

It can be very helpful to preface intimate questions with an explanation about their importance in the individual's health care and with reassurances (when they can be made honestly) of confidentiality: "People are at risk for different diseases and need different tests depending on what activities they're engaging in now and in the past. I will need to ask you some personal questions that I ask all of my patients about sexual activity to help give you the best possible care. Everything you tell me will be kept confidential." This can then be followed by more detailed questions regarding the age at onset of sexual activity, number and genders of past and present partners, specific behaviors engaged in, and knowledge of and compliance with guidelines for risk reduction.

As with all patients, an individual's support system should be explored. When appropriate, and when desired by the patient, this support system should be included in the patient's health care. Research has shown (contrary to some popular myths) that many lesbians enjoy consistent support from strong partner relationships and friends (Bradford and Ryan 1988). It is important for practitioners to be aware that lesbian women often turn to friends as their primary source of support, unlike heterosexuals, who consider both family members and friends as equally supportive (Kurdek and Schmitt 1987).

Health care providers can follow these very concrete suggestions to convey to patients that they are in a safe environment in which they can relax and trust their practitioner (Rankow 1995c, 1997c; J. C. White 1995):

- Include a patient's partner or friend if desired by the patient
- Discuss issues of confidentiality, including how disclosed information will be treated in the written medical record
- Display magazines, brochures, and images that reflect the full diversity of the patient population, including lesbian women
- Post a nondiscrimination policy in the office waiting room: *"We do not discriminate on the basis of race, national origin, gender, language, income, age, education, sexual orientation, or disability."*
- Use inclusive language for all health education materials and for patient history and intake forms

## Health Concerns of Lesbian Women

The health concerns of lesbians have only recently begun to be studied in any systematic way. Previously, research funding had not been awarded to study whether lesbian women had any specific, unique health care issues (Stevens 1992). The earliest studies were performed with sample sizes so small and narrow that the relevance of the results was unknown. Most of the early work involved surveys of self-identified lesbians and primarily sampled those who were young, white, middle class, and well educated. Many opportunities for data collection and research were missed. For example, the Centers for Disease Control recorded little data early in the HIV epidemic about the sexual orientation or activity of women diagnosed with AIDS. This supported the belief that lesbians were at low risk for HIV/AIDS because a woman who reported any heterosexual behavior after 1978 was grouped with heterosexual women (Peterson et al. 1992). In addition, many possible sources of data were neglected, because researchers often did not ask questions that allowed stratification of results by sexual orientation or behavior.

Clearly, better research with larger numbers and more diversity among respondents is necessary to better define the health care needs of lesbian women (Hollibaugh et al. 1993; Rankow 1998; Solarz 1999; J. C. White 1998). Results from newer research are starting to be published, including how to perform research that includes lesbians (Bradford et al. 1997; Herek et al. 1991), and several large multicenter prospective studies include information that will allow stratification by sexual orientation (e.g., Women's Health Initiative, Harvard Nurses' Study). Health practitioners will need to follow the relevant literature for results of new research regarding lesbian health.

## Breast Cancer

No research findings comparing the risk of breast cancer in lesbian women with that in heterosexual women are available, although some are under way (S. A. Roberts et al. 1998). Some studies have suggested that risk factors for breast cancer such as nulliparity, childbearing after age 30, never having breastfed, and increased alcohol consumption exist more frequently in lesbian women (Biddle 1993; Bradford and Ryan 1988; Bradford et al. 1994; Bybee 1991; Johnson et al. 1987b; McKirnan and Peterson 1989; Rankow 1995a, 1995b; Rankow and Tessaro 1998a; W. F. Skinner 1994). Some researchers have also noted that lesbians appear to receive fewer mammograms and clinical breast examinations and are less likely to perform regular breast self-examinations in keeping with recommended standards of care (Biddle 1993; Bradford and Ryan 1988; Bybee 1991; Haynes 1992; Johnson et al. 1987a; O'Hanlan 1993; Rankow and Tessaro 1998b). There are also concerns that lesbian women who are estranged from their families because of their disclosure of their sexual orientation may not have access to family medical records, including history of breast cancer (Rankow 1995c). Current research may help clarify risk factors. Lesbians should follow guidelines for all women, including regular self breast examinations, yearly breast examinations by a health care provider, and mammogram schedules based on age and known risk factors.

## Sexually Transmitted Diseases

Early research showed that sexually transmitted diseases did not occur frequently in lesbian women (Robertson and Schachter 1981), and many clinicians believed that sexually transmitted diseases appeared in lesbians only if they had been sexually active with men. Several researchers (Johnson et al. 1981; Robertson and Schachter 1981) noted that rates of infection with sexually transmitted diseases such as gonorrhea, syphilis, genital herpes, and chlamydia are very low among lesbians who are sexually active exclusively with other women. J. C. White and Levinson (1993) found the rate of transmission of human papillomavirus (HPV) between women to be quite low, although HPV is transmissible from one female partner to another. However, clinical experience suggests that a number of infectious agents can be passed between female sexual partners, including *Candida, Gardnerella vaginalis, Trichomonas, Chlamydia,* and hepatitis A. Newer research is starting to show that genital HPV infection and squamous intraepithelial lesions are not uncommon among women who have sexual intercourse with women and do occur in those who have never been sexually active with men (Carroll et al. 1997; Marrazzo et al. 1998; O'Hanlan and Crum 1996).

The limited research on infectious disease transmission between women greatly hampers clinicians' ability to define cost-effective guidelines for treatment of female partners of women with various gynecologic infections and for prevention of sexually transmitted diseases in lesbians. The following recommendations are based on current knowledge and experience (Rankow 1995c, 1997a; J. C. White 1997):

- Routine screening for sexually transmitted diseases in the absence of signs or symptoms is probably not cost effective in women who are exclusively sexually active with other women.
- When a woman has a recurrent infection, or certainly if her partner is symptomatic, the partner should be examined and cultured as well. Recurrent or resistant vaginal infections may indicate the presence of HIV.
- Lesbians need Pap smears and pelvic exams; how frequently they need them depends on their individual history of sexual behavior, previous sex-

ually transmitted diseases, and number of partners and should follow current guidelines for all women (Marrazzo et al. 1998).

- Because some lesbians may have regular or occasional sex with men, all routine standards of care for both prevention and treatment of infection should apply. Adolescents may be at particular risk of engaging in unprotected activity with both male and female partners.
- To know what anatomic areas require culturing (vagina, throat, anus), the practitioner must have knowledge of what sexual activities have been practiced. Assumptions should not be made.
- Anticipatory guidance about "safer sex" can serve as a less threatening introduction to sensitive topics. Providers should be knowledgeable about the full range of human sexual behavior and be comfortable discussing this in language appropriate for the patient.

Most HIV-positive lesbians are reported to have acquired the infection through intravenous drug use or unprotected heterosexual activity (often with gay or bisexual men or intravenous drug users). Bevier et al. (1995) reported that women who report both drug use and sexual activity with other women were likely to engage in multiple high-risk behaviors, including unprotected vaginal or anal intercourse with bisexual or drug-using male partners, sex for money or drugs, sex while high, and sharing of injection materials. Intravenous drug–using women who reported having intercourse with women were significantly more likely to test positive for HIV than drug-using women who reported having intercourse with men only. Because this is counter to the widespread assumption that lesbians are at low risk for HIV disease, it is especially important to explore the full range of risk behaviors with women who have sex with women.

Only a few incidents of woman-to-woman HIV transmission have been reported in the literature (Chu et al. 1990; Greenhouse 1987; Marmor et al. 1986; Monzon and Capellan 1987; Perry et al. 1989; Rich et al. 1993; Sabatini et al. 1984). However, grassroots lesbian AIDS projects are documenting growing numbers of HIV-positive women whose only apparent risk factor is unprotected sexual activity with an HIV-positive female partner. Because it is known that HIV and other sexually transmitted diseases are transmissible through exchange of body fluids such as cervical or vaginal secretions and menstrual blood, it is imperative that practitioners provide all of their patients with up-to-date guidelines for safer sex (Rankow 1995c): 1) Direct genital-to-genital stimulation between women may allow mucosal exposure to blood, sexual fluids, or genital lesions and may therefore be an unsafe practice. 2) Sexual partners should use latex barriers, male or female condoms, or household plastic wrap to protect against oral contact with vaginal fluids, menstrual blood, blood resulting from traumatic penetration, fecal-borne pathogens, HPV, herpes virus lesions, and breast milk. Although intact skin is usually thought to be adequate protection, latex gloves or finger cots may be worn if one partner has cuts on the fingers or hands. 3) Only water-based lubricants should be used with latex or plastic wrap because oil-based products (including food products that contain oils) may degrade the integrity of the barrier. 4) Ideally, sex toys should not be shared. Alternatively, such objects should be well cleaned and/or covered with a fresh condom between partners or prior to moving from rectum to vagina. 5) Lesbian women engaging in sexual activity with men should follow standard guidelines for "safer sex," including the use of condoms and spermicide for each encounter.

It is essential that public health education messages reflect the reality that lesbian and bisexual women do contract HIV/AIDS and other sexually transmitted diseases. Clinicians need to be aware that the current information in medical literature regarding lesbians may be neither complete nor accurate. Prevention efforts must be comprehensive and should include harm reduction information for female-to-female transmission, heterosexual activity, and drug-related risks.

## Gynecologic Care and Screening

Several researchers have studied the issue of lesbian women and Pap smears (Biddle 1993; Buenting 1992; Bybee 1991; Johnson et al. 1981; Kunkel and Skokan 1998; Marrazzo et al. 1998; Rankow and Tessaro 1998a; Robertson and Schachter 1981). It appears that lesbians are less likely to get pelvic examinations and Pap smears and more likely to wait longer than the recommended interval between such exams. Furthermore, some practitioners have erroneously informed patients that they do not need Pap smears in the mistaken belief that lesbian women do not get cervical cancer (Ferris et al. 1996).

The risk factors for cervical dysplasia and cancer in lesbian women are the same as in heterosexual women, including sexually transmitted disease infection at an early age, multiple sexual partners, smoking, diethylstilbestrol exposure, and exposure to HPV, HIV, or herpes simplex virus. It is important that a practitioner ascertain an individual patient's history to determine an appropriate schedule for pelvic examination and Pap smears. Practitioners should make sure that patients have an accurate understanding of their own risk status, as well as knowledge about the importance and recommended frequency of screening.

Although no full-scale research has been performed on the incidence of gynecologic cancers in lesbian women, it is known that various factors, such as nulliparity and nonuse of oral contraceptives, may increase a woman's risk of endometrial and ovarian cancer. This increases the importance of regular pelvic examinations for these women. Furthermore, women who do not see a practitioner regularly for such screening may also miss the opportunity to receive other important preventive care, including blood pressure checks, cholesterol screening, examination of stool for occult blood, and health education.

## Reproductive Issues

Among the assumptions that a practitioner must work to avoid is the belief that a lesbian woman does not have or is not planning to have children (Patterson 1992). In fact, many lesbians parent children from previous heterosexual relationships and many are creating families with children through adoption, fostering, or conception via donor insemination or heterosexual intercourse. It is vital that practitioners advise women who intend to use insemination that privately obtained semen (as opposed to semen obtained through a licensed sperm bank) may put them at risk of contracting HIV. Licensed sperm banks carefully screen their donor sperm, and fresh sperm donated by a friend or acquaintance will not have been screened and could therefore transmit HIV or other organisms. There is, however, little likelihood of HIV infection if the sperm donor test results are negative for HIV, he abstains from all sexual activity with any possibility of HIV transmission for 6 months, and he is then retested and results are again negative.

To provide optimal prenatal care, a practitioner must continue to provide an open, safe environment in which a patient can freely express her needs. Asking a patient about whom she might like to include in prenatal visits or at the birth (as opposed to asking whether the father will be present) helps convey to the woman that she is in a supportive environment. Asking whether the woman will be a single parent or will be coparenting allows the patient to communicate her family's structure honestly and comfortably. Information about parenting issues, support, and other resources is often available to women from their health care providers. Therefore, it is helpful to know whether a patient has any children or is involved in any parenting relationships.

Although all patients should be encouraged to file a durable power of attorney to designate individuals who have emergency decision-making powers, this process is particularly important for women involved in same-sex relationships. These relationships often do not have the legal protections or rights assumed by a heterosexual spouse. Complications and emotional devastation can occur when partners are denied access, information, or involvement in the care of a loved one. Similarly, legal documents should be drawn up and available to health care providers to allow a nonbiologic parent to have medical authority over her children.

## Mental Health Issues

In any health care practice providing primary or gynecologic care, various psychosocial and mental health issues may need to be addressed. Compared with physical health issues, the literature available about mental health and lesbians is extensive. A recently published book, *Textbook of Homosexuality and Mental Health* (Cabaj and Stein 1996), summarizes current knowledge. Little research is available, however, about the prevalence and incidence of major mental illnesses in lesbians, although no mental illnesses are known to occur more often in lesbians than in other women (Rothblum 1994b). In most contexts, the psychosocial issues that lesbian women bring up with their health care providers are similar to those of heterosexual women and cover the spectrum of depression, anxiety, problems with families (children, parents, partners), work-related problems, substance abuse, loneliness, losses, past or present physical or sexual abuse, and other traumatic events and include significant mental illnesses that should be referred for psychiatric evaluation or treatment (Rothblum 1990, 1994a; Trippett 1994).

Bradford et al. (1994) summarized the mental health information obtained from the National Lesbian Health Care Survey. They reported that rates of depression and suicide attempts in the lesbian women in their sample were similar to rates in heterosexual women. However, more lesbians had participated in counseling at some time during their life than had heterosexuals. Rates of physical abuse, sexual abuse, and incest were high but not significantly different than similar reports for all women. This survey also suggested that substance abuse might be more frequent and eating disorders less frequent in lesbians. Earlier research, which primarily used samples of lesbians found in bar settings, did show that lesbians had significantly higher rates of alcohol abuse, often three times more than heterosexual women (Cabaj 1996; Diamond and Wilsnack 1978; Hall 1993; Lewis et al. 1982).

Newer research, with better sampling, identification, and methods, showed no significant difference in current drinking when comparing lesbian and heterosexual women. However, more lesbians reported past problematic drinking and participation in 12-step recovery programs (Hughes and Wilsnack 1997; Hughes et al. 1997).

Some unique stressors exist for lesbian women. Issues such as social isolation, homophobia, discrimination, fear of hate crimes, "coming out," and the experience of "being different" are complex and potentially alienating. Bradford and Ryan (1988) outlined some of the social abuses suffered by lesbians, which included verbal and physical attacks and lost employment. Members of most minority groups learn about coping with discrimination and difference from their families of origin, who usually share the minority status (DeMonteflores 1986). The effects of discrimination and difference are increasingly complicated for those who are members of more than one minority.

Disruption of relationships with the family of origin may also occur with disclosure of one's sexual orientation or because of fears of the response to disclosure. Rejection by family, friends, religious community, coworkers, or fellow students can be devastating. Lesbians in many states may be denied or lose housing, custody of children, employment, health care, or legal representation solely on the basis of sexual orientation. Such constant blows and threats from all corners of an individual's personal and professional life can result in chronic fear, depression, and damaged self-esteem. Some women respond by internalizing this hatred and directing it against themselves. Abuse of cigarettes, food, alcohol, and other drugs may occur in the face of these types of stress. Furthermore, other sequelae of continual stress may include physical symptoms such as gastric complaints, headaches, or pain syndromes.

Some lesbian women attempt to avoid these stresses by withholding information about their sexual orientation from family, friends, and coworkers. The individual begins living a kind of double life, in which she presents herself publicly as heterosexual while secretly considering herself (or living) as a lesbian. J. Smith (1988) has suggested that the energy invested in such a double life and the experience of living with the constant threat of exposure could take an emotional toll that results in an increased chance for dysthymia and depression.

Practitioners may be presented with various issues related to trauma, especially if nonjudgmental, routine questions are included to elicit current and past traumatic events. Acknowledging the trauma and providing support may be all that is necessary, although providing referral to resources or treatment options experienced with lesbians may be helpful. For instance, lesbian women share with heterosexual women a similar likelihood (about 38%) of being survivors of childhood sexual abuse (Klinger and Stein 1996). Those providing gynecologic health care to survivors of childhood sexual abuse need to be particularly sensitive to these patients' emotional issues (Rankow et al. 1998). Although identification, symptoms, complications, and treatment are similar to those of heterosexual women, knowledge of lesbian-only resources where available is often helpful.

As in any relationship, lesbian relationships may be complicated by domestic violence. However, community resources available to heterosexual women with abusive partners, such as shelters and the legal system, may be homophobic and may deny that lesbian battering exists. As with heterosexual women, discussion of the abuse, strategies for safety, and referral to appropriate resources may be necessary steps in helping the victim (Klinger and Stein 1996; Renzetti 1989).

Any of the life events that may need to be explored with some patients may have different ramifications for lesbians. Loss of a partner (through either death or separation) may be a uniquely difficult trauma for lesbians because the normal social supports available for heterosexual couples are absent. Some lesbians choose to acknowledge the permanence of their relationships with marriage or other commitment ceremonies, whether or not these are supported by their families or faith communities. Finding a faith community accepting of homosexuality is not always easy. Lesbians may have nowhere to find support for issues related to their children and school. Health care practitioners should have an awareness of local, regional, and national resources that may provide needed information, support, and experience.

Some researchers have expressed particular concern about the effect of psychosocial stresses on lesbian women at the extremes of the age spectrum. Teenage women—whether lesbian or unsure of their sexual orientation—and older women may have special concerns. Specific issues may depend on the individual's age, age when she acknowledged her homosexuality, and her social, cultural, and political milieus.

Because adolescence is an intense period during which an individual's identity is explored and begins to gel, lesbian youths have a potentially difficult path. The adolescent tasks of defining self, individuating from family, developing social skills, and finding one's place within society are more complex for lesbians, who must struggle with issues of adolescence without the benefit of supportive societal institutions, role models, and the rituals of passage and celebration available to their heterosexual peers (Kreiss and Patterson 1997). Some studies have found that gay and lesbian youths are at significant risk for suicidality (Moscicki et al. 1995; Proctor and Groze 1994). Gibson (1989) suggested that this risk represents three times the risk for heterosexuals. Homosexual adolescents are also at greater risk for homelessness and its attendant risks of exposure to violence, rape, drug and alcohol use, and sexually transmitted diseases, including HIV/AIDS.

Health care practitioners can alleviate some of the stresses on lesbian teens by providing an environment in which they can expect nonjudgmental care. Inclusive and comprehensive information on risk-reduction guidelines should be offered to all young patients. It is important to allow for the possibility of the full spectrum of behavior, to avoid judgments or assumptions about sexual identity, and to assure confidentiality. Practitioners should be well aware of the painful pressures affecting lesbian adolescents, including social isolation, rejection by family and/or peers, and resulting depression and self-hatred (Kourany 1987).

Older lesbian women may also have an increased risk of social isolation. "Coming out" may have been essentially impossible within their lifetimes, and the result may be intense alienation. Some authors have written about the triple challenge faced by older lesbian women who must struggle against ageism, sexism, and homophobia (Gentry 1992). For women who were unable to disclose themselves as lesbians when they were young, these burdens can become particularly heavy. Some researchers have suggested that older lesbian women are less likely to be involved in the greater lesbian community (Bradford and Ryan 1988). Practitioners should be alert and sensitive to the structure of an individual's support system. The practice environment should be supportive of disclosures that an individual may choose to make but patients should not feel pressured to disclose.

## Summary

Health care practitioners need to be sensitive to the possibility that any of the issues discussed here may affect their lesbian patients. However, it is equally important that practitioners realize the limitations of current research in this field. No assumptions can be made based solely on a patient's sexual orientation. Thorough, methodic, nonjudgmental history-taking is the only way to explore these kinds of issues with each patient individually. In the future, carefully designed epidemiologic studies will provide better information so that practitioners have better resources to guide their care of lesbian patients.

Good health care for lesbian women strongly resembles good health care for any group: a nonjudgmental atmosphere that allows the patient to guide personal disclosures, is respectful of the amazing variety of human behavior and experience, is free of all assumptions, is mindful of the importance of language in defining the dynamics of a relationship, and pays careful attention to the needs of the specific individual being served. Antilesbian biases throughout society in general and the medical profession in particular point to the importance of very consciously working to create an atmosphere of security and respect that will allow the health care needs of nonheterosexual women to be defined and addressed.

Furthermore, epidemiologic studies will help define whether lesbian women have a greater incidence of particular medical problems. Such studies are also needed to help practitioners draw up reasonable guidelines for protecting their patients from exposure to infectious diseases, treating patients who have acquired such diseases, and preventing the spread of infection to partners. Concerns regarding substance use and depression need to be explored, with studies designed to adequately represent the truly diverse lesbian population. Furthermore, many of the issues that are important in both obstetrics/gynecology and psychiatry involve family and couple dynamics and require an understanding of an individual patient's personal psychologic milieu and social supports.

Good (1976) wrote of the importance of gynecologists understanding a patient's sexual and psychosexual orientation in order to provide sound holistic care. He commented that the specialty of obstetrics and gynecology treats conditions and deals with anatomy that is always subject to intense emotional and psychosocial implications. Lesbian women face a complex overlay of issues because of their sexual orientation. Excellent health care for lesbian women takes these issues, and their potential effect on the patient's life, into account.

# References

Banks A, Gartrell N: Lesbians in the medical setting, in Textbook of Homosexuality and Mental Health. Edited by Cabaj RP, Stein TS. Washington, DC, American Psychiatric Press, 1996

Bevier PJ, Chaisson MA, Hefferman RT, et al: Women at a sexually transmitted disease clinic who report same-sex contact: their seroprevalence and risk behaviors. Am J Public Health 85:1366–1371, 1995

Biddle BS: Health Status Indicators for Washington-Area Lesbians and Bisexual Women: A Report on the Lesbian Health Clinic's First Year. Washington, DC, Whitman Walker Clinic, 1993

Bradford J, Ryan C: The National Lesbian Health Care Survey: Final Report. Washington, DC, National Lesbian and Gay Health Foundation, 1988

Bradford J, Ryan C, Rothblum ED: National lesbian health care survey: implications for mental health. J Consult Clin Psychol 62:228–242, 1994

Bradford J, Honnold JA, Ryan C: Disclosure of sexual orientation in survey research on women. Journal of the Gay and Lesbian Medical Association 1:169–177, 1997

Buenting J: Health life-styles of lesbian and heterosexual women. Health Care Women Int 13:165–171, 1992

Bybee D: Michigan Lesbian Health Survey. Lansing, MI, Michigan Organization for Human Rights, 1991

Cabaj RP: Substance abuse in gay men, lesbians, and bisexuals, in Textbook of Homosexuality and Mental Health. Edited by Cabaj RP, Stein TS. Washington, DC, American Psychiatric Press, 1996, pp 783–799

Cabaj RP, Stein, TS (eds): Textbook of Homosexuality and Mental Health. Washington, DC, American Psychiatric Press, 1996

Carroll N, Goldstein R, Lo W, et al: Gynecological infections and sexual practices of Massachusetts lesbian and bisexual women. Journal of the Gay and Lesbian Medical Association 1:15–23, 1997

Chafetz J, Sampson P, Beck P, et al: A study of homosexual women. Social Work 19:714–723, 1974

Chaimowitz GA: Homophobia among psychiatric residents, family practice residents, and psychiatric faculty. Can J Psychiatry 36:206–209, 1991

Chu SY, Buehler JW, Fleming PL, et al: Epidemiology of reported cases of AIDS in lesbians, United States 1980–89. Am J Public Health 80:1380–1381, 1990

Deevey S: Older lesbian women: an invisible minority. J Gerontol Nurs 16:35–39, 1990

DeMonteflores C: Notes on the management of difference, in Contemporary Perspectives on Psychotherapy with Lesbians and Gay Men. Edited by Cabaj RP, Stein TS. New York, Plenum, 1986, pp 73–101

Diamond DL, Wilsnack SC: Alcohol abuse among lesbians: a descriptive study. Journal of Homosexuality 4:123–142, 1978

Douglas CT, Kalman CM, Kalman TP: Homophobia among physicians and nurses: an empirical study. Hospital and Community Psychiatry 36:1309–1311, 1985

Ferris DG, Batish S, Wright TC, et al: A neglected lesbian health concern: cervical neoplasia. J Fam Pract 43:581–584, 1996

Garfinkle EM, Morin SF: Psychologists' attitudes toward homosexual psychotherapy clients. Journal of Social Issues 34:101–112, 1978

Gentry S: Caring for lesbians in a homophobic society. Health Care Women Int 13:173–180, 1992

Gibson P: Gay male and lesbian youth suicide, in ADAMAHA Report of the Secretary's Task Force on Youth Suicide. DHHS Publication No. ADM 89-1623. Washington, DC, Government Printing Office, 1989, pp 110–142

Good R: The gynecologist and the lesbian. Clin Obstet Gynecol 19:473–481, 1976

Greenhouse P: Female-to-female transmission of HIV. Lancet 2:401–402, 1987

Hall JM: Lesbians and alcohol: patterns and paradoxes in medical notions and lesbians' beliefs. J Psychoactive Drugs 25:109–119, 1993

Haynes SG: Are lesbians at high risk of breast cancer? Presented at the 14th National Lesbian and Gay Health Foundation Conference, Los Angeles, CA, July, 1992

Hepburn C, Gutierrez B: Alive and Well: A Lesbian Health Guide. Freedom, CA, Crossing Press, 1988

Herek GM, Kimmel DC, Amaro H, et al: Avoiding heterosexist bias in psychological research. Am Psychol 46:957–963, 1991

Hollibaugh A, Vazquez C, Plumb M: Lesbian Health Issues and Recommendations. Washington, DC, National Gay and Lesbian Task Force Policy Institute, Health Policy Project, 1993

Hughes TL, Wilsnack SC: Use of alcohol among lesbians: research and clinical implications. Am J Orthopsychiatry 67:20–36, 1997

Hughes TL, Hass AP, Avery L: Lesbians and mental health: preliminary results from the Chicago Women's Health Survey. Journal of the Gay and Lesbian Medical Association 1:137–148, 1997

Hume BJ: Perspectives on women's health: disclosure decisions, needs, and experiences of lesbians. Unpublished master's thesis, Yale University, New Haven, CT, 1983

Johnson S, Guenter S: The role of "coming out" by the lesbian in the physician–patient relationship. Women and Therapy 6:231–238, 1987

Johnson S, Guenther S, Laube D, et al: Factors influencing lesbian gynecological care: a preliminary study. Am J Obstet Gynecol 140:20–28, 1981

Johnson SR, Smith EM, Guenther SM: Comparison of gynecologic health care problems between lesbians and bisexual women. J Reprod Med 21:805–811, 1987a

Johnson SR, Smith EM, Guenther SM: Parenting desires among bisexual women and lesbians. J Reprod Med 32:198–200, 1987b

Klinger RL, Stein TS: Impact of violence, childhood sexual abuse, and domestic violence and abuse on lesbians, bisexuals, and gay men, in Textbook of Homosexuality and Mental Health. Edited by Cabaj RP, Stein TS. Washington, DC, American Psychiatric Press, 1996, pp 801–818

Kourany RFC: Suicide among homosexual adolescents. Journal of Homosexuality 13:111–117, 1987

Kreiss JL, Patterson DL: Psychosocial issues in primary care of lesbian, gay, bisexual, and transgender youth. J Pediatr Health Care 11:266–274, 1997

Kunkle LE, Skokan LA: Factors which influence cervical cancer screening among lesbians. Journal of the Gay and Lesbian Medical Association 2:7–15, 1998

Kurdek LA, Schmitt JP: Perceived emotional support from family and friends in members of homosexual, married, and heterosexual cohabiting couples. Journal of Homosexuality 14:3–4, 1987

Lewis CE, Saghir MT, Robins E: Drinking patterns in homosexual and heterosexual women. J Clin Psychiatry 43:277–279, 1982

Marmor M, Weiss LR, Lyden M, et al: Possible female-to-female transmission of human immunodeficiency virus (letter). Ann Intern Med 105:969, 1986

Marrazzo JM, Koutsky LA, Stine KL, et al: Genital human papillomavirus infection in women who have sex with women. J Infect Dis 187:1604–1609, 1998

Mathews WC, Booth MW, Turner JD, et al: Physicians' attitudes towards homosexuality: survey of a California county medical society. West J Med 144:106–110, 1986

McKirnan DJ, Peterson PL: Alcohol and drug use among homosexual men and women: epidemiology and population characteristics. Addict Behav 14:545–553, 1989

Michaels S: The prevalence of homosexuality in the United States, in Textbook of Homosexuality and Mental Health. Edited by Cabaj RP, Stein TS. Washington, DC, American Psychiatric Press, 1996, pp 801–818

Monzon OT, Capellan JMB: Female-to-female transmission of HIV. Lancet 2:40–41, 1987

Moscicki EK, Muehrer P, Potter LB, et al (eds): Research Issues in Suicide and Sexual Orientation. Suicide and Life-Threatening Behavior 25(suppl):1–94, 1995

Muller MJ, White JC: Medical student attitudes towards homosexuality: evaluation of a second-year curriculum. Journal of the Gay and Lesbian Medical Association 1:155–159, 1997

O'Hanlan KA: Lesbians in health research. Presentation to the Office of Research on Women's Health, National Institutes of Health scientific meeting on the recruitment and retention of women in clinical studies (NIH publication No. 95-3756). Washington, DC, U.S. Department of Health and Human Services, 1993

O'Hanlan KA, Crum CP: Human papillomavirus-associated cervical intraepithelial neoplasia following lesbian sex. Obstet Gynecol 88:702–703, 1996

Olsen CG, Mann BL: Medical student attitudes on homosexuality and implications for health care. Journal of the Gay and Lesbian Medical Association 1:149–154, 1997

Patterson CJ: Children of lesbian and gay parents. Child Dev 63:1025–1042, 1992

Perry S, Jacobsberg L, Fogel K: Orogenital transmission of human immunodeficiency virus (letter). Ann Intern Med 111:951–952, 1989

Peterson L, Doll L, White C, et al: No evidence for female-to-female HIV transmission among 960,000 female blood donors. J Acquir Immun Defic Syndr 5:853–855, 1992

Proctor CD, Groze VK: Risk factors for suicide among gay, lesbian, and bisexual youths. Journal of Social Work 39:504–513, 1994

Randall CE: Lesbian phobia among BSN educators: a survey. J Nurs Educ 28:302–306, 1989

Rankow EJ: Breast and cervical cancer among lesbians. Women's Health Issues 5:123–129, 1995a

Rankow EJ: Lesbian health issues for the primary care provider. J Fam Pract 40:486–493, 1995b

Rankow EJ: Women's Health Issues: Planning for Diversity. Washington, DC, National Lesbian and Gay Health Association, 1995c

Rankow EJ: Addressing the HIV care needs of women who have sex with women. Innovations: Issues in HIV Service Delivery Spring:10–11, 1997a

Rankow EJ: Lesbian health issues and cultural sensitivity training for providers in the primary care setting: results of a pilot intervention. Journal of the Gay and Lesbian Medical Association 1:235–242, 1997b

Rankow EJ: Primary care concerns of the gay or lesbian patient. N C Med J 58:92–98, 1997c

Rankow EJ: Applying principles of cultural competency to research on lesbian health. Journal of the Gay and Lesbian Medical Association 2:135–138, 1998

Rankow EJ, Tessaro I: Cervical cancer risk and papanicolaou screening in a sample of lesbian and bisexual women. J Fam Pract 47:139–143, 1998a

Rankow EJ, Tessaro I: Mammography and risk factors for breast cancer in a sample of lesbian and bisexual women. Am J Health Behav 22:403–410, 1998b

Rankow EJ, Cambre KM, Cooper K: Health care seeking behavior of adult lesbian and bisexual survivors of childhood sexual abuse. Journal of the Gay and Lesbian Medical Association 2:69–76, 1998

Renzetti CM: Building a second closet: third party responses to victims of lesbian partner abuse. Family Relations 38:157–163, 1989

Rich JD, Buck A, Tuomala RE, et al: Transmission of human immunodeficiency virus presumed to have occurred via female homosexual contact. Clin Infect Dis 17:1003–1005, 1993

Roberts SA, Dibble SL, Scanlon JL, et al: Differences in risk factors for breast cancer: lesbian and heterosexual women. Journal of the Gay and Lesbian Medical Association 2:93–101, 1998

Robertson M: Lesbians as an invisible minority in the health services arena. Health Care Women Int 13:155–163, 1992

Robertson P, Schachter J: Failure to identify venereal disease in a lesbian population. Sex Transm Dis 8:75–76, 1981

Rothblum ED: Depression among lesbians: an invisible and unresearched phenomenon. Journal of Gay and Lesbian Psychotherapy 1:67–87, 1990

Rothblum ED: Introduction to the special section; mental health of lesbians and gay men. J Consult Clin Psychol 62:211–212, 1994a

Rothblum ED: "I only read about myself on bathroom walls": the need for research on the mental health of lesbians and gay men. J Consult Clin Psychol 62:213–220, 1994b

Sabatini MT, Patel K, Hirschman R: Kaposi's sarcoma and t-cell lymphoma in an immunodeficient woman: a case report. AIDS Res 1:135–137, 1984

Saunders JM, Tupac JD, MacCulloch B: A Lesbian Profile: A Survey of 1000 Lesbians. West Hollywood, CA, Southern California Women for Understanding, 1988

Shatz B, O'Hanlan K: Anti-Gay Discrimination in Medicine: Results of a National Survey of Lesbian, Gay, and Bisexual Physicians. San Francisco, CA, Gay and Lesbian Medical Association (formerly American Association of Physicians for Human Rights), 1994

Skinner WF: The prevalence and demographic predictors of illicit and licit drug use among lesbians and gay men. Am J Public Health 84:1307–1310, 1994

Smith J: Psychopathology, homosexuality, and homophobia. Journal of Homosexuality 15:59–73, 1988

Solarz AL (ed): Lesbian Health: Current Assessment and Directions for the Future. Washington, DC, National Academy Press, 1999

Stevens PE: Lesbian health care research: a review of the literature from 1970 to 1990. Health Care Women Int 13:91–120, 1992

Stevens PE, Hall JM: Stigma, health beliefs, and experiences with health care in lesbian women. Image: Journal of Nursing Scholarship 20:69–73, 1988

Stevens PE, Hall JM: Abusive health care ineteractions experienced by lesbians: a case of institutional violence in the treatment of women. Response: To the Victimization of Women and Children 13:23–27, 1990

Townsend MH: Gay and lesbian issues in graduate medical education. N C Med J 58:114–116, 1997

Townsend MH, Wallick MM: Gay, lesbian, and bisexual issues in medical schools, in Textbook of Homosexuality and Mental Health. Edited by Cabaj RP, Stein TS. Washington, DC, American Psychiatric Press, 1996, pp 633–644

Trippet SE: Lesbians' mental health concerns. Health Care Women Int 15:317–323, 1994

Trippet SE, Bain J: Reasons American lesbians fail to seek traditional health care. Health Care Women Int 13:145–153, 1992

Wallick MM: Homophobia and heterosexism: out of the medical school closet. N C Med J 58:123–125, 1997

Wallick MM, Cambre KM, Townsend MH: How the topic of homosexuality is taught at U.S. medical schools. Acad Med 67:601–603, 1992

White JC: HIV risk assessment and prevention in lesbians and women who have sex with women: practical information for clinicians. Health Care Women Int 18:127–138, 1997

White JC: Challenges and opportunities in clinical research on lesbian health. Journal of the Gay and Lesbian Medical Association 2:55–57, 1998

White JC, Dull VT: Health risk factors and health-seeking behavior in lesbians. J Womens Health 6:103–112, 1997

White JC, Levinson W: Lesbian health care: what a primary care physician needs to know. West J Med 162:463–466, 1995

White JC, Levinson W: Primary care of lesbian patients. J Gen Intern Med 8:41–47, 1993

White TA: Attitudes of psychiatric nurses toward same sex orientations. Nurs Res 28:276–281, 1979

Zeidenstein L: Gynecological and childbearing needs of lesbians. J Nurse Midwifery 35:10–16, 1990

# Ethics and Women's Health

CAROL C. NADELSON, M.D.

Despite their basis in rationality, ethical principles are influenced by personal values and beliefs and by societal context. In medicine, as new technologies have emerged and health care delivery systems have changed, beliefs about the responsibilities, obligations, and relationships between health care providers and patients have been challenged, and some have changed (Nadelson 1996).

The increasing complexity and cost of technology, coupled with limited resources to provide care, create new ethical dilemmas related to the need to make decisions based on competing priorities, often without established guidelines about processes or guiding principles. Values and ethical systems also vary widely among cultures and individuals and often conflict.

As health care delivery systems evolve, decisions about medical care are increasingly being made by those whose training and ethical frameworks are not in health care but in business and economics. Thus, their perspective and priorities may differ from those with medical training who traditionally were responsible for these decisions. For example, the chief executive officers (CEOs) of profit-making managed care organizations do not expect to deliver care in the same way as if they were running nonprofit organizations. They must be focused on the interests of their investors. Their *primary* concern is not the public good, although they may provide public benefit. They might decide whether or not to include a specific procedure as a benefit of a partic-ular health plan based more on economic factors than on clinical indications. Likewise, in the interest of efficiency and better information transfer, they might decide to institute computerized medical records and require disclosure of patient diagnostic and treatment information, thus making confidential patient information more accessible to a range of people, many of whom have no involvement in patient care. Although patients may consent to this release of information, they do so under duress, because they fear losing health care coverage if they do not. The concept of informed consent is altered by this practice; it is not truly informed consent if the patient has no alternative. Physicians may also favor having data more available to them, not being cognizant of implications for patients in terms of their privacy concerns or their risk of losing future insurability if certain information is not treated confidentially.

These issues have ethical implications for all involved in health care delivery. This chapter describes general principles of medical ethics and focuses on those that have special consequence for women's health.

## Changing Codes of Medical Ethics

Codes of medical ethics have existed since ancient times and have varied with culture and era. Currently, as guiding principles, most Western countries emphasize the autonomy or self-determination of patients, a concept of beneficence that implies doing good rather than merely doing no harm, a concept of justice related to access to resources, and the physician's primary responsibility to his/her individual patient (Nadelson 1991).

Different priorities are placed on these principles in different countries and systems of care. Thus, patient autonomy might be considered less important than equitable access to resources, and limiting the availability of a particular procedure or medication may be a policy based on socioeconomic, age, or prognostic factors. Patient autonomy might also be considered less important than family interests (so that another person, such as a spouse or parent, might be required to consent to a procedure), or than government interests (so that the government might make a specific treatment or procedure unavailable, such as contraception or abortion, contrary to the desire of the woman involved). "Paternalism is the intentional limitation of the autonomy of one person by another, where the person who limits autonomy justifies the action exclusively by the goal of helping the person whose autonomy is limited. Paternalism seizes decision-making authority by preventing persons from making or implementing their own decisions" (Beauchamp 1995, pp. 1914–1915). Thus, paternalism is a fundamental concern in medical ethics; whether and when it can be morally justified has been the subject of much debate.

In the United States, the locus of paternalism in health care has shifted with changes in delivery systems. Many of the manifestations of paternalism observed in physicians in the past are less evident in the practices of individual physicians today and more apparent in health care systems themselves. These systems, like all bureaucracies, are even less likely to be empathic with the needs or autonomy of individuals than many physicians were in the past or to take account of differences between patients (Nadelson 1994), and they are more likely to consider societal interests as primary in order to predict and control costs and health outcomes.

Debates about confidentiality and informed consent often involve paternalism and autonomy, as the earlier example of the company CEO making a decision to abrogate patient confidentiality illustrates. These issues have been most striking in debates about whether managed care organizations and the physicians they employ must inform patients of all appropriate treatments for their medical conditions and, in addition, notify them of the limits imposed by their particular health care contract.

Decisions about the availability of a particular type of care are often dealt with paternalistically, although ostensibly the patient may seem to have some choice. The patient may be asked to pay a high copayment for certain procedures, or care may be denied based on gatekeeping policies, the nature of which are often not disclosed to the patient or physician. For example, although psychiatric care may be covered with specific guidelines regarding number of visits allowed or the payment per visit, indirect limits can be imposed by limiting approved providers, not providing options for patients to receive partial benefits if they wish to seek care outside of their particular health care plan, not allotting all visits written into the plan by setting up exclusionary criteria for each visit, or by limiting approved services, such as psychotherapy, to a certain number of visits. These decisions are often made by gatekeepers who may have no mental health background, have not seen the patient, and who are following a rigid protocol that determines the number of visits allocated to a particular symptom or diagnosis.

Pellegrino and Thomasma (1988) have indicated that the conflicting ethical principles in contemporary health care are based on business, contractual, preventive, covenantal, and beneficence models. From the business perspective, they suggest that medicine has come to be seen as a commodity and that the ethical obligation of doctor to patient has become that of businessman to consumer. The contractual model is an extension of the business model whereby a contract formalizes the relationship, which could protect the patient from excessive physician paternalism or economic self-interest, but could also limit the commitment and responsibility inherent in the physician–patient relationship. The preventive or public health model obligates the health care provider to protect many "healths" and does not place as high a priority on the individual doctor–patient relationship. Current health care delivery systems involving managed care organizations, including health maintenance organizations, use various combinations of these models and focus less on individual patients and more on the groups of patients or "lives" they cover.

A somewhat different perspective is the covenantal model, which is grounded in the trust and obligation between the physician and the patient. In reemphasizing the importance of the principle of beneficence inherent in this model, Pellegrino and Thomasma (1988) have suggested that the physician and patient are joined because of the patient's needs and that both partners recognize the patient's dependence on the physician and the physician's responsibility for making good and moral judgments on the patient's behalf. This model acknowledges that the patient who is ill may not be capable of totally free and informed consent or autonomy by virtue of anxiety, fear, or lack of knowledge, and he/she expects that the physician will act beneficently.

The nature of the covenantal relationship and the principle of beneficence call into question the ethics of many current medical practices, including the role of physician as a gatekeeper or guardian of society's resources in the rationing of health care (Nadelson 1986; Pellegrino and Thomasma 1988). Serious ethical questions arise if the physician cannot be trusted to act in his/her patient's best interests. If the physician becomes a double or triple agent, acting for a managed care organization, the government, an insurance company, an employer, and presumably for the patient as well, the convanental relationship is compromised.

Physicians in today's society find it increasingly difficult to differentiate their roles and responsibilities as agents of their patients from their roles as agents of those with interests beyond those of the individual. Conflict between these roles is particularly evident in laws requiring that confidentiality be breached, such as by reporting child abuse, threats of harm to another individual, or certain illnesses, such as sexually transmitted diseases. Protecting the confidentiality of physician–patient relationships runs counter to societal concern about the public good in these situations, and confidentiality may not be upheld as an overriding ethical principle in courts of law (Freudenheim 1991). The earlier illustration regarding the confidentiality of medical records is another example of a breach of confidentiality not necessarily based on the wishes or concerns of the individual patient.

Compromising confidentiality has many potential repercussions, including the possibility that patients will no longer trust their physicians with certain types of information or seek appropriate or necessary care. Requirements for reporting HIV-positive individuals for the purpose of tracing contacts and advising them about risks or for reporting patients who have made threats of violence or committed child abuse or other crimes of violence are of particular concern to patients. Use of genetic testing raises additional concerns about confidentiality because of the potential that this information might be used to exclude people from health insurance or employment or for other discriminatory practices.

Another aspect of the conflicting roles of physicians that has important ethical considerations is the pressure to make decisions based on nonclinical indications. For example, for economic reasons such as increasing reimbursement or decreasing cost, a physician may be pressured to recommend one treatment rather than another, to use an alternative medication instead of one that he or she might ordinarily prescribe, or to discharge a patient from the hospital when, in his or her clinical judgment, these are not the best decisions for the patient. Although physicians are held accountable for their medical decisions and can technically override the decisions of health care organizations and insurance companies, the decision of whether to pay for a treatment effectively precludes certain types of care for many patients. Insurance and managed care companies have argued that they are not practicing medicine and are justified in making decisions about reimbursement, an opinion that is increasingly not shared by the courts and legislatures.

Physicians may also be asked to take responsibility for treatments they have not personally recommended or administered because other personnel, who may not be legally qualified, have been the direct caretaker of the patient. This request places the physician in an ethical (and legal) dilemma and potentially harms the patient, often without his or her knowledge or consent (Nadelson 1986).

## Ethical Issues: Women Patients

In the United States, many of the practices described above affect women more than men because women are more often poor, uninsured or underinsured, and have had more limited access to comprehensive health insurance (Institute of Medicine 1991). In addition, many insurers do not cover gender-specific preventive care, such as mammograms or Pap smears, and may not pay for specific medications such as hormone therapy or certain antidepressants. Failure to reimburse for medications more adversely affects women because they are prescribed more medications, including psychotropic medications, than are men (National Institutes of Health 1992; Taggart et al. 1993).

Women are also higher users of health care services generally, are more likely to use home health care because they have more chronic illness, more often live alone (especially as they age), and pay more out-of-pocket than do men because their coverage is less adequate (Commonwealth Fund 1997). Higher copayments or other restrictions on access to care are likely to further increase costs and limit services available to women.

Policies related to reproduction, including availability of sterilization or abortion, and allocation of resources for new reproductive technologies clearly affect women more than men and decisions about them are often paternalistic. For example, the decision in the United States to prohibit development or use of RU 486, an abortifacient with other possible medical uses, was based on the values and beliefs of those with decision-making authority, not those of the women who would be most affected. Other examples include decisions about insurance coverage for infertility treatments, funding birth control or abortion services, and banning the use of fetal tissue for research, the latter of which occurred because it was felt that more women would seek abortions if they felt there was a justification for it or that "good" use could be made of the products of conception (Hilts 1991).

The special characteristics of women's reproductive roles lead to specific ethical considerations. Because decisions about childbearing, contraception, abortion, sterilization, and surgery involving reproductive organs have profound social consequences, the autonomy of a woman in deciding these questions is often challenged. In many cultures, woman have not been in a position to achieve their own goals if those goals are distinct from those of their family and society. Decisions about medical care or surgical procedures that have an impact on sexuality and childbearing are often made by others and reflect the personal, cultural, or religious values of the physician, family, or society (Nadelson 1994). For example, whether sterilization or abortion is funded can determine whether a woman can make that choice. In these cases, assumptions are made and actions are taken that compromise a woman's autonomy. As Nelson (1992) stated,

> Social response to women's reproductive abilities typically has made their bodies part of the public domain in a way that men's are not . . . And as wombs have become increasingly public spaces medically, they have also be-

come increasingly public politically; women's choices, not only about how they manage their pregnancies, but also about how they will manage their work, their leisure, their use of both legal and illegal drugs, and their sexuality, are further subject to society's scrutiny and to the law's constraints. (p. 13)

One of the more troubling contemporary ethical dilemmas concerns the purposes and uses of prenatal testing. When used to diagnose fetal disorders, prenatal testing may lead to a decision to have an abortion, which may be counter to public policy. Even those who support the right to choose abortion, however, may be uncomfortable about the potential use of abortion for social reasons including family finances, unmarried status, or even gender selection. From an ethical perspective any restriction can be said to limit a woman's autonomy and place the interests of the mother in opposition to those of the fetus, but the limits of fetal, maternal, and paternal rights have not been clearly defined.

Because prenatal testing can reveal the gender of a fetus, abortion could occur because that gender is undesired. In addition to the ethical problem this raises, other potential consequences exist. In families and cultures in which male children are more valued than female children, major changes in population demographics could occur and have been reported. The argument has also been made that once these new technologies are available, control of their use is not possible. Thus, unethical or coercive practices could result, including forced abortion and even infanticide. Debate about a particular abortion procedure, called *partial birth abortion* in the popular press and federal and state legislatures, has raised concerns about legislating medical procedures, the ethics of overriding the clinical judgment of a physician in determining medical indications, and the autonomy of both physician and patient in making medical decisions.

Extensive use of reproductive technologies, including requests from elderly, unmarried, and homosexual people, also raises ethical dilemmas. Paternalism is evident in biases about what constitutes "legitimate" families and who should be accorded use of new technologies. Gender bias about motherhood for elderly women is clearly demonstrated by the lack of similar concern about the high numbers of elderly men becoming fathers (Angell 1997). New technologies, Brody (1988) notes, "raise the specter of reproduction totally controlled by females . . . Patriarchal dominance and male lineage are suddenly at risk. Affiliative rights and knowledge of parenthood, particularly of fatherhood as an aspect of identity, become unsure. Even the social mother can no longer state with certainty that this is her biological offspring" (p. 203).

These techniques and their use raise questions about the role of biologic versus social parents, the rights of children born from these procedures, and the nature of informed consent by all parties. A woman donating ova or making a surrogate contract, for example, may have been coerced, especially if financial recompense is part of the decision. She may not able to make an informed decision because she cannot predict her feelings after gestation. The advent of surrogacy has also brought into focus questions about whether women can be used as incubators and whether fetuses have become commodities, raising the specter of forced pregnancy presented by Margaret Atwood in her novel *The Handmaid's Tale*. Certainly, contractual surrogacy and ovum donation place pressure on poor women to rent their bodies or parts of their bodies.

Mental health professionals are often called on with the expectation that they can predict outcomes and psychologic risks despite the absence of data on psychologic impact. Not only is information lacking on how men and women involved in these technologies will fare, but no data are available on the outcome for children born into these families. In addition, no guidelines or criteria for selection of surrogate mothers and families have been formed, although there has been a great deal of polarized debate.

Additional ethical questions involving the rights and status of children born through these new techniques remain unsettled. The right to know one's genetic, family, and medical background has been controversial in cases of adoption; it is also controversial in cases of surrogacy or other types of reproductive technologies. A potential conflict exists between the privacy interests of the parents and the right of the child to know. In many instances records are altered or simply not kept.

Use of embryo freezing with potential for later use raises additional ethical dilemmas and legal problems when couples divorce, die, or seek to terminate the "life" of the embryo. A new kind of paternalism also arises when procedures and technologies are reserved for specific types of individuals or situations (e.g., only where there is an organic impediment to conception, or when the women requesting the techonology are married heterosexuals or within certain age boundaries) (Van Hall 1988). These decisions are often made by practitioners, with their own biases and expectations, rather than as a result of an informed and deliberative decision-making process.

Substance abuse during pregnancy is another subject of ethical and legal controversy. Historically, the fetus was more often viewed as a potential threat to the mother's life and health because pregnancy and childbirth resulted in substantial morbidity and mortality rates. In recent years, as the physical dangers have decreased, mothers have come to be seen as potential threats to their offspring. Thus, pregnant alcohol- and drug-addicted women have been subjected to legal action and even prison sentences. This pits the autonomy of the mother against the interests of the fetus. In addition, it changes the nature of the obstetrician–patient relationship, because the obstetrician is treating both the mother and the fetus as "the patient" rather than just the mother. As in the case of abortion, the fetus is accorded the same rights and personhood as the mother despite the total physiologic dependency of the fetus on the mother. Ethicists have long debated when and whether the personhood of the fetus can be differentiated from that of the mother (Blank 1986; Bowes and Selgestad 1981; Cole 1990; Harrison 1990; Johnsen 1987; Lenow 1983; McNulty 1987–1988; Murray 1987; Nadelson 1994; Rhoden 1987).

Another controversy involving pregnant women relates to consent for in utero treatment of their fetuses and whether failure to consent constitutes fetal abuse. Here, a distinction between moral and legal responsibilities of the mother has been made. It has generally been held that a pregnant woman cannot be coerced into accepting a treatment to benefit her fetus. The physician's ethical duty according to the American Medical Association Board of Trustees (1990) is to be noncoercive and accept the informed decision of the patient.

The emergence of AIDS in all segments of our society has also raised ethical considerations regarding HIV testing, the right to privacy, and the protection of others. This has increasingly emerged as an issue for women because the AIDS rate in young women is rapidly rising, often related to coercive sexual practices, and women have not benefited from some of the successful new treatments (Benderly 1997).

## Physician–Patient Sexual Interaction

Concern is increasing about sexual interaction between physicians and other health care providers and their patients. Although the incidence of these sexual contacts is difficult to accurately document, reports suggest that it is a significant problem (American Medical Assocation 1990). In the past, sexual activity with patients was defended by some physicians as not necessarily harmful and possibly therapeutic, but the profession has judged it to be categorically exploitative and unethical, compromising the ability of the physician to be objective and to give necessary care. Studies have also determined that it is damaging to patients and may have acute as well as long-term consequences. In addition to the shame, guilt, and mistrust patients experience, they have been reported to suffer from posttraumatic stress disorder, anxiety and depressive disorders, sexual symptoms, sleep disorders, and substance abuse. Reports have also been made of increased suicide risk and psychiatric hospitalization (American Medical Association 1990; American Psychiatric Association 1989; Bouhoutsos et al. 1983; Burgess 1981; Feldman-Summers and Jones 1984; Gabbard 1989; Herman et al. 1987; Kluft 1989; Pope and Bouhoutsos 1986; Simon 1991).

Several reasons exist for the decision to consider doctor–patient sexual intercourse to be unethical. First, it breaches the fundamental trust of this fiduciary relationship. Second, it casts doubt on the physician's capacity for objective professional judgment. Third, it must take account of the patient's psychologic involvement with the physician inherent in the clinical situation. Patients rapidly develop feelings toward their doctors, called *transference,* which involves the displacement of feelings derived from past relationships onto the current doctor–patient relationship. The doctor can thus be viewed as an all-knowing parent, and a great deal of power is turned over to the doctor by the patient (Gabbard and Nadelson 1995).

Although some believe that a relationship might not be unethical in certain circumstances, for example, when the clinical encounter is brief such as occurs in an emergency room, or when the care provided does not involve an intense interpersonal relationship, as occurs when a patient receives anesthesia. However, there is reason to be cautious even in these circumstances. The patient may overidealize the physician as a savior and succumb to a seduction. Likewise, questions have been raised about when a patient ceases to be a patient and how long can one assume that the transference would be operative. No clear guidelines exist, and certainly questions about paternalism can be raised by the restrictiveness of many current ethical and legal standards and procedures.

Efforts to enforce ethical guidelines forbidding sexual activity between doctor and patient have been hampered by concerns about confidentiality and public exposure that have made it difficult for patients to register formal complaints (Marmor 1976). Substantial progress, however, has been made in the past decade. Civil actions have been brought in the courts, and several states have adopted criminal, civil, and licensing regulations that specifically proscribe sexual contact with patients on the part of psychotherapists, physicians, other health care providers as well as others in positions of authority such as teachers and employers (Jorgenson et al. 1991). Between 5% and 10% of psychiatrists and psychologists have reported sexual contact with patients

(Gartrell et al. 1989). Some data available on sexual interaction between patients and nonpsychiatric physicians suggest that the figures are comparable in the United States and other countries. For psychiatrists in the United States, it has been estimated that about 88% of reported incidents of sexual misconduct involve male psychiatrists and female patients; 7.6% involve male psychiatrists and male patients; and 3.5% involve female psychiatrists and female patients (Gartrell et al. 1989; Simon 1989). In a series of over 2,000 cases of therapist–patient sex, Schoener et al. (1989) noted that approximately 20% of cases involved a same-sex dyad, and 20% of the therapists were female.

## Conclusion

This chapter considers the basic principles of medical ethics and briefly touches on some contemporary and emerging ethical issues, including those that especially affect women. For the physician, the complex dynamics of the relationship with the patient demand continual vigilance in order to maintain clarity about his or her role as the patient's advocate as opposed to the agent of society and about the special nature of the boundary of professional and personal relationships. For society, the changing role of women and the emergence of new technologies, especially those involving reproduction, have raised questions with profound ethical implications. It is also clear that culturally determined ethical values often clash. At this time, medical decision making and the processes for resolving some of the dilemmas discussed here are inconsistent. It will likely take some time to resolve these ethical issues.

## References

American Medical Association: Sexual misconduct in the practice of medicine: report of the Council on Ethical and Judicial Affairs of the American Medical Association. Presented to and passed by the House of Delegates, Miami, FL, December 19, 1990

American Medical Assocation Board of Trustees: Legal interventions during pregnancy: court-ordered medical treatments and legal penalties for potentially harmful behavior by pregnant women. JAMA 264:2663–2670, 1990

American Psychiatric Association: The Principles of Medical Ethics (with annotation especially applicable to psychiatry). Washington, DC, American Psychiatric Association, 1989

Angell M: Pregnant at 63? Why not? New York Times, 25 Apr 1997, p A31

Beauchamp TL: Paternalism, in Encyclopedia of Bioethics, Vol 4, 2nd Edition. Edited by Reich WT. New York, Simon & Schuster Macmillan, 1995, pp 1914–1920.

Benderly BL: In Her Own Right: The Institute of Medicine's Guide to Women's Health Issues. Washington, DC, National Academy Press, 1997

Blank R: Emerging notions of women's rights and responsibilities during gestation. J Leg Med 7:441–469, 1986

Bouhoutsos J, Holroyd J, Lerman H, et al: Sexual intimacy between psychotherapists and patients. Professional Psychology: Research and Practice 14:185–196, 1983

Bowes W, Selgestad B: Fetal versus maternal rights: medical and legal perspectives. Obstet Gynecol 58:209–214, 1981

Brody E: Culture, reproductive technology and women's rights: an intergovernmental perspective. J Psychosom Obstet Gynaecol 9:199–205, 1988

Burgess A: Physician sexual misconduct and patients' responses. Am J Psychiatry 138:1335–1342, 1981

Cole H: Legal interventions during pregnancy. JAMA 264:2663–2670, 1990

Commonwealth Fund: Selected Facts on U.S. Women's Health. New York, Commonwealth Fund, 1997

Feldman-Summers S, Jones G: Psychological impacts on sexual contact between therapists or other health care practitioners and their clients. J Consult Clin Psychol 52:1054–1061, 1984

Freudenheim M: Business and health: guarding medical confidentiality. New York Times, 1 Jan 1991, p 1

Gabbard G: Sexual Exploitation in Professional Relationships. Washington, DC, American Psychiatric Press, 1989

Gabbard G, Nadelson C: Professional boundaries in the physician-patient relationship. JAMA 273:1445–1449, 1995

Gartrell H, Herman J, Olarte S, et al: Prevalence of psychiatrist-patients sexual contact, in Sexual Exploitation in Professional Relationships. Edted by Gabbard G. Washington, DC, American Psychiatric Press, 1989, pp 3–13

Harrison M: Psychological ramifications of "surrogate" motherhood, in Psychiatric Aspects of Reproductive Technology. Edited by Stotland NL. Washington, DC, American Psychiatric Press, 1990, pp 97–112

Herman J, Gartrell N, Olarte S, et al: Psychiatrist–patient sexual contact: results of a national survey, II. Psychiatrists' attitudes. Am J Psychiatry 144:164–169, 1987

Hilts P: Groups set up panel on use of fetal tissue. New York Times, 8 Jan 1991, p 24D

Institute of Medicine: Assessing Future Research Needs: Mental and Addictive Disorders in Women. Washington, DC, Institute of Medicine, 1991

Johnsen D: A new threat to pregnant women's autonomy. Hastings Cent Rep 17:33–40, 1987

Jorgenson L, Randles R, Strasburger L: The furor over psychotherapist–patient sexual contact: new solutions to an old problem. William and Mary Law Review 32:645–732, 1991

Kluft R: Treating the patient who has been exploited by a previous therapist. Psychiatr Clin North Am 12:483–500, 1989

Lenow J: The fetus as a patient: emerging righs as a person? Am J Law Med 9:1–29, 1983

Marmor J: The seductive psychiatrist. Psychiatry Digest 31:10–16, 1976

McNulty M: Pregnancy police: the health policy and legal implications of punishing pregnant women for harm to their fetuses. New York University Review of Law and Social Change 16:277–319, 1987–1988

Murray T: Moral obligations to the not-yet born: the fetus as patient. Clin Perinatol 14:329–343, 1987

Nadelson CC: Presidential address. Health care directions: who cares for patients? Am J Psychiatry 143:949–955, 1986

Nadelson CC: Emerging issues in medical ethics. Br J Psychiatry 158(suppl):9–16, 1991

Nadelson CC: Health care: is society empathic with women? in The Empathic Practitioner: Empathy, Gender, and Medicine. Edited by More ES, Milligan MA. New Brunswick, NJ, Rutgers University Press, 1994, pp 190–204

Nadelson CC: Ethics and empathy in a changing health care system. Pharos 59:29–32, 1996

National Institutes of Health: Opportunities for Research on Women's Health (NIH Publication No. #92-3457). Washington, DC, US Department of Health and Human Services, 1992

Nelson JL: Comment. Hastings Cent Rep 22:13, 1992

Pellegrino E, Thomasma D: For the Patient's Good. New York, Oxford University Press, 1988

Pope K, Bouhoutsos J: Sexual Intimacy Between Therapists and Patients. New York, Praeger, 1986

Rhoden N: Cesareans and samaritans. Law, Medicine, and Health Care 15:118–125, 1987

Schoener G, Milgrom J, Gonsiorek J, et al: Psychotherapists' Sexual Involvement with Clients: Intervention and Prevention. Minneapolis, MN, Walk-In Counseling Center, 1989

Simon R: Sexual exploitation of patients: how it begins before it happens. Psychiatr Ann 9:104–112, 1989

Simon RI: Psychological injury caused by boundary violation precursors to therapist-patient sex. Psychiatr Ann 21:614–619, 1991

Taggart LAP, McCammon SL, Allred LJ, et al: Effect of patient and physician gender on prescriptions for psychotropic drugs. J Womens Health 2:353–357, 1993

Van Hall E: Manipulation of human reporduction. J Psychosom Obstet Gynaecol 9:207–213, 1988

# The Male Perspective

MICHAEL F. MYERS, M.D., F.R.C.P.C.

Scanning the table of contents of this book on the health care of women, one sees that the substance of every chapter in each of the three sections affects (and is affected by) men—men as husbands or boyfriends, men as other family members (e.g., fathers, brothers, sons), men as friends, and men as clinicians to women. Furthermore, the notion of "men in relation to women" (Bergman and Surrey 1992) forms a critical element in understanding many of the illnesses and problems described here: the presenting symptoms, the etiology of the symptoms, how openly and comfortably the woman communicates her distress, how significant men in her life react or do not react, the ways in which male and female physicians interview, diagnose, and treat women patients, and what is taught and granted ascendancy in our medical schools and training settings. Our time-honored biopsychosocial model of assessing and treating patients demands an in-depth appreciation of the role of gender in the exemplary care of women.

It is impossible to do an exhaustive analysis of the male perspective in all of the areas covered by this text. I have selected only certain clinical situations in the hope that many of my observations and those of others extend further. My "data" are the stories of men and women patients seen over my 25 years of psychiatric practice as both an individual therapist and marital therapist; my professional liaison with colleagues in obstetrics and gynecology who refer patients (individuals and couples) to our marital therapy teaching clinic; my clinical research on the male patient; my insights from a course on gender issues taught to residents in psychiatry; and, where applicable, my review of published literature on men in relation to the health care of women.

Men and Pregnancy

Most men feel a tremendous surge of satisfaction, happiness, and validation of their masculinity on learning that their wife or partner is pregnant. These emotions are quickly confounded by others, however, if the pregnancy is un- wanted, unplanned, or threatening to health or relationship equilibrium. Di- amond (1986) described other needs and conflicts that are triggered for men by pregnancy: envy toward the prospective mother; concerns of responsibil- ity, adulthood, and aging; competition and a need for connection with one's own father; wishes to revitalize the relationship with one's parents; jealousy toward the developing fetus, who is the object of his partner's rapt attention; and unresolved conflicts in the couple's marriage or partnership. Because men cannot become physiologically pregnant, many express their needs cre- atively (e.g., building a nursery, saving money for the "new addition," writing a children's book, constructing a playground) (Diamond 1992).

Ross (1982) has called the father the "forgotten parent" in psychoanalytic literature. He observed 65 boys between the ages of 3.5 and 10 years and not- ed various intense wishes among them both to have and to care for babies (Ross 1983). He felt that the paternal identity of an adult man does not just exist in a vacuum but begins much earlier in life and is merely activated or crystallized by the birth and presence of his children. Cath's (1986) emphasis on the dynamic interplay between the man and woman and how they view each other as prospective and actual parents of their children is significant. He calls this the *alliance of couplehood*—that is, the positive and negative contribu- tions to family mutuality that begin long before conception. How the couple nurtures each other ensures the nurturance of their offspring. Greenberg and Morris (1974) have used the term *engrossment* to describe the excitement, joy, and fascination that fathers manifest with their newborn infants.

As clinicians, we are likely to witness and be asked to assist with the more unfortunate male concomitants of pregnancy—men who are completely against the pregnancy and who demand termination; men who become vio- lent during their partner's pregnancy (Gazmararian et al. 1996); men who withdraw from their partners both emotionally and sexually; men who over- work and neglect their partners; men who act out sexually with other women (and sometimes other men), including beginning an affair; men who drink to excess and/or abuse other drugs; men who become anxious (May 1994) or clinically depressed; and men who threaten abandonment or who actually do leave the relationship. Many of these situations present as emergencies and require urgent medical and psychiatric attention to protect the health and well-being of the pregnant woman and her relationship.

## Men and the Postpartum Period

Feelings of exclusion, diminishment, and alienation are not uncommon in new fathers. Some men have a delayed reaction to the baby's birth. They behave as if no change has occurred in their lives and make little or no effort to assist with the baby. They may also resent giving up their freedom or independence to share the workload at home. Some men feel inept at or anxious about child care and may feel threatened by the competence and facility with which their wives adapt to motherhood and may feel belittled when their wives try to teach them basic skills of bathing and feeding their new daughter or son (and these feelings may be warded off by defensiveness, rigidity, and offense). Some men regress into childlike behavior, demanding attention from their busy, tired, and often beleaguered wives, whereas other men may feel guilty about their competitive, jealous, and resentful feelings toward their new baby. Classically, men do not talk about these emotions until (or if) they are blurted out during a fight or when the man is disinhibited by alcohol.

Marital problems are not uncommon in couples during the postpartum period. Anticipating and accepting the realities and responsibilities of parenthood are much easier for couples who are older, reasonably mature as individuals, and who are informed and prepared. However, many couples have an unplanned pregnancy, are very young, and have not had much time to get to know each other. Hence, their ability to communicate, to trust and count on the other, and to feel and expect commitment to the family are tenuous. Miscommunication and misunderstandings abound and soon both partners feel disillusioned, resentful, and unhappy.

Navigating their way through the stormy passages of new parenthood can be tough when people cannot really talk well with each other. Both partners are coming to terms with giving up much of the freedom and self-interest that they enjoyed before the baby was born. They are both adapting to the new roles of mother and father (Marks and Lovestone 1995). Lovemaking must be scheduled around the baby's sleep–wake cycle and not uncommonly the fatigue that new mothers feel eclipses their libido. Few husbands truly understand this; they may develop angry, hurt, rejected, and confused feelings. Furthermore, their concerns about birth control may not be in harmony, and one partner or the other may be terrified of another pregnancy so early, especially when postpartum psychiatric disorders have occurred (Peindl et al. 1995).

The most common marital symptoms are poor communication (both quantitative and qualitative); frequent arguments and fights, perhaps with physical violence; lack of sexual desire in one or both; overwork in the man with corresponding loneliness, resentment, and increased exhaustion in his partner; financial worries; misuse of alcohol or other drugs; and an undiagnosed psychiatric illness in one or both of them (Areias et al. 1996; Merchant et al. 1995). Dual-career and two-paycheck couples may have the additional problem of never seeing each other except when they are exhausted, especially if they work opposing shifts to ensure that one of them is always the caregiver. These couples may feel tremendous friction because of gender-role rigidity and ambiguity; their stated goal may be to share domestic and childcare responsibilities equally, but each may end up feeling overburdened or shortchanged. In traditional marriages, exhaustion is equally as common in both partners.

## Men and Infertility

How do men react to and cope with infertility (Meyers et al. 1995a)? Mourning of one's anticipated or assumed ability to have a child always accompanies the threat or the reality of infertility (Myers 1990). All stages of bereavement are common (e.g., denial, shock, anger, bargaining, depression, and acceptance), and because men tend to be less openly expressive than women, their distress may not be evident. They may also be suppressing feelings to remain supportive and "strong" for their wives, although this stance can backfire when or if the man's wife misinterprets his controlled manner as disinterest or coldness. Speaking privately with each partner often clarifies that the man does indeed have many feelings about their difficulty conceiving a child.

Mourning may be accentuated if the man learns that the infertility resides within him. "Shooting blanks," the common colloquial expression for azoospermia, covers up the underlying pain and assault to gender identity (one's inner sense of masculinity and maleness). Clinically, these men may manifest their distress by withdrawing from their wives (both emotionally and sexually), brooding, overworking, preoccupying themselves with sports, becoming irritable, drinking, or acting out sexually with other partners. Their need for privacy may be heightened and their wives may feel that they are not free to talk about their infertility problem with trusted friends and family members. Marital strain is not uncommon (Meyers et al. 1995b).

Men may also find that the diagnostic procedures and investigations that they must undergo are stressful. "I have never felt so naked in my life" were the words of one man as he described his experience of being asked so many questions about his medical history and sexual life, of undergoing an extensive physical and genital examination, of submitting to laboratory tests, and of providing a specimen for semen analysis. Attempting pregnancy by scheduling intercourse at the time of ovulation each month can become difficult after some time, no matter how much couples try to relax, be versatile, or use humor. Many husbands begin to feel the pressure of intercourse on demand; they feel objectified or that they are machines that deposit sperm on schedule once a month. Engaging in sex becomes a chore or work and is no longer erotically pleasurable.

How do men react to the new reproductive technologies? Few gender-specific data are available (Edelmann et al. 1994; Laffont and Edelmann 1994), but it would seem that the more information that both partners have the better. This includes lectures, reading material, consultations with various specialists, and a sense of freedom and opportunity to ask questions. Husbands must be encouraged to ask questions about costs, invasive procedures, success rates, timelines, time involvement, medical and psychologic complications, and any possible religious or moral conflicts that they may have about the technology. Relinquishing control and trusting physicians and their procedures may be challenging for some men living with an infertility problem, possibly in opposition to their wives who do not share their reservations.

## Men and Abortion

Although men do not actually experience termination of a pregnancy, they certainly have a host of feelings about abortion. I restrict my discussion here to clinical situations in which men are faced with an unwanted pregnancy in a loved one (as opposed to male beliefs, feelings, polemics, and political views on abortion). Although the decision to end a pregnancy is ultimately the woman's, many couples agonize over coming to that point and rarely is the man completely neutral about the decision. A continuum of male ideology seems to exist, ranging from absolute conviction that the pregnancy must be terminated to absolute horror or revulsion at the mention of therapeutic abortion.

What are some of the attitudinal determinants in men regarding abortion? Some young men, much like their female counterparts, are very clear that they are not psychologically ready to become fathers (e.g., they are adolescents, students, unemployed, undergoing psychiatric or substance dependence treatment, not ready for a committed relationship). Some men are clear that they cannot afford a child or another child. They have the maturity to recognize the economic responsibility of being a father and take the matter seriously rather than renounce this onto their partner or the state. Some happily married men who have had a family and who are just beginning to feel freed up (or who have long-range plans for more protected time with their wives) will fight hard against an unwanted pregnancy. Their wives, however, may privately want another child or may at least be open to becoming pregnant. Because their marriage is strong and they can afford another child, these women may be aghast at and threatened by how vehemently opposed their husbands are toward continuing with the pregnancy. Some men are conscious of negative or ambivalent feelings about their relationship or marriage before learning of the pregnancy and thus have no desire for fatherhood when considering separation or marital therapy.

A range of psychologic determinants may be operative in men who want their partner's pregnancy to continue. Some men have religious or spiritual prohibitions against abortion that influence their wishes and beliefs about their partner's pregnancy. This includes men without current religious affiliation but whose rearing included religious observance. They may experience a resurgence of strong antiabortion feelings when faced with an unwanted pregnancy. Some may have had one or more previous partners become pregnant and have therapeutic abortions; they have reflected on these experiences and do not believe that they can support another termination. For some men, impregnating a woman is narcissistically driven; becoming a father regulates their gender identities as men. Such men will resist their partner's wish to end the pregnancy by abortion. When their partners have shaky self-worth, assertiveness, and autonomy, men who are controlling will ensure against a therapeutic abortion by cajoling, coercion, threats of abandonment, sexual acting out with others, and abuse (physical, verbal, sexual, emotional).

## Men's Reactions to Breast Cancer

Women who are diagnosed with and treated for breast cancer are far from monolithic and so are their partners or husbands. What is known, however, is that these men do have a reaction when their loved one is faced with cancer. One study of women and their partners over a 1-year period following surgery showed improvement in negative emotions, psychologic distress, psychologic well-being, and performance of vocational, domestic, and social roles for both partners (Hoskins 1995). Studies indicate that younger women experience more emotional distress than do older women, although the inverse relationship between age and emotional distress is not consistent across all studies (Northouse 1994). Younger husbands reported more problems carrying out domestic roles and a greater number of life stresses than did older husbands. Even when women with breast cancer have good helping relationships with others, research findings suggest that the partner plays a huge role in their adaptation, particularly when communication is characterized by high empathy and low withdrawal (Pistrang and Barker 1995). Studies of women with recurrent breast cancer show that partners have a mutual influence on one another (Northouse et al. 1995a), that one or both members of more than 50% of the couples scored outside the normative range on either depressed mood or marital adjustment (Lewis and Deal 1995), and that women reported more emotional distress than did their husbands (although each had a similar number of psychosocial role problems) (Northouse et al. 1995b).

It is well known that women with breast cancer worry about their partners' reaction to their physical appearance; however, this focus on cosmetics is not always an issue for women alone. It is not unusual to learn of men who cannot look at the scarred or missing breast or who no longer feel sexual with their wives. At least one study has shown significant emotional distress and depression in husbands 4 months after their wives' surgery (Omne-Ponten et al. 1993). There was little scored difference between men whose wives had had mastectomies and men whose wives had had breast-conserving surgery. What may be more important in how a man copes with breast cancer in his partner are other variables, such as his personal health status; his subjective sense of happiness with and commitment to the marriage prior to the diagnosis; his coping resources, including a capacity for living with threat, uncertainty, and loss; his psychologic maturity; the nature and number of his supportive relationships outside the marriage; his occupational and/or financial security; his preexisting healthy relationship with children; and his religious and/or spiritual leanings.

## Men and Menopause

Menopause is one of the critical stages in the individual life cycle (Erikson 1963). Life cycle stages in both men and women correspond closely to critical stages in marriage. Although the actual prevalence of marital dysharmony during menopause is not known, we do know that a peak in divorce occurs after 20–25 years of marriage (Cherlin 1981). Clinically, many men and women seek marital therapy at this stage of life and marriage, and many unhappily married women and men leave their marriages.

Menopause is characterized by normal unrest and struggle, a transitional stage that is common in most marriages. Furthermore, menopause corresponds with middle adulthood, including a restabilizing and reordering of one's priorities. The marital task is to resolve conflicts and to strengthen the marriage for the long haul. Despite enormous conflict and tremendous unhappiness in couples coming for marital assistance at this time of life, what is not always understood is the tenacity of marital bonding in the face of adversity, the commitment to the marriage covenant ("for better and for worse"), and the toughness and resilience of people who have been together for a long time.

Husbands and wives may differ in their rates and directions of emotional growth at menopause. Problems with loss of youthfulness may arise that contribute to feelings of depression, extramarital affairs, or both in either partner. In enduring marriages, intimacy may be threatened by the aging process and by boredom despite stability and security. Children leaving the family home may increase or decrease intimacy; the empty nest syndrome—that is, dissatisfaction and unhappiness when children leave the home—is not universal (Bernard 1982) and is identified in both men (Scher 1992) and women. Menopause is a time of new beginnings when women, who have put many of their personal needs and wishes on hold for their husbands and children, are now free to pursue their own goals. This may include leaving a loveless, empty, or grim marriage.

What about male menopause? This term has become a pejorative descriptor applied to men in their middle years who suddenly do something out of character or indicative of a problem with aging. Examples might include training for triathlons; becoming a vegetarian; visiting an ashram; getting a hair transplant; having a facelift; buying a jazzy sports car; or taking up with a much younger woman. Sometimes menopause in a woman is juxtaposed with a midlife crisis in her husband, a combination that can threaten marital equilibrium. We live in a youth-oriented society, and many men in their middle years are attracted to younger women and not to their female contemporaries (Myers 1989). We are products of the culture in which we live, a culture of menopausal myths and myths that erode women's self-esteem (Notman et al. 1991).

# When Male Physicians Treat Female Patients

Gender is merely one of the many variables (age, socioeconomic level, race, ethnicity, sexual orientation, marital status, language, and so forth) that contribute to the unique and dynamic interplay when male physicians treat female patients. I only wish to emphasize some basic facts that form the bedrock of all male physician–female patient encounters and inform diagnosis and treatment. Left unrecognized, these factors can lead to omission, error, biologic reductionism, scientific inaccuracies in research, and treatment noncompliance.

It must first be acknowledged that gender discordance exists within the physician–patient relationship. Male physicians must accept that because they are men they will be viewed differently than if they were women. Being viewed differently is value neutral; it should not be misconstrued as being viewed more positively or negatively. The transference feelings that the woman patient brings to the professional relationship will be centered in her early and current relationships with men and women, her previous experience with male and female physicians (especially ones who work in obstetrics and gynecology or other branches of medicine related to women's illnesses), her ideology about male and female gender roles, including men and women in the professions, and her personal and family history (mother absence, father absence, sexual abuse or assault, males or females as role models, and so forth). These factors may contribute to the various transferences (e.g., dependent, mistrustful and guarded, hostile, regressive, erotic) that can occur when women are treated by men.

Second, male physicians must respect the concept of countertransference when they treat women patients. In other words, they must be open to identifying and reflecting on their feelings, attitudes, beliefs, and values toward women in general and their women patients in particular. This requires a nondefensive and sometimes emotionally laden (anxiety, guilt, shame, anger, hurt) inner appraisal of personal and family-of-origin issues, especially one's lifetime relationships with females. If physicians are under strain at home (e.g., living with marital conflict, separation, isolation, or depression), they must be encouraged to seek help. They must also be open to new concepts and gender-specific research that exposes outdated scientific inaccuracies, flawed experimental design and methodology, and sexism in academia and medical centers. Physicians must be able to embrace the evolving directives concerned with gender-neutral language in our work with patients and colleagues as being respectful and professional. They should also keep abreast of new developments in sexual harassment policies in the workplace and the ethical guidelines issued by licensing bodies and medical institutions to respect and preserve the boundaries of the doctor–patient relationship.

Third, many male physicians are interested in and could learn from formalized teaching about the myriad transference and countertransference issues when men treat women. These are elementary and central features of the physician–patient relationship, and yet they are not well taught in medical school or residency programs. Teaching methods include didactic lectures, assigned readings, seminars, videotapes, and role-playing exercises of common clinical situations. When possible, this teaching is best done by other physicians, both men and women, who practice the same branch of medicine as the trainees (importing nurses, psychologists, or psychiatrists to teach obstetrics and gynecology residents about transference and countertransference issues may fail). The best teachers in each discipline are male clinicians who are everyday role models and whose treatment of women patients and colleagueship with women health professionals are exemplary.

## Conclusion

Men are significant characters in the lives of all women and key players in the psychologic aspects of women's health care. In this chapter, I have selected only a small number of obstetric, gynecologic, and other disorders to examine how men influence and are influenced by women. I hope that some of these observations are generalizable to other clinical situations and, furthermore, that physicians who treat women extend their reach to the men who are so important in their patients' lives.

## References

Areias ME, Kumar R, Barros H, et al: Correlates of postnatal depression in mothers and fathers. Br J Psychiatry 169:36–41, 1996

Bergman SJ, Surrey J: The woman-man relationship: impasses and possibilities. Stone Center Document #5. Wellesley, MA, Stone Center, 1992

Bernard J: The Future of Marriage, 2nd Edition. New Haven, CT, Yale University, 1982

Cath SH: Fathering from infancy to old age: a selective overview of recent psychoanalytic contributions, in Toward a New Psychology of Men: Psychoanalytic and

Social Perspectives. Edited by Friedman RM, Lerner L. New York, Guilford, 1986, pp 65–75

Cherlin AJ: Marriage, Divorce, Remarriage. Cambridge, MA, Harvard University, 1981

Diamond MJ: Becoming a father: a psychoanalytic perspective on the forgotten parent, in Toward a New Psychology of Men: Psychoanalytic and Social Perspectives. Edited by Friedman RM, Lerner L. New York, Guilford, 1986, pp 41–64

Diamond MJ: Creativity needs in becoming a father. Journal of Men's Studies 1:41–45, 1992

Edelmann RJ, Connolly KJ, Bartlett H: Coping strategies and psychological adjustment of couples presenting for IVF. J Psychosom Res 38:355–364, 1994

Erikson EH: Childhood and Society, 2nd Edition. New York, WW Norton, 1963

Gazmararian JA, Lazorick S, Spitz AM, et al: Prevalence of violence against pregnant women. JAMA 275:1915–1920, 1996

Greenberg M, Morris N: Engrossment: the newborn's impact upon the father. Am J Orthopsychiatry 44:520–531, 1974

Hoskins CN: Adjustment to breast cancer in couples. Psychol Rep 77:435–454, 1995

Laffont I, Edelmann RJ: Psychological aspects of in vitro fertilization: a gender comparison. J Psychosom Obstet Gynaecol 15:85–92, 1994

Lewis FM, Deal LW: Balancing our lives: a study of the married couple's experience with breast cancer recurrence. Oncol Nurs Forum 22:943–953, 1995

Marks M, Lovestone S: The role of the father in parental postnatal mental health. Br J Med Psychol 68:157–168, 1995

May KA: Impact of maternal activity restriction for preterm labor on the expectant father. J Obstet Gynecol Neonatal Nurs 23:246–251, 1994

Merchant DC, Affonso DD, Mayberry LJ: Influence of marital relationship and child-care stress on maternal depression symptoms in the postpartum. J Psychosom Obstet Gynecol 16:193–200, 1995

Meyers M, Diamond R, Kezur D, et al: An infertility primer for family therapists, I: medical, social, and psychological dimensions. Fam Process 34:219–229, 1995a

Meyers M, Weinshel M, Scharf C, et al: An infertility primer for family therapists, II: working with couples who struggle with infertility. Fam Process 34:231–240, 1995b

Myers MF: Men and Divorce. New York, Guilford, 1989, pp 94–110.

Myers MF: Male gender-related issues in reproduction and technology, in Psychiatric Aspects of Reproductive Technology. Edited by Stotland NL. Washington, DC, American Psychiatric Press, 1990, pp 25–35

Northouse LL: Breast cancer in younger women: effects on interpersonal and family relations. J Natl Cancer Inst Monogr 16:183–190, 1994

Northouse LL, Dorris G, Charron-Moore C: Factors affecting couples' adjustment to recurrent breast cancer. Soc Sci Med 41:69–76, 1995a

Northouse LL, Laten D, Reddy P: Adjustment of women and their husbands to recurrent breast cancer. Res Nurs Health 18:515–524, 1995b

Notman MT, Klein R, Jordan JV, et al: Women's unique developmental issues across the life cycle, in Review of Psychiatry Volume 10. Edited by Tasman A, Goldfinger SM. Washington, DC, American Psychiatric Press, 1991, pp 556–577

Omne-Ponten M, Holmberg L, Bergstrom R, et al: Psychosocial adjustment among husbands of women treated for breast cancer: mastectomy vs. breast-conserving surgery. Eur J Cancer 29A:1393–1397, 1993

Peindl KS, Zolnik EJ, Wisner KL, et al: Effects of postpartum psychiatric illnesses on family planning. Int J Psychiatry Med 25:291–300, 1995

Pistrang N, Barker C: The partner relationship in psychological response to breast cancer. Soc Sci Med 40:789–797, 1995

Ross JM: In search of fathering: a review, in Father and Child. Edited by Cath SH, Gurwitt AR, Ross JM. Boston, MA, Little, Brown, 1982, pp 21–32

Ross JM: Father to the child: psychoanalytic reflections. Psychoanal Rev 70:301–320, 1983

Scher M: The empty nest father. Journal of Men's Studies 1:195–200, 1992

# Collaborations Between Psychiatry and Obstetrics and Gynecology

NADA L. STOTLAND, M.D., M.P.H.

This book addresses the psychiatric issues related to obstetrics and gynecology and the women's reproductive health issues relevant to psychiatry. This chapter is about process. Given the many clinical, educational, and research areas in which psychiatry and obstetrics/gynecology have important collaborative contributions to make, how does the collaboration take place? Sites range from the laboratory bench and classroom to the delivery room and the halls of government. Methods include written materials, formal lectures, conjoint or consultative work in the office or at bedside, joint committees, and the formation of multispecialty organizations that develop programs, activities, and publications of mutual interest. Although I am most familiar with activities and circumstances in the United States, this chapter attempts to acknowledge, at least, the differences among countries with respect to service organization.

## History

Reproductive organs, functions, and events have always aroused scientific curiosity and evoked powerful affects. The history of psychosomatic medicine and consultation psychiatry arose in large part at the intersection of psychiatry and obstetrics/gynecology. The ancient Greek word *hysteria* denoted a disease in which otherwise unexplainable physical symptoms were thought to be caused by the wanderings of an unmoored uterus (*hyster-*) from its normal position in the pelvis to the body sites manifesting the symptoms (Pomeroy 1975). Freud (1931/1961) conceptualized development in terms of psychosexual stages and considered the formation of a successful heterosexual relationship, including procreation, to be the sine qua non of normal maturity. Freud also understood many psychologic symptoms as the disguised expression of unfulfilled, repressed sexual desires.

One of the landmark psychosomatic collaborations of the twentieth century was that of Benedek, a psychiatrist and psychoanalyst, and Rubinstein, a gynecologist. They studied women during the course of psychoanalysis undertaken for reasons unrelated to the object of their research. The patients kept track of their menstrual periods, the gynecologist monitored urinary levels of the then newly discovered female hormones, and the psychoanalyst recorded evidence of the patients' moods and thought content in their dreams and associations (Benedek and Rubinstein 1942). These collaborators concluded that hormonal changes characteristic of the ovulatory phase were associated with affects and thoughts of nurturance and interest in sexual intercourse. It seemed to them that cyclic changes of this kind would enhance the likelihood of conception and therefore the preservation of the species.

During the 1940s and 1950s, psychoanalysis was a (or *the*) dominant force in American psychiatry. The power of psychodynamics to explain human feelings and behaviors was impressive, and attempts were made to use it in arenas ranging from international relations to preschool education. Because many or most psychoanalysts were also physicians, considerable interest arose in applying psychoanalytic knowledge and technique to medical diagnosis and treatment and thereby also in enhancing the integration of psychiatry into the rest of medicine. Such an integration was otherwise somewhat threatened by psychoanalysts' distance from and even rejection of the traditional authoritarian approaches of clinical medicine (Alexander 1950; Dunbar 1954). Psychoanalytic technique was used in the study of patients with various medical illnesses (Alexander 1950; Dunbar 1954). Authors described constellations of personality traits and unconscious conflicts that characterized sufferers from several major diseases. Physical symptoms were conceptualized in terms of neurotic compromise—for example, the asthmatic patient's wheezing was a cry for the mother; the hypertensive patient's cardiovascular changes resulted from repressed rage; infertility was the result of an unconscious terror of motherhood. Therapeutic interventions based on these etiologic formulations were reported to have positive effects. In some major medical centers, psychiatrists and psychoanalysts were assigned to some or all medical units to work with medical colleagues and patients on a regular basis.

Over the years, for various reasons, these arrangements eroded. Improvements in research methodology called previous conclusions into question. Many of the patients studied had already suffered from their diseases for many years. There was no way to know whether the psychodynamics revealed in their diagnostic interviews were the cause or the result of their years of pain and disability. Suppressed feelings of neediness and anger were to be expected under the circumstances. Imputed causal connections between personality types and medical disorders did not hold up to scientific scrutiny. Researchers discovered genetic, infectious, and other etiologic factors for hitherto mysterious signs and symptoms. For example, the ability to examine the fallopian tubes through laparoscopy and microscopy sometimes revealed evidence of surgically repairable tubal damage that had resulted from prior pelvic infections. These discoveries led some clinicians to conclude that psychodynamic explanations for infertility, for example, were a "wastebasket," an etiologic last resort, for conditions not yet conquered by "real" science and that these explanations stigmatized already suffering patients as being somehow responsible for their own conditions.

Other factors that played roles in the decline of psychiatric and psychodynamic involvement in medical care included funding, personnel, the development of other mental health disciplines, and the burgeoning of biologic approaches to psychiatry (Fenton and Guggenheim 1981). Some of these approaches, such as the dexamethasone suppression test, were expected to supplant the need for the understanding of childhood experience and current conflicts. Increasingly effective psychoactive medications were developed and quickly adopted into the armamentarium of nonpsychiatric physicians, including obstetrician/gynecologists (OB/GYNs).

At the same time, evidence of synergistic relationships between biologic and psychosocial factors in the genesis and phenomenology of illness continued to appear. We now know, again, that mind and body are inextricably interrelated, but in ways more numerous and complex than earlier supposed (Sharpe et al. 1996). Life events can precipitate mood and neurohumoral changes that affect immune responses. Eating disorders and reproductive dysfunctions are related. Psychosocial factors exist in infertility; some infertile couples are not having sexual intercourse or are using a schedule or technique that precludes conception for reasons of ignorance or inhibition. Situations like these continue to baffle clinicians and patients and lead to needless medical interventions and expenditures (Christie 1997). The consulting psychiatrist can help by encouraging the infertility team to incorporate a few simple screening questions into the initial diagnostic process (Christie and Pawson 1987).

Consultation-liaison psychiatry reinforces and uses the medical identity of psychiatry (Lipowski 1986). Several organizations and publications are devoted to psychosomatic and consultation-liaison issues. Subspecialty groups address issues related to specific medical conditions: oncology, nephrology, AIDS, and obstetrics/gynecology. The latter is discussed below. However, few if any medical care institutions support the assignment of a psychiatrist to each clinical specialty service. Most of the clinical problems discussed in this book are handled by general psychiatrists or psychiatrists in another subspecialty (child and adolescent, forensic, geriatric) or in general consultation-liaison psychiatry rather than by psychiatrists who spend much or all of their time working with OB/GYNs. This chapter provides an overview of issues and activities for the psychiatrist working with obstetrics and gynecology.

# Clinical and Cultural Substrate of Obstetric/Gynecologic Practice

Psychiatric consultation to another medical specialty is facilitated by familiarity with the content and style of that specialty's practice (Stotland and Garrick 1990). Although OB/GYNs share many issues with all other physicians, they also face some challenges unique to their specialty. Most of the subspecialties, as well as the general practice, of obstetrics and gynecology attract practitioners who enjoy active intervention and expect their interventions to result in relatively prompt and positive clinical outcomes. This stance serves them well for much of their clinical work but leads to frustration in many of the situations in which psychiatric consultation is sought: failure of the patient to comply with medical recommendations, behavior that is actively self-destructive and/or threatens the well-being of the fetus or newborn, grief responses to procreative losses, physical complaints without diagnosable physical foundation, and intense transference reactions to the gynecologist (Stotland 1988).

In 4 years of training, residents in obstetrics and gynecology must master a huge and explosively growing body of medical information as well as an array of techniques, including ultrasonography, amniocentesis, chorionic villus sampling, normal and complicated childbirth, and several kinds of macroscopic and microscopic surgery. Some of these techniques, such as induced abortion and the use of reproductive technologies, are highly contentious.

This field of study overlaps significantly not only with general surgery and oncology but also with pediatrics, urology, and infectious disease. The designation of obstetrics and gynecology as a primary care specialty has protected the field from some of the more draconian cuts in educational funding, but has also added a whole new burden to training and practice: mastery of the whole body of general office practice.

This load of clinical and academic work involves the care of patients whose problems and treatments carry a tremendous emotional valence. Obstetrics and gynecology involves not only routine pelvic examinations and normal deliveries, which are in themselves emotionally demanding on patient and staff, but also the care of patients who have been raped; who have given birth to extremely small and/or damaged infants; who seek to terminate pregnancies at various stages; whose pregnancies are highly desired but threatened by medical or psychiatric illness; who have sexually transmitted diseases that threaten their fertility, health, or survival; who have malignancies; and who have difficulties with their sexual and/or reproductive functions. Little or no time is available for OB/GYNs, especially residents, to talk to these patients at length; to learn about the emotional dimensions of these clinical problems; to acquire skills for diagnosing, referring, and treating the psychiatric complications of these conditions; or to acknowledge and accept the profound feelings that these conditions engender in the treating physician (Adler 1972).

In addition to the clinical, technical, and emotional complications, many of the most vexing ethical conflicts in clinical medicine are faced by the OB/GYN (Strong et al. 1997): Should a pregnant woman be forced to undergo an obstetric intervention in the interest of her fetus or be punished if her behavior results in fetal damage? Which patients, if any, should be admitted to artificial insemination, in vitro fertilization, or surrogate mother programs (Lantos 1990)? Are physicians obligated to provide induced abortions, and at what stages of gestation and under what circumstances? What constitutes informed consent for sterilization? Legal and social standards vary widely from culture to culture.

Not uncommonly, OB/GYNs must repair medical damage caused by behavior that they find personally repugnant (e.g., cocaine abuse during pregnancy) or that they must provide services of which they do not fully approve (e.g., contraceptives for early adolescents). When these ethical and emotional demands are placed on a sleep-deprived resident who is struggling to develop technical skills and who chose this specialty in the hope of facilitating expeditious and happy outcomes, the result may be avoidance, depression, and rage.

These emotions are often reflected in requests for psychiatric consultation and in the functioning of the health care team requesting them (Karasu et al. 1977).

Recent changes in the social context of medical practice in the United States have had a particularly problematic impact on OB/GYNs. The proliferation of malpractice litigation has hit obstetricians especially hard. In the state of Illinois, for example, nearly 100% of obstetricians will be sued by patients at some point duirng their careers. Charles and Kennedy (1985) have documented the interruption of practice, avoidance by colleagues, loss of self-esteem, changes in practice patterns, and suspicion of future patients caused by malpractice suits even for the majority of doctors who will be found innocent of the charges brought against them. Physicians feel constrained to perform diagnostic and therapeutic interventions on preventive legal, rather than medical, grounds. This tends to warp cognition as well as emotion.

Obstetrics is also legally perilous because any allegedly damaged infant and its family make a wrenching spectacle in the courtroom, because the life-long care of such an infant is so costly, and because the statute of limitations on bringing a lawsuit does not apply until the infant has reached the age of majority and has had the opportunity to realize the nature and cause of his or her disability. Advances in reproductive technology and obstetric technique constitute a two-edged sword (Hummel and Kettel 1997; Mahowald et al. 1996): the public expects the medical profession to be able to solve any problem and to produce a perfect outcome in every case, whereas the very patients who are at higher risk because of delayed childbearing are those who are most likely to seek legal recourse for any frustration. These problems are of less concern in countries other than the United States, where the proliferation of lawsuits of every type is a significant social challenge.

Consumer criticism of medicine has also been highly focused on obstetrics and gynecology. Finding physicians wanting in knowledge and attitude, a group of mothers in the Chicago area founded the La Leche League to promote breastfeeding (La Leche League International 1987). Chapters were founded in countries all over the world, and the demographics of infant feeding changed; the proportion of mothers breastfeeding on leaving the hospital rose from a small minority to a significant majority. Unfortunately, manufacturers of infant formula were doing extensive marketing in countries where breastfeeding was the normal mode of infant feeding at the same time. Formula feeding was associated with sophistication, but many families lacked the resources to sterilize the bottles and refrigerate the formula. Many infants died as a result.

At about the same time, physical therapists, nurses, and nonmedical persons began to teach prepared childbirth classes that educated expectant parents about the anatomy and physiology of pregnancy, labor, delivery, and the postpartum period (Bing 1973). These classes also, however, brought women and their significant others together to question and defy traditional medical authority (Chalmers and McIntyre 1994). They encouraged patients to believe that they could and should comprehend medical questions and make informed choices about their own care and substitute relaxation and distraction techniques, over which they had control, for dependence on analgesics and anesthetics administered by professionals that could lead to iatrogenic complications. They also encouraged the participation of significant others in the experience of labor and delivery, diminishing to a significant degree the central emotional role of the physician (Seiden 1978). Organizations and articles in the popular press questioned routine repeat cesarean delivery and the indications for the enormous number of hysterectomies performed in the United States as compared with other affluent countries. Books like *Our Bodies, Ourselves*, which was written by a women's collective, explained issues that had been the exclusive domain of OB/GYNs (Boston Women's Health Collective 1984).

All of these developments, such as the increase in sensational malpractice litigation, aroused or gave voice to suspicion and hostility between patients and doctors (Arms 1975), at least in the United States. OB/GYNs found it ironic that, despite the enormous efforts they expended acquiring and applying knowledge and skills in the interest of women's health, they should be viewed in the press and the consulting room as purveyors of needless and often damaging interventions and as dismissive of women and their autonomy over their reproductive organs and functions (Leppert et al. 1996). There was, however, significant clinical and documentary foundation for women's complaints (Friedman 1986; Hellerstein 1984; Scully and Bart 1973). No empirical foundation existed for many obstetric and gynecologic practices, such as episiotomy, prohibitions against intercourse for 6 weeks after childbirth, or the removal of healthy ovaries along with diseased uteri. Textbooks sometimes implied, or even stated, that women who were in menopause or pregnant were emotionally and cognitively incapacitated and that their physicians would have to guide them paternalistically through this reproductive stage.

With a few exceptions, the people complaining about OB/GYN care were female, and the people complained about were male. Since the first edition of this book was prepared, a revolution has occurred in the gender composition of North American obstetrics and gynecology training programs.

Some residency classes are entirely female and male applicants feel they have to justify their interest in the field. Yet the academic and organizational leadership of the specialty is still largely male; the second woman president in the history of the American College of Obstetricians and Gynecologists completed her term in 1998. It is not clear whether changes in gender composition at the entry level have had a significant impact on attitudes and practices, at least to date. The ethos of the field is passed along and strongly colors not only clinical practice but also the personal experiences of newer practitioners. If a trainee is never exposed to patients who labor and deliver happily and successfully without medical intervention, he or she is likely to demand maximum intervention for his or her own deliveries. Another factor driving styles of practice is managed care, diminishing hospital stays, length of outpatient visits, and continuity of care. The American College of Obstetricians and Gynecologists has convinced the United States Congress to mandate that women have access to OB/GYNs as primary care providers rather than requiring specialty referral. In many other countries, access to specialty care is still at the discretion of a family practitioner.

## Consultation-Liaison Mechanisms

The realities of practice and developments in knowledge and technique in obstetrics and gynecology can be assimilated by the liaison psychiatrist by attending grand rounds and other conferences in the obstetrics and gynecology department. The psychiatrist can also use the occasion of the conference to meet members of the department and to make comments on psychiatric aspects of the cases and issues discussed. "Curbside" consultations can be sought and referrals made for formal inpatient and outpatient consultations. Attendance at obstetrics and gynecology meetings is tangible evidence of interest, involvement, availability, and credibility.

The psychiatrist may also elect to participate in inpatient-care rounds regularly or to be present at or available to one or more outpatient clinics (Nickels and McIntyre 1996). On rounds or in a clinic, the psychiatrist can get an excellent sense of the ethos of the service and the personalities and level of psychologic sophistication of the students, residents, and attending staff as well as the typical psychosocial and psychiatric problems of the patients. The psychiatrist's participation underscores the integration of psychiatric with medical concerns and offers the opportunity for helpful comments and interventions without the necessity for formal psychiatric consultation. The psychiatrist can help members of the service learn to recognize early signs of psychiatric disorders before they develop into difficult management problems or emergencies as well as to decide when and how to call for formal consultation. Psychiatrists occasionally amaze obstetrics and gynecology staff by using interviewing skills to obtain information crucial to diagnosis and treatment (the patient is upset because her husband is not the biologic father of the child she is about to deliver; the patient with prepartum bleeding is noncompliant with the order for bed rest because she has had attention deficit/hyperactivity disorder since childhood, not because she is bad or stupid; the patient doesn't follow medical recommendations because she is deaf and cannot hear them; the patient will not give consent for surgery because a relative died during an operation).

Services in most academic and large community hospitals include family planning, sometimes with separate sections for adolescents, normal and high-risk prenatal care, infertility diagnosis and treatment, general gynecologic care, urogynecology, gynecologic cancer diagnosis and treatment, and services in other subspecialty areas. In a busy department, there will be far too many services and clinics for even the most energetic and dedicated psychiatrist. Interested residents, fellows, and even medical students taking senior electives in consultation psychiatry can add to the psychiatric presence, get valuable experience, and develop subspecialty practice and research interests. This sort of program requires an investment of time by faculty or senior consultants that is approximately equivalent to the time that would be required for the direct provision of services. In addition, the liaison is disrupted by the inevitable rotation and graduation of trainees unless permanent staff maintain a clinical presence.

Formal teaching is an important component of the substance and technique of liaison work. While busy OB/GYNs seldom seek classroom hours, the staff members in charge of resident conferences and grand rounds are almost always eager to fill time slots, and now that obstetrics and gynecology is a primary care specialty, training programs are under pressure to include psychosocial issues in the curriculum. The audience, although wary of unrealistic demands on physicians' time and psychologic sophistication, is generally interested in scientifically stimulating and clinically useful information about common psychiatric problems such as anxiety and affective disorders. It is best to come prepared both with new findings about neurotransmitters, imaging, or psychopharmacology and with specific and easily implemented suggestions for screening, diagnosis, referral, and treatment. Nonpsychiatric physicians are often uncertain about how to distinguish among the various categories of mental health professionals and when to refer to each, so it is worthwhile to detail the different trainings and practices of counselors, social workers, psychologists, and psychiatrists.

It is not enough to recommend that screening for major psychiatric illness be a part of obstetric and gynecologic care. Obstetricians appreciate, and are more likely to use, a short list of questions to add to their admission history ("Have you ever been referred or referred yourself to see a psychiatrist, psychologist, or social worker?"; "Have you ever been admitted to a hospital for psychiatric treatment?"). Other suggestions include the wording of questions about sexual practices ("What is the nature of your sexual practices in the past and at this point in time?" rather than "Are you gay?") and exposure to sexually transmitted diseases; criteria for prescription of antidepressants and referral for psychiatric care; assessment for organic brain syndromes; and assessment of competence to consent for surgery, care for oneself, and care for an infant. Brief standardized and validated assessment instruments that can be completed by the nurse or the patient in the waiting room are increasingly popular; the psychiatrist should bring copies and information about how to obtain them; screening questionnaires are available for depression, domestic violence, and alcohol abuse. Simple charts of antidepressant names, dosages, and side effects are useful. Many OB/GYNs are also interested in the psychologic aspects of issues in their areas of expertise: induced and spontaneous abortion; pregnancy, labor, and delivery; new reproductive technologies; and malignancies and in how to approach and support patients facing these events.

## Interdisciplinary Organizations and Activities

Issues in psychosomatic obstetrics and gynecology are discussed in many forums today. Symposia can be found on the programs of any major psychiatry or obstetrics and gynecology meeting; the keynote address at the 1998 Annual Clinical Meeting of the American College of Obstetricians and Gynecologists was on depression. National and international organizations devoted entirely to the field include the International Society for Psychosomatic Obstetrics and Gynecology, which publishes the *Journal of Psychosomatic Obstetrics and Gynaecology* and has member societies in many countries, including North America (the North American Society for Psychosocial Obstetrics and Gynecology). The North American Society holds yearly meetings in early spring; the International Society holds meetings approximately every 3 years.

Groups devoted to specific topics such as postpartum psychiatric illness (the Marcé Society) and menopause (the North American Menopause Society) can also be found. Participation in these organizations acquaints members with the range of work being done and the people who are doing it. Membership consists of professionals in both mental health and obstetrics and is interdisciplinary, including physicians, psychologists, nurses, social workers, and midwives. Similar organizations exist in Europe, Asia, South America, and Australia/New Zealand.

The American College of Obstetricians and Gynecologists has founded the Jacobs Institute for Women's Health, which offers periodic symposia on policy and practical issues related to women's health and publishes the quarterly journal *Women's Health Issues*. Members of many professional and consumer groups have also come together to address the policy and legislative implications of several interdisciplinary issues that are discussed in the next section. For example, the American Medical Association, the American Psychiatric Association, and the American College of Obstetricians and Gynecologists were among the participants in an *amicus curiae* brief in the *Webster v. Reproductive Health Services* abortion law case decided by the Supreme Court in 1989 (*Webster v. Reproductive Health Services* 1989).

## Issues for the Future

At the interface of psychiatry and obstetrics and gynecology lie a number of emerging and emergent social, policy, and ethical as well as medical problems. These include the impact of the abuse of alcohol and crack cocaine on the fetus, with its attendant issues of maternal versus fetal rights, autonomy, punishment, and care; the unknown and sometimes notoriously problematic implications of surrogate motherhood and embryo freezing and transfer; the legislative and judicial restrictions on induced abortion, as mentioned previously; AIDS as a heterosexually and prenatally transmitted disease; and many others.

Interdisciplinary research in some of these areas has been significantly diminished by governmental restrictions on funding and even on the nature of the research performed. For example, very little research has been done on contraception for the past 10 or more years despite the continued high incidence of unintended pregnancy. Too little work has been published about induced abortion despite allegations and misinformation about its psychosocial concomitants. Research involving fetal tissue has been banned in the United

States, Canada, the United Kingdom, and parts of Europe.

At the level of clinical practice, funding is again a major issue, at least in the United States. No longer do hospital and academic departments have the luxury of hiring psychiatric liaison-consultants to teach and spend time in clinical service areas. Patients' health insurance policies often severely limit their access to psychiatric services. Mental health care is increasingly "carved out" for management by companies that limit the choice and availability of services. Carveouts may mean that the insurance that funds a patient's obstetric and gynecologic care in a given facility requires that her psychiatric care be provided in another facility. These constraints are, fortunately, not characteristic of many other countries.

Similarly, both faculty and trainees in United States medical schools are under increasing constraints to generate clinical income to pay their salaries and support the teaching enterprise, often while trying to fulfill a mission to care for the medically indigent and uninsured. Some subspecialty care, such as infertility diagnosis and treatment, is lucrative. Once a good liaison relationship has been formed, the psychiatrist may be able to convince the infertility, oncology, or other service that psychiatric screening and support are important for clinical care and that they can be built into funding for the programs, or that patients and their insurance companies can be expected to pay for them (Frankel and Hall 1996). Governmental and private funding for research at the interface of psychiatry and obstetrics/gynecology is available in adolescent sexual behavior, psychosocial factors in cancer prognosis, treatment of premenstrual dysphorias, and well-being at and after menopause. The National Institutes of Health, National Institute of Mental Health, and the Public Health Service have offices dedicated to women's health. Information about research opportunities is available from them.

Psychiatric consultation to obstetrics and gynecology is rich in breadth and depth. The consulting psychiatrist can participate in scientific developments at the cutting edge of human genetics and reproduction, in human events from the conception to the end of life, and in the most tragic and wrenching to the most heroic and joyous experiences. An awareness of the social context and the clinical realities facing the OB/GYN will help the consultant develop a consultative style and content that the consultee will appreciate and use in the interests of patients. Participation in interdisciplinary organizations and activities offers the interested psychiatrist the opportunity to meet and work with colleagues in other fields, to advance knowledge and care, and to act in concert in the public arena.

# References

Adler J: Helplessness in the helpers. Br J Med Psychol 45:315–326, 1972

Alexander F: Psychosomatic Medicine. New York, WW Norton, 1950

Arms S: Immaculate Deception: A New Look at Women and Childbirth in America. Boston, MA, Houghton Mifflin, 1975

Benedek T, Rubinstein B: The sexual cycle in women, in Psychosomatic Medicine Monographs, Vol 3. Washington, DC, National Research Council, 1942

Bing E: Six Practical Lessons for an Easier Childbirth. New York, Bantam, 1973

Boston Women's Health Collective: The New Our Bodies, Ourselves. New York, Simon & Schuster, 1984

Chalmers B, McIntyre J: Do antenatal classes have a place in modern obstetric care. J Psychosom Obstet Gynaecol 15:119–123, 1994

Charles SC, Kennedy E: Defendant: A Psychiatrist on Trial for Medical Malpractice. New York, Free Press, 1985

Christie GL: The management of grief in work with infertile couples. J Assist Reprod Genet 14:198–191, 1997

Christie GL, Pawson ME: The psychological and social management of the infertile couple, in The Infertile Couple. Edited by Pepperel RS, Hudson B, Wood C. New York, Churchill Livingstone, 1987, pp 35–50

Dunbar HF: Emotions and Bodily Changes: A Survey of Literature on Psychosomatic Interrelationships. New York, Columbia University Press, 1954

Fenton BJ, Guggenheim FG: Consultation-liason and funding: why can't Alice find Wonderland. Gen Hosp Psychiatry 7:255–260, 1981

Frankel BL, Hall RC: The value of consultation-liaison interventions to the general hospital. Psychiatr Serv 47:418–420, 1996

Freud S: Female sexuality (1931), in The Standard Edition of the Complete Psychological Works of Sigmund Freud, Vol 21. Translated and edited by Strachey J. London, England, Hogarth, 1961, pp 223–243

Friedman EA: The obstetrician's dilemma: how much fetal monitoring and cesarean section is enough? N Engl J Med 315:641–643, 1986

Hellerstein D: The training of a gynecologist: how the "old boys" talk about women's bodies. Ms., November 1984, pp 136–137

Hummel WP, Kettel LM: Assisted reproductive technology: the state of the ART. Ann Med 29:207–214, 1997

Karasu TB, Plutchnik R, Conte H, et al: What do physicians want from a psychiatric consultation service. Compr Psychiatry 18:73–81, 1977

La Leche League International: The Womanly Art of Breastfeeding. Franklin Park, IL, Interstate Publishers, 1987

Lantos JD: Second-generation ethical issues in the new reproductive technologies: divided loyalties, indications and the research agenda, in Psychiatric Aspects of Reproductive Technology. Edited by Stotland NL. Washington, DC, American Psychiatric Press, 1990, pp 87–96

Leppert PC, Partner SF, Thompson A: Learning from the community about barriers to health care. Obstet Gynecol 87:140–141, 1996

Lipowski ZJ: Consultation-liaison psychiatry: the first half century. Gen Hosp Psychiatry 8:305–315, 1986

Mahowald MB, Levinson D, Cassel C: The new genetics and women. Milbank Q 74:239–283, 1996

Nickels MW, McIntyre JS: A model for psychiatric services in primary care settings. Psychiatr Serv 47:522–526, 1996

Pomeroy S: Goddesses, Whores, Wives, and Slaves: Women in Classical Antiquity. New York, Schacken, 1975

Scully D, Bart P: A funny thing happened on the way to the orifice: women in gynecology textbooks, in Changing Women in a Changing Society. Edited by Huber J. Chicago, IL University of Chicago, 1973, pp 283–288

Seiden A: The sense of mastery in the childbirth experience, in The Woman Patient, Vol 1. Edited by Notman M, Nadelson C. New York, Plenum, 1978, pp 87–105

Sharpe M, Gill D, Strain J, et al: Psychosomatic medicine and evidence-based treatment. J Psychosom Res 41:101 107, 1996

Stotland N: Social Change and Women's Reproductive Health Care. New York, Praeger, 1988

Stotland NL, Garrick TR: Manual of Psychiatric Consultation. Washington, DC, American Psychiatric Press, 1990

Strong C, Miller BE, Photopulos GJ, et al: An approach to teaching ethical, legal, and psychosocial aspects of gynecologic oncology in a residency program. Obstet Gynecol 89:142–144, 1997

Webster v Reproductive Health Services, 109 S.Ct. 3040 (1989)

# What Is a Minority?

## Issues in Setting and Dialogue

MINDY THOMPSON FULLILOVE, M.D.

In the complex social organization of the human, the dominance of the societal factors becomes most patent. The physiological processes of fertilization and incubation, although the same in all societies, take place in social settings that vary historically, leading to damage, death, or survival of the foetus. In any one period of history, the supportive or destructive conditions in which fertilization and incubation take place vary with the class or social group to which the adults belong. Nurturance is accomplished by widely diversified procedures, depending on the society and the group within the society to which the child and parents belong. *It is no longer easy to generalize about the three processes as they occur in a particular species.* The physiology of reproduction in people is comparable in all settings. Different societal settings increase or decrease the probability of the survival of the offspring, as well as behavioral patterns involved in reproduction. It is possible that with the increased mastery by humans over environmental factors by means of improved technology, the very physiology of the processes of fertilization, incubation and nurturance may change.

Ethel Tobach, American Museum of Natural History, 1971

Preparation of this chapter was supported in part by a fellowship from the Open Society Institute.

# What is a Minority?

What is a minority? This chapter suggests that the label *minority* is an arbitrary political construction that has life meaning because it indicates the economic, social, and cultural opportunities available to individuals. Specifically, the political construction of majorities and minorities is reflected in the construction of social spaces that vary in the nature and quantity of resources they possess. The social construction of habitat by human groups in conflict with each other creates the conditions within which girls mature into womanhood, have babies, and raise children. Tobach, in the analysis quoted above, reminds us that the physiology of reproduction is the same in all settings, but as the settings vary, so too will the health and welfare of mother and infant be altered (Tobach 1971). This chapter considers the problem of minority status as a major factor shaping the patterns of health and disease among women in the United States.

In a country obsessed with race, it is typically assumed that we know what we mean when we say "minority"—is it not a synonym for the minority racial and ethnic groups? Furthermore, because those groups are stigmatized and subject to discrimination, "minority" carries the connotation "despised by the majority."

Because "minority" signals that we are talking about racial groups, it is helpful to examine the concept of race. Racial classification is a pseudoscientific system based on the premise that human beings can be visually sorted into groups. In practice, these groups are assigned relative biologic superiority or inferiority that in turn is incorporated into a social system giving political and social supremacy—as well as better health outcomes—to the allegedly superior group (Cooper and David 1986).

The racial system of classification is so fundamental to our thinking in the United States that we often forget to examine and challenge its flawed assumptions. In reality, racial classification is a crude system that lumps disparate peoples with different language, culture, and history into a small number of groups (see Table 28–1). It does not match well with the identities that people ascribe to themselves. What, for example, would be the identity of a woman flute player with one Vietnamese and one Senegalese parent, born Catholic, but currently a practicing Buddhist, who lives in Oakland, California with her husband and sees her girlfriend on alternate Fridays? In the spirit of the Bay Area, such a woman might well inform you that she is a Sagittarian, a vegan, and was Marie Antoinette in a past life just to complicate matters.

**TABLE 28–1.**  We are not one people

It is difficult to speak of sexuality issues among Latinos in the United States as if they were just one homogeneous group of individuals. The U.S. Latino population—estimated to be more than 20 million people—includes individuals who speak many different languages and come from different regions, races, classes, and cultures of the Americas.

Ernesto de la Vega (1990)

The number and sheer depth of stereotypes about Indians create stress and anxiety for many Native Americans. At the root of such stereotypes is the mistaken view that we are *one* people. Like Europeans, Native Americans are not one people, although our experiences with the outside world have helped to create a pan-Indian identity. One's tribe (nation)—Choctaw, Peoria, Tlingit, Malecite, Arikara, Okanagan, Snohomish, Caddo—is where one's primary ethnic identity lies. Each tribe has developed its own language, customs, and beliefs; each has had a different history; and each has exercised its own strategy for dealing with the relentless invasion of new peoples and with the catastrophic changes that have taken place in their traditional lifestyles.

Ronald M. Rowell (1990)

One must be sensitive to the lumping of Asians and Pacific Islanders together as one homogenous group. In addressing the health care/AIDS information and education needs of Asians and Pacific Islanders in the United States, it is necessary to recognize the cultural diversity of this population. There are at least 43 different Asian and Pacific Islander groups, from more than 40 countries and territories, who speak more than 100 different languages and dialects (some unwritten). Each group has a distinct culture and heritage.

Deborah A. Lee and Kevin Fong (1990)

People with black skin share a common motherland in Africa but, as a result of the diaspora, have lived on many continents and under many governments. Haiti, the West Indies, the United States, as well as all the countries of Africa, have been home to black people. Emerging from each homeland are people with cultures, beliefs and history that are as different as they are alike.

Robert Fullilove,<br>American Public Health Association Annual Convention,<br>October, 1990, New York, NY

Let us consider, as well, the concept of minority. By definition, a *minority* is the numerically smaller of two groups. In the United States, groups are formed along many lines of demarcation: race, sexual orientation, religion, ethnicity, country of origin, social class, and many others. The small groups—homosexuals as compared with heterosexuals, Catholics as compared with Protestants, independently wealthy as compared with working people—are called minority. Of course, a person's affiliation may include many groups. A single individual might belong to the majority racial group but a minority religious group, as did President John F. Kennedy, who had to overcome prejudice against Catholics in his bid to become president.

Minorities might be considered weak and helpless, but minority groups have learned how to get and keep power; in South Africa under the apartheid system it was possible for a very small white minority to control the wealth and power of a massive country. Minorities might be considered inferior and despicable, but that is not inherently so; in the United States, a shrinking percentage of the population controls an expanding proportion of the country's wealth. The small size of the power elite is taken as proof of its special status. The members of the *Fortune* 500 are not a minority, therefore: they are the elect.

Because minority signifies a relational category, minority status may disappear when the referent is changed. In the Central Harlem neighborhood of New York, 86% of the residents are African American. When whites are outnumbered by people of color—an event demographers say will happen in the twenty-first century—they will be considered a minority.

In the analysis of health problems, race and minority are treated not as flawed and fluid concepts but as rigid and meaningful representations of reality. The assumption that we can measure race permits us to compile mountains of data specifying disease by racial and ethnic categories. That such analyses regularly inform us that minorities have more health problems than the majority confirms its meaning as an important variable. The thinking is that because we find racial differences, race is important and we must continue to measure race.

Several recent studies have helped to challenge this circular reasoning. Greenberg and Schneider (1994) answered the issue directly in an article titled "Violence in American Cities: Young Black Males is the Answer, but What was the Question?" This tongue-in-cheek title is meant to draw the reader's attention to the analysis that points to violence as a problem of young black men. The authors cited a number of articles drawing this association and noted:

Black male homicide is an extremely serious problem. But near singular concern, or giving the appearance of singular concern, with solving the crisis of urban violence by focusing on assaultive violence by young black males begs the question of what are the roots of urban violence. Focusing on any one population, no matter how serious its problem, leads critics, such as psychiatrist Peter Breggin, to charge that a narrow age/race/sex focus leads to asking narrow questions, such as genetic causes of violence. It leads away from asking broad questions, such as if other populations, old and young, whites and Hispanics, and females living in environments similar to young black males might also be highly susceptible to violence. (pp. 179–180)

To address these larger issues, Greenberg and Schneider focused on the process of marginalization that has altered the landscape in many American cities. They noted that pariah land uses were increasingly concentrated in certain inner-city areas of New Jersey. They called these pariah land uses TOADS, standing for Temporarily Obsolete Abandoned Derelict Sites, and LULUS, standing for Locally Unwanted Land Uses. They proposed a marginalization hypothesis, that is, that marginalization of people and land use exacerbates violence.

In examining three marginalized New Jersey cities, Newark, Camden, and Trenton, as compared with the rest of the state, they found strong support for their hypothesis. Of particular importance is the finding that marginalization affects all the populations living in the distressed areas. "The reality of Camden, Newark, and Trenton is that young white males have virtually the same probability of manifesting a violent cause of death as young black males" (Greenberg and Schneider 1994, p. 185). The authors concluded that "Violence flourishes in unstable personal, neighborhood, and regional environments . . . . If we want to try to explain high rates of urban violence, we must stop equating violence with homicide, and we must focus on the macro, neighborhood, and personal environments of all the people that reside in these marginal places" (p. 185).

The influence of location is demonstrated in two important studies from the cardiovascular literature. In the first of these, Fang and colleagues (1996) examined the death rates from cardiovascular disease of blacks and whites living in the city of New York but born in various parts of the country. Interestingly enough, death rates vary for each group, and the patterns differ for different forms of heart disease. Death rates from coronary heart disease for blacks born in the Northeast were similar to those for whites born in that area. Blacks born in the South had a rate of death from coronary heart disease that was 30% higher than that of Northeastern-born blacks. A third group of blacks, born in the Caribbean, demonstrated significantly lower death rates from coronary heart disease than those born in the Northeast. The authors concluded, "If the favorable survival patterns of Caribbean migrants were conferred on other blacks, the current interracial pattern would be reversed, and mortality from cardiovascular disease among blacks would be well below that among whites" (p. 1551).

In the second study, Geronimus et al. (1996) studied excess mortality among blacks and whites in the United States. The team studied mortality among blacks in selected areas of New York city, Detroit, Los Angeles, and Alabama (in one area of persistent poverty and one higher-income area each) and among whites in areas of New York city, metropolitan Detroit, Kentucky, and Alabama (in one area of persistent poverty and one higher-income area each). Sixteen areas were studied in all. Obviously, if race were the overriding factor determining health outcomes, then blacks would have had higher mortality than whites in all areas, with little difference across sites. The actual findings presented a more complicated picture. The authors summarized by saying,

> Our findings are generally consistent with the association between race and excess mortality in the United States that is often reported. However, the poverty rate and the location of a groups (urban and northern vs. rural and southern) are also important. White residents of Detroit fared as poorly as residents of some black areas that we studied. One black comparison group (that in Queens-Bronx) had a mortality rate only slightly higher than the national average for whites. (p. 1555)

These studies present a clear pattern in which location and resources shape health outcomes. Three issues need to be examined at this point. First, it is important to understand that groups, and the individuals in groups, are related to each other. The relational processes are quite specific to historical and geographic factors. Second, the construction of particular ecosystems is the culmination of the great forces of time and place. Understanding features of ecosystems can give us important insights into the health process in a given area. Third, the health process in a given area is integrated into the individual's lifestory in characteristic ways. Based on an understanding of relational process, ecosystem, and lifestory, it is possible for the care provider to understand and assist in resolving health problems of women from minority groups.

# The Relational Process

Waves of migrants have come to or been dragged to the United States over the past four centuries. Some of the incoming groups have been welcomed into the workforce and into the power structure. Others have struggled for the very survival of their group. The stakes have been high: control over the wealth and bounty offered by a huge, well-endowed continent. Among the weapons of the battle have been those "isms"—such as racism and religious intolerance—that allowed people to deny the humanity of their competitors. In 1903, W. E. B. Du Bois, the foremost black historian and commentator, said, "The problem of the color line is the problem of the 20th century—the relation of the darker to the lighter men in Asia and Africa, in America, and the islands of the sea" (Du Bois 1967, p. 23). Almost 100 years later, despite battles for equality that have attracted international concern and attention, we still live in a world in which race, ethnicity, religion, and gender determine one's chance to live a healthy and productive life. In fact, the barriers of stigma create an ecology for minority people that is distinctly different from that of majority people.

When the barriers of culture intersect with the barriers of oppression—and even of genocide—we face additional barriers of anger, fear, dissembling, and contempt. The characteristics of the intersection of culture with oppression are shaped by the history of the meeting. The story of Japanese people in the United States includes their internment in concentration camps in World War II, when Americans did not trust the loyalty of Japanese to their new country. Chinese men came to America to work on the railroads and were forbidden to bring their wives. The old single men remain part of the story of Chinatown in San Francisco and elsewhere. The almost complete annihilation of Native Americans by war and disease beginning immediately on contact with white civilization ranks with the Holocaust as a horrific story of genocide.

Within most groups, women have relatively less power than men. However, the status of women differs from group to group. In the 1990s, the ascension to power of the Taliban in Afghanistan threatened the very survival of women, arousing international concern for their safety. This is in marked contrast to accomplishments of women in the United States, where they have gained a large measure of social and political freedom and decreased the differentials in economic opportunity. The meeting of groups is often an opportunity for women to rethink culturally defined status and roles in a creative and unceasing process of balancing attachment to ethnic traditions with the pursuit of women's liberation.

Thus, intergroup relations provide an opportunity for women to question received tradition about their social status. One of the most remarkable struggles to have come out of this intergroup contact is the struggle against female circumcision, which is practiced in many countries in Africa. This ancient ritual is a rite of passage for girls on the threshold of womanhood. Because it is thought to ensure a woman's purity, it increases a woman's marriageability in many cultures. However, the practice is a dangerous one that can have serious, even life-threatening consequences for women. The struggle against female circumcision is spurred by contact between African women and women from other countries. Increasing recognition of the health cost of the ritual is empowering women to call for the banning of the custom. Yet because it challenges traditions that are centuries old and are endorsed by the patriarchal societies in which they are practiced, the struggle to eliminate female circumcision is likely to be bitter and protracted.

Women who immigrate from one country to another are also exposed to differing traditions of women's status. Women immigrating to the United States largely find themselves given more opportunity than they experienced at home. This is both exciting and stressful. One implication of the new freedom is that women can step into American-style gender roles. This "Americanization" of women is often deeply disturbing for their husbands and can lead to tension, strife, and in some cases violence. It also poses challenges for women, who are often given opportunity on the one hand but deprived of traditional sources of support on the other. This new balancing act has important implications for childbearing and childrearing as well as for women's health overall.

## Ecologic Settings

In this section, I describe three ecologic settings. These brief accounts are not meant to provide an exhaustive description of the settings in which minority people live and work. Rather, they are meant to enable the reader to compare and contrast the life of people living in each of these settings and the health care problems that occur there.

### Inner-City Disintegration and the Growth of the Underclass

The growth of the underclass has been described as a form of "American Apartheid" (Massey 1990), created by an interaction between rising rates of poverty and high levels of residential segregation. Where these social forces have intersected—for example, among blacks and Puerto Ricans in large urban areas of the Northeast and Midwest—they have acted to create an urban underclass that is persistently poor, spatially isolated, and disproportionately minority. Furthermore, the structures and social networks that enabled the poor to survive poverty have been weakened, if not decimated, by the same forces that have created the underclass itself.

As Sampson (1990), Wallace (1990), and others have pointed out, the growth of the underclass is not simply a result of economic decline but rather economic collapse in conjunction with the collapse of other complex social policies on housing, fire protection service, and transportation networks. Sampson cites as an example the decision in Chicago to concentrate poor blacks in massive federal housing projects. He notes,

> with the concentration of poor blacks in housing projects, social transformation of the ghetto became profound . . . . Undeniably, family disruption in the black community is concentrated in public housing. In 1980, of the 17,178 families with children living in Chicago public housing projects, only 11% were married couple families. Teen-age pregnancy and out-of-wedlock births are similarly high. (p. 529)

Whereas Sampson's work focused on the association between housing policies and crime rates, D. Wallace and Wallace (1990) provided similar analysis on the association between housing policies and health. Characteristic of the areas housing the urban underclass is a process of "contagious housing destruction," in which a significant proportion of the residential housing is destroyed through neglect, abandonment, and inadequate municipal services. The Taylor Homes in Chicago or the Latrobe Homes in New Orleans have a "snaggle-toothed" appearance characteristic of this contagious process. In the South Bronx, contagious housing destruction was responsible for massive displacement of the poor. According to the authors,

> People had to move in such large numbers in so short a time that local communities were destroyed and local essential services imbalanced with respect to utilization . . . . These changes have two meanings: the breaking up of communities by forced migration and the crowding of the poor into the remaining housing . . . The old social networks which had coped with the effects of poverty and overcrowding had been destroyed in the migrations. Churches, social clubs, and political organizations died. The effects of overcrowding and increased poverty from rising rents had (and have) few mitigating influences. (p. 268)

In sum, the structure of families, of social networks, and of neighborhoods—that is, all aspects of the social networks of the poor—have been undermined.

A great deal of scholarship from many disciplines makes it clear that social networks are important for the maintenance of health. The social networks of the poor have several specific functions that ensure survival. First, the network acts as a "resource bank," in which members share whatever they have. These banks are critically important because they provide a mechanism to "tide you over" in times of scarcity. Second, the network collectively acts to raise the children. Parents are thus freed to solve the economic problems of the family without having to worry about inadequate supervision for the young ones. Third, the network acts to provide "reality testing" counterbalancing the stress, trauma, and negative messages that the poor receive. Social reality testing mitigates the potential narcissistic wound of a racist attack by reframing it. For example, black people will commonly say to each other, "White people will be white people," which acts to discount a racist act or message. In the aftermath of urban desertificaton, what is left of the social and cultural capital that had ensured survival for area residents?

An important paper by Kelly (1994) examined these issues in the life of a young woman living in the declining West Baltimore community. As described by Kelly, "Arson and abandonment are frequent, as evidenced by the abundance of charred and boarded-up buildings which often become safe houses for drug dealers . . . Business opportunities are puny, with the exception of as myriad of grocery stores and liquor shops inherited by Korean immigrants from an earlier cohort of Jewish entrepreneurs" (p. 91). Kelly was drawn to the area because of the high rates of adolescent pregnancy. Contact over several years with Towanda Forrest, who gave birth to her first child at age 14, provided Kelly with insights into the process of early pregnancy in a distressed setting.

Kelly linked the impoverishment of the setting with Towanda's choice to have a child. Although Towanda was aware of the value of education in an abstract fashion, she herself was unable to read above the second grade level. The "education" available to her in overcrowded, underfunded ghetto schools offered little hope for decent employment. Furthermore, she did not know people with good education or good jobs, adding to her suspicion that such options were beyond her reach. Yet within a context that set such serious limitations on life choices, childbearing was viewed as important and life affirming. Viewed from within the context of her life setting, Towanda's choice to have a child—Kelly even called it her "triumph"—is quite rational.

Kelly made the point that policymakers outside of the inner city view early childbearing with suspicion and contempt. She challenged such an assessment as inadequately informed from the "emic,"—that is, the insider–perspective. Health care providers are just as likely as others from the outside to argue for behaviors that are unrealistic given the context. Campaigns for condom use and delay of pregnancy and to "just say no to drugs" have all fallen short of their goals, in large measure because the implementation of such preventive actions is not consonant with external constraints on behavior. In the impoverished setting of urban desertification, the pursuit of better health depends on contextual interventions that rebuild the housing and economic infrastructure of the area.

## Health Care at the Mexican-American Border

Warner (1991), a researcher at the Lyndon B. Johnson School of Public Affairs at the University of Texas in Austin, described the United States–Mexico border as transborder metropolitan areas that have grown from sparsely populated deserts into a region with 10 million inhabitants. The transborder cities include Tucson, Arizona, and Nogales, Mexico, with a population of 1 million; San Diego, California, and Tijuana, Mexico, with a current population of 3.5 million; Rio Grande Valley and El Paso, Texas, and Juarez, Mexico, with a population over 1 million; and Laredo, Texas, and Nuevo Laredo, Mexico, with 400,000 people. The region has a unique character because of its increasing interdependence: many of the region's problems cannot be solved by local municipalities without assistance from both federal governments or binational cooperation.

The disparities between the United States and Mexico create conditions that have an enormous impact on the area. Of the many Mexicans who cross the border to find work in the United States, most are poor, and many are illegal entrants. The receiving communities are taxed to supply health care, especially because few provisions have been made for funding the health needs of illegal immigrants. As noted earlier, many Mexican-American mothers deliver their babies out of the hospital. Warner (1991) points out the serious consequences of the major gaps that exist in the services available to the poor: "In 1980, of the births occurring in Texas border counties, 6,215 of the 28,645 births to persons giving a Texas residence were out of the hospital, while 2,550 of the 4,216 listing a Mexico residence were out of the hospital" (p. 245).

Communicable diseases, including sexually transmitted diseases (STDs), are a significant threat to the health of the population in the border area.

STDs have long been a problem because of the cross-border use of red light districts and the increased difficulty of contact tracing. Of 1,502 cases of AIDS reported in Mexico through mid-1988, roughly 20% were thought to come from the six Mexican border states.

Finally, the border communities show all of the problems attendant to rapid growth, uncontrolled development of industry, poverty, and instability. At the most extreme, the border residents live in *colonias*, or unincorporated settlements on both sides of the border. As Warner noted, "These communities often lack septic tanks, sewers, or running water, and outdoor privies commonly abut water wells, making most of the water unfit for consumption" (p. 242).

## Caribbean Immigrants in the New South

DeSantis, a researcher at the University of Miami, has written extensively on the problems of women arriving from Cuba and from Haiti in 1980 (DeSantis 1989). She points out that

> The mass arrival in 1980 of 125,000 Cubans during the Mariel Sealift or "Freedom Flotilla" and the 36,000 Haitians who entered during the same year overwhelmed the health care, social, political, and economic systems of Southeast Florida. Community agencies were already straining to meet the needs of other low-income groups in the area. The influx of Cuban "Marielitos" and Haitian "Boat People" caused health care professionals to become increasingly frustrated by the sheer numbers requiring curative and preventive health care. The frustration also resulted from lack of knowledge about the new immigrants who differed from previous groups of Cubans and Haitians in their health care orientations, educational backgrounds, socioeconomic status, and social support systems. (p. 70)

These two groups entered the United States at the same time but differed on almost every other measure of education and economic prospects. Cuban refugees comprised several subgroups, including families, gay men, and people with criminal histories or mental illness. Although poorer than earlier refugees from that country, all came from a society with universal literacy and an aggressive health care system based on Western biomedical medicine. The Cubans had received appropriate preventive health care—including vaccinations—while in Cuba, and had learned to value a system of health care similar to that in the United States. Finally, Cuban refugees for the most part felt secure that they would be able to stay in the United States.

DeSantis (1989) observed that the Cuban immigrant parents shared decision making and tended to bring the extended family into decisions about the child's health care. She hypothesized that efforts of the Cuban government toward sexual equality in the domestic realm had led to this male–female sharing of household functions. Cuban mothers felt empowered to act on their children's behalf. If a child became ill, the mothers said, "It's the parents' fault. They did not love him enough" (p. 80).

The Haitian boat people, by contrast, came from one of the poorest countries in the world. They were often illiterate, rural people, with a long tradition of folk medicine and little access to Western biomedical care. The Haitians as a group had a less secure status in the United States and feared they might be deported back to Haiti where they faced death, torture, or other kinds of abuse. This group, although willing to use the American health care system, did not share the philosophy of the system. Haitian mothers, historically responsible for child care in Haiti, continued to carry alone most of the responsibility in this domain. Few older women were available to assist these women in carrying out their responsibilities. In contrast with their Cuban counterparts, DeSantis found that Haitian women felt relatively powerless to affect their child's health. Although they did not believe illness was preventable, once signs and symptoms were present, they quickly sought treatment for the child.

## Lifestory

Ecologic settings are locations within which the lifestory unfurls. Well-being and mental health are dependent on the presence or absence of a health-promoting environment as well as the individual's ability to extract goods from that environment. Stories of women's experiences provide insight into these processes. McDowell's (1996) beautiful memoir of growing up in Bessemer, Alabama, *Leaving Pipe Shop: Memories of Kin*, is occasioned by the need to understand the possible contribution of asbestos to her father's untimely death. As she examines her family story, she realizes that many of her relatives died at early ages. In a sense, she lived through, on a personal basis, the excess mortality from heart disease that Fang et al. (1996) studied in a more theoretical manner. These early deaths meant that she was orphaned before she had entered graduate school. By her mid-40s, only one of the relatives from her parents' generation was still surviving. It is worth considering the relationship between the early orphaning in this story and the early parenting in the story of Towanda Forrest mentioned earlier.

In both cases, the warp of family life is shaped by the trials and tribulations of everyday life in a poor, segregated industrial community. *In* is perhaps the key word to understanding McDowell's story. The problems of racism are, in many ways, external to Pipe Shop. McDowell does not open her memoir by talking about race. Rather, she starts with a line that is all-too-familiar to many adult children: "You got to come home" (p. 17). Although offered at the outset as a simple intergenerational interaction between aunt and niece, this family summons leads her to a deeper understanding of the context of her home community. For example, the problem of asbestos hovers in the background of the story—did her father die of asbestos poisoning? It is only when she has broadened her view of Pipe Shop past the interior world of childhood that she can begin to appreciate the problems faced by black industrial workers in the deep South.

The sense of *in* is profoundly present in the chapter "Restriction and Reclamation: Lesbian Bars and Beaches of the 1950s" by Joan Nestle (1996), in the book *Queers in Space: Communities, Public Spaces, Sites of Resistance.* Nestle's struggle, however, is profoundly different from McDowell's. As a lesbian trying to find spaces in New York city within which to be a lesbian, Nestle is constantly reminded of the outside forces arrayed in opposition. She writes,

> Silenced and policed, we congregated in allotted spaces. Borders were marked and real: vice laws, police, and organized crime representatives controlled our movements into and out of our "countries." But what could not be controlled was what forced the creation of these spaces in the first place—our need to confront a personal destiny, to see our reflections in each other's faces and to break societal ostracism with our bodies. What could not be controlled was our desire. (p. 61)

Nestle's narrative illuminates the search to create safe space that occupied gay men and lesbian women at that time. This search evolved from furtive meetings in hidden places to open displays of gay and lesbian political activity, such as the gay pride marches that have become a regular occurrence in many cities. Despite the new openness, the policing of gay/lesbian life continues in modern times and influences many social interactions, not least of which is the search for health. Cochran and Mays (1988) have pointed out that many lesbian women are afraid to reveal their sexual orientation to their physicians, indicating that the doctor's office is not yet a part of the gay-positive space Nestle and others have sought to master.

Lifestories are quite particular and belie the generalizations that words like *minority* and *race* seek to imply. Understanding the health of the individual is absolutely dependent on a willingness to understand the individual's unique path through life regardless of how that path differs from one's own. The minority woman, in her capacity for procreative and recreative sexuality, does not differ from her majority counterpart, but because she lives under more adverse conditions, her ability to realize her wishes and dreams is more limited. Given her risk for ill health, the chances are great that she will have contact with the health care system. At that moment, when the health care provider and the patient meet, the provider faces the challenge of establishing a dialogue that can assist in the diagnosis and treatment of illness. This dialogue is at the heart of health care. Through that communication must come accurate information about the patient's symptoms, behaviors, and attempts at self-care. Eventually, it must enable the provider to convince the patient to follow a prescription for care. Finally, the dialogue is most truly a healing interaction if both provider and patient have felt affirmed and respected.

As we speak across differences, we face barriers created by the differences in values and traditions. Hussain (1990) described an encounter at the Afghan Mission Hospital with a young man who appeared to be dying. A member of the Puthan tribe from the mountainous area of Pakistan, the dying man feared the taint to his honor that a death away from home would bring. His family decided to take him home, a decision adamantly opposed by Hussain, who thought hospital-based care was the patient's only hope. Despite the doctor's grim prognosis, the man survived and returned to bring a gift to the doctor—a second gift, in fact, the first being the lesson in respecting others' values.

## Implications for Practice

Writers speaking on minority issues emphasize, almost without cessation, the variation that characterizes minority populations and that must be the first assumption one makes in addressing another human being. The task, given the diversity of human cultures and human experiences, is not to assume that any survey of "minority" cultures can prepare the practitioner for the task of cross-cultural communication. Rather than approach the situation with assumptions about behavior or attitudes, the practitioner must have a strategy for data collection.

First, the practitioner must be aware that 1) the patient has cultural expectations about roles and greetings and 2) the patient from a stigmatized minority group will be sensitive to signs of disrespect. Because we cannot know the assumptions of all the cultures with which we will interact, it is useful to behave toward the patient as one would behave toward an honored member of one's own culture. It will never hurt the practitioner's image for the translator to clarify an act by saying, "That is how they show great respect in their culture." By contrast, it will be particularly injurious to the developing relationship for patients to discover they have been slighted or treated discourteously. Dr. Muriel Pettione, a senior attending physician at Harlem Hospital Center, a major hospital serving the black community in New York City, often points out how offensive it is for young residents to show signs of disrespect, such as calling an older woman patient by her first name. Indeed, that kind of impropriety will destroy trust and injure communication.

Second, practitioners, who perforce must act without a manual of cultures, should use the services of "key informants," as anthropologists call those members of the community who help them to understand culture. Social workers, nurses, typists, taxi drivers—in fact, anyone with a command of the two cultures—can help the practitioner to understand the words and actions of the patient. With the help of the guide, the practitioner can assemble a working understanding of the life-setting of the patient. Is the patient well-to-do or poor? Educated? Fluent in many languages and cultures? Living in adequate housing and in a safe neighborhood? Involved in stable social and sexual relationships? Because such questions are a routine part of the biomedical examination taught to health care practitioners, it is not important to elaborate in more detail on what to ask. Rather, it is important to underscore that such questions provide information and prevent unwarranted—and perhaps stigmatizing—assumptions.

Finally, practitioners must be aware that they act in the context of cultural conflict. We have not, in the United States, succeeded in being a melting pot. Rather, some people have been incorporated into the dominant culture, whereas others have been blocked out. Therefore, individuals from different cultures do not necessarily meet as equals. The health care provider must take the responsibility for establishing a dialogue of equality. When that occurs, the provider–patient relationship will have a capacity for respect, for understanding, and for healing.

It is, in any event, rare that we have empathy for each other. Purdy, a pathologist in California, described living through a serious earthquake (Purdy 1990); just before the earthquake he had struggled to diagnose a specimen that eventually was identified as metastatic ovarian cancer. After the earthquake, he found (unusual for him) that he wanted to meet the patient. For Purdy, the earthquake, which had shaken his belief in the world as secure, allowed him to empathize with the young woman with terminal cancer. He wrote,

Like all of us, [Sarah] had plans for the summer, for next year, for many years to come. Now she would have to plan for something else. She reminded me of the child I saw during the earthquake, screaming at God to ease up on it. A couple of nurses hugged him and tried to console him, but he was too shaken for human comfort, too aware that no human was mightier than what had just shaken the earth. He was alone in his fear, as I was, as Sarah is, each of us complacent about the security of our routine lives, taking everything—our health, our safety on terra firma—for granted, never knowing when the earth might all of a sudden shake the life from us or when the faults beneath our own surface may begin a unique, solitary, and frightening slippage. (p. 2883)

It seems that these transcendent human experiences have a unique importance, because they allow us to see across all the barriers of difference and to understand the samenesses in human existence. As health care providers, we will encounter many of these powerful human events. With attention and concern, we can make many effective and emphatic encounters.

## Conclusion

What is a minority? This chapter has sought to suggest that *minority* takes on meaning for health practitioners because it implies powerlessness. A corollary of powerlessness is the relegation to less desirable habitat. A corollary of poor habitat is poor health.

Perhaps the fundamental implication of this analysis is that those concerned with the health of minority women have two obligations. The first is obvious: to deliver decent care in a respectful manner. The second obligation is less often recognized and is rarely part of the curriculum in health professions schools: to challenge the distribution of resources that makes for bad habitat. This implies challenging the right of powerful groups to an unequal share of the world's goods. It also implies challenging—within all groups—the oppression of women and the limitations on their freedom.

On another level, close inspection of the concept of minority teaches us that we are each a member of the minority of one and the majority of humankind. It is this deeper reality of humanness and individuality that should guide practitioners as they help women stay healthy.

References

Cochran SD, Mays VM: Disclosure of sexual preference to physicians by black lesbian and bisexual women. West J Med 149:616–619, 1988

Cooper R, David R: The biological concept of race and its application to public health and epidemiology. J Health Polit Policy Law 11:97–116, 1986

DeSantis L: Health care orientations of Cuban and Haitian immigrant mothers: implications for health care professionals. Med Anthropol 12:69–89, 1989

Du Bois WEB: The Souls of Black Folk. Greenwich, CT, Fawcett, 1967

Fang J, Madhavan S, Alderman MH: The association between birthplace and mortality from cardiovascular causes among black and white residents of New York city. N Engl J Med 335:1545–1551, 1996

Geronimus AT, Bound J, Waidmann TA, et al: Excess mortality among blacks and whites in the United States. N Engl J Med 335:1552–1558, 1996

Greenberg M, Schneider D: Violence in American cities: young black males is the answer, but what was the question? Soc Sci Med 39:179–187, 1994

Hussain SA: A parting gift. JAMA 263:1254, 1990

Kelly MPF: Towanda's triumph: social and cultural capital in the transition to adulthood in the urban ghetto. International Journal of Urban and Regional Research 4:88–111, 1994

Massey DS: American apartheid: segregation and the making of the underclass. Am J Sociol 96:329–357, 1990

McDowell DE: Leaving Pipe Shop: Memories of Kin. New York, Scribner, 1996

Nestle J: Restriction and reclamation: lesbian bars and beaches of the 1950s, in Queers in Space: Communities, Public Places, Sites of Resistance. Edited by Ingram GB, Bouthillette A, Retter Y. Seattle, WA, Baypress, 1996, pp. 31–45

Purdy LJ: Aftershock. JAMA 263:2883, 1990

Sampson RJ: The impact of housing policies on community social disorganization and crime. Bull N Y Acad Med 66:526–533, 1990

Tobach E: Some evolutionary aspects of human gender. Am J Orthopsychiatry 41:710–715, 1971

Wallace D: Roots of increased health care inequality in New York. Soc Sci Med 31:1219–1227, 1990

Wallace D, Wallace R: The burning down of New York city. Anthropos 9:256–272, 1990

Warner DC: Health issues at the US-Mexican border. JAMA 265:242–247, 1991

# Index

*Page numbers printed in **boldface** type refer to tables or figures.*

Breast cancer *(continued)*
  pregnancy following, 27
  psychiatrist's role in reducing
    psychologic distress and,
    471–472
  recurrence of, 470–471
  treatment of, 460–461, 465–467
Breastfeeding. *See also* Lactation
  decision making about, 119
Bromocriptine, for infertility, 209
Bulimia nervosa, 444. *See also* Eating
    disorder(s)
  menstrual cycle and, 185
Bupropion (Wellbutrin)
  for depression associated with
    gynecologic cancer, **322**
  sexual behavior and, 393
Buspirone, for posttraumatic stress
    disorder, 520
Butyrophenones, during pregnancy, **73**

C

Cancer. *See* Breast cancer; Gynecologic
    cancer
Carbamazepine, during pregnancy, **74,**
    80–81
Cardiovascular disease, in pregnancy,
    20
Caregivers, perinatal loss and, 157–158
Caribbean immigrants, 622–623
CD4+ T lymphocytes, decline in, in
    HIV infection, 338–339
Cervical cancer, 307–308
  among lesbian women, 558
Cervical conization, for human
    papillomavirus infection, 280
Cervical dysplasia
  in HIV infection, 339
  among lesbian women, 558
"Cervical factors," infertility due to,
    210
Chemotherapy, for breast cancer, 461
  psychologic reactions to, 467
Child abuse
  of malformed children, 44–45
  neurologic consequences of, 486

  sexual
    definition of, 479
    history of, in women abused as
      adults, 481
Childbirth, posttraumatic stress
    disorder due to, 55
Childbirth classes, 603
Childlessness, 370
Children
  fear of loss of custody of, in
    schizophrenic pregnant women,
    52
  long-term effects of maternal drug
    therapy on, 77, 81–82
  as motivator for marriage, 369
  planning for, after being diagnosed
    with HIV infection, 351–352
  social importance of producing,
    366
China, induced abortion in, 224
Chinese Americans, 617
Chlordiazepoxide, gender differences
    in, 411
Chlorpromazine, gender differences in,
    409
Chorionic villus sampling (CVS), **37,**
    39
  genetic termination following, 42
  psychologic consequences of, 40
  time issues with, **38**
Chromosome abnormalities, 34
Chromosome analysis, prenatal, **37**
Chromosome translocations, 34
Chronotherapy, menstrual cycle and,
    192–193
Cigarette smoking, teratogenicity of,
    426, **427**
Cleft lip/palate, anxiolytics and, 82
Client-therapist relationship, for treating
    victims of violence, 505–509
Clinician Administered PTSD Scale
    (CAPS), 499
Clomiphene, for infertility, 209
Clomipramine
  gender differences in, 411
  sexual behavior and, 393
Clozapine, during pregnancy, **73**